NURSING ISSUES
in Leading and Managing Change

JEANETTE LANCASTER, RN, PhD, FAAN

Sadie Heath Cabaniss Professor of Nursing and Dean
School of Nursing
University of Virginia
Charlottesville, Virginia

with 64 illustrations

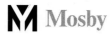

Mosby

St. Louis Baltimore Boston Carlsbad Chicago Minneapolis New York Philadelphia Portland
London Milan Sydney Tokyo Toronto

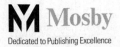

Dedicated to Publishing Excellence

A Times Mirror
Company

Publisher: Sally Schrefer
Editor: Michael S. Ledbetter
Developmental Editor: Lisa P. Newton
Project Manager: John Rogers
Production Editor: Betty Hazelwood
Design Manager: Amy Buxton
Designer: Pati Pye
Manufacturing Supervisor: Karen Boehme

Copyright © 1999 by Mosby, Inc.

Composition by the Clarinda Company
Printing/binding by R.R. Donnelley & Sons Company

Mosby, Inc.
11830 Westline Industrial Drive
St. Louis, Missouri 63146

Library of Congress Cataloging in Publication Data

Nursing issues in leading and managing change / [edited by] Jeanette
   Lancaster.
        p.   cm.
     Includes bibliographical references and index.
     ISBN 0-323-00250-1
     1. Nursing services—Administration.   2. Organizational change.
   3. Medical care—United States.   I. Lancaster, Jeanette.
     [DNLM: 1. Nursing—organization & administration.   2. Nurse
   Administrators.   3. Organizational Innovation.   4. Leadership.
   5. Delivery of Health Care—organization & administration.   WY
   105N97473 1998]
   RT89.N793   1998
   362.1′73′068—dc21
   DNLM/DLC
   for Library of Congress   98-26134
                                                         CIP

98 99 00 01 02 / 9 8 7 6 5 4 3 2 1

Contributors

Charles Braun, PhD
Assistant Professor of Management
Lewis College of Business
Marshall University
Huntington, West Virginia

John G. Bruhn, PhD
Provost and Dean
Penn State Harrisburg
Middletown, Pennsylvania

Angeline Bushy, RN, PhD, CNS
Bert Fish Endowed Chair
Community Health Nursing
University of Central Florida
Daytona Beach, Florida

Ann H. Cary, RN, MPH, PhD, A-CCC
Professor and Coordinator, PhD in Nursing Program
George Mason University
College of Nursing and Health Science
Fairfax, Virginia;
Scholar in Residence
American Nurses Credentialing Center
Washington, DC

Sheryl Feutz-Harter, RN, MSN, JD
Attorney
Shughart, Thomson, and Kilroy
Kansas City, Missouri

Mattia J. Gilmartin, RN, MSN, MBA
Doctoral Candidate
School of Nursing
University of Virginia
Charlottesville, Virginia

Doris F. Glick, RN, PhD
Associate Professor and Director, Primary Care
    Community Nursing Center
School of Nursing
University of Virginia
Charlottesville, Virginia

Margaret R. Grier, RN, FAAN, FACMI
Professor
College of Nursing
University of Kentucky
Lexington, Kentucky

Cheryl Bland Jones, RN, PhD, CNAA
Expert
Center for Primary Care Research
Agency for Health Care Policy and Research
Rockville, Maryland

Shannon D. Kennedy, BA
MBA Candidate in Health Organization Management
Texas Tech University
Lubbock, Texas

Eric G. Kirby, MBA, PhD
Assistant Professor of Management and Health
  Organization Management
College of Business Administration
Texas Tech University
Lubbock, Texas

Pamela A. Kulbok, RN, DNSc
Associate Professor of Nursing
School of Nursing
University of Virginia
Charlottesville, Virginia

Clinton E. Lambert, Jr., RN, PhD, CS
President and Counselor
Lambert Counseling Services, Inc.
Thomson and Waynesboro, Georgia;
Clinical Professor
Department of Mental Health–Psychiatric Nursing
Medical College of Georgia
School of Nursing
Augusta, Georgia

Vickie A. Lambert, RN, DNSc, FAAN
Dean and Professor
Medical College of Georgia
School of Nursing
Augusta, Georgia

Melinda Lancaster, BSBA
Marketing Coordinator
Southcorp Packaging USA, Inc.
Atlanta, Georgia

Wade Lancaster, PhD
King Fahd University of Petroleum & Minerals
College of Industrial Management
Department of Management and Marketing
Dhahran 31261
Saudi Arabia

P.J. Maddox, RN, MSN, EdD
Coordinator, Health Systems Management
College of Nursing and Health Sciences
George Mason University
Fairfax, Virginia

Russell C. McGuire, RN, MSN, CNOR
Doctoral Student
College of Nursing
University of Kentucky
Lexington, Kentucky

Lynn Noland, PhD, NP
Assistant Professor
University of Virginia School of Nursing;
Nurse Practitioner
University of Virginia Kidney Center
Charlottesville, Virginia

Richard A. Ridge, RN, MBA
Doctoral Student
School of Nursing
University of Virginia
Charlottesville, Virginia

Juliann G. Sebastian, RN, PhD, CS
Associate Professor and Assistant Dean for Advanced
  Practice Nursing
College of Nursing
University of Kentucky
Lexington, Kentucky

Jean Sorrells-Jones, RN, PhD, FAAN
Executive Director and Chief Nurse
University of Texas Medical Branch Hospitals;
Associate Professor
University of Texas School of Nursing at Galveston
Galveston, Texas

Marcia Stanhope, RN, DSN, FAAN, C
Associate Dean and Professor
College of Nursing
University of Kentucky
Lexington, Kentucky

Karen MacDonald Thompson, RN, MSN
Doctoral Candidate
University of Virginia;
Healthcare Consultant, The Epsilon Group
Charlottesville, Virginia

Sharon Williams Utz, RN, PhD
Associate Professor and Chair
Division of Adult Health, Acute & Critical Care
    Nursing
School of Nursing
University of Virginia
Charlottesville, Virginia

Reviewers

Sharon Minton Kirkpatrick, RN, MN, PhD
Vice President and Dean of Nursing
Graceland College
Independence, Missouri

Linda S. Smith, RN, MSN
Assistant Professor
State University of West Georgia
Department of Nursing
Carrollton, Georgia;
Doctoral Student
University of Alabama at Birmingham;
Special Government Employee for HHS/FDA

Preface

When the forerunner of this book, *Concepts for Advanced Nursing Practice: The Nurse as a Change Agent,* was written in 1982, it did seem as though society, health care, and nursing practice were engaged in significant, unprecedented change. Now, some 16 years later, that earlier rate of change is considered a mere preamble to the rate, scope, and radicalness of present day change. The terms used in the original title have different connotations now as well. Advanced practice nursing currently refers to nurses with master's preparation as clinical specialists, nurse practitioners, or certified nurse midwives. In 1982 that term was used with less precision and definitiveness. Similarly, *change agent* was a popular and often used term in the 1980s to refer to people who were catalysts for change. Now we talk about change management or change leadership more than catalyzing change.

Like the title of the book, in so many ways the actual paradigm for thinking about change is entirely different. In the 1980s we talked about "planned change" and the key phrases of systematic, orderly, and evolutionary change were used. In the 1990s we talked about system redesign, downsizing, and restructuring. Now we talk about fast-paced, strategic, and revolutionary change. Speed is of the essence. Organizational stability and predictability are no longer part of the contemporary institution, and the relationship of the employer to the employee is markedly different from what it was in earlier times.

Instead of talking about categories of adopters, today those who resist change because they have concerns about the direction the organization is going, are afraid they cannot meet the new performance expectations, or are unwilling to learn new skills are increasingly seen as "dispensable employees." Phrases such as "you are either on the train or on the tracks" and "move on or move out" convey our current view of change, organizations, and employees.

Hospitals and health agencies are facing the same challenges that other types of organizations are facing. They must restructure to become competitive and either partner with other agencies through alliances, mergers, or acquisitions or assume a larger portion of the market share previously held by someone else. These same agencies must simultaneously operate more efficiently with smaller staff, especially at the management level, and must learn new skills of including more of the staff in the decision-making process. Further, technology is no longer an option. Although costly to purchase and complex to operate, technology is essential for effective health care management.

Each time major changes occur in the structure of health care and particularly in how it is financed, the domino effect is enormous. With managed care, several major shifts have occurred that dramatically affect nursing. First, although nurses have always been mindful of the effectiveness of their care, we have historically talked about the process of care. We taught students to "give the best possible care" and use whatever resources were needed to assure the best result for the client. Now we must hold nurses accountable for achieving the best possible outcome while using the least possible resources. Our world now is filled with words like *restructuring, reengineering, delegation, unlicensed assistive personnel, substitution, collaboration, data management, risk management, accountability,* and *team work.*

Nurses have never been more critical to the success of the health care system than they are now. The education and practice of nursing is based on a range of scientific principles from both the physical and behavioral sciences. Nurses know how to assess, plan, implement, and evaluate. They know how to communicate, collaborate, and work in teams. However, because nursing is heavily occupied by women, nurses must learn new skills for dealing with change that include leadership and management of the process. For years, nurses have too often followed orders rather than taken the initiative; taken their place within an existing system that they did not create rather than designed an innovative system for effectively delivering care; and hesitated to describe exactly what they did and the outcomes that their work had for patients and the organization. Nurses must learn skills from successful business women and men about how they manage change and also how they communicate the value and effectiveness of their work.

What then is needed? Nurses must understand the principles and mechanisms for leading as well as participating in a changing health care world. This book provides a range of information about change; the context in which it occurs; the skills needed to make change happen efficiently; the environmental challenges in which change must occur; and some useful tools for those who lead, follow, and evaluate change. Each chapter is written by an expert in the area and is presented in a practical and easy-to-read manner so that readers can readily apply the information to the level and type of change in which they find themselves. No area of nursing and health care is exempt from change, and nurses, who represent the largest group of health care providers, must become expert in leading and managing change.

Jeanette Lancaster

Contents

xiii

PART **III**   EFFECTING CHANGE IN THE HEALTH
                 CARE SYSTEM

Detailed Contents

NURSING ISSUES
in Leading and Managing Change

THEORETIC FOUNDATIONS FOR CHANGE

The Evolution of Health Care Delivery Systems

Eric G. Kirby and Shannon D. Kennedy

INTRODUCTION

This chapter focuses on the evolution of health care delivery systems in the United States. Health care in the United States is delivered through a variety of systems, each serving a different segment of the population. Because of changing social conditions, these health care delivery systems have also changed.

In its earliest beginnings, health care was so crude and rudimentary that people had low expectations. As medical understanding and technology improved, people began to expect that they would receive the best care possible, provided in state-of-the-art facilities and delivered in a medically appropriate manner. Lately, there has been a growing awareness of the financial costs of providing care. As a result, the current trend is to provide appropriate care in a cost-effective manner.

All facets of health care delivery have been affected by changing social norms. Both private and public health care delivery systems have changed. The role of health care professionals also has changed. By considering changing social norms, this chapter examines the past, present, and future of the major components of the health care delivery system in the United States, including the changing role of nursing.

There is no single health care delivery system in the United States. Instead, there are many separate components, each serving different segments of the population in different ways. Although these components occasionally overlap, they are frequently separate from one another. Some are governmental agencies, supported by public funds, and others are either for-profit or not-for-profit corporations that rely on income generated from operations. Occasionally several different components use the same facilities and personnel, but often they use facilities and personnel that are completely separate from one another (Torrens, 1993).

An examination of historical roots shows why the United States has many different health care delivery systems. In the earliest days, health care was entirely a private matter. People generally took care of themselves, obtained the services of private physicians and nurses when needed, and purchased medications from chemists' shops. There were no insurance companies so all medical services were paid out-of-pocket. For those people who could not afford care or did not have a family member to care for them, charitable hospitals were established as voluntary, nonprofit corporations to provide health

3

care. These were usually located in larger towns and cities.

In the early 1900s, a new element was added with the development of municipal hospitals. Local governments established these hospitals to care for poor people in their area who were not capable of caring for themselves or could not receive care from the voluntary nonprofit charity hospitals. These public facilities were generally large, acute care general hospitals with busy clinics and emergency rooms. At the same time, state governments were developing mental hospitals. The cities had previously been responsible for the care of mentally ill persons, but after 1900, state governments began to assume this responsibility. Every state soon had at least one mental hospital where emotionally disturbed individuals were offered what little care was available.

As the cost of health care began to rise rapidly after World War II, health insurance plans became popular in the United States. The first were the Blue Cross/Blue Shield plans developed during the Great Depression by hospitals and physician associations to ensure that they received payment for services rendered. These plans were followed by labor union health and welfare trust funds, established to provide benefits negotiated by union members. At the same time, private, for-profit insurance companies expanded their efforts to insure employees of companies as well as individuals. Finally, large, government-sponsored and government-supervised health insurance plans evolved, such as Medicaid and Medicare.

Private medical practitioners, voluntary nonprofit hospitals, municipal and state hospitals, and a multitude of health insurance plans all developed during the same period, independent of each other and for different purposes. The result was a rich diversity of opportunities and approaches to providing care in a manner most appropriate to meeting the needs of a range of people and situations. At the same time, the result can be described as a chaotic, uncoordinated, and inefficient use of valuable health care resources (Torrens, 1993).

OBJECTIVES

After reading this chapter, you will be able to:

1. Understand the fragmented nature of the U.S. health care delivery system
2. Describe the concept of external environment
3. Know what is driving change in health care delivery systems
4. Understand the evolution of private health care delivery systems
5. Know the main types of managed care organizations
6. Understand the evolution of public health care delivery systems
7. Evaluate the impact the evolution of health care delivery systems is having on the role of nursing

■ THE IMPACT OF THE EXTERNAL ENVIRONMENT

The preceding discussion illustrates the impact of changing external environmental conditions on health care organizations. The United States was growing and developing; social values were changing; and a multitude of demographic social groups were becoming more vocal. As a result, health care delivery systems evolved to meet the new challenges.

What is the external environment? In common usage, the term *environment* generally conjures up visions of green trees, babbling brooks, fuzzy squirrels, and spotted owls. These are all parts of the *physical environment,* which is but one factor in an organization's external environment. External environment is *all* phenomena that are outside an organization and have the potential to influence the or-

ganization. An organization's external environment comprises *everything* outside its doors. This includes customers, suppliers, competitors, labor unions, governmental agencies, economic conditions, social norms, physical environment, population demographics, and levels of technology.

Put simply, all organizations exist within an external environment that affects their operations. The external environment is the source of resources, such as patients, personnel, and medical supplies necessary for survival. However, as factors in the external environment change, organizations also must change. This is necessary for continued acquisition of resources. Organizations that fail to evolve will have difficulty recruiting and retaining physicians and nurses, attracting patients, and obtaining profitable managed care contracts. In other words, as the external environment changes, organizations also must change to survive.

■ DRIVING FORCES

To be effective, health care organizations must understand the external environment in which they operate so they can anticipate and respond to the significant shifts that take place within this environment. A key to organizational survival is understanding what changing factors within the external environment are driving the need for organizations to change. Driving forces are those changing factors in the external environment that cause an organization to change in response. In other words, they are those factors that are "driving" change. Significant driving forces affect health care delivery systems.

In the United States, one of every seven people employed currently works in the health care industry, and more than 14% of the gross domestic product (GDP) is spent on health care services. Over time, this percentage of the nation's economic activity allocated to health-related services has increased dramatically.

Key terms	
Term	**Definition**
Health care delivery system	A collection of people and organizations working together to provide health care to the population
Organization	Two or more people working together within identifiable boundaries to accomplish a common goal
External environment	All phenomena that are outside an organization and have the potential to influence the organization
Physical environment	The flora, fauna, and geologic factors influencing an organization's actions

From the beginning of the twentieth century through the 1960s, health care expenditures were at relatively moderate and reasonable levels (Williams, 1995). Beginning in the late 1960s and continuing through today, U.S. health care expenditures have increased significantly. In 1960, 5.3% of the GDP was spent on health care–related services (Health Care Financing Administration, 1993). This figure had climbed to 7.4% in 1970, 9.2% in 1980, and 12.2% in 1990. In 1993, 14.2% of the GDP went to health care–related services. This represents a compounded annual increase of 11.8%, compared with a compounded annual growth rate of 8.5% for the GDP as a whole during the same period (Harris, 1994).

No country in the history of the world has ever allocated so much of its economic resources to health care as the United States currently does. Resources allocated to the health care sector of the economy must be taken from other sectors. As an illustration of this, it has been estimated that American automobile manufacturers spend $700 per car providing health care for their employees, a cost passed on to customers (Kaplan, 1993). With health care accounting for a growing percentage of the economy, consumers and politicians must increasingly make spending allocation decisions between health care and other areas, such as consumption, savings, and debt reduction. As long as the United States is willing to spend more on health care and less for other sectors of the economy, the increasing health care costs can be accommodated. However, many policymakers, employers, and individuals worry that the United States will soon reach the limits of what society will tolerate in allocating resources to health care needs (Williams, 1995).

At the same time, U.S. society has some general expectations for the manner in which health care is delivered. Among those factors considered to be the most important—in addition to low fees—are having a choice about which physicians and hospitals to patronize and having access to care when needed (Taylor & Morrison, 1993). Other important factors include the "social right" of access to medical care; the ability to obtain enough information to better understand treatment options; and the desire to have medical care providers who are communicative, are helpful, and possess effective interpersonal skills (Harris, 1994). Although this list is not exhaustive, it does provide some insight into people's expectations for "appropriate care."

Thus health care delivery systems need to do things inexpensively *and* correctly: care providers must keep costs down without cutting corners. To better understand this dilemma, it is useful to distinguish between two classes or types of environments in which organizations must operate: economic and institutional (Kirby, 1996). Economic environments are those within which a product or service is exchanged in a market such that organizations are rewarded with increased legitimacy for effective and efficient control of the work process. In an economic environment, rationalized structures and procedures are developed to efficiently coordinate and evaluate the necessary work. In other words, the focus is on outcomes.

Institutional environments, on the other hand, are characterized by rules, requirements, values, and norms to which an organization must comply to receive legitimacy and support. In institutional environments, organizations are rewarded with enhanced legitimacy for using "proper" structures and following "appropriate" procedures, not for quantity and efficiency of output. In other words, the focus is on processes (Figure 1-1).

Through various institutional systems, society defines what goals are appropriate and how organizations should pursue them. Such belief systems provide the appropriate means of pursuing goals. These institutional systems, or control mechanisms, can include educa-

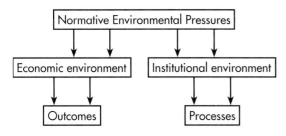

Figure 1-1 ■ Environmental pressures for process and outcomes.

tional systems, public opinion, laws, ideologies, professions, regulatory agencies, certifications, awards, and endorsements. One group of such systems that has a significant impact on health care delivery systems is normative institutional systems (DiMaggio & Powell, 1983).

Normative systems comprise values and norms that specify what is desirable and how things should be done (Scott, 1995). Normative systems place constraints on organizational actions by defining acceptable goals, such as reducing health care costs, and they also specify appropriate ways to pursue the goals, such as following accepted medical practices. Normative control mechanisms are derived from the values of society as a whole and from notions such as commonly accepted ideas of what is "right" and "appropriate."

Given the importance of normative systems, the goal of any organization is to gain and maintain legitimacy in the eyes of society. Legitimacy reflects normative support and alignment with accepted values, as well as an organization's compliance with social obligations (Scott, 1995). The loss of legitimacy can result from failure to conform to accepted practices, values, and norms. This may lead to more coercive mechanisms being used to control an organization's behavior. In other words, if social obligation cannot adequately control an organization's actions, legal and regulatory sanctions may be needed to achieve the desired results.

All organizations exist in both economic and institutional environments to some extent, but one is generally stronger and more important than the other (Meyer & Scott, 1983). Automobile manufacturers, for example, operate in a strong economic environment with pressures for low-cost, high-quality cars and in a weak, although still extant, institutional environment with pressures such as pollution control and workplace safety issues. Religious organizations, on the other hand, generally operate in a strong institutional environment characterized by expectations for compassion and charity but in a weak economic environment in which efficient salvation is not a primary goal.

Health care delivery organizations are in a relatively unique environment in which both institutional and economic environments are strong (Alexander & Amburgey, 1987). The institutional environment, reflecting values governing the provision of necessary and appropriate care, safety, easy access to care, societal welfare, and prolonged life, has been a primary part of the medical care environment since the time of Hippocrates. However, changes in the health care environment have brought about conditions in which cost containment, cost reduction, and improved efficiency in the utilization of effective services are also very important (Shortell & Kaluzny, 1994). The relative strength of technical and environmental forces is shown in Figure 1-2.

The current situation was not always the case. The balance between institutional and economic forces in health care is relatively new. Numerous examples of the supremacy of institutional forces over economic forces can be found in the recent past.

Past

American health care delivery systems have evolved through several phases. In the beginning, health care delivery in the United States consisted of individual services functioning in-

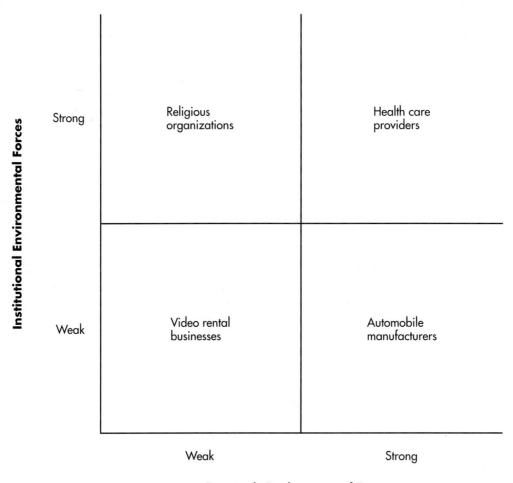

Figure 1-2 ■ Relative strength of environmental forces. (Modified from Scott, W.R. [1992]. *Organizations: Rational, natural, and open systems* [3rd ed.]. Englewood Cliffs, N.J.: Prentice-Hall.)

dependently and without much interaction. This isolation changed with the development of the first large hospitals in the mid-1800s. The advent of hospitals marked the beginning of some form of organized health care system, and the development of a health care system continued to grow primarily as a series of hospitals until the mid-1900s (Torrens, 1993).

With the advent of World War II, the United States saw major changes in the social, political, and technologic aspects of health care delivery. Interest grew in the social and organizational structure of health care. For the first time, attention was directed toward the financing of health care through insurance plans. Power over health care delivery was also increasingly concentrated in the federal government, as witnessed by the Hill-Burton Act, by the huge research budgets of the National Institutes of Health, and by the creation of Medicare (Torrens, 1993).

A key development during this time, in terms of environmental forces, was a shifting perception of health care from a privilege of wealthy persons to a social right of all people. People were no longer content to receive whatever charity was given to them but instead expected quality care to be delivered appropriately and consistent with accepted practices. In other words, the period immediately following World War II witnessed the birth of the current institutional environmental forces facing health care organizations.

Present

In the early 1980s, people began to question the uncontrolled growth of health care delivery. People started to realize that the limits of society's resources were being reached and that health care systems had to consider more cost-effective options for delivering care. Limited resources and restricted growth were forcing a reorganization of the methods of financing and delivering care. In terms of driving forces, the 1980s witnessed the birth of public awareness of the current economic environmental forces facing health care organizations.

In recent public opinion polls, random members of the U.S. adult population were asked about many environmental factors thought to be important to health care organizations. Among those factors rated the most important by the respondents were having a choice about which physicians and hospitals they patronized, access to care when needed, and low financial costs to themselves (Taylor & Morrison, 1993). The general public is also concerned that administrative costs have become too high because of inefficiency and waste (Woolhandler & Himmelstein,

1991). Finally, when asked about utilization of medical services, approximately 75% of Americans favored coordination and control over expensive and marginally effective medical care (Louis Harris & Associates, 1983; Yankelovich, Skelly, & White, Inc., 1984).

Most employers are interested in holding down their cost in providing health insurance to employees (Levit et al., 1994). As a result they are particularly interested in managed care organizations (MCOs) that can offer reduced monthly premiums through mechanisms such as providing cost-effective care and efficient administrative practices (Taylor & Morrison, 1993).

A meta-analysis of public opinion surveys identified the following beliefs of Americans about their health care: (1) access to medical care should be a social right; (2) out-of-pocket expenses should be minimized; (3) freedom to choose physicians and facilities should exist; (4) patients should be able to obtain enough information to better understand treatment options; (5) care providers should be communicative and helpful and should possess effective interpersonal skills; (6) access to high-quality medical care should be available; and (7) bureaucratic and administrative overhead should be reduced (Harris, 1994).

Although public opinion is not an exact science, evidence suggests it does impact health care organizations (Blendon & Altman, 1984). While there are many ways to conceptualize environmental forces, these surveys reflect the strong elements of both economic and institutional forces operating in the health care environment.

As a direct result of these beliefs, many new models of health care delivery systems are emerging and the ideas of MCOs are spreading throughout the United States. A variety of new health care delivery organizations have appeared to provide medical care and other services to patients in their homes. New intermediary organizations are appearing to review patient care quality and utilization of services. Physicians are moving away from solo practices and into large group practices to obtain greater bargaining power for negotiating with insurance companies. Hospitals are rapidly purchasing or establishing freestanding surgical centers, outpatient clinics, and other low-overhead facilities. In short, because of increasing economic and institutional environmental pressures, virtually no health care organization has remained untouched and unchanged. To survive and remain competitive, all health care delivery systems have had to conform to prevailing environmental forces (Kirby & Sebastian, 1998).

Future

As we have seen, health care delivery systems have always faced pressure from institutional environmental forces to provide all necessary medical care in the most appropriate manner possible. Since the 1980s, economic forces facing all aspects of health care delivery have grown significantly stronger. This focus on the fiscal nature of care provision has been achieved, to some extent, at the expense of the provision of appropriate care. In all likelihood, in the foreseeable future, institutional forces will again be stronger. Although cost effectiveness will still be important, it will need to be achieved through mechanisms that do not adversely impact the quality and delivery of care.

A good way to visualize this process is to picture a pendulum (Figure 1-3). In the past, the pendulum arm was far over to the institutional side of the continuum. As time has passed, the arm has swung in the other direction, toward the economic side. In the future, the arm will probably hang in the middle, reflecting a balance between institutional and economic environmental forces.

In fact, there is already a movement away from favoring economic forces over institutional forces. Initiatives to curb actual or perceived de-

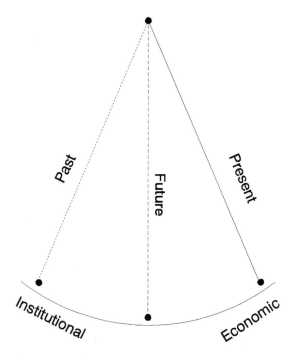

Figure 1-3 ▪ Balance between institutional and economic forces.

ficiencies in managed care have arisen at the federal level and in every state legislature. Because of the perception by most people that MCOs are overemphasizing cost containment at the expense of the provision of care, legislative action has focused on access to appropriate care, availability of information, and freedom of choice. In fact, the most draconian of these measures would have outlawed capitation as a payment mechanism in Oregon (Savage et al., 1997).

The following sections focus on the evolution of private and public health care delivery systems in response to driving forces in the economic and institutional environments.

▪ PRIVATE HEALTH CARE ORGANIZATIONS

The term *private health care organization* refers to nongovernmental organizations designed to provide health care to the populus. These can

Key terms	
Term	**Definition**
Driving forces	Key factors in the external environment that are causing organizational change
Institutional forces	Forces in the external environment that are defining how things should be done
Appropriate care	Medical care provided in a way that society believes to be proper
Economic forces	Forces in the external environment that are pushing for things to be done efficiently
Cost-effective care	Medical care provided in a way that balances the possibility of positive outcomes with the expense of providing the care
Legitimacy	The social right to exist; respect
Managed care organization	An organization that contracts to provide health care to a defined population of patients

be not-for-profit organizations, such as the religious-based health care systems of the Methodist and Catholic churches. They can also be for-profit corporations, such as Columbia/HCA or Blue Cross/Blue Shield. Private health care delivery systems comprise hundreds of different varieties and specializations of medical care providers, facilities, and insurance companies. The key idea behind private health care delivery organizations is that they provide basic and specialty care to anyone who is willing and able to pay the required fees.

Past

Perhaps the most significant organization in the evolution of private health care delivery has been the hospital. Although originally developed as locations to provide rudimentary care for poor people, in the late 1800s hospitals began to emerge as leaders in medical care provision. Before this time wealthy people in society received the best care in their homes. After this time, hospitals became accepted as the best setting for the care of serious illness and injury. To better illustrate this transformation, in 1873 there were only 178 hospitals with 35,604 beds in the United States. By 1929, 6665 hospitals provided 907,133 beds. This rapid growth was brought about by advances in medical knowledge and technology that rapidly changed the hospital's role from a "holding pen" of poor and sickly individuals to a desirable location to receive the finest care available. This transformation has been characterized as an evolution from a social welfare facility to an institution of medical science (Starr, 1982).

In this new role, the hospital assumed an increasingly important position in health care delivery. As medical care technology advanced, the hospital became the central repository for its costly equipment. Physicians competed for privileges at prestigious hospitals. People expected to receive quality care in a hospital, and home care generally was considered to be second rate. If medical care was to be given in an appropriate manner, it had to be given in a hospital. However, with increased pressure from economic environmental forces, all of this changed in the late 1980s and 1990s.

Present

Compared with the dominance of the hospital in private health care delivery systems of the past, today the large freestanding hospital is akin to a dinosaur. For example, as managed care penetration in an area reaches approximately 30% (i.e., 30% of the people living within an area are enrolled in some form of managed care plan), the demand for hospital beds is approximately one half of what it was before the introduction of managed care. Because hospitals are expensive to equip, staff, and maintain, more and more hospitals are downsizing or shutting down entirely. Increasing integration of health care systems and the need to provide comprehensive services for purposes of contracting with employers and insurers have forced hospitals into many other related businesses, such as ambulatory care and home health services (Ermann & Gabel, 1985).

As mentioned, new strategies are being developed to deliver health care in an appropriate and cost-effective manner. In general, the current private health care delivery system can be characterized as a series of close relationships among various components of the delivery system. The most prevalent strategy at this time is managed care. In fact, MCOs have assumed the dominant position previously held by hospitals in private health care delivery systems.

■ OVERVIEW OF MANAGED CARE

Managed care has had a significant influence on the nature and delivery of health care within the United States. MCOs attempt to manage the cost and quality of health care. MCOs operate on the assumption that traditional fee-for-service models do not provide adequate financial controls and utilization incentives for physicians and hospitals to contain the costs of providing health care. The desire to restructure the incentive system to discourage excessive use of costly resources was one of the driving forces resulting in the development and evolution of managed care (Williams, 1995).

Under managed care, patients' needs are balanced with efforts to provide cost-effective care. Typically, MCOs enroll subscribers by promising to provide all necessary medical care in exchange for a fixed monthly premium. The MCO also contracts with hospitals, physicians, and other medical care providers to dispense the necessary medical care to its enrollees at a discounted reimbursement rate. In exchange for accepting reduced fees, the caregivers gain access to the MCO's enrollees.

MCOs use various mechanisms to achieve the objectives of cost containment, maintain the quality of care, and manage patient needs. Primary care gatekeepers are an important control mechanism; they are primary care physicians (PCPs) or mid-level providers (e.g., nurse practitioners, physician assistants) who provide most necessary primary health care. Referrals to specialists require the approval of the gatekeeper. Utilization reviews are used to control the physicians' prescribed use of services and oversee the appropriateness of care prescribed by physicians. Contractual arrangements are established with individual physicians and physician groups to provide care at a discounted price and with some oversight in exchange for access to the MCO's patient base. Financial mechanisms, such as co-payments and deductibles, are created to provide enrollees with a financial incentive to avoid seeking unnecessary care. Case managers are often assigned to high-risk, high-volume patients to coordinate all facets of care provided, thus reducing costly duplication of efforts. Predetermined rates are set for reimbursing physicians for the care they provide to patients. Through these and other mechanisms, MCOs seek to control the costs and utilization of care provided to patients while meeting patients' needs for quality care.

The methods of managing care have evolved over time (Findlay, 1993). Initially, managed care was oriented toward limiting benefits and providing utilization reviews, such as second opinions for surgery. Later, managed care involved provider networks and utilization management through arrangements such as health maintenance organizations (HMOs) and preferred provider organizations (PPOs). The most sophisticated MCOs use quantitative quality measures, patient care management teams, and elaborate physician selection and monitoring techniques. These organizations increasingly involve the vertical integration of services ranging from family-oriented primary care to tertiary hospital care, nursing homes, and home health agencies.

This evolution of MCOs reflects a growing awareness of the impact of financial aspects of health care. Increasingly, MCOs are developing cost-containment methods, constraints on unnecessary utilization, performance evaluation criteria, and other techniques for oversight. All the while, the fundamental objective has been to enhance cost containment, maintain quality, and facilitate the management of patient care needs (Williams, 1995).

So far, the term *managed care* has been used to describe any type of health plan that tries to control costs associated with providing medical care to its enrollees. There are literally hundreds of variations of managed care plans (Wagner, 1996). In an effort to make some sense of this alphabet soup, they can be grouped into three basic types: HMOs, PPOs, and IDS/Ns (Box 1-1).

Health Maintenance Organizations

HMOs are health care organizations that are responsible for both the provision of care and the

B O X 1 - 1

Managed Care Acronyms

Acronym	Term
FFS	Fee for service
HMO	Health maintenance organization
IDS/N	Integrated delivery system/network
IPA	Independent practice association
MCO	Managed care organization
PCP	Primary care physician
POS	Point of service
PPO	Preferred provider organization

financing of care. In essence, they are a combination of a health insurance company and a health care delivery system. Whereas the old fee-for-service (or indemnity) insurers, such as Blue Cross/Blue Shield, were responsible for paying for the treatment patients received from virtually any health care provider, HMOs are responsible for actually providing care to their enrollees. As a result, HMOs must seek to balance the economic and institutional environmental forces by ensuring the appropriateness, quality, and cost effectiveness of all care provided. One of the ways HMOs do this is by requiring all enrollees to first see a PCP before seeing a specialist. Because specialists are generally more expensive than PCPs, referrals can be made only through these PCP gatekeepers, thus reducing the demand for costly services by medical specialists. Other ways HMOs seek to meet environmental pressures are through utilization reviews and other cost-containment measures.

Of the many different forms of HMOs, five are discussed here. Basically, they differ from one another in the way the HMO relates to the physicians. From the perspective of the enrollee, there is little difference among the various types of HMOs. In fact, unless the enrollee discusses financial incentives with his or her physician (which some HMOs forbid their physicians doing), the enrollee may not know the particular form of HMO.

Staff Model HMO In a staff model HMO, the physicians are employees of the HMO. They typically receive a salary plus incentive bonuses based on their performance. This type of plan gives the HMO a great deal of control over the actions of the physicians, making it easier for the HMO to control costs and utilization of medical services. On the down side, staff model HMOs are expensive to maintain. Given the high salaries most physicians earn, the overhead expenses of employing a large number of physicians from a variety of specialties can make it difficult to establish a staff model HMO. Staff model HMOs usually provide patients with little choice in the physician they are allowed to select. As a result, these HMOs often fail to conform to prevailing institutional forces.

Group Model HMO In a group model HMO, the HMO contracts with an independent physician group to provide care for the plan's enrollees. The physicians are employees of the group practice rather than employees of the HMO. Depending on the specifics of the contract binding the group practice and the HMO, the physicians may or may not be able to see patients who are not members of the HMO, in addition to the plan's enrollees. Group models provide the HMO with the ability to control cost and medical care utilization, without having to bear the expense of paying physician salaries. Instead, the HMO agrees to pay the physician group a set fee for the treatment of a specific ailment (this is referred to as *capitation*). Like staff models, group models often are cited for failing to conform to institutional pressures because of limited choice of physicians by enrollees.

Network Model HMO A network model HMO is similar to a group model HMO in that the HMO contracts with physicians rather than employs them. The difference between the two types is in the number of physician groups under contract to the HMO. In a network model, the HMO contracts with many physician groups to provide care to its enrollees. In other words, the enrollees can receive care from a wide network of physicians (hence the name) instead of only from a limited number. Often, HMOs employing a network model contract with a multitude of group practices, each specializing in a different type of medicine. For example, the HMO may contract with a couple of primary care groups, a pediatrics group, a few obstetrics/gynecology groups, and so on. Like the group model, the physician groups are generally reimbursed under capitation. In a net-

work model, the HMO gives up some control over cost and utilization in exchange for providing the enrollee with more choices.

Independent Physician Association Model HMO From the outside, the independent physician association model HMO (IPA HMO) looks very much like a large network model HMO. The difference is that the physicians are not employees of physician groups but are instead individual practitioners with separate offices who are members of an association. The HMO contracts with this association of independent physicians to provide all necessary care to its enrollees. Like the group and network models, the physicians are generally compensated under capitation. Of all the HMO models, the IPA HMO provides the most challenges in terms of effectively controlling cost and utilization rates. However, it has the lowest overhead of all the HMO models as well. An IPA HMO also provides enrollees with the widest number of physicians from which to choose, which can be a powerful tool for recruiting new enrollees.

Point-of-Service HMO Point-of-service (POS) plans are an attempt by insurance companies to better meet institutional pressures for choice and quality of care. Basically, a POS plan is a hybrid of a traditional HMO. It functions exactly as an HMO (of any model), except that the enrollee has the option of receiving medical care from any provider. Generally, as long as the enrollee stays "in network" (i.e., the enrollee receives care through the traditional HMO network), he or she pays only a small co-payment (typically less than $25). However, if an enrollee elects to receive care "out of network," there is a financial penalty. Often the enrollee must pay a deductible (e.g., $500), and then the HMO will reimburse the enrollee for only 80% of "reasonable and customary charges." This means that the enrollee may have to pay the deductible, a percentage of reasonable and customary charges, and 100% of the amount billed by the physician that the HMO considers to be too high. In short, it can be quite expensive to go out of network under a POS plan, However, the option is available.

Preferred Provider Organizations

Preferred provider organizations (PPOs) are similar to group or network HMOs in that the insurance company contracts with physicians and hospitals to provide care to their enrollees. PPOs differ from HMOs in one key area: choice. Enrollees of PPOs are generally allowed to see any physician they wish. They are not limited to an exclusive set of physicians. The physicians and hospitals with which the insurance company contracts are termed *preferred providers.* Patients receiving care through a preferred provider pay low deductibles and co-payments. When an enrollee chooses to see a physician who is not a preferred provider, he or she pays considerably higher deductibles and co-payments. Although enrollees are not required to see a preferred provider, there is a considerable financial incentive to do so. PPOs also differ from HMOs in that they do not require enrollees to go though a PCP gatekeeper before receiving care.

Integrated Delivery Systems/Networks

The latest organizational model designed to meet institutional and economic environmental forces is the integrated delivery system/network (IDS/N). There are three major components in health care delivery: medical care providers, hospitals, and insurance companies. The logic behind an IDS/N is that all three components combine to form one integrated system. The goal is to achieve better conformity to economic and institutional environmental forces through greater economies of scale, more effective utilization of clinical resources, greater influence over provider behavior, and reduced administrative overhead.

IDS/Ns typically have organizational structures that vertically integrate medical care providers, hospitals, and health plans to provide a coordinated continuum of care. This type of health care delivery organization is often willing to be held clinically and financially accountable for the outcomes and health status of the enrollees it serves. A key principle of IDS/Ns is the alignment of incentives to encourage cooperation rather than adversarial relationships among physicians, hospitals, and health plans (Blair et al., 1995). The emergence of these

Key terms	
Term	**Definition**
Private health care delivery system	Collection of nongovernmental people and organizations providing care to anyone willing and able to pay the fees
Indemnity insurance	Insurance based on reimbursing providers or patients for care received
Managed care	Coordinated health care system based on prepayment and oversight of services
Utilization review	After-the-fact oversight of medical services prescribed by physicians
Capitation	Reimbursement system based on predetermined fees
Gatekeeper	Primary care physician responsible for a patient's needs
Enrollee	A person who is a member of a managed care plan

types of organizational forms requires that all components—medical care providers, hospitals, and health plans—adapt to the ever-increasing economic and institutional environmental pressures.

■ **TREND TOWARD INCREASED COST CONTAINMENT**

As has been shown, private health care provision is increasingly emphasizing cost-containment mechanisms. However, many researchers, physicians, and health care administrators have begun to argue that cost controls are being implemented at the expense of the provision of appropriate care (Clancy & Brody, 1995).

It has been noted that the best health care organizations, in terms of providing high-quality and appropriate care while still controlling costs, are usually the older organizations (Kassirer, 1995). Such organizations were generally established in the 1940s through the 1960s, "when cost containment was an unexpected benefit rather than the central purpose" (Clancy & Brody, 1995, p. 338). In contrast, MCOs, for example, that fail to conform to appropriate external standards of medical care are more commonly found among the newest MCOs. Rather than controlling costs through means such as the use of generic drugs (which generally do not affect clinical outcomes), newer MCOs often use alternative means, such as "exclusion of sicker patients, rationing by inconvenience, burdensome micro-management of clinical decisions, or denial of beneficial but expensive care to some patients, either by micro-management or by perverse incentives for providers" (Clancy & Brody, 1995, p. 338).

MCOs have been accused of violating many accepted health care values, such as undermining patients' trust of physicians' motives, recruiting only the healthiest patients and refusing care to truly sick patients, forcing physicians to withhold costly treatments, and increasingly promoting the use of less-skilled medical staff (Kassirer, 1995). Managed care has also been attacked for harming academic medical centers and other medical research establishments (Kassirer, 1995), causing an increase in the percentage of the population without health care coverage, and even contractually forbidding physicians disclosing the existence of services not covered by the managed care plan (Rodwin, 1995).

A recent example of this trend toward increased emphasis on cost containment rather than the provision of appropriate care can be found at Kaiser Permanente. Kaiser Permanente circulated an internal memo in 1995 pushing for 8-hour postobstetric hospital stays as a means of reducing expenditures in routine childbirths. This was being proposed even though most physicians claimed it violated accepted notions of necessary and appropriate medical care.

As a direct result of such emphasis on cost containment at the expense of "appropriate care," many legislative bodies are taking action. For example, effective January 1, 1998, a new federal law ended such "drive through" deliveries by prohibiting MCOs from discharging patients less than 48 hours after natural childbirth and less than 96 hours after cesarean delivery (Savage et al., 1997). As of December 1996, 30 states had already passed similar measures (Savage et al., 1997).

Future

The current trend in health care delivery systems indicates that vertical integration is the best way to meet environmental pressures. Health care delivery systems will certainly become far more integrated in the future. However, will this be enough to provide a competitive advantage and promote survival? It is unlikely. Responding to the need for more coordination in response to changing environmental conditions should not be an isolated act that is independent of the organization's overall strategic purpose. As discussed at the beginning of this chapter, each of the health care delivery subsystems was formed to meet the unique needs of a distinct segment of the population. Organizational managers must be careful not to lose sight of the population they are trying to serve. Although integration provides an exceptional method for reducing administrative redundancies, it can also lead to the organization trying to be everything for everybody. If there is one lesson to be learned from other industries, it is that under extremely dynamic environmental conditions, unfocused expansion and integration, more often than not, lead to failure instead of success. Integration can make an organization sluggish and unable to respond rapidly to environmental changes and prevent it from using state-of-the-art technologies not available within the organization—all characteristics necessary for success in turbulent environments.

Because of these potential disadvantages, some health care delivery systems are turning to virtual integration instead of vertical integration. The logic of creating an efficient continuum of care through alignment of incentives is still the same. The difference comes in ownership and governance mechanisms. Instead of purchasing components to create an IDS/N, virtual integration uses long-term strategic alliances (or very close partnerships). This creates a loosely coupled network capable of achieving objectives not possible by any single organization. Emphasis is placed on communication, commitment, participation, and stability. The objective is not only to achieve similar goals as in the vertically integrated systems, but also to provide the organization with greater flexibility. It is far easier to sever an unproductive alliance than to divest an underperforming division.

Key terms	
Term	**Definition**
Competitive advantage	Being more profitable than most organizations in the industry
Strategic alliance	Very close business partnership
Vertical integration	Owning different types of medical care facilities
Virtual integration	Linking different types of medical care facilities through strategic alliances instead of ownership

■ PUBLIC HEALTH CARE ORGANIZATIONS

Private health care delivery systems are only one facet of our complex health care system. Another important component is the public health care delivery system. Unlike private health care organizations, which have historically focused primarily on providing acute care, public health care organizations have traditionally focused on the prevention of disease. Public health agencies at the state and local levels form the first line of defense against disease and illness. Additional support is provided at the federal level through the national Centers for Disease Control and Prevention, as well as other agencies and even at the international level through the World Health Organization. However, like private health care organizations, public health care organizations are facing similar economic and institutional forces. How public health organizations have dealt with these pressures in the past and present and some likely actions for the future are detailed in the following discussions.

Past

Public health care delivery has its origin in the prevention of infectious diseases. Epidemics of smallpox, bubonic plague, cholera, typhoid fever, venereal disease, malaria, tuberculosis, and other diseases have had a significant impact on human population throughout history. The industrialization of U.S. society, with its accompanying influx of people to urban areas, increased the risk of infectious diseases. The urbanization of America created a greater need for safe water and food supplies. Increased modernization has also brought about "new" diseases and epidemics (e.g., mental illness, heart disease), as well as health risks caused by unsafe working conditions, vehicular accidents as a result of increased traffic, and rodent and sanitation problems arising from crowded living conditions (Williams, 1995).

In response to these issues, most large communities had public health departments by the late 1800s. These bureaucracies grew as the problems they faced through industrialization also grew. By 1900, most states had their own health departments to oversee laboratories, coordinate health education, and regulate food and water supplies (Shonick, 1993).

At the same time, the federal government was involved in public health care delivery, such as operating hospitals in various ports. Following the passage of the Social Security Act of 1935, federal involvement in public health expanded substantially. Subsequently the National Institutes of Health, the Food and Drug Administration, and other governmental agencies, all designed to prevent the spread of disease, were developed (Shonick, 1993).

Present

At present, the federal, state, and local governments, through public health agencies, oversee a broad range of issues, from the prevention of the spread of tuberculosis and measles to violence, drug abuse, teen pregnancy, and homelessness. Public health agencies even focus on prevention of tooth decay. The logic is that all these problems have deeply rooted social determinants and have affected the health of the public (Sommer, 1995). Public health care has grown to encompass a host of marginal issues and problems for virtually every fragmented segment of society; anything that impacts society's health status is covered under some public health program, regardless of where the determinants of the problem lie.

Many governmental agencies share control for these various aspects of public health. The reason for this shared control is that, since the 1960s, a growing number of responsibilities have been developed and assigned to various agencies. The assignment of health care delivery issues to other agencies has occurred, in part, because of a public perception of public health agencies as technically inadequate and managerially inefficient. In addition, there are special interest groups seeking to increase the power and responsibility of their "pet" agencies.

Whatever the cause, the current state of public health care delivery is generally one of disarray, chaos, and a lack of coordination. Multiple agencies are responsible for multiple facets of care, with corresponding bureaucratic and administrative inefficiencies and redundancies. Because of the economic and institutional forces impacting the system, there is a great deal of pressure to improve the delivery of public health care in terms of cost, quality, and access.

Given the environmental pressures, it would be wrong to assume that the entire system is a disjointed quagmire. It is not. In fact, an increasing movement toward greater integration of primary prevention, general preventive services, and primary care has been evident for a number of years. However, there is still much room for improvement.

Future

The role of public health care organizations in the future will depend, in part, on the further development of managed care and health care reform and on beliefs about personal responsibility. There is currently a strong movement to hold individuals more accountable for their actions. As resources become scarcer, a growing number of people are unwilling to subsidize individuals who have made a series of bad choices in their life or simply refused to accept responsibility for their actions. The creation of finite welfare benefits aimed at ending welfare as a life-style is one of the first outcomes of these beliefs. In another example, Proposition 187, passed by a large margin in California in 1995, sent a clear signal that the public was unwilling to pay for illegal aliens to receive public services. These same values are going to have a significant impact on the entire public health care delivery system. Is it an appropriate role for the government to spend precious resources protecting people from themselves (i.e., regulating smoking, alcohol, fatty foods, vehicle passenger restraints), or should the role of public health be scaled back to its original goals (i.e., prevention of infectious disease, oversight of water and food purity)?

However this debate plays out, with increasing control over the full range of expenditures for health-related activities, further integration among these services will be necessary. Greater integration with private health care delivery systems is also coming, one example of which is the growing number of Medicare recipients being given incentives to enroll in private MCOs. As with private health care delivery, increased use of vertical and virtual integration is coming. However, given the greater diversity of interests

Key terms	
Term	**Definition**
Public health care delivery system	Collection of governmental agencies focusing on disease prevention and other issues impacting the health of the population
Bureaucracy	A large organization designed around specialization of tasks and division of labor
Medicare	A federal insurance program for elderly people
Medicaid	A federal insurance program for poor people

in the public sector and the limited availability of funds, the roles of individuals, employers, MCOs, and governmental agencies need to be clarified during this period of integration and collaboration (Shonick, 1993).

A more integrated and comprehensive approach to public health care delivery will yield greater benefits in preventing and treating disease and in protecting the population. In those areas where prevention is cost effective, reductions in overall health care costs can be significant.

■ ROLE OF NURSING

For centuries, the primary role of nursing has been to provide patient care. Nurses have carried out medical regimens, provided nursing care, and assessed and treated patients. They have also functioned as aides to physicians. However, this is changing. The nursing profession and the role of nursing have evolved over the years.

Past

Before the mid-1800s, nursing care was provided by volunteers, generally men and women of various religious orders who had little or no formal training. During the Crusades, for example, some military orders of knights, most notably the Knights Hospitalers, provided nursing care. By the end of the eighteenth century, nurses were working in hospitals but they were commonly people who had been imprisoned for drunkenness or who could not find work elsewhere. Hospitals during the time the United States was born were dirty and pestilent and were considered unsuitable environments for "proper" young women.

Like many other facets of the health care delivery system, modern nursing began in the mid-1800s with the advent of schools for training nurses modeled on the principles of Florence Nightingale. In the United States, the Spanish-American War and World War I established the need for more nurses. As a result, nursing schools increased their enrollments and several new experimental programs were developed. In 1920, a study funded by the Rockefeller Foundation recommended that nursing schools be independent of hospitals and students no longer be exploited as cheap labor. As a result, several university schools of nursing were opened. In 1934, another widely read study recommended a decrease in the supply of nurses and an increase in the quality of educational programs.

During the Great Depression, large numbers of nurses were unemployed, and the number of nursing schools declined. World War II brought about another surge in demand. The Cadet Nurse Corps, begun in 1943, subsidized nursing education for thousands of young people (mostly women) who agreed to become military

nurses for the duration of the war. Since the end of World War II, technologic advances in medicine and health care have required nurses to become better educated and more sophisticated in the provision of care.

The history of the nursing profession reflects changing institutional environmental forces and how the profession evolved to face them. Initially, nursing care provided little more than solace for dying patients, and thus it was a role best suited for religious personnel. As sick persons began migrating to rather primitive hospitals, they expected some rudimentary routine care. However, given the awful physical conditions of these facilities, the very low expectation for quality of care (and correspondingly low expectation for successful outcomes), and the social norms of the time, this care was clearly not a role for professionals; thus the role of nursing evolved into a low-skilled, little-respected task.

Beginning in the mid-1800s, through the actions of Florence Nightingale and others, nursing began to be recognized as a discipline that involved skills and thus demanded trained practitioners. In the United States, this was driven in large part by the recognition of Civil War veterans of the value of skilled nurses in reducing fatalities. With 600,000 men fighting in the war, out of the total U.S. population of 31 million, social norms abruptly changed. Suddenly nursing was no longer a menial occupation, but a somewhat honorable profession. Thus the role of nursing evolved into one of trained professionals. However, the profession was unable to completely shake its old image as a low-skilled, little-respected task—a perception still present today.

As technology improved, the skills needed by nurses increased. Patients began expecting to receive care from highly skilled professional nurses. This drove a need for better training facilities and better trained professionals. Again, with the changing institutional forces, the profession evolved. College-educated nurse graduates became common.

Present

Nursing professionals are struggling to shed their historical stereotype as underpaid female hospital laborers. In the process, considerable controversy has been created both inside and outside the profession. For example, when attempts are made to unionize nurses, these efforts force to the surface the tension many nurses feel between being highly skilled health care professionals versus underpaid employees in a bureaucratic health care organization (Williams, 1995).

The nursing profession is attempting to change its role in the health care delivery system. With a large number of highly educated practitioners, the leaders of the profession have called for an expansion of the independent role of the nurse within the hospital and the creation of new professional roles outside hospitals. Nurses are also seeking to clarify their relationship to physicians, particularly within the context of clinical decision making in the hospital (Aiken, 1982).

Many new roles have emerged for the registered nurse (RN), including positions as clinical nurse specialist, nurse practitioner, nurse anesthetist, nurse clinician, and case (or care) manager. These positions involve working in a multitude of different settings, such as ambulatory care clinics, nursing homes, and home care programs. Career opportunities are also available in utilization and quality review roles, in which nurses participate in inspection of clinical records (Mick & Moscovice, 1993).

Future

"The question for the future of nursing is not whether nursing will exist but rather how it will evolve in the changing health care environment" (Korniewicz & Palmer, 1997, p. 112). As just discussed, the driving forces of the institutional and economic environments are forcing all aspects of the health care system to evolve. The nursing profession is no different. The role of nursing in the foreseeable future will be considerably different from what it was even 10 years ago. One trend is the development of a two-tiered profession, with relatively low-skilled (and lesser-paid) practical nurses and nurses' aides performing traditional routine patient care and highly skilled, highly educated (and considerably higher-paid) professional nurses focusing heavily on managerial duties and the care of critically ill patients. Perhaps the biggest change currently facing the nursing profession is the need for nurses to combine the traditional role of being primarily patient caregivers with the new role of patient care managers.

A variety of new roles for nurses, particularly for those with master's and doctoral preparation, will evolve in response to environmental forces. Among these new roles are case managers, public health/public policy leaders, independent nurse practitioners, clinical research managers, health care administrators, genetic consultants, health care prevention coordinators, telemedicine professionals, and bioethics consultants (Korniewicz & Palmer, 1997). Many of these roles require increased administrative and managerial skills. As a result, the demand for nurses trained in business management as well as nursing will grow.

Many universities are gearing up to better prepare students to meet these new demands. For example, Texas Tech University has begun a joint program between the schools of nursing and business administration, in which a student can earn an MSN and an MBA in Health Organization Management in less time than it would take to pursue each degree separately. Although Texas Tech is at the forefront of academe in this respect, it is not unique. Other universities are offering or are preparing to offer similar programs. Traditional nursing programs prepare students who are well equipped to meet the institutional forces but often leave them ill prepared to deal with the economic aspects. The goal of these new programs is to provide nurse administrators with the business training to successfully meet the coming challenges driven by the economic environment.

■ SUMMARY

This chapter focuses on changing health care delivery systems in the United States. Health care in the United States is delivered through a variety of different systems, each serving a different segment of the population. Driven by changing economic and institutional environmental forces, these health care delivery systems have changed.

In its earliest beginnings, health care was so crude and rudimentary that people had low expectations for successful outcomes. As medical understanding and technology improved, institutional environmental forces developed. People began to expect that they would receive the best care possible, provided in state-of-the-art facilities and delivered in a medically appropriate manner. Lately, awareness of the financial costs of providing care has been growing. As a result of strong economic environmental forces, the current trend is to provide appropriate care in a cost-effective manner.

All facets of health care delivery have been impacted by these changing social norms. Private health care delivery systems have evolved from hospital-focused, indemnity insurance–based care to integrated delivery systems with capitated payments. Public health care delivery systems have changed, too. Since its inception, the role and responsibility of the public health care system have expanded tremendously. With the new cost-conscious mentality, people are struggling to define appropriate goals and roles

for public health care agencies. Because of these changes in delivery systems, the role of nursing has changed from exclusively providing patient care to balancing care provision and care management. In short, the environment in which health care delivery systems and health care professionals exist is evolving. To survive and meet the new challenges, health care organizations and professional roles must also evolve.

■ KEY POINTS

- Health care in the United States is delivered through a variety of systems, all of which are in a state of flux, and changes in these systems are being driven by changing environmental forces.
- The financial costs of delivering health care are major drivers in the changes that are sweeping this industry.
- Private health care delivery systems have evolved from hospital-focused indemnity insurance to fee-based care and more recently to integrated delivery systems with capitated systems of payment.
- The external forces that surround health care are major drivers in the way in which the current health care delivery system is being redesigned. There is more emphasis on cost effectiveness; more health care plans are for profit; there is a greater emphasis on community-based care; and the role of the family has grown as patients have gone home from hospitals with more urgent health care problems than would have been the norm in the past.
- In an era of cost cutting, the impact of institutional environments is significant. That is, institutional environments are characterized by rules, requirements, values, and norms to which the organization must comply.
- The role of the hospital in the current health care system has changed remarkably from the role that institutions played in the past. For

much of the history of U.S. health care, the hospital was central to the system. Now the system is more decentralized with much more care given in outpatient and ambulatory settings.

- Managed care organizations and the concepts that guide them have changed the way in which health care is delivered and also have changed the locus of decision making. Currently, many health care plans and managed care organizations require that a primary care gatekeeper determine which type of specialist the patient needs to see. Patients who choose to make arrangements for care other than those sanctioned by their health plan may be required to pay more out-of-pocket expenses.

- Nursing, like all other aspects of the health care system, has also changed, with more nurses choosing jobs outside the hospital and also outside the traditional public health role. Nurses increasingly are working in community settings and in businesses related to health care but that do not provide direct patient care.

■ CRITICAL THINKING QUESTIONS

1. Given all the changes in health care described in this chapter, design the ideal health care system, taking into account these components:

   A. Would the system be a national system or remain in the private sector?

   B. How would the system be financed?

   C. What would the role of the physician be?

   D. What types of roles would nurses assume?

   E. What would the advantages of the ideal system be compared with the system that we currently have? What would the disadvantages be?

2. Consider the community that you know the most about (i.e., where you grew up, where you have lived, or where you currently live).

Describe the way in which the health care delivery system is organized. What would you change if you had the ability to do so?

3. As you consider the health care system in your community, whose vested interests are being served by the current system? Who would gain, and in what way, if the system were changed? Who would lose if the system were changed?

4. If you were involved in setting health policy, what changes in health care would you support? How would you go about doing this? What coalitions would you build?

5. Describe a new health care system in which nurses are the gatekeepers and take a leadership role in designing the system, triaging patients, and evaluating the outcomes of the organization.

■ REFERENCES

Aiken, L. (1982). The impact of federal health policy on nurses. In L. Aiken (Ed.). *Nursing in the 1980s: Crises, opportunities, and challenges.* Philadelphia: Lippincott.

Alexander, J.A., & Amburgey, T.A. (1987). The dynamics of change in the American hospital industry: Transformation or selection. *Medical Care Review, 44,* 279-321.

Blair, J.B., Fottler, M.D., Paolino, A.R., & Rotarius, T.M. (1995). *Medical groups face the uncertain future: Challenges, opportunities, and strategies.* Englewood, Colo.: Center for Research in Ambulatory Health Care Administration.

Blendon, R.J., & Altman, D.E. (1984). Public attitudes about health-care costs: A lesson in national schizophrenia. *New England Journal of Medicine, 311,* 613-616.

Clancy, C.M., & Brody, H. (1995). Managed care: Jekyll or Hyde? *Journal of the American Medical Association, 273,* 338-339.

DiMaggio, P.J., & Powell, W.W. (1983). The iron cage revisited: Institutional isomorphism and collective rationality in organizational fields. *American Sociological Review, 48,* 147-160.

Ermann, D., & Gabel, J. (1985). The changing face of American health care: Multihospital systems, emergency centers, and surgery centers. *Medical Care, 23,* 401-420.

Findlay, S. (1993). Networks of care may serve as a model for health care reform. *Business & Health, 11*(2), 27-31.

Harris, J.S. (1994). *Strategic health management: A guide for employers, employees, and policy makers.* San Francisco: Jossey-Bass.

Health Care Financing Administration, U.S. Department of Health and Human Services. (1993). *1993 HCFA statistics* (Pub. No. 03341). Washington, D.C.: U.S. Government Printing Office.

Kaplan, R.M. (1993). *The Hippocratic predicament: Affordability, access, and accountability in American medicine.* San Diego, Calif.: Academic Press.

Kassirer, J.P. (1995). Managed care and the mortality of the marketplace. *New England Journal of Medicine, 333,* 50-52.

Kirby, E.G. (1996). The impact of social norms and economic requirements of the strategic marketing of managed care organizations. *Health Marketing Quarterly, 14*(4), 45-54.

Kirby, E.G., & Sebastian, J.G. (1998). The effect of normative social forces on managed care organizations: Implications for strategic management. *Journal of Healthcare Management, 43*(1), 81-95.

Korniewicz, D.M., & Palmer, M.H. (1997). The preferable future for nursing. *Nursing Outlook, 45,* 108-113.

Levit, K.R., Cowan, C.A., Lazenby, H.C., McDonnell, P.A., Sensenig, A.L., Stiller, J.M., & Won, D.K. (1994). National health spending trends, 1960-1993. *Health Affairs, 13*(5), 14-31.

Louis Harris & Associates. (1983). *The Equitable healthcare survey: Options for controlling costs.* New York: Equitable Life Assurance Society.

Meyer, J.W., & Scott, W.R. (1983). *Organizational environments: Ritual and rationality.* Beverly Hills, Calif.: Sage.

Mick, S.S., & Moscovice, I. (1993). Health care professionals. In S.J. Williams & P.R. Torrens (Eds.). *Introduction to health services* (4th ed., pp. 269-296). Albany, NY: Delmar.

Rodwin, M.A. (1995). Conflicts in managed care. *New England Journal of Medicine, 332,* 604-607.

Savage, G.T., Kirby, E.G., Cochran, C.E., Friedman, L.H., & Purtell, D. (1997, August). *Health care at the crossroads: Managed care and the two faces of state reforms.* Paper presented at the meeting of the Academy of Management, Boston.

Scott, W.R. (1995). *Institutions and organizations.* Thousand Oaks, Calif.: Sage.

Shonick, W. (1993). Public health agencies and services: The partnership network. In S.J. Williams & P.R. Torrens (Eds.). *Introduction to health services* (4th ed., pp. 73-107). Albany, N.Y.: Delmar.

Shortell, S.M., & Kaluzny, A.D. (1994). Organization theory and health services management. In S.M. Shortell & A.D. Kaluzny (Eds.). *Health care management: Organization design and behavior* (3rd ed., pp. 3-29). Albany, N.Y.: Delmar.

Sommer, A. (1995). W(h)ither public health? *Public Health Reports, 110,* 657-661.

Starr, P. (1982). *The social transformation of American medicine.* New York: Basic Books.

Taylor, H., & Morrison, J.I. (1993). Public opinion: Attitudes toward managed healthcare. In P. Boland (Ed.). *Making managed healthcare work: A practical guide to strategies and solutions* (pp. 51-69). Gaithersburg, Md.: Aspen.

Torrens, P.R. (1993). Historical evolution and overview of health services in the United States. In S.J. Williams & P.R. Torrens (Eds.). *Introduction to health services* (4th ed., pp. 1-28). Albany, N.Y.: Delmar.

Wagner, E.R. (1996). Types of managed care organizations. In P.R. Kongstvedt (Ed.). *The managed health care handbook* (3rd ed., pp. 33-45). Gaithersburg, Md.: Aspen.

Williams, S.J. (1995). *Essentials of health services.* Albany, N.Y.: Delmar.

Woolhandler, S., & Himmelstein, D.U. (1991). The deteriorating administrative efficiency of the U.S. health care system. *New England Journal of Medicine, 324,* 1253-1258.

Yankelovich, Skelly, & White, Inc. (1984). *Health and health insurance: The public's view.* Washington, D.C.: Health Insurance Association of America.

Systems Theory and Analysis in Health Care and Nursing

Richard A. Ridge and Cheryl Bland Jones

INTRODUCTION

Six blind men, located at different parts of an elephant, set about to analyze and describe the elephant. Upon completion of each man's task, findings were reported as follows: the man at the tail described the elephant as ropelike; the man at the trunk concluded that the elephant was similar to a snake; and the man at a leg described the elephant as a tree. The other men reached similar conclusions based upon their location relative to the elephant and the limited information available. After a discussion of each man's findings, the men could reach no consensus about the elephant's description. Their ability to understand the whole elephant was impeded by each man's limited perspective and by an inability to agree upon or synthesize information obtained separately. The moral of this story is that a clear identification of the system or subsystem under consideration is a crucial prerequisite to a clear understanding of the whole.

This ancient Hindu fable, converted to verse by John Godfrey Saxe (1868), is often cited in systems texts (Churchman, 1968) to highlight the importance of perspective and the inherent faulty logic associated with focusing on a single, isolated part of a whole. Knowledge and appreciation of the elephant, in its entirety, would have undoubtedly led these men to consensus

on the elephant's description and to a better description than any of the men could have reached alone.

There is an ongoing demand for nurses to understand and respond to challenges, threats, and opportunities within the profession and within the larger health care system. These challenges include the following:

- Transformation of the health care financing and delivery systems
- Increasing competition among health care providers
- Expansion and proliferation of managed care
- Restructuring of practice and service delivery to meet changing societal demographics and needs
- Increasing pressure to downsize care delivery systems
- Shifting from hospitals as locus of care delivery to a continuum of care services ranging from prevention to the home and beyond
- Providing cost-effective, affordable, and accessible care to individuals in need

Successful resolution of these challenges will require increased intradisciplinary and interdisciplinary collaboration, further clarification of professional roles, continued formation and development of health care networks, continued effective work redesign, and close attention to identifying and meeting health care needs. These numerous interrelated issues in health care and nursing are probably not amenable to separate and isolated solutions, which may improve one aspect of a problem at the expense of another. Rather, integrated and cost-effective solutions that consider all aspects of a situation are required to resolve the myriad of complex issues facing nursing and health care.

Systems theory provides a framework for conceptualizing and defining many issues and problems in nursing and health care. An inherent premise of systems theory is that appreciating a system and relationships between its components—within the context of its environment—will increase the likelihood that the system will function more efficiently and effectively. Systems theory is the foundation of systems science, a discipline whose domain of inquiry includes the study of principles and characteristics of systems (Klir, 1991). Systems science provides the basis for understanding systems in a broad range of applications, including nursing and organizational contexts.

This chapter introduces systems theory as a philosophy and framework for understanding, analyzing, and changing systems in health care organizations and nursing. A brief chronology of general systems theory (GST) development is presented within the context of systems science, and an overview of systems is provided. A discussion of systems theory in organizations is presented, with special emphasis on health care organizations. The King Systems Theory of Nursing (King, 1971, 1981), the Neuman Systems Model (Neuman, 1995; Neuman & Young, 1972), and applications of systems approaches in nursing and health care are presented to illustrate how systems theory has been used. A method of systems analysis is introduced, followed by application of the method to a nursing issue, to demonstrate how systems theory can be extended to systematically evaluate complex problems within evolving health care systems.

OBJECTIVES

After reading this chapter, you will be able to:

1. Describe the development and principal aspects of general systems theory
2. Identify general systems as a model for understanding organizations
3. Analyze the major components of general systems
4. Cite health care and nursing examples of open and closed systems
5. Relate principles of systems theory and analysis to nursing practice and management
6. Evaluate the use of systems theory and analysis in health care organizations

■ DEVELOPMENT OF GENERAL SYSTEMS THEORY AND SYSTEMS SCIENCE

GST emerged from the organismic perspective in biology during the 1920s and 1930s (Bertalanffy, 1968). This perspective recognized the living organism as an aggregate of cells, not fully understandable by analytic reduction into smaller and smaller parts. The competing mechanistic perspective, on the other hand, held that reality can be best understood by isolating parts of the organism to determine individual causal chains (Bertalanffy, 1968). Whereas Bertalanffy pursued the empiric, inductive approach of studying individual systems to form generalizations, Ashby (1958) took the deductive approach of considering all possible systems, real and theoretic, to further refine the theory. The philosophy, meaning, and significance of systems theory were summarized by Laszlo (1972) as a unitary framework for understanding and studying complex hierarchic systems.

Systems theory was further developed and generalized for application across other disciplines, including the social sciences. A classic example from biology is Miller's Living Systems model (1978). This model incorporates principles and concepts from GST in a hierarchic model of living systems, ranging from the cellular level to organizational and societal level systems. Other disciplines incorporating GST include operations research and engineering (Churchman, 1968), economics (Boulding, 1956), management science (Kast & Rosenzweig, 1972), and sociology (Parsons, 1951).

Systems Assumptions and Components

Merriam-Webster's Collegiate Dictionary (1994, p. 1199) defines a system as "a set or arrangement of things so related as to form a whole." This definition is consistent with GST, albeit incomplete, and provides a good starting point for discussing the assumptions and components of systems theory and analysis. For this discussion, a system is defined as an interrelated set of subsystems that interacts to optimize system output (Bertalanffy, 1968).

Systems Assumptions Several assumptions are necessary for understanding and applying systems theory in organizations, nursing, and health care. The first assumption is that systems comprise components that function and interrelate to form a whole with a purpose, goal, or objective (Bertalanffy, 1968). Churchman (1968) emphasizes the importance of defining a system's purpose, which reflects the overall objectives of the system in relation to its environment, and specific objectives ranked in order of importance to the system.

Additional assumptions relate to the system's relationship with the environment and internal organization. The second assumption in systems theory is that systems can be open or closed. According to Bertalanffy (1968), systems that interact with the environment are open, whereas systems that do not interact with, or are isolated from, their environments are considered closed. Through interactions, open systems receive input from and provide output to the environment. Hence, living, social, and organizational systems interact with the environment, at least to some degree, and are considered open. It can be argued that completely closed systems do not exist in living, social, or organizational contexts (Bertalanffy, 1968) but exist only in controlled or isolated situations.

The notion of an open or closed system can be further expanded by considering openness as a continuum rather than a simple dichotomy. Thus a system could interact more or less with its environment, and the interaction of a system with its environment could vary across time. In addition, different types of systems (e.g., social, mechanical) may vary by degree of openness. Kast and Rosenzweig (1972) note that most social organizations and their subsystems are partially open and partially closed.

Key terms	
Term	**Definition**
System	A set of interrelated components that serve a greater purpose or objective than the singular components (Bertalanffy, 1968)
Systems theory	A philosophy and conceptual framework for understanding and analyzing systems
Systems analysis	Problem-solving method for systems issues, based on systems theory
Open system	Systems that interact with their environments
Closed system	Systems that do not interact with their environments

The third assumption of GST is that systems increase their internal structure and communication as a result of interacting with the environment (Bertalanffy, 1968). As energy enters the system, the components self-organize within certain prescribed structures and functions that serve to move the system toward goal attainment. Subsystems emerge and relationships are formed in an overall effort to satisfy the goals and objectives of the system as a whole (Bertalanffy, 1968; Kast & Rosenzweig, 1972; Miller, 1965, 1978).

The concept of *differentiation* expands on the assumption that systems increase their internal structure and communication in response to environmental interaction. Increased interaction with the environment results in an increase of input and output, which necessitates higher levels of system function (Miller, 1965, 1978). Differentiation refers to the degree to which the system has developed in size and complexity. In a discussion of societal organization and differentiation, Laszlo (1972) asserts that open, adaptive systems evolve toward higher levels of complexity (i.e., differentiation) as they interact with their environments in pursuit of goals and objectives. A system well matched with its environment becomes increasingly complex, creating subsystems and establishing or modifying throughputs. Within organizations, for example, differentiation occurs as internal structures and communication increase in terms of complexity (i.e., levels and specialization), formalization (i.e., reliance on formal policy and procedures), and centralization (i.e., locus of decision making) (Robbins, 1990).

Systems Components A typical open system (Figure 2-1) provides a reference for further discussion of systems components. The system comprises four subsystems, interconnected by feedback loops and surrounded by a boundary that separates the system from its environment. Input (i.e., resources) and output, targeted toward a purpose, exist in the environment and are connected to the system via feedback loops. Each subsystem also serves a limited intent or objective related to the system's overall purpose.

The *boundaries* of a system are the points of interaction between the system and the environment (Bertalanffy, 1968) (see Figure 2-1). The boundary operates like a set of limitations or parameters under which a specific system functions. The system resides within the boundary, and the external environment exists outside the boundary. System boundaries also serve to differentiate the system from its environment, and internal boundaries function to differentiate subsystems within a system and relations within the system as a whole. For example, boundaries in a social system, such as an organization, may denote organization, department, or unit levels. Boundary definition is important because it distinguishes the system from its environment and the subsystem from the system. Figure 2-1

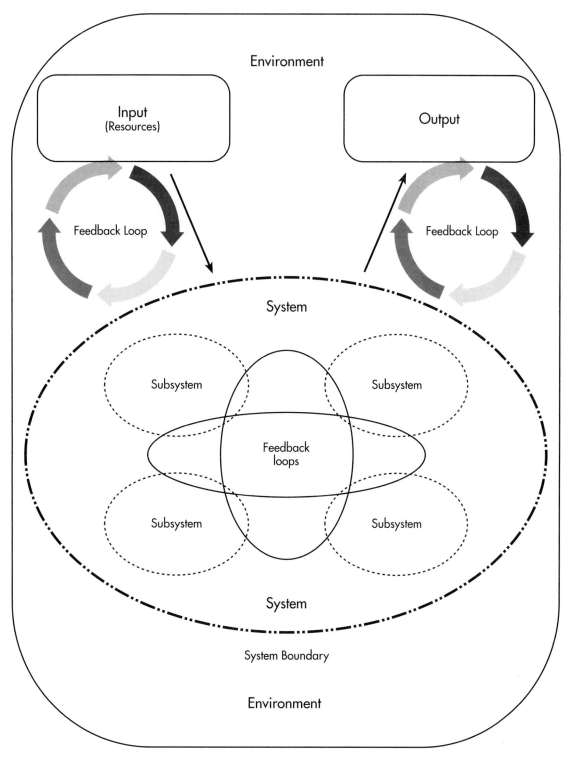

Figure 2-1 ▪ **Typical open systems.** (From Richard A. Ridge and Cheryl B. Jones, 1997.)

Key terms	
Term	**Definition**
Differentiation	Continuous interaction between systems and environments leading to increasingly complex interdependence within and between systems and an evolution toward greater levels of sophistication and organization (Miller, 1978)
Boundaries	Points at which open systems interact with the external environment and individual subsystems interact with the internal environment (Kast & Rosenzweig, 1972)
Throughput	Process applied to resources within the system components (Klir, 1991)
Input	Resources from the environment that are incorporated into system, such as oxygen into a cell (Miller, 1978)
Output	Matter, energy, or information that emerges from the system for some purpose or value to the environment (Miller, 1978)
Environment	The context within which the system exists (Bertalanffy, 1968)

shows a system that distinguishes its four individual subsystems, the environment, and its boundaries.

An example of a system is the hospital, with individual departments such as patient care,

pharmacy, radiology, and laboratory as subsystems. The hospital resides within the overall environment, described in terms of social, political, cultural, and economic terms. The input of the hospital system includes patients and resources, with the output consisting of health care services.

Defining that which is internal and external to the system boundary further facilitates the identification of system components. The distinction between environment and system can be further explicated by identifying factors that serve to limit or enhance system activity but remain outside the sphere of influence by the system (Boulding, 1956). For example, social and political factors outside the control of an organization are considered to be part of the environment. Churchman (1968) notes that a system exists not only within an environment but also by means of its environment. In other words, systems must be defined, to some extent, in relation to environments. The distinction will vary depending on the nature of a system at any time. Generally, the environment includes factors that are predefined, given, and not amenable to system manipulation, such as external, political, social, and economic factors. On the other hand, the system consists of components that can be modified in response to the environment.

Open systems are commonly characterized as having input, throughput, and output. *Input* is the entire set of resources entering a system, which includes information, matter, and energy (Bertalanffy, 1968). Figure 2-1 shows input as resources within the environment but existing outside the system boundary. Input should be described in terms of its salient attributes. For example, information related to size, type, category, and quantity of a given resource is essential to describe and evaluate the system relative to its goals, objectives, and purpose. The labor market pool, which can be specified in terms of number, skill level, extent of experience, and salary, is an illustration of an organizational input.

Throughput refers to processes within a system or individual subsystem used to transform inputs and move the system toward reaching established goals and objectives (Miller, 1965, 1978). Throughput is the intermediary and necessary system component that links input and output. In Figure 2-1, throughputs include all processes that occur within system and subsystem boundaries. For example, a throughput in a human resource subsystem of an organization is the payroll process.

Output, an essential element of open systems, is the end product of a system's efforts. In this case, inputs of matter, energy, or information enter the system and are transformed within subsystems and exported to the environment as output (Bertalanffy, 1968; Miller, 1965, 1978). Output is intended to meet the system's purpose, goals, and objectives. Organizational output may include goods, products, and services, as well as less tangible outcomes, such as reputation with the community, relationships with other systems in the environment, and financial status.

The output of a system is directly related to the input and may be described on at least three dimensions: (1) desirable or undesirable, (2) intended or unintended, and (3) primary or secondary. First, the desirability of an output is related to the extent to which the particular output facilitates the attainment of system goals. Output that interferes with or does not contribute to the desired goals is considered undesirable. For example, the paper waste of an organization generated as a result of inefficient processes is undesirable. Second, output may be the intended result of the system throughput when it is foreseen and planned or the unintended result of throughput, in which case the output is unanticipated. To continue the paper waste example, waste produced as a result of prescribed procedures and standard processes

would be considered intended, whereas unnecessary waste incurred through faulty equipment or deficient personnel performance would be considered unintended. Third, output may be referred to as primary, when it is related to the principal purpose of a system, or as secondary, in which case the output is related to lower priority goals and objectives. For example, if the waste paper output were used to generate revenue that supported the overall organization, this would be considered secondary output, since it is beneficial to the organization but it is not directly related to the primary organizational purpose. Finally, it should be noted that these categorizations of output are not mutually exclusive, and output may be described in any or all of these dimensions.

Constraints, as described by Klir (1991), are factors within the environment or system that serve to limit subsystem activity. Constraints relate to each system component and are beyond the scope of system control: input constraints influence availability of resources; throughput constraints affect subsystem processes; and output constraints are environmental factors that limit output. Examples include availability of personnel or supplies (input constraints), organizational policies and procedures that directly affect subsystems (throughput constraints), and environmental factors such as market demand (output constraints).

Feedback serves as communication and control mechanisms within the system, and between the system and its environment, whereby output-related information is appropriately relayed. Feedback loops (see Figure 2-1) coordinate and integrate system activity, regulate flow of input and output, and control interactions between the system and its environment (Miller, 1978). Although many complex internal and external feedback processes have been described, simple feedback serves as a prototype. Bertalanffy (1968) describes feedback as a circular and continuous process that involves a stimulus, re-

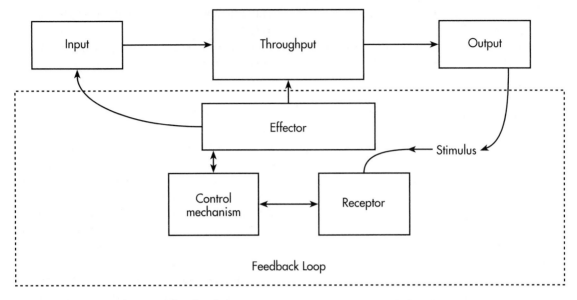

Figure 2-2 ■ Typical feedback loop. (From Richard A. Ridge and Cheryl B. Jones, 1997.)

ceptor, control mechanism, and effector (Figure 2-2). The feedback process occurs when a receptor receives a stimulus (i.e., information related to the output) from a subsystem or the environment and then forwards a signal to the control mechanism. The control mechanism, in turn, communicates with the effector regarding system output. The effector interacts with system input and throughput to regulate system activity by increasing or decreasing system output. Feedback loops, which serve as communication links, can occur on many levels within a system, and between the system and its environment (see Figure 2-1). An example of a feedback loop within a system is the communication between departments within an organization required to deliver a service to customers. An example of feedback between a system and its environment is a customer satisfaction survey process.

Hierarchy is the notion that systems range in degree of structure and function from simple to complex (Bertalanffy, 1968). Systems with less structure and function are lower on the hierar-

chy, whereas systems with greater complexity are higher. Inherent in the idea of hierarchy is the progressive and graded nature of systems in which successive levels build on previous subordinate ones. The idea of hierarchic order allows comparison of different systems and generalizations of system theory across a wide range of system types. For example, within the hierarchy of a health system network, individual hospitals consist of individual departments, which in turn comprise specific multiple units.

Classifying Systems The idea of hierarchic systems has been expanded and formalized within several classification schemata of systems. The classification of systems provides additional insight into applying systems theory, understanding system structure and function, conducting systems analysis, and ultimately modifying system processes. Specifically, by classifying systems, their components, relationships, and boundaries are more readily identified. Classification schemata provide a method to describe and compare systems for study, al-

Key terms	
Term	**Definition**
Constraints	Factors within the environment or system that serve to limit throughputs or subsystem activity (Klir, 1991)
Feedback	Information or output from one subsystem to another or from the environment to the system that serves to adjust the system's internal processes or throughputs (Bertalanffy, 1968)
Hierarchy	Ranking and defining of systems and subsystems in terms of their relative interdependence and complexity in terms of structure and function (Bertalanffy, 1968)

though no single classification schema is all inclusive. Table 2-1 presents an overview of three systems classifications.

The first classification, developed by Boulding (1956), is a nine-level model designed to form a common systems language across multiple disciplines and to serve as a guide for studying systems. Boulding's classification begins at the level of static structure and progresses along a dimension of increasing organizational complexity to the highest level of transcendental systems. Lower-level systems function as simple feedback mechanisms, whereas higher-level systems become progressively larger and incorporate an increasing number of subsystems and feedback loops. Higher-level systems become more complex, and as a result, multiple and potentially conflicting goals and objectives become a concern. The highest level in this classification, transcendental, is the most abstract and is intended to include systems

that are beyond the current level of systems knowledge.

Miller's living systems theory (1965, 1978), developed within a biologic framework, contains a seven-level hierarchy of living systems, including organizations. Incorporating some of Boulding's higher levels, the classification emphasizes the general nature of living systems, uniting elements of biology and social organization. This model further develops systems classification by specifying aspects of input, throughput, and output that characterize each level. In this taxonomy, the lowest level of a living system is the cell, and each successive level is a system that comprises lower-level subsystems. Hence, a system of cells makes up an organ, a system of organs makes up an organism, a system of organisms makes up a group, and so forth, until the highest level of supranational is achieved.

Klir's five-level classification of systems (1969, 1985) is the most abstract classification system presented here. Developed from an engineering perspective, this schema was designed as an all-inclusive general classification for describing and studying all systems. Although there are similarities between Klir's classification and that of Miller (1965, 1978), Klir defines levels in terms of three relationships: (1) the investigator (observer) and the environment, (2) the investigated object and its environment, and (3) the interaction between investigator and object. The levels in this taxonomy are further defined in terms of system complexity, degree of interaction with the environment, and the ability of the system to adapt to external forces. At the lowest level, input and output are nonexistent and the system is essentially closed (Bertalanffy, 1968). Higher levels include systems that interact more with the environment, with descriptions that focus on boundaries and the relationship of the system with its environment. These higher-level systems often require data modeling and interpretation for

T A B L E   2 - 1

Classification Schemata for Determining System Levels

Boulding's Systems Hierarchy (1956)	Miller's Living Systems (1965, 1978)	Klir's Systems Hierarchy (1969, 1985)
1. Static structures	1. Cell	1. Source system
2. Simple dynamic systems	2. Organ	2. Data system
3. Cybernetic	3. Organism	3. Generative system
4. Open/self-maintaining	4. Group	4. Structure system
5. Genetic-social	5. Organization	5. Meta-systems
6. Lower animal	6. Society	
7. Human	7. Supranational	
8. Social		
9. Transcendental		

complete systems description. The highest level, meta-systems, includes large-scale systems comprising multiple systems that function independently but are linked together through relationships in the environment.

■ SYSTEMS THEORY AS A MODEL FOR STUDYING ORGANIZATIONS

Insofar as organizations are systems, methods for analyzing, understanding, and managing organizations are grounded in systems theory. The integration of organizational behavior and systems theory presented in the works of Katz and Kahn (1966), Thompson (1967), Kast and Rosenzweig (1972), Nadler and Tushman (1982), Senge (1990), and Banner and Gagne (1995) illustrates the natural linkages.

In a discussion of organizations and systems theory, Katz and Kahn (1966) recommend a shift away from describing organizations solely as isolated or closed systems and toward characterizing organizations as open systems. Katz and Kahn point out at least three significant problems that result when organizations are treated as closed systems. First, the closed systems view fails to recognize the dependency of the system on its environment for input and that input may vary across time and space. Second, the closed systems view does not recognize that there are often multiple approaches to achieve a given objective. In reality, organizations must adapt to their environments through the formation of subsystems and feedback loops to examine current approaches and create new approaches to meet goals and objectives. Third, the closed systems view fails to allow for system differentiation and the development of subsystems that serve to monitor conditions in the environment and facilitate changes in input or output.

Thompson (1967) compares and contrasts the closed and open systems perspective in organizations. The closed system is described as a rational model, whereas the open system is viewed as a natural-systems model for organizations. The rational model is based on the notion that environmental conditions are fixed or at least highly predictable and certain. The natural-systems model recognizes and incorporates environmental uncertainty as a necessary condition for designing flexible and adaptive systems. Thompson emphasizes that organizations function as open systems with subsystems specifically developed for interaction with the input and output elements of the environment. The technical core, or throughput, of the organization becomes connected to the environment through the subsystems.

Kast and Rosenzweig (1972) suggest that systems theory is a necessary conceptual framework in organizational behavior and management science, providing the basis for a contingency view of organizations. The contingency view recognizes the organization's relationship with its environment and the need for an organization to adapt to a changing environment for survival. Subsystems are delineated from the environment by specific boundaries, and flexible management and operational subsystems are developed in response to the environment. This viewpoint provides additional perspective by emphasizing that organizational systems exist and interact on at least three levels—the environment, the social organization, and the human or participant level. Kast and Rosenzweig believe that the full use of systems theory in organizations is limited by a lack of organizational subsystems knowledge, leading to the implementation of a partial systems approach in highly complex systems. For example, in a hospital context, relationships among nursing units and between nursing units and other departments must be taken into consideration to address system-wide issues.

Nadler and Tushman (1982) also view organizations as systems and advocate a congruence approach to organizational effectiveness. In this model, emphasis is on the "fit" between and among system input, throughput, and output and the degree to which the input, throughput, and output interact as a whole. Their definition of input includes not only resources but also environmental factors, historical issues, and strategic plans. Throughput occurs within and among system tasks, individuals, organizational structures, and informal arrangements.

Output is described in terms of goal attainment, resource utilization, and adaptability to the environment. The hypothesis in this model is that organizations with higher levels of congruence will be more effective, as measured by the degree to which actual output meets expected performance. The model recognizes that various combinations of system components may facilitate maximal output. In addition, the model recognizes the importance of time and current function in determining future organizational performance.

Senge (1990) regards organizations as systems in which individuals interact in such a way as to accomplish the organization's goals and objectives. In this model, effective organizations comprise people who function interdependently as a team, with an emphasis on the acquisition and development of new skills and processes. Leadership within what Senge calls "the learning organization" strives toward supporting the interdependencies of people and teams in an effort to develop new capabilities in response to the environment.

In writing about learning organizations, Senge (1990) characterizes systems thinking as a powerful problem-solving language that guides understanding of complex issues within organizations. Beyond simply understanding issues or organizations as being made up of parts, systems thinking reflects interrelationships and patterns within organizations rather than discrete structures and components. Systems thinking is a perspective that reflects the ability to see and appreciate the "big picture" and provides the "sensibility for the subtle interconnectedness that gives living systems their unique character" (Senge, 1990, p. 69). The identification and understanding of major relationships of variables within a system and between a system and its environment are prerequisites for a valid conceptualization of the system as a whole. As characterized by Senge (1990), systems thinking is an art and science that includes but is not limited to the large set of methods derived from systems theory.

An example in nursing practice is provided by comparing the patient care perspective of case management with traditional episode-of-care approaches. In the traditional approach, the nurse might focus on the acute needs of the patient at the time of hospitalization, with little attention to health behavior, disease prevention, and health promotion issues that may be amenable to nursing intervention. In the case management approach, which reflects systems thinking, nursing care is restructured to include the care of the patient along a continuum of time outside the limited period of hospitalization to provide maximum impact.

Banner and Gagne (1995) characterize postcontingency theory as being complementary to systems theory. In this model, organizations are viewed as infinitely complex systems within environments defined in terms of economic, political, and cultural factors. These authors suggest that although it remains important to understand the interconnectedness of subsystems, it is often difficult, if not impossible, to identify and quantify all significant system variables. Hence, postcontingency theory places less emphasis on predicting and controlling system processes and greater attention on creating organizational cultures that promote creativity in the pursuit of common goals.

In effect, systems theory has provided the foundation for the development of significant and valuable perspectives in the study of organizational effectiveness. The systems perspective illustrates the evolution in organizational theory from the closed view to the open systems model, which clarifies two significant implications. First, the emphasis on internal control within organizations has shifted to a recognition of the value and necessity of participation among system components and members. Second, the focus on internal organizational functioning has

Key terms	
Term	**Definition**
Learning organization	Striving of leadership within learning organizations toward supporting the interdependencies of people and teams in an effort to develop new capabilities in response to the environment
Systems thinking	A powerful problem-solving language that guides understanding of complex issues within organizations, based on the assumption that organizations are made up of parts with patterns of interaction, rather than discrete structures and components
Postcontingency theory	Views organizations as infinitely complex systems within complex environments defined in terms of economic, political, and cultural factors

been transformed to an ever-expanding appreciation of the importance of the organization's relationship within the greater social context.

■ SYSTEMS THEORY IN HEALTH CARE AND NURSING

Systems theory is particularly useful in health care and nursing, since nursing is an interactive social system within health care organizations and the greater health care industry (Hazzard, 1971). Further, systems theory has been widely used in health care and nursing as a foundation for theory development, to study organizational and professional practice issues, and to develop practice innovations. This section provides a brief overview of major works in these areas, including health care systems management and conceptual models of nursing based on systems theory.

Systems Theory in Health Care Systems Management

Howland (1963a, 1963b) and Howland and Mc-Dowell (1964) integrated systems theory and health care management to construct a systems approach in the design and operation of patient care and hospital systems. Specifically, Howland and McDowell described a model that related the design of a hospital system to its operations, emphasizing the management of patient care objectives. Although this work was published more than 30 years ago, it has important implications in health care today. Specifically, this work shifted the focus within hospitals from disciplines (i.e., nursing, medical, and the resulting "hospital" care) to the outputs of care, or patient outcomes. Howland and colleagues advocated the use of traditional criteria, such as nursing hours per patient day, to augment additional standards related to patient education and discharge.

In a discussion of factors driving major health care delivery changes and the reinvention of the hospital, Shortell et al. (1995) envision the need for hospitals to undergo significant change. These authors foresee a shift from the hospital as the focal point of health care delivery to an integrated health care system, whereby health care delivery occurs across a continuum of services. The transition from single hospital to health care systems is characterized as a shift from hospital independence to system integration. Shortell et al. draw upon systems theory for insight into understanding this transition from the multihospital systems formed in the

1980s (i.e., horizontal integration) to the formation of health care networks incorporating organizations that provide a variety of health care services (i.e., vertical integration) (Box 2-1). The authors describe the 1980s multihospital systems as being based primarily on achieving administrative economies of scale and not well integrated in terms of sharing common purpose, goals, and objectives. Current health system networks, on the other hand, have formed in response to a redefinition of the primary organizational objective via the social environment from the delivery of acute care to the management of population health. Networks, in turn, restructured to align services with the new purpose, goals, and objectives, driven by societal need and market forces.

The ability of an organization to function more effectively when structured as a system rather than as separate individual components is further explicated by Shortell and Hull (1996). They examined factors that promote integration and the formation of organized health care delivery systems. Financially viable and efficient systems were able to provide more accessible and cost-effective care across the continuum than nonintegrated hospitals. Key system factors related to the alignment of physician services with the overall hospital mission and the alignment of the entire enterprise with community needs. Specific factors included a synthesis of physician and hospital organization structures, the implementation of physician incentives aligned with the overall objectives, and the systematic vertical integration of clinical services.

On a small scale, an example of the benefit from integration of systems is situations where the acute care hospital has been integrated with home health care services. On an optimal level, patients would perceive high levels of consistency and continuity of care as they transferred between systems of care.

As health care networks emerge in response

Types of System Integration

Horizontal

Horizontal integration refers to the joining of two or more systems (i.e., organizations or business entities) that produce either the same or similar products or services.

Examples
- The merger of several physician practices
- The merger of two or more community hospitals
- An acquisition of many specialty hospitals with similar services, such as the establishment of national chains of rehabilitation, psychiatric, or substance abuse treatment facilities
- Alliances or networks of specialty services, such as day surgery centers or hospices

Vertical

Vertical integration refers to the joining of two or more systems whose products or services are inputs to, or outputs from, one another.

Examples
- The merger of physician practices and hospitals
- The acquisition of home care agencies, long-term care facilities, or nursing homes by an acute care facility
- The acquisition of physician primary care practices by an acute care hospital

Data from Conrad, D.A., & Shortell, S.M. (1996). Integrated health systems: Promise and performance. *Frontiers of Health Services Management, 13* (1), 43-45.

to environmental factors, additional challenges arise. Welton et al. (1997) used a systems-based approach to describe the integration of primary care and public health systems into a community health system that increases the accessibility to and the delivery of cost-effective health care. The common goals and objectives of both primary care and public health systems were identified, consistent with the *Healthy People 2000 Review 1993* (National Center for Health Statistics, 1994), including the concern for population health; and opportunities for shared infrastructures (i.e., subsystems) were explored. The resulting integrated community health system would, theoretically, better meet the overall objectives of population health than would either primary care or public health services alone and would function more effectively.

Systems theory has provided a basis for understanding health care delivery systems within the context of organizational effectiveness (i.e., the ability to attain system goals) and environmental change. The systems approach supports the integration of health care delivery services and the shift away from hospital-based care.

Systems Theory as a Model For Nursing Practice

Systems theory has been used in the development of several nursing theories. Two widely used models, King's Systems Theory (King, 1981) and the Neuman Systems Model (Neuman, 1995; Neuman & Young, 1972), illustrate how systems theory has been and can be used in nursing. These models have been developed, researched, and applied across settings and within multiple areas of nursing practice, education, administration, and research.

King's Systems Theory of Nursing (1971, 1981) is based on the belief that nursing is an open system within a dynamic and interactive environment. Based in part on the work of Boulding (1956) and Kast and Rosenzweig (1972), the model incorporates two fundamental assumptions: (1) nursing involves concern for the health of individuals and groups; and (2) human beings interact with their environment. Concepts of the model reflect these basic assumptions and are defined within the three levels of individual systems, interpersonal systems, and social systems. At the individual level, a nurse or patient functions as a total system, with the concept of self being central to the formation of system boundaries. The self is considered to be goal oriented, with physical and emotional boundaries. Perception is the individual's primary connection to the external environment and serves to establish the individual's view of the environment.

Each individual interacts with other individuals, thus forming the next level of interpersonal system. In this level, two individuals form a dyad, three form a triad, and four or more constitute a group. The relationships between and among individuals and groups become central to the model and provide the focus for a detailed description of the communication and interaction processes. The concept of role is also central to this system level and is based on the idea that individuals establish relationships with others in the system depending on their perception of the role they will fill and behavioral expectations. The development of roles is consistent with the concept of differentiation within systems, whereby subsystems evolve in response to environmental needs. At the social system level, the system comprises individuals and groups functioning as subsystems, with the overall system defined as society. The concept of organization within the social system is used to reflect integration of the structure, functions, and resources present and available to individuals and groups within the system.

Within King's framework, nurses promote change within social systems by participating in decisions related to the formulation and attainment of organizational goals. Nurses are uniquely positioned to synthesize organizational, professional, and consumer goals and objectives and to participate in the formation of organizational structures and operational processes. Nurses develop and attain positions of power and authority from which effective systems-related decision making may occur.

King's conceptual framework has been applied to numerous issues and problems in nursing (King, 1996). Nursing research applications include the development of a model of social support and family health (Frey, 1989), a study of the use of nursing diagnosis (Byrne-Coker et al., 1990), and an analysis of nurse-patient interactions (Nagano & Funashima, 1995). Each of these studies provides support for King's levels of personal systems, including the relationship between perception and self, and the ability to pursue and attain goals.

In practice, King's framework emphasizes interactions between the provider and patient and between the patient-provider dyad and the environment. Nursing practice applications include the development of a model for ambulatory care of patients with cancer (Porter, 1991), the organization of hospital-based managed care (Hampton, 1995), and the development of a community-based AIDS case management program (Sowell & Grier, 1995). King's framework has also been applied as the conceptual basis for the implementation of theory-based nursing practice in an academic health center (King, 1996). Specifically, the framework was used to promote systematic change within the nursing department by integrating the development of practice standards, documentation systems, patient and nurse satisfaction evaluation systems, and continuing education strategies.

The *Neuman Systems Model* (Neuman, 1995; Neuman & Young, 1972) synthesizes concepts from systems and adaptation theory and emphasizes the integration of mind, body, and spirit into a patient system in constant interaction with a changing environment. The purpose of nursing in this model is to facilitate integration of the whole person and the achievement of maximal functioning within the environment, including the cultural context. Nursing activities are focused on adaptation of the individual to the environment through stress reduction. The model specifies elaborate lines of defense and resistance, which serve as system boundaries between the individual and the environment. Nursing activities focused on reducing stressors and enhancing resistance lead to adjustments in system boundaries. In turn, the health of the individual is improved. Health is measured by the extent to which the individual achieves health-related goals and objectives, either from the individual patient's or nurse's perspective.

Essential concepts in the Neuman model include three levels of environmental stress and three levels of nursing intervention. Stressors are present within the patient and the external environment and are described as intrapersonal, interpersonal, or extrapersonal. The actual and potential reactions of the individual patient to the stressors provide the basis for nursing intervention. The model emphasizes the holistic nature of the individual and the interaction of various stressors within the individual. Nursing interventions serve to stabilize the individual within the environment by creating or preserving linkages among the patient, environment, health, and nursing (Neuman, 1995; Neuman & Young, 1972). The three levels of nursing intervention—primary, secondary, and tertiary—reflect the extent to which stressors have permeated the boundary of the patient system: primary interventions focus on maintaining and preserving patient health; secondary interventions manipulate individual and environmental stressors and resources; and tertiary interventions focus on the preservation of health gains achieved and stabilization of the individual within the environment.

The Neuman Systems Model also has been used extensively in research, practice, and education within nursing and in allied health disciplines, such as physical and occupational therapy (Neuman, 1995). The model has provided the conceptual framework for at least 85 nursing research studies between 1989 and 1993 across a broad range of substantive areas (Neuman, 1995). For example, Moody (1996) demonstrated how the model can be applied to the study of nursing faculty job satisfaction. In this study, the university was viewed as an open system with five subsystems: goals and values; technology; structure; psychosocial; and management. These subsystems were used to examine the effects of demographic and managerial variables on staff satisfaction. The model has also served as a basis for the development of nursing practice models in multiple specialties, including psychiatric nursing (Stuart & Wright, 1995), critical care nursing (Bueno & Sengin, 1995), gerontologic nursing (Peirce & Fulmer, 1995), community nursing (Buchanan, 1987), and perinatal nursing (Trépanier et al., 1995). Applications in education include baccalaureate and associate degree nursing curriculum development (Lowry & Newsome, 1995), student clinical evaluation (Strickland-Seng, 1995), and physical therapy curriculum development (Toot & Schmoll, 1995).

Systems Theory and Shared Governance

Porter-O'Grady has published widely on shared governance, first as a model for nursing and later as a model for system-wide governance. Porter-O'Grady defines governance as an organizational model that incorporates the values of interdependence, shared decision making, and accountability into a system design that empowers professional staff at the levels of service and administration (Porter-O'Grady, 1994b). Shared governance incorporates systems principles to provide an organizational context that empowers nurses and other staff as close to the point of service as possible, in an overall effort to meet the health service mission. This intention is predicated on the belief that the person or persons closest to the point of service (i.e., care delivery) have the best available information on which to base decisions related to patient care and service delivery. Effective underlying linkages and relationships (i.e., subsystems) are prerequisites for the implementation of shared governance. In a shared governance system, subsystems and feedback loops are specifically tailored to the immediate needs of care delivery staff.

Within nursing, shared governance has been linked to improved staff communication, increased job satisfaction, decreased costs within nursing care units (Motz & Lewis, 1994), improved staff nurse perception of management style, increased staff nurse job satisfaction, and decreased staff turnover (Jones et al., 1993). The decentralized approach to decision making encourages staff to participate in the transformation of organizations within the dynamic and changing environment to better meet the organization's mission. As a method of organizational change, shared governance has been implemented and developed in more than 1000 hospitals in the United States (Porter-O'Grady, 1994b).

An example of successful shared governance is provided by Westrope et al. (1995). Initially proposed as a solution to high staff turnover and low nursing staff morale, the model addressed nurses' commitment to the organization, job satisfaction, and intent to stay. By the mid-implementation point, they were able to demonstrate significant positive changes in job satisfaction, commitment to the organization, and turnover.

In whole systems shared governance, linkages for shared decision making are created at all levels within and across disciplines and structures in health care. The evolution of shared governance from nursing-specific to system-wide structures is necessary for full integration and collaboration across disciplines and between administrators and clinicians (Porter-O'Grady, 1994b). In the fully developed whole systems model, roles in the organization shift from a state of isolated subsystems to a system of integrated relationships. This evolution of shared governance provides the foundation for whole systems change through the development of community-focused partnerships of providers, hospitals, and health professionals (Evan et al., 1995; Porter-O'Grady, 1994a). Whole systems shared governance provides a viable approach to successfully address issues related to the restructuring of practice and service delivery and increasing pressure to downsize acute care organizations.

Other Systems Approaches in Health Care and Nursing

A wide variety of systems approaches have been applied in nursing and health care beyond the development of nursing theory. A review of the literature reveals a number of studies referring to systems approaches and systems analysis. However, there is variability in the extent to which systems theory is truly applied. For example, some studies use the term *systems analysis* to describe the critique of a system without the use of a theoretic systems framework (Banfield, 1987; DeWoody & Price, 1994). These studies illustrate how the systems approach might be expanded, further developed, and applied within nursing and health care. Appropriate methods should include a theoretic systems framework and an emphasis on the identification of input, throughput, output, environment, and their interrelationships to achieve maximal benefit of the systems approach.

Leape et al. (1995) used a systems analysis to identify and evaluate failures contributing to actual and potential adverse drug events on medical and surgical nursing units. Four subsystems were identified: physician ordering, transcription and verification, pharmacy dispensing and

TABLE 2 - 2		
Van Slyck's Nursing Management System Levels		
Level	**System Outcome**	**Specific Objective**
Belief system	Philosophic foundation	Clear identification of philosophy of nursing and patient care
Patient classification system	Patient acuity	Identification of individual patient acuity levels
Staffing system	Staffing standards	Staffing standards for each acuity level are established
Productivity monitoring system	Staffing variance	Variances are identified, monitored, and evaluated in terms of significance and acceptability
Audit system	Validation of acuity	Verification of the validity and reliability of the acuity system
Costing system	Cost of services	Actual costs of nursing at each acuity level are identified
Billing system	Patient charges	Services are billed as nursing charges per patient day

Data from Van Slyck, A. (1991). A systems approach to the management of nursing services. I. Introduction. *Nursing Management, 22*(3-9).

delivery, and medication administration. Errors were categorized by subsystem, and underlying causes were identified for each error. A total of 15 system failures were identified, relating to feedback loops between the four subsystems and between the four subsystems and the external hospital environment. Examples of system failures include deficiencies in drug knowledge dissemination, noncompliance with dosing and administration procedures, and inadequate staffing. The use of systems analysis in this case allowed the identification of system failures associated with multiple subsystems and feedback loops and provided a more comprehensive review of medication administration processes and objectives than would have been possible by focusing on a single, isolated subsystem.

A hierarchic system of nursing services was developed by Van Slyck (1991a, 1991b, 1991c, 1991d, 1991e, 1991f, 1991g) to develop, implement, utilize, and evaluate patient acuity systems. The initial problem was conceptualized as

a lack of reliable and valid data related to patient status and nursing services, as evidenced by widespread misuse and nonuse of patient care acuity data. After identifying and stating specific systems goals and objectives, the cause of the problem was identified as unrealistic expectations of the patient acuity subsystem within the organization: patient classification, productivity, and staffing were expected to be outputs of a system designed solely to produce acuity data. Equally important, the acuity system could not function in a valid and reliable manner without the input of a clear philosophy of patient care and nursing services. A hierarchic set of goals was established that included objectives related to risk management, staffing assignments, and staff allocation. The further specification of system needs related to these objectives led to the identification and classification of the seven required subsystems and their interrelationships (Table 2-2). To illustrate the hierarchic nature of the model, for example, the development of a nursing resource management system clarified the insufficiencies of the single patient acuity subsystem. Subsequently, each subsystem was identified and designed with the output at one level functioning as the input for the next level. GST allowed for the recognition of the interrelationships between subsystems that impacted the development, implementation, and evaluation of patient acuity systems. Van Slyck was able to decrease the likelihood that a narrow focus on one single subsystem would occur by carefully considering the acuity system's context.

Parillo (1993) conducted a systems analysis of an occupational health department within a large urban health maintenance organization (HMO) to increase organizational effectiveness. In this case, specific systems components were identified and described within the context of GST. The occupational health department was viewed as a system within an environment consisting of legislative, economic, sociocultural, and political variables. A comprehensive and exhaustive list of inputs included management, employees, physicians, supplies, and clinical and management information systems. Throughputs covered the range of services provided within the occupational health department, including direct care, administration, and organizational program activities, such as the infection control and safety functions. Outputs, defined in terms of goals and objectives, related to the four environmental variables and included an increase in medical and safety report compliance, a reduction in the number of lost workdays, and a decrease in employee anxiety after blood or body fluid exposure. Major feedback loops between the internal system and the external environment were analyzed for effectiveness and efficiency. Effectiveness related to the extent that the objectives were met by the output, and efficiency related to the amount of resources required to produce the output. Recommendations for systems improvement focused on

evaluating each internal system process for its relative value in producing desired system outputs. By incorporating the systems perspective into this analysis, Parillo was able to fully identify and critique the system in relation to its input, output, and environmental context.

Soderberg and Walter (1991) used systems analysis to design physical therapy clinical research centers. A two-step process was used to identify the essential components of a research center. First, through a review of the literature, essential components of existing clinical centers in other disciplines, such as medicine and nursing, were identified. Goals and objectives, subsystems, and feedback loops and resources were proposed. Second, in a Delphi study, managers and clinicians from 118 academic institutions were surveyed using open-ended questions derived from the systems analysis. Subsequently, essential environmental and system components were identified, including (1) organizational factors that facilitate center development; (2) specific levels of required resources; and (3) essential program elements and desirable outputs expected from consumers, administrators, and external funding sources. This study demonstrates a systems approach in the program design mode that benefited from the systematic identification of goals, objectives, and system requirements.

Pedersen (1997) used a work redesign approach to reengineer patient care delivery in a multiple-unit, 467-bed community hospital. In this systems-based approach, the boundaries of subsystems were defined by individual inpatient care units, with the focus on processes within, but not between, individual units. Analysis of nursing activities focused on differentiation of levels of practice and determining the optimal skill mix. Environmental factors were limited to personnel cost constraints. The top 10 nursing activities for each skill level, such as patient assessment, medication administration, patient education, bathing, and vital signs, were monitored over a 3-year period. Targets for registered nurse (RN) and non-RN activities were established and used as indices of performance during the work redesign project. In this case, the environmental context beyond the unit level was essentially excluded; however, the in-depth analysis of work within the unit-level system was facilitated by the narrow focus.

Finally, a more comprehensive systems approach was used by Tunick et al. (1997) in the reengineering of a multidisciplinary cardiovascular surgery service in an academic medical center. Systems analysis principles guided the project: goals and objectives were first established, and then subsystems and their interrelationships were redefined. The overall goals of improving customer satisfaction and increasing profitability related to this service line provided the basis for redesigning all aspects of patient care, from preadmission to posthospital care. The systems perspective facilitated the interdisciplinary approach to the complex task of redesigning the entire set of clinical processes associated with the care of this patient population.

These studies illustrate the wide range in the application of systems theory, as well as the benefits achieved through its use. The systematic approach to organization-related problem solving that begins with the identification of goals and objectives and proceeds to focus on subsystems and feedback loops increases the validity of the problem identification and the likelihood that appropriate solutions will be developed, implemented, and evaluated.

■ SYSTEMS THEORY AND CHANGE

Certain aspects of organizational change theory are necessary to appreciate the contributions and potential of applied systems theory and analysis within nursing and health care. Organizational change theory, grounded in the work of Lewin (1951) and Parsons (1951), introduced concepts of psychology into the de-

velopment of models for understanding and promoting change in organizations. Change theory provides a framework for understanding individual and group behavior relative to promoting and adapting to change within social structures. Individuals and groups are viewed as patient systems within social environments. Whereas change theory provides the sociopsychologic perspective, general systems theory provides an overarching compatible understanding of systems.

Chin and Benne (1985) place systems theory and analysis within the context of general strategies for effecting planned change in human systems, whereby knowledge of systems is used and applied to modify practice. According to Chin and Benne (1985), systems analysis is an organizational change strategy that is based on empiricism and rational thought. Quantitative methods are coupled with behavioral science to design and implement systems that meet organizational goals and objectives. Systems analysis is used by management to analyze internal structures and processes and assess important elements of the environment. The focus of systems analysis is on improving interactions between subsystems and between the system and its environment.

■ SYSTEMS ANALYSIS

Whereas systems classification provides a rudimentary link between systems theory and the description of systems, systems analysis is the link between problem-solving processes within organizations and designing, changing, and evaluating systems. This section presents a method of systems analysis derived from the works of Churchman (1968), Klir (1969), and Gibson (1991) to initiate and facilitate change within nursing and health care. The method is especially applicable to nursing and health care because it reflects (1) the presence of multiple and often conflicting goals, (2) the assumption that there often are many ways to achieve the same goals and objectives, and (3) the notion of available and constrained resources.

Systems analysis is defined by Churchman (1968) as the application of systems theory to the study of system function. The process involves the identification of indicators of change, the planning of systematic solutions, the implementation of solutions (i.e., change), and the development of evaluation methods (Churchman, 1968). Systems analysis examines the system as a whole and as an interactive set of subsystems in relation to relevancy, effectiveness, and efficiency. Relevancy means that the system is analyzed to determine its purpose and congruence with the environment. Effectiveness is the extent to which the system meets its established objectives. Efficiency refers to the level of resources (or input) required to meet the objective (or output). Churchman emphasizes that systems analysis may be used to study the assessment, design, implementation, or evaluation of an issue, project, program, or organization. As a problem-solving process, systems analysis may be used before systems are created, as in the design mode, or subsequent to system implementation, as in the evaluation mode.

According to Gibson (1991), systems analysis is a problem-solving method with eight characteristics (Box 2-2). Gibson stresses that all eight characteristics should be present and incorporated throughout the systems analysis process. These characteristics provide the foundation on which the actual analysis should be based. The first of these characteristics, the *top-down approach,* refers to the need to begin the analysis of a system from a general, broad perspective before focusing on specific components. Clear identification of environmental assumptions and policy concerns before examining subsystem processes increases the likelihood that the analysis will be valid. A *goal-oriented focus*

B O X 2 - 2

Characteristics of Systems Analysis

1. Top-down approach
2. Goal-oriented focus
3. Rational and objective basis
4. Policy component coupled to the quantitative component
5. Generalized problem
6. System optimization
7. Explicit recognition of the values of the client, investigator, and system users
8. Focus on the problem from the client perspective

Data from Gibson, J.E. (1991). *How to do a systems analysis.* Charlottesville, Va: University of Virginia Press, Department of Systems Engineering.

---

emphasizes the importance of identifying a system's goals, objectives, subsystems, and processes that are necessary for optimal functioning. The analysis should be based on a conceptual framework, providing a *rational and objective basis,* and should focus solely on the system and environment under study without external bias. The systems analysis should also include a *policy component* that considers social, cultural, and political factors in the environment that influence input, throughput, and output. The problem should be *generalized* to environmental factors that impact the system, including the identification of all stakeholders, system users, and nonusers. *System optimization* refers to the achievement of specific goals and objectives, as operationalized by critical parameters and indices of performance. *Explicit recognition of the values of the patient, investigator, and system users* serves to validate the goals and objectives of a system, increasing the likelihood that a meaningful system will be developed. The eighth and final component, a *fo-*

cus on the problem from a patient perspective, further ensures that meaningful and valid analyses will be obtained.

In this framework, the individual designing or evaluating the system assumes the role of systems analyst. The systems analyst oversees the entire process, including the identification and recruitment of stakeholders, facilitation of group processes, and other aspects of project management. The analyst ensures that the change process is based on a comprehensive and systematic problem-solving approach by incorporating the eight elements identified above.

Expanding on these requirements, Gibson (1991) presented a method for analyzing systems that incorporates these eight characteristics throughout a multiphase process. The five phases in the analysis process (Box 2-3) are goal development, definition of indices of performance, development of alternate solutions, rank ordering of alternate solutions, and iteration and transition.

The first phase of systems analysis focuses on a review of the system's general goals and objectives. Goals and objectives are stated in general terms from the perspective of individuals or subsystems, suppliers of input, and consumers of output within the environment. Overall goals are stated, prioritized, and then used to generate specific goals and objectives for performance measurement. In the design mode, goals and objectives are used as targets, whereas in the evaluation mode, goals and objectives provide the basis for performance assessment and problem identification.

The second phase of systems analysis is the definition of performance indices. These indices are specific measures derived from system goals and objectives. Indices of performance should be meaningful, understandable, and measurable. In other words, each performance index should be quantifiable, valid, and reliable. The use of meaningful measures is critical to facilitate col-

---

BOX 2-3

Major Phases of Systems Analysis

Phase	Description
Goal development	The overall purpose, goals, and objectives are identified.
Definition of indices of performance	Criteria by which the overall system and its components will be evaluated are specified.
Development of alternate solutions	Potential alternate systems for achieving the stated purpose, goals, and objectives are identified.
Rank order of alternate solutions	Each alternate system is evaluated and ranked according to the ability to meet the stated goals and objectives.
Iteration	The plan is reviewed with all stakeholders and refined as needed.

Data from Gibson, J.E. (1991). *How to do a systems analysis.* Charlottesville, Va: University of Virginia Press, Department of Systems Engineering.

---

laboration and cooperation from individuals involved in system design or evaluation. In the evaluation mode, performance indices are used to conduct a systematic assessment of current system performance. Variances among goals, objectives, and performance are stated in terms of each measure, thereby identifying specific system problems.

Once problems are identified, the third phase of systems analysis begins—the development of alternate solutions. Each solution is a system that may potentially meet established system goals and objectives. Alternate solutions are generated through brainstorming, literature review, and the use of expert consultants. At this point, the development of alternate solutions demands creativity and should not reflect environmental constraints. Instead, plausible systems are identified. The alternatives in most analyses should include maintaining the current program or system (i.e., the status quo). Revisions of the current system become additional alternatives to be evaluated. This approach enhances the assessment of the current system, providing an objective basis for the planning and implementation of changes.

Identified alternatives are then used in the fourth phase of analysis—a ranking of alternatives. This ranking is made in terms of (1) ability of the system to meet the goals and objectives, as measured by the indices of performance; (2) potential for adverse effects to occur; (3) resources required for implementation and operation; and (4) sensitivity to parameter violations. Alternatives are also evaluated in terms of system constraints. The relative advantages and disadvantages of each alternative are compared, contrasted, and rank ordered. Ranking methods may range from simply rating the alternatives in relation to one or more performances to more elaborate economic analyses of resources.

In the fifth phase—iteration and transition— the overall problem or issue is conceptualized as a whole to include all important system components; each system component is evaluated and reevaluated in relation to the problem, to other components, and to the system as a whole. The system is examined from input to output, with special attention placed on the ability of subsystems to function and interact effectively. Feedback loops within the system, and between the system and its environment, are scrutinized for effectiveness and efficiency. In brief, the system is assessed for its overall ability to meet goals and objectives subject to environmental constraints.

The iteration and transition phase begins with a review of the systems analyst's perspectives by the stakeholders. Systems constraints, resources, goals, and objectives are validated with the stakeholders, and the analysis continues with a repetition of the five phases until the costs of additional analysis outweigh expected benefits. As an iterative process, most analyses of complex systems require multiple cycles of the five phases (Gibson, 1991). Specific and detailed systems are then designed or redesigned with respect to input, throughput, and output. Transition from design or evaluation to actual implementation should be a concurrent process throughout this phase. Gibson (1991) emphasizes the relationship between early planning for implementation and successful performance. This requirement increases the likelihood that all assumptions related to system requirements will be validated and verified with all stakeholders before actual implementation.

A Nursing Example

Essential aspects of the five-phase systems analysis process can be demonstrated with an example from nursing: the transition from the traditional model of care delivery to case management. The implementation of case management in a hip replacement population is used in this example because this population has been widely studied as a model for process improvement. The scenario begins with a question raised about the current processes of care delivery given recent changes in health care and the state of knowledge related to care of the hip replacement population: to what extent is the care being provided to patients undergoing hip replacement relevant, effective, and efficient? After discussions among team members reveal unsatisfactory answers to this question, a systems analyst is assigned. This role may be assumed by the nurse manager, clinical specialist, or another staff member.

T A B L E 2 - 3

Phases of Systems Analysis: Case Management of the Total Hip Replacement Patient Population

	Phase	Activity
Phase 1	Goal development	Identify the overall purpose and the specific goals and objectives expected with the care of the hip replacement population.
Phase 2	Definition of indices of performance	Identify specific criteria by which the overall program, and specific components, will be evaluated.
Phase 3	Development of alternate solutions	Identify possible program or system models.
Phase 4	Rank ordering of alternate solutions	Rank each model, including the current system, according to the extent that it is forecast to meet the indices of performance.
Phase 5	Iteration and transition	Review the selected plan with all stakeholders, and refine it in accordance with the desired goals and objectives, and constraints.

The analysis is described here in terms of the basic elements of each phase (Table 2-3), with each successive phase building on the previous one. The process within each phase is not meant to be exclusive, and an actual analysis might include greater detail in all phases of the process.

In phase 1, the individual assuming the role of systems analyst identifies and recruits all stakeholders and facilitates the group to identify the overall purpose of the program. In this case, stakeholders would include administrative and interdisciplinary clinical staff members, patients, and payers. The purpose is specified as follows: to provide cost-effective, quality care to patients undergoing hip replacement. Box 2-4 delineates goals and specific objectives that reflect program priorities as stated by the stakeholders. The objectives are specified to a level of detail that allows for objective measurement. For example, the goal *to provide quality care* is vague, ambiguous, and immeasurable. This program goal is further defined in more measurable terms: ensuring optimal clinical outcomes, minimizing adverse events and complications, and ensuring optimal patient and family satisfaction. Each goal, in turn, is clarified in terms of specific objectives, which are further refined for measurement in the next phase. In this example, a general sense develops among all persons involved that the program objectives are not being fully met by the current system.

In phase 2, specific criteria by which each goal and objective will be measured are identified (Table 2-4). Indices of performance for the system are defined that relate to each objective as identified in phase 1. The particular levels or targets for each index are established. For example, various compliance, incidence, and satisfaction rates may be established based on historical experience or external benchmarks derived from best practice models. Ideally, the indices are then used as measures of the systems' success and become fully integrated into subsequent quality improvement activities. In this example, it is clear that the current program is in need of change; the status quo does not address any of the indices of performance, and specific variances between objectives and performance are identified and specified.

Case Management of the Total Hip Replacement Patient Population:
Phase 1 of Systems Analysis: Goal Development

The purpose of this program is to provide cost-effective quality care to patients undergoing total hip replacement.

Specific Goals and Objectives

A. Provide quality care
1. Ensure optimal clinical outcomes
   a. Provide appropriate preparation before admission
   b. Provide appropriate care during hospitalization
   c. Provide appropriate care after hospital discharge
   d. Improve preoperative functional status
2. Minimize adverse events and complications
   a. Ensure effective pain management
   b. Prevent deep vein thrombosis and pulmonary embolus
   c. Promote bowel and bladder elimination
3. Ensure optimal patient and family satisfaction

   a. Provide appropriate support and communication
   b. Provide opportunities for communication with all members of the team before, during, and after hospitalization

B. Maximize cost efficiency
1. Ensure appropriate use of diagnostic techniques
   a. Ensure necessity of laboratory tests
   b. Ensure necessity of radiologic procedures
2. Ensure appropriate hospital length of stay
   a. Maintain hospital length of stay within Medicare guidelines
   b. Ensure ongoing preparation and planning for discharge
3. Ensure payer satisfaction
   a. Comply with hospital-stay limits
   b. Maintain communication with payers regarding unforeseen and unplanned events

In phase 3, the focus shifts to an examination of the system itself and the identification of alternate subsystems, as measured by the indices of performance. The development of alternate solutions forces the consideration of different approaches and increases the likelihood that objectives and the system will be well matched. In this case, four alternatives are identified (Box 2-5, p. 54): maintain the current program, implement an acute care clinical pathway, implement full-continuum case management, and implement payer-based case management.*

In phase 4, each of the four alternatives is evaluated in terms of performance indices. In

this example each alternative is rated as potentially having no impact, a positive impact, or a negative impact on each index (Table 2-5). This process incorporates educated and "best" guesses, along with variable degrees of probability as each index is rated. Ratings are used to rank order the alternatives. The acute care clinical pathway addresses almost all the indices, and the payer-based case management model has less impact. In this case, the full-continuum case management model is given the best ranking and, in turn, is considered the best choice based on available knowledge and data.

In phase 5, all assumptions related to goals and objectives, resources, constraints, and alternate solutions are reviewed with all stakeholders. In this phase, the chosen alternative is recommended on the basis of how well it meets the

---

* See Powell (1996) for a comprehensive description of case management and Bower (1992) for a description of various case management models.

Text continued on p. 54.

TABLE 2 - 4

Case Management of the Total Hip Replacement Patient Population: Phase 2 of Systems Analysis: Definition of Indices of Performance

Specific Goals and Objectives		Indices of Performance
General Goal: Provide Quality Care		
Ensure optimal clinical outcomes	Provide appropriate preparation before admission	Cancellation rate because of inadequate preparation before surgery (e.g., identification of unresolved medical issues at time of surgery)
	Provide appropriate care during hospitalization	Compliance rates with specific standards of care for physician and nursing care, and for physical and occupational therapy, as measured by documentation audits
	Provide appropriate planning for care after hospital discharge	Incidence of patients with needs identified after hospitalization
		Patient satisfaction with posthospitalization plans
		Readmission rates
	Improve preoperative functional status	Functional status measures before surgery and at 3 and 12 mo after surgery
Minimize adverse events and complications	Ensure effective pain management	Patient's report of pain on 0-10 scale each hospital day, on discharge, and on third follow-up day
	Prevent deep vein thrombosis and pulmonary embolus	Incidence rates of deep vein thrombosis across the continuum (i.e., including after discharge)
		Incidence rates of pulmonary embolus across the continuum (i.e., including after discharge)
	Promote bowel and bladder elimination	Compliance with bowel elimination protocols as measured by documentation audits
		Incidence of constipation on day of discharge

Case Management of the Total Hip Replacement Patient Population: Phase 2 of Systems Analysis: Definition of Indices of Performance—cont'd

Specific Goals and Objectives		Indices of Performance
Ensure optimal patient and family satisfaction	Provide appropriate support and communication	Ratings of patient satisfaction related to support and communication with staff
		Ratings of patient education responses
		Incidence of patient complaints
	Provide positive overall experience for patients, families, and significant others	Ratings of overall patient satisfaction related to support and communication with staff
General Goal: Maximize Cost Efficiency		
Ensure appropriate use of diagnostic techniques	Ensure necessity of laboratory tests	Utilization rates of complete blood count (CBC), prothrombin time (PT), and partial thromboplastin time (PTT) compared with external benchmark rates and institutional standards
	Ensure necessity of radiologic procedures	Utilization rates of diagnostic radiology procedures before and after surgery compared with external benchmark rates and institutional standards
Ensure appropriate hospital length of stay	Maintain hospital length of stay within Medicare guidelines	Hospital length of stay, in days
	Ensure ongoing preparation and planning for discharge	Compliance rates with daily discharge conferences
		Incidence of patients without discharge plan by hospital day 3
Ensure payer satisfaction	Comply with hospital-stay limits	Variance with payer-prescribed hospital length of stay
	Maintain communication with payers regarding unforseen and unplanned events	Compliance with regular and ongoing conferences between payers and caregivers

TABLE 2 - 5

Case Management of the Total Hip Replacement Patient Population: Phase 4 of Systems Analysis: Rank Order of Alternate Solutions*

	Alternatives (Program Options)			
	Maintain Current Program	Acute Care Clinical Pathway	Full-Continuum Case Management	Payer-Based Case Management
Indices of Performance				
Cancellation rate because of medical issues identified at time of surgery	No change	No change	+	No change
Compliance rates with specific standards of care for physician and nursing care and for physical and occupational therapy	No change	+	+	No change
Incidence of patients with needs identified after hospitalization	No change	+	+	−
Rates of patient satisfaction with posthospitalization plans	No change	+	+	−
Functional status measures at 3 mo and 1 yr after surgery	No change	+	+	+
Patient-reported pain on 0-10 scale each hospital day, on discharge, and on 30-day follow-up	No change	+	+	No change
Incidence rates of deep vein thrombosis across the continuum (i.e., including after discharge)	No change	+	+	No change
Incidence rates of pulmonary embolus across the continuum (i.e., including after discharge)	No change	+	+	No change
Compliance with bowel elimination protocols	No change	+	+	No change

*Plus sign reflects a predicted improvement in the specific index, and negative sign reflects a decline.

Case Management of the Total Hip Replacement Patient Population:
Phase 4 of Systems Analysis: Rank Order of Alternate Solutions*—cont'd

	Alternatives (Program Options)			
	Maintain Current Program	Acute Care Clinical Pathway	Full-Continuum Case Management	Payer-Based Case Management
Incidence of constipation on day of discharge	No change	+	+	No change
Ratings of patient satisfaction related to support and communication with staff	No change	+	+	No change
Incidence of patient complaints	No change	+	+	+
Ratings of overall patient satisfaction related to support and communication with staff	No change	+ (in-hospital only)	+	No change
Utilization rates of complete blood counts (CBC), prothrombin time (PT), and partial thromboplastin time (PTT)	No change	+ (in-hospital only)	+	+
Utilization rates of diagnostic radiology procedures before and after surgery	No change	+ (in-hospital only)	+	+
Hospital length of stay, in days	No change	+	+	+
Compliance rates with daily discharge conferences	No change	+	+	No change
Compliance with payer-prescribed hospital length of stay	No change	+	+	+
Compliance with regular and ongoing conferences between payers and caregivers	No change	+	+	+
Overall Rank	4	2	1	3

BOX 2-5

Case Management of the Total Hip Replacement Patient Population: Phase 3 of Systems Analysis: Development of Alternate Solutions

Alternatives	Description
Maintain current program	Maintain current status quo of program processes
Acute care clinical pathway	Implement an acute care clinical pathway that prescribes significant activities to occur in a day-by-day sequence during hospitalization
Full-continuum case management	Implement a case management model that includes patient/provider involvement from point of decision to have surgery to appropriate follow-up in the posthospital setting
Payer-based case management	Case management by payer, with emphasis on case monitoring and cost control

program's purpose, goals, and objectives within the environmental context of resources and constraints, as predicted by its impact on specific indices.

Specifically, the next step is for the stakeholders to determine input requirements for each alternative and then, from a cost/benefit point of view, select the best alternative. In comparing the two top alternatives, the case management model might require the greatest short-run increase in resources with the additional salary requirements of a case manager. If

this additional resource exceeds constraints, possibly the next best alternative, the clinical pathway, would be selected. The iterative process continues with the comparing and contrasting of each alternative with respect to all system factors until a decision is made regarding the selection and specifications for the system alternative. In this case, there is sufficient commitment and support throughout the system to develop and implement full-continuum case management for the hip replacement population. At this point, the implementation plan is further defined and specific system changes are enacted in a coordinated and integrated manner.

■ LIMITATIONS

GST and systems analysis are based on the classical, traditional paradigm that incorporates principles of prediction, control, and stability into a linear model of organizational study and change. Problems and issues are identified, causal relationships are established, solutions are implemented, and results are evaluated. In complex nursing and health care systems, linear models of specific causes and effects may be oversimplifications of reality, thus leading to ill-defined or misunderstood issues, problems, and solutions. The validity of the traditional paradigm and methods has been challenged in the context of highly complex, dynamic systems and environments, as discussed below. Links between system components may not be limited to one-way causal relationships but may, in fact, be nonlinear, given that system constraints and desired outputs are in constant transition. Specific limitations of traditional models, coupled with knowledge developed through systems application, provide insight into future directions in systems thinking.

■ FUTURE DIRECTIONS FOR NURSING

Koerner (1996) proposes that nursing in the postmodern world requires alternatives to quantitatively driven, predictive systems–based models that offer only partial understanding of increasingly complex systems issues. She outlines four aspects of systems that should be viewed differently: self-organization, self-regulation, self-generation, and self-renewal. *Self-organization* emphasizes interdependence and interrelationships of subsystems with flexible and loose boundaries. *Self-regulation* implies that systems do not achieve equilibrium with their environment and that internal stability enhances a system's ability to respond proactively to environmental factors. *Self-generation* reflects the idea that in the postmodern world, the organization must relate to information in new and different ways. Patterns and trends of behavior and means of data collection become less important than the focus on behavioral paradoxes and inconsistencies and data fluctuations and distributions. *Self-renewal* refers to the extent to which the creative capacity of individuals and organizations leads to the spontaneous creation of systems that were not predicted or planned. In summary, a systems analysis should reflect an understanding of loose and flexible system boundaries, less emphasis on system stability as a goal, less reliance on linear mathematic models, and increased awareness of the spontaneous creation of subsystems. Thus embracing a post–modern world view that recognizes complex interactions within and across systems strengthens nursing.

McDaniel (1997) offers further criticism of traditional systems-based approaches in nursing from the view of quantum and chaos theories. Although it is beyond the scope of this chapter to fully discuss either of these theories, it is necessary to introduce them as a basis for enhancing the understanding of systems theory and analysis. Quantum theory supports the notions that the world (i.e., systems, environments) is unpredictable and that current measurement methods are fundamentally flawed. Because the

world is unpredictable, accurate information derived from historical or present data does not improve the ability to predict subsequent events. Also, the world is interdependent with the observer, leading to interactions between the analyst and the observed, which threatens the validity of causal relationships.

Chaos theory provides further insight into how complex systems, such as organizations, change over time and directly challenges the validity of the traditional equilibrium-seeking systems approach. Chaos theory describes dynamic or non-equilibrium-seeking entities that may more closely approximate complex organizational systems (Mark, 1994). A fundamental presumption in chaos theory is that positive and negative feedback mechanisms interact constantly (i.e., dynamically) and that although organizational outcomes are often unpredictable, patterns of behavior may emerge over time. This challenges the validity of traditional causal relationships between system interventions and outcomes. In addition, small differences in initial conditions may lead to large overall organizational changes. Systems analysis of the future should recognize and incorporate the unpredictability of the system and the environment, the relationship between the observer and the observed, and the likelihood of multidirectional causal relationships. By embracing this expanded systems view, nursing will be better positioned to deal effectively with complex changes within nursing and the health care environment.

An illustration of the limitations of traditional approaches and the additional value of chaos theory is offered by Mark (1994) in her example of nursing staff turnover. In traditional approaches, causal models of nursing turnover typically include turnover as a dependent variable in relation to individual, job-related, organizational, and economic and labor market variables. Assumptions of this approach include the notion that some optimal level of turnover exists and that it can be modeled and predicted using the set of independent variables. Chaos theory allows for the possibilities that there is no single optimal turnover level and that the turnover rate itself may impact the independent variables under study in a nonlinear manner.

Porter-O'Grady (1997) relates the nonlinear principles to system leadership and organizational change in nursing. In the quantum view, several nonlinear systems assumptions depart from the traditional linear model. First, relationships between system components are more important than control. Second, the interdependencies of system components can be addressed only within the context of their relationship to each other. Third, healthy systems are in a constant state of disequilibrium with the environment, ensuring their ability to respond to ongoing change. Thus organizational change is an ongoing, unpredictable, and multidirectional process that occurs in response to point-of-service interactions of subsystems with the environment. In response to these limitations, the systems analysis should emphasize the importance of the interrelationships between subsystems, consideration of all relationships as a whole, and the effect of point-of-service interactions on the system's ability to adapt to its environment. Porter-O'Grady argues that nursing and health care leadership should facilitate the shift to a system in which decisions and leadership are supported within point-of-service groups and the role of the nurse as a knowledge worker is reaffirmed.

Further work needs to be done in the refinement of GST and systems analysis; however, systems analysis, as an iterative and dynamic process, can incorporate many of the propositions of the nonlinear models. It may be that, on some levels of analysis, the linear approach is valid, whereas on other levels, the nonlinear view may be more appropriate. In a discussion of systems thinking and postmodernism, Jackson (1995) suggests that to minimize potential limitations, systems analysis should proceed with an inherent skepticism of its assumptions and methods at each step in the process. In other words, the validity of using traditional methods to analyze increasingly uncertain and unpredictable systems and environments is enhanced by continuously reassessing the methods and assumptions of systems analysis.

■ SUMMARY

Systems theory provides a foundation for conceptualizing and defining many issues and problems within nursing and health care. Issues and problems defined in terms of systems and the environment are likely to be addressed in an integrated manner that fosters organizational success. The unpredictability and the dynamic nature of the health care environment and health care organizations underscore the need to approach organizational change from a systems viewpoint. The use of systems theory and systems analysis minimizes the likelihood that isolated, fragmented, ineffective, and potentially harmful organizational changes will be proposed or implemented.

Traditional systems approaches, however, must be applied within the context of emerging paradigms for understanding organizational change. Quantum theory and chaos theory provide additional and valuable perspectives within which systems theory and analysis can be further developed and applied. In a truly systematic approach, these new theories will contribute to a greater understanding of issues and concepts within systems and their environments and within their interrelationships. The enhancement and refinement of the traditional systems methods should allow for a proactive and transformational approach to achieving organizational effectiveness within nursing and health care.

■ KEY POINTS

• Systems theory provides a framework for conceptualizing and organizing the way to examine problems, issues, and plans within health care. By using systems theory, which by its very nature takes into account the environment, issues and problems can be addressed in an integrated manner.

• Systems theory is especially useful as a way to structure thinking and planning in a time of change and uncertainty because of the structure this framework adds to the process and because it calls attention in a systematic way to the parts or components of the process or group.

• Although traditional systems approaches form the background for the work being done today, both quantum theory and chaos theory provide valuable perspectives for looking at organizations that are trying to transform themselves in the midst of rapid change.

• A well-used adaptation of systems theory is that developed by Peter Senge, in which he describes organizations as systems in which people interact to accomplish the goals and objectives of the organization. He calls organizations *learning organizations* and says that systems thinking is one way for people to see the big picture.

• Systems theory can be applied to health care in a variety of ways. One is the multicomponent health care system that consists of a hospital and its related practices. Each component separately can also be viewed as a system.

• Several nursing theories are built on systems thinking, including those of King and Neuman and the more recent work by Porter-O'Grady.

• Systems analysis is used to plan, critique, or evaluate a system. It adds structure to the process of looking closely at the way that a system functions. It is essentially a problem-solving process with a set of sequential steps.

■ CRITICAL THINKING QUESTIONS

1. Consider a nursing unit with which you have had experience. Describe the systems components of the unit. Evaluate the functioning of the unit from a systems perspective. Answer these questions from a systems perspective about the unit:
   A. What are the boundaries of this unit system?
   B. Describe on a given day the input, output, and throughput that you observe in this system.
   C. Identify at least three constraints on the effective functioning of this system.

2. Using the learning organization concept developed by Peter Senge, analyze a group or organization of which you are a member. How is systems thinking used in the system? If the system does not function like a learning organization, what changes are needed to establish it as such?

3. Using one of the nursing theories that are built on systems theory discussed in this chapter, evaluate a patient care situation, identifying how you could use or explain the care given from the perspective of that theory.

4. Identify a problem in a clinical area with which you are familiar. Using the concept of shared governance, outline a plan for intervening in the problem.

5. Take a clinical problem with which you have recently been confronted. Using systems analysis, evaluate the way in which the system functions and the changes that could be effected to lead to a more effective system.

■ REFERENCES

Ashby, W.R. (1958). General systems theory as a new discipline. *General Systems Yearbook, 3,* 1-6.

Banfield, S. (1987). A management systems analysis of Huguley Home Health Agency. *Caring, 6*(7), 45-50.

Banner, D.K., & Gagne, T.E. (1995). *Designing effective organizations: Traditional and transformational views.* Thousand Oaks, Calif.: Sage.

Bertalanffy, L. von (1968). *General system theory.* New York: George Braziller.

Boulding, K.E. (1956). General systems theory: The skeleton of science. *Management Science, 2,* 197-208.

Bower, K.A. (1992). *Case management by nurses.* Washington, D.C.: American Nurses Publishing.

Buchanan, B.F. (1987). Human-environment interaction: A modification of the Neuman systems model for aggregates, families, and the community. *Public Health Nursing, 4*(1), 52-64.

Bueno, M.M., & Sengin, K.K. (1995). The Neuman systems model for critical care nursing: A framework for practice. In B. Neuman (Ed.). *The Neuman systems model* (pp. 275-292). East Norwalk, Conn.: Appleton & Lange.

Byrne-Coker, E., Fradley, T., Harris, J., Thomarchio, D.C., & Caron, C. (1990). Implementing nursing diagnosis within the concepts of King's conceptual framework. *Nursing Diagnosis, 1*(3), 107-114.

Chin, R., & Benne, K.D. (1985). General strategies for effecting changes in human systems. In K.D. Benne & R. Chin (Eds.). *The planning of change* (pp. 22-45). New York: CBS College Publishing.

Churchman, C.W. (1968). *The systems approach.* New York: Dell.

Conrad, D.A., & Shortell, S.M. (1996). Integrated health systems: Promise and performance. *Frontiers of Health Services Management, 13*(1), 43-45.

DeWoody, S., & Price, J. (1994). A systems approach to multidimensional critical paths. *Nursing Management, 25*(11), 47-51.

Evan, K., Aubry, K., Hawkins, M., Curley, T.A., & Porter-O'Grady, T. (1995). Whole systems shared governance: A model for the integrated health system. *Journal of Nursing Administration, 25*(5), 18-27.

Frey, M. (1989). Social support and health: A theoretical formulation derived from King's conceptual framework. *Nursing Science Quarterly, 2*(3), 138-148.

Gibson, J.E. (1991). *How to do a systems analysis.* Charlottesville, Va.: University of Virginia Press, Department of Systems Engineering.

Hampton, C.C. (1995). King's theory of goal attainment: A framework for managed care implementation in a hospital setting. *Nursing Science Quarterly, 7*(4), 170-173.

Hazzard, M.E. (1971). An overview of systems theory. *Nursing Clinics of North America, 6*(3), 385-393.

Howland, D. (1963a). Approaches to the systems problem. *Nursing Research, 12*(3), 172-174.

Howland, D. (1963b). A hospital system model. *Nursing Research, 12*(4), 232-236.

Howland, D., & McDowell, W.E. (1964). The measurement of patient care: A conceptual framework. *Nursing Research, 13*(1), 4-7.

Jackson, M.C. (1995). Beyond the fads: Systems thinking for managers. *Systems Research 12*(1), 25-42.

Jones, C.B., Stasiowski, S., Simons, B.J., Boyd, N.J., & Lucas, M.D. (1993). Shared governance and the nursing practice environment. *Nursing Economics, 11*(4), 208-214.

Kast, F., & Rosenzweig, J. E. (1972). General systems theory: Applications for organization and management. *The Academy of Management Journal, 15*(6), 447-465.

Katz, D., & Kahn, R.L. (1966). *The social psychology of organizations.* New York: John Wiley & Sons.

King, I.M. (1971). *Toward a theory for nursing: General concepts of human behavior.* New York: John Wiley & Sons.

King, I.M. (1981). *A theory for nursing: Systems, concepts, process.* New York: John Wiley & Sons.

King, I.M. (1996). The theory of goal attainment in research and practice. *Nursing Science Quarterly, 9*(2), 61-66.

Klir, G.J. (1969). *An approach to general systems theory.* New York: Van Nostrand Reinhold.

Klir, G.J. (1985). The emergence of two-dimensional science in the information society. *Systems Research, 2*(1), 33-41.

Klir, G.J. (1991). *Facets of system science* (vol. 7). New York: Plenum.

Koerner, G.J. (1996). Imagining the future for nursing administration and systems research. *Nursing Administration Quarterly, 20*(4), 1-11.

Laszlo, E. (1972). *Introduction to systems philosophy.* New York: Gordon & Breach, Science Publishers.

Leape, L.L, Bates, D.W., Cullen, D.J., Cooper, J., DeMonaco, H.J., Gallivan, T., Hallisey, R., Ives, J., Laird, N., Laffel, G., Nemeskal, R., Petersen, L.A., Porter, K., Servi, D., Shea, B.F., Small, S.D., Sweitzer, B.J., Thompson, B.T., & Vliet, M.V. (1995). Systems analysis of adverse drug events. *Journal of the American Medical Association, 274*(1), 35-43.

Lewin, K. (1951). *Field theory in social science.* New York: Harper.

Lowry, L.W., & Newsome, G.G. (1995). Neuman-based associate degree programs: Past, present, and future. In B. Neuman (Ed.). *The Neuman systems model* (pp. 197-214). East Norwalk, Conn.: Appleton & Lange.

Mark, B.A. (1994). Chaos theory and nursing systems research. *Theoretic and Applied Chaos in Nursing, 1*(1), 7-14.

McDaniel, R.R. Jr. (1997). Strategic leadership: A view from quantum and chaos theories. *Health Care Manage Review, 22*(1), 22-37.

Merriam-Webster's collegiate dictionary (10th ed.). (1994). Springfield, Mass.: Merriam-Webster.

Miller, J.G. (1965). Living systems: Structure and process. *Behavioral Science, 10,* 337-379.

Miller, J.G. (1978). *Living systems.* New York: McGraw-Hill.

Moody, N.B. (1996). Nurse faculty job satisfaction: A national survey. *Journal of Professional Nursing, 12*(5), 277-288.

Motz, D., & Lewis, J. (1994). Shared governance: Is it a catalyst of change? *Journal of Burn Care & Rehabilitation 15*(4), 375-385.

Nadler, D.A., & Tushman, M.L. (1982). A model for diagnosing organizational behavior: Applying a congruence perspective. In D.A. Nadler, M.L. Tushman, & N. Hatvany (Eds.). *Managing organizations.* Boston: Little, Brown.

Nagano, M., & Funashima, N. (1995). Analysis of nursing situations in Japan using King's goal attainment theory. *Quality Nursing, 1*(1), 74-78.

National Center for Health Statistics. (1994). *Healthy people 2000 review, 1993.* Hyattsville, Md.: Public Health Service.

Neuman, B.M. (1995). *The Neuman systems model* (3rd ed.). East Norwalk, Conn.: Appleton & Lange.

Neuman, B.M., & Young, R.I. (1972). A model for teaching total person approach to patient problems. *Nursing Research, 21*(3), 264-269.

Parillo, V.L. (1993). Systems analysis of an occupational health department: Recommendations to increase effectiveness. *AAOHN Journal, 41*(5), 220-227.

Parsons, T. (1951). *The social system.* Glencoe, Ill.: The Free Press.

Pedersen, A. (1997). A data driven approach to work redesign in nursing units. *Journal of Nursing Administration, 27*(4), 49-54.

Peirce, A.G., & Fulmer, T.T. (1995). Application of the Neuman systems model to gerontological nursing. In B. Neuman (Ed.). *The Neuman systems model* (pp. 293-308). East Norwalk, Conn.: Appleton & Lange.

Porter, H. (1991). A theory of goal attainment and ambulatory care oncology nursing: An introduction. *Canadian Oncology Nursing Journal, 1*(4), 124-126.

Porter-O'Grady, T. (1994a). Building partnerships in healthcare: Creating whole systems change. *Nursing & Health Care, 15*(1), 34-38.

Porter-O'Grady, T. (1994b). Whole systems shared governance: Creating the seamless organization. *Nursing Economics, 12*(4), 187-195.

Porter-O'Grady, T. (1997). Quantum mechanics and the future of healthcare leadership. *Journal of Nursing Administration, 27*(1), 15-20.

Powell, S.K. (1996). *Nursing case management: A practical guide to success in managed care.* Philadelphia: Lippincott-Raven.

Robbins, S.P. (1990). *Organization theory: Structure, design, and application* (3rd ed.). Englewood Cliffs, N.J.: Prentice-Hall.

Saxe, J.G. (1868). *The poems of John Godfrey Saxe.* Boston: Ticknor & Fields.

Senge, P.M. (1990). *The fifth discipline: The art and practice of the learning organization.* New York: Doubleday/Currency.

Shortell, S.M., & Hull, K.E. (1996). The new organization of the health care delivery system. In S.H. Altman & U.E. Reinhardt (Eds.). *Strategic choices for a changing health care delivery system* (pp. 101-148). Chicago: Health Administration Press.

Shortell, S.M., Gillies, R.R., & Devers, K.J. (1995). Reinventing the American hospital. *The Millbank Quarterly, 73*(2), 131-159.

Soderberg, G.L., & Walter, J.M. (1991). Modeling physical therapy clinical research centers. *Physical Therapy, 71*(10), 734-745.

Sowell, R.L., & Grier, J. (1995). Integrated case management: The AID Atlanta model. *Journal of Case Management, 4*(1), 15-21.

Strickland-Seng, V. (1995). The Neuman systems model in clinical evaluation of students. In B. Neuman (Ed.). *The Neuman systems model* (pp. 215-225). East Norwalk, Conn.: Appleton & Lange.

Stuart, G.W., & Wright, L.K. (1995). Applying the Neuman systems model to psychiatric nursing practice. In B. Neuman (Ed.). *The Neuman systems model* (pp. 215-225). East Norwalk, Conn.: Appleton & Lange.

Thompson, J.D. (1967). *Organizations in action.* New York: McGraw-Hill.

Toot, J.L., & Schmoll, B.J. (1995). The Neuman systems model and physical therapy educational curricula. In B. Neuman (Ed.). *The Neuman systems model* (pp. 231-246). East Norwalk, Conn.: Appleton & Lange.

Trépanier, M. J., Dunn, S.I., & Sprague, A.E. (1995). Application of the Neuman systems model to perinatal nursing. In B. Neuman (Ed.). *The Neuman systems model* (pp. 309-320). East Norwalk, Conn.: Appleton & Lange.

Tunick, P.A., Etkin, S., Horrocks, A., Jeglinski, G., Kelly, J., & Sutton, P. (1997). Reengineering a cardiovascular surgery service. *Journal on Quality Improvement 23*(4), 203-216.

Van Slyck, A. (1991a). A systems approach to the management of nursing services. I. Introduction. *Nursing Management, 22*(3), 16-17.

Van Slyck, A. (1991b). A systems approach to the management of nursing services. II. Patient classification system. *Nursing Management, 22*(4), 23-25.

Van Slyck, A. (1991c). A systems approach to the management of nursing services. III. Staffing system. *Nursing Management, 22*(5), 30-34.

Van Slyck, A. (1991d). A systems approach to the management of nursing services. IV. Productivity monitoring system. *Nursing Management, 22*(6), 18-20.

Van Slyck, A. (1991e). A systems approach to the management of nursing services. V. The audit system. *Nursing Management, 22*(7), 14-15.

Van Slyck, A. (1991f). A systems approach to the management of nursing services. VI. Costing system. *Nursing Management, 22*(8), 14-16.

Van Slyck, A. (1991g). A systems approach to the management of nursing services. VII. Billing system. *Nursing Management, 22*(9), 18-21.

Welton, W.E., Kantner, T.A., & Katz, S.M. (1997). Developing tomorrow's integrated community health systems: A leadership challenge for public health and primary care. *The Millbank Quarterly, 75*(2), 261-289.

Westrope, R.A., Vaughn, L., Bott, M., & Taunton, R.L. (1995). Shared governance: From vision to reality. *Journal of Nursing Administration, 25*(12), 45-54.

3

Effects of Health Care Economics and Financing on Nursing and Health Care Delivery

Cheryl Bland Jones and Mattia J. Gilmartin

INTRODUCTION

The system for financing health care in the United States can be characterized as complex, value laden, and, in recent years, turbulent. Subsequently, this turbulence permeates the entire health care system, including its structure, processes, and outcomes and any individual or group who comes in contact with the system. An understanding of the health care financing system, therefore, is imperative for visualizing and implementing the role of the advanced practice nurse in the evolving health care system.

This chapter provides an overview of the system for financing health care in the United States, presents milestones in the development of health care financing, and highlights anticipated changes in health care financing. Ultimately, this chapter provides answers to important questions such as *why* the system has evolved as it has, *how* providers are paid for services delivered, *who* is reimbursed, *what* services are covered, and *where* the money comes from. A discussion of these issues will enable nurses to prepare for further change in the U.S. health care financing system, to recommend strategies for shaping the future system, and to more clearly define the role of nursing in the health care system of the future.

OBJECTIVES

After reading this chapter, you will be able to:

1. Describe the system for financing health care in the United States
2. Compare and contrast mechanisms for provider reimbursement
3. Evaluate major health care funding sources
4. Analyze specific health care financing issues at the level of the overall economy, the industry, organizations, providers, and consumers
5. Examine incentives within the health care financing system
6. Evaluate the cost of change

61

Key terms	
Term	**Definition**
Economics	The study of allocating scarce resources to satisfy desires (Wonnacott & Wonnacott, 1982)
Finance	The study of money and capital markets, investments, and management of resources (Finkler & Kovner, 1993)
Macroeconomics	"Big picture" view—the behavior of the economy as a whole, or an aggregate-level perspective; for example, gross domestic product, employment (Boyes, 1991)
Market	Buyers and sellers within a particular industry who exchange goods and services (Folland et al., 1993)
Microeconomics	"Small picture" view—the behavior of units within an economy; for example, industries, firms, households, consumers (Mansfield, 1988)
Economic efficiency	Maximizing productive efforts (Wonnacott & Wonnacott, 1982)
Time value of money	Financial concept that reflects the notion that "a dollar today is worth more than a dollar tomorrow" (Brigham & Gapenski, 1989)

■ THE BIG PICTURE: MACROECONOMICS

The 1990s represent the economic era of health care, with the current health care financing system shaped by market forces. Most recently, these forces have brought to bear pressures to contain costs and have brought about a rush to merge health care organizations (HCOs), integrate and align services, downsize or reengineer operations, develop new partnerships, and engage in joint ventures—all in an effort to achieve efficiencies within organizations and across the system as a whole.

Market forces are not only changing the ways in which health care is delivered, but also shifting the focus of health care: from the hospital to health care systems; from episodic and inpatient care to continuous and outpatient care; from individual-based to population-based care; from a "product" to a "service" perspective; from market share of admissions to covered lives; from independence to integration; from management of the particulars to systems thinking; from a focus on management and coordination to quality improvement; from a national to a global perspective; and most important, from illness treatment to health promotion and disease prevention (Shortell et al., 1995).

From an historical perspective, the mechanisms for financing health care have been a driving force behind the structure of the health care industry, health care technology, and health care delivery in the twentieth century. Table 3-1 illustrates this point. For example, during the 1960s technologic advances focused on "hardware" technologies (i.e., equipment or durable technologies) versus advances in the provision of health care services; at the same time, health care was financed through a retrospective payment system, whereby reimbursement was based on the amount providers billed for a particular service. This retrospective payment system contributed to and enabled the development of these hardware technologies—since providers were paid for the bill they submitted, the bill often included the costs of developing and using these hardware technologies. Moreover, this system did not demand efficiencies in service delivery because the bill was paid, regardless of the cost. On the other hand, technologic advances in the 1990s have shifted more toward the service aspects and innovations in delivery of health care services, primarily driven by prospective payment, managed care, and capitation; these mechanisms necessitate efficiencies in "producing" health care services versus supporting the delivery of increasingly expensive equipment.

The U.S. government exerts tremendous influence over the health care system, through both its direct expenditures and its policymaking. As noted in Table 3-1, the federal government became a major player in the health care industry between 1930 and 1950, with the enactment of the Social Security Act (set up a U.S. public insurance program for retirees), the Hill-Burton Act (provided public funds for constructing hospitals in rural areas), and other acts. The government became an even bigger player in the health care market with the introduction of Medicare and Medicaid legislation in the 1960s. State governments also influence the health care system through their allocation of block grants and other resources. Given that federal and state governments pay for approximately 40% of U.S. health care, governmental actions play a key role in the health care economy.

The U.S. government also influences health care in other important ways (Cleland, 1990): first by establishing the federal budget and second by setting interest rates. In the process of determining the nation's budget, spending increases and decreases are set. Included in these spending decisions is the amount of money the government will allocate to federal health care programs. In addition, the government—through the Federal Reserve—sets interest

rates; these rates in turn affect borrowing costs for individuals, consumers, organizations, and other groups. Increased interest rates retard spending on new health care programs, facilities, research, and other investments in health care. Increased interest rates also impact the amount of money consumers and other groups are willing to spend on health care consumption. Decreased interest rates would, obviously, have the opposite effect, that is, to promote spending and consumption.

Although recent developments noted above are moving the health care system forward developmentally (and certainly in a way that is philosophically congruent with nursing's focus on disease prevention and health promotion), it is important to consider the primary force behind these changes, namely, the escalating costs of health care during the last quarter of the twentieth century. In fact, health care expenditures during this period have grown at a faster pace than the overall economy, with hospital costs and physician services comprising well over half of health care expenditures in 1994 (Health Care Financing Administration [HCFA], 1996).

Figure 3-1 illustrates the progressive, upward trend in U.S. health care expenditures—from approximately $41 billion in 1965 to approximately $949 billion in 1994 (HCFA, 1996).* Concomitantly, the amount of money spent on health care by each individual within the United States increased, on average, from $172 in 1965 to $3074 in 1994 (HCFA, 1996). If one looks across this time period, total and per capita health care expenditures in the United States have increased, on average, approximately 11% annually over this period, roughly a doubling every 7 years (Jones, 1996).

---

* The year 1965 is often used as a baseline of comparison for health care cost statistics by the HCFA and other groups because that date predates the implementation of Medicare and Medicaid.

T A B L E   3 - 1

An Historical Overview of Twentieth Century Health Care Delivery in the United States

	1900-1920s	1930-1950s	1960-1980s	1990s
Financing Mechanism	Private payment for physician, hospital, and nursing services Philanthropic-sponsored hospitals	Blue Cross/Blue Shield formed Social Security Act Hill-Burton and Lantham acts National Mental Health Act	Medicare legislation Tax Equity and Financial Responsibility Act	Managed care financing/health care reform Balanced budget amendment limiting Medicare/Medicaid funding
Industry Structure	Specialty hospitals for specific diseases Proliferation of general hospitals; 1 bed to every 304 persons	AMA-created hospital ownership designations JCAH established	Rise of for-profit hospitals and multihospital chains	Mergers, alliances, partnerships, and acquisitions Growth of for-profit and managed care delivery organizations
Medical Technology	Germ theory, aseptic technique, and anesthesia developed Blood transfusions Stethoscopes, thermometers, and microscopes in use	Sulfa drugs, penicillin, and vaccines EKGs and EEGs available Intensive care units established University hospital system established	Cardiac care units Chemotherapy, electronic monitoring, renal dialysis, open heart surgery, organ transplantation, computerized scanners developed	Second-generation scanners Telemedicine and information systems Clinical guidelines Service technologies AIDS therapies
Leading Causes of Mortality	Influenza, pneumonia, tuberculosis, gastritis, heart disease, stroke, personal injury, chronic nephritis, cancer, "diseases of early infancy," diphtheria	Heart disease, cancer, stroke, personal injury, respiratory disease, diabetes mellitus, suicide, chronic liver disease, homicide	Heart disease, cancer, stroke, personal injury, pneumonia, chronic liver disease, diabetes mellitus, suicide, homicide	Heart disease, cancer, stroke, personal injury, chronic obstructive pulmonary disease, pneumonia and influenza, diabetes mellitus, suicide, chronic liver disease and cirrhosis, HIV

Nursing Profession	Nurse's training schools established ANA founded First nurse registration law	Federal legislation funding nursing education State boards for nursing license examinations University-based nursing education advocated Practical and associate degree nursing programs established NLN founded ANF founded First issue of *Nursing Research* published	ANA position paper on nursing education Commonwealth Fund and Nurse Training Act for advanced nursing education First doctorate of nursing science (DNS) program Prescriptive authority for nurse practitioners in some states National Center for Nursing Research established	Pew Foundation's report on the health professions National Institute of Nursing Research
Organization of Nursing Services	Functional nursing in hospitals by student nurses Private duty, public health/visiting nursing careers for graduates	Team nursing Professional nursing moves into hospital setting	Primary care nursing Shared governance practice models introduced	Introduction of unlicensed assistant personnel Trend toward multidisciplinary care teams

Data from Kalish, P.A., & Kalish, B.J. (1995). *The advance of American nursing* (3rd ed.). Philadelphia: J.B. Lippincott Co.; Kovner, A.R., (1990). *Jonas's health care delivery in the United States* (4th ed.). New York: Springer; National Center for Health Statistics (1982). *Health in the United States.* Department of Health and Human Services publication no. (PHS) 83-1232, Public Health Service. Washington, D.C.: U.S. Government Printing Office; Stevens R. (1989). *In sickness and in wealth: American hospitals in the twentieth century.* New York: Basic Books.
AMA, American Medical Association; *JCAH,* Joint Commission on Accreditation of Hospitals; *EKG,* electrocardiogram; *EEG,* electroencephalogram; *AIDS,* acquired immunodeficiency syndrome; *HIV,* human immunodeficiency virus; *ANA,* American Nurses Association; *NLN,* National League for Nursing; *ANF,* American Nurses Foundation.

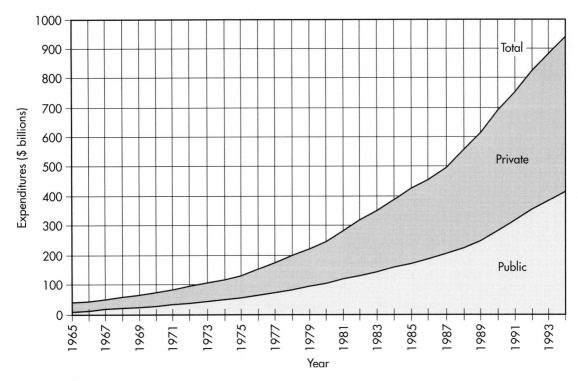

Figure 3-1 ■ **National health care expenditures, 1965 to 1994 (in billions of dollars).** (From Health Care Financing Administration [1996]. *1996 Data compendium.* Baltimore: U.S. Department of Health and Human Services, Health Care Financing Administration.)

To further explore increases in health care spending, inflation-adjusted expenditures are compared with unadjusted expenditures in Figure 3-2. After accounting for the effects of inflation, 1994 health care expenditures are approximately four times greater than 1965 spending figures, that is, $41 billion in 1965 compared with $148 billion in 1994.* During this period, overall inflation averaged approximately 3%, while the costs of physician and hospital services increased 6% and 7%, respectively—approximately twice the general rate of inflation

(HCFA, 1996).* Levit et al. (1996) note, however, that the rate of growth in health care spending was slower in 1994 than in the three previous decades.

---

* If calculated in 1994 dollars, these comparison figures become $249 billion in 1965 and $949 billion in 1994.

---

* Inflation, or a general increase in prices, is measured by the consumer price index (CPI). The CPI reflects inflation by measuring the prices of a fixed basket of goods and services during a given period of time. Throughout the late 1980s and early 1990s increasing concern has been expressed at the federal level about the CPI calculation methodology and its overstatement of inflation. Effective January 1999 a new formula, the geometric mean estimator, will be used to calculate certain CPI index categories to correct for the reported overestimation (see http://stats.bls.gov/cpigmo2.htm). The impact of this change on health care and other spending tied to the CPI likely will mean smaller future increases.

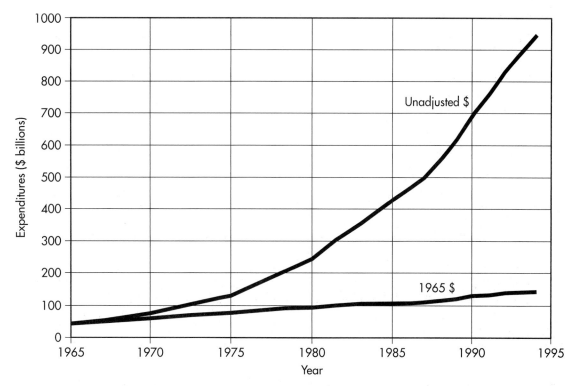

Figure 3-2 ■ National health care expenditures, adjusted for inflation (in 1965 dollars). (From Health Care Financing Administration [1996]. *1996 Data compendium.* Baltimore: U.S. Department of Health and Human Services. Health Care Financing Administration.)

The last indicator typically discussed in relation to health care spending is the percentage of gross domestic product (GDP), or the value of all goods and services produced in the United States during a 1-year period, that can be attributed to health care. Figure 3-3 shows that national health care expenditures as a percentage of the GDP increased from 5.9% in 1965 to 13.6% in 1994 (HCFA, 1996). Although one might argue that there is nothing wrong with spending this proportion of the GDP on health care, the real concern is over the spending *trend*: if health care comprises 14% of the GDP in 1994, what does the future hold? For comparison purposes, consider that the United Kingdom and Japan spend 6.9%, Germany and Canada spend 9.5%, and France spends 9.7% of GDP on health care (Abraham, 1997; Health Canada, 1997).

An examination of the reasons behind increases in health care spending is essential to appreciate and anticipate the future. A number of reasons are typically cited to explain increased health care spending (Folland et al., 1993; Newhouse, 1993).

First, the U.S. population has increased from approximately 200 million in the mid-1960s to more than 300 million in the 1990s; an increase

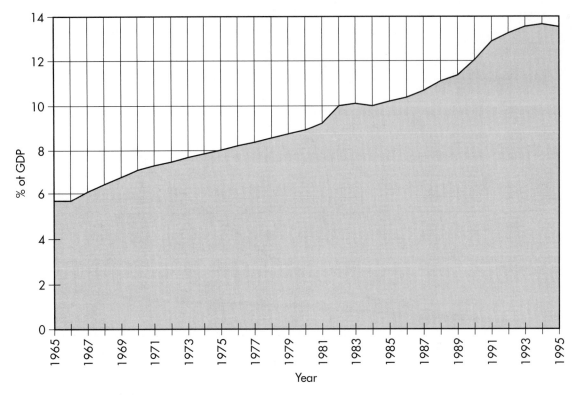

Figure 3-3 ■ National health care expenditures as a percentage of gross domestic product. (From Health Care Financing Administration [1996]. *1996 Data compedium.* Baltimore: U.S. Department of Health and Human Services. Health Care Financing Administration.)

in the population means that there are more people to consume the services. Second, people are living longer; in 1965 approximately 10% of the population lived to age 65 years or older, compared with 12.5% today. It might be expected that as people age, so too does their likelihood of developing a chronic illness or consuming health care services. Third, supplier-induced demand and unnecessary procedures, whereby physicians and other providers actually encourage the use of medical services for their own economic gain, play a role. On a similar note, the practice of defensive medicine (out of fear of being sued) could also contribute to

increased health care spending. Fourth, the U.S. public and private health care financing systems have encouraged past increases in spending; the retrospective payment system and fee-for-service payment actually provided incentives for overtreating and overspending. Fifth, consumer expectations place increased demands on the health care system; as a society Americans want the biggest and best and constantly demand a "magic pill" as a remedy for their ailments. Sixth, the cost of providing care to indigent persons has placed increased demand on the system and contributed to cost shifting, in which certain groups are charged and pay

BOX   3 - 1

Why Have Health Care Costs Increased?

- Larger population
- Population living longer
- Supplier-induced demand
- Financing system
- Patient expectations
- Indigent care
- TECHNOLOGY!!

Data from Folland, S., Goodman, A.C., & Stano, M. (1993). *The economics of health and health care.* New York: Macmillan; Newhouse, J.P. (1993). *Health Affairs, 12*(supplement), 152-171.

higher prices to cover the costs of those who cannot afford to pay for health care (Box 3-1).

Although these and many other reasons can be cited to explain the rise in health care spending, Newhouse (1993) systematically argues that, in fact, *technology,* or the "march of science," is primarily responsible for health care spending increases during the final quarter of the twentieth century. Thomas (1974) linked technology and health care spending and categorized health care technology into three levels. The first level, "nontechnology," is expensive, but necessary, care provided at the bedside by nurses, physicians, and other health care providers. This level of care is palliative and required when diseases are not well understood, as with acquired immunodeficiency syndrome (AIDS) in the late 1980s. The second level, "halfway technology," again is extremely expensive and reflects a state of knowledge about a particular disease that is somewhat better than the nontechnology level yet the disease is still poorly understood. What sets this level of technology apart from nontechnology is that technology at this level focuses on dealing with diseases after the fact and often aims at postponing death (e.g., heart disease). Thomas offers, however, that this level of technology is necessary for knowledge development to progress to the next level—"high technology." This level of technology is the least costly and results from a true understanding of a particular disease process. Examples of high technology include immunizations and antibiotics.

Based on Thomas's classification of technology, the escalation of health care costs is somewhat more understandable as one looks back over time. During the final quarter of the twentieth century, emphasis has been placed on dealing with many diseases (e.g., AIDS), and the U.S. health care financing system in retrospect has supported that perspective. As people become increasingly knowledgeable about many disease processes that confront society and develop high technologies, costs may actually decrease.

Although the retrospective payment system facilitated the development of halfway and high technologies, it did so in a manner that promoted the inefficient use of resources. Efforts to eliminate inefficiencies from today's health care system are being made in a climate where new diseases are emerging and the system is constantly faced with new challenges. Meeting these challenges requires health care to integrate knowledge and information from other elements of society and to strive for the efficient development of new health care technologies. As Thomas (1974) notes, however, the only way to achieve the efficiencies of high technology is through knowledge development obtained through a true understanding of disease processes brought about through research (which requires long-term investment by the health care system). The key is to carefully consider resource allocation, recognizing that different types of technologies may be more efficient. As Thomas illustrates, all technology is not the same, and the benefits and limitations of technologies should be distinguished whenever possible.

A closer examination of increasing health care expenditures illuminates other, perhaps more pragmatic, considerations within the system that contribute to increasing health care costs: the number of people requiring health care; the severity, or nature, of illness; the availability of technology to prevent or treat illnesses; the availability of a source to pay for the care; and finally, but no less important, whether persons (patients and their families) are aware of and demand the latest technology and treatments. It is interesting to note that health care consumption is based on choices made at the individual level, yet payment is typically made at another level altogether. The bottom line is that, regardless of other occurrences within the market, economic and financial issues affect every other aspect of the health care industry.

■ **SOURCES OF PAYMENT: THE PAYERS**

Although the money that goes into health care can be traced to individuals, the payment for health care services typically comes from a public or private group or a third party rather than from the individual who receives a particular service. Public third-party payers include the local, state, and federal governments, whereas private third-party payers include insurers, employers, individuals, and private groups or associations (Knickman & Thorpe, 1995).

The proportion of funding coming from public and private sources has changed over time (Figure 3-4; HCFA, 1996). In 1965, approximately 25% and 75% of health care funding came from public and private sources, respectively. In 1994, approximately 44% of health care funding came from public source and the remaining 56% came from private sources. Figure 3-4 also illustrates that the percentage of public spending increased rather sharply after 1965 and has remained fairly constant since that time.

The change in public and private funding sources is more clearly documented in Figure 3-5. On close examination, the gradual growth in health care funding from public sources and the gradual decline in private health care spending since 1965 are apparent. Of particular interest is the fact that personal, out-of-pocket spending for health care also decreased from 56% in 1965 to 20% in 1994, whereas private insurance and public contributions are increasing on a percentage basis (HCFA, 1996; Box 3-2, p. 73). Each of the health care funding sources is discussed in more detail below; in addition, types of payment strategies used by funding sources are presented.

Public Health Care Funding

The federal government funds health care primarily through two programs, Medicare and Medicaid, both implemented in 1966. *Medicare* is the federal government's health insurance program that covers individuals who are 65 years of age or older, who are disabled, or who have chronic kidney disease. This program, the nation's largest health insurance program (covering more than 38 million Americans), is administered through the Health Care Financing Administration (HCFA, 1997). Medicare has two components, known as Parts A and B. Part A, or hospital insurance (HI), covers 80% of inpatient hospital services, skilled nursing facilities, home health services, and hospice care. The income to fund Part A comes from the HI trust fund; this trust fund is maintained through contributions from payroll taxes, railroad retirement funds, enrollee premiums, interest on investments, and other general revenues (HCFA, 1997). Part B, or supplemental medical insurance (SMI), is voluntary and pays for the cost of physician and outpatient services, medical equipment, supplies, and other health services. This component of Medicare is funded through the SMI trust fund, made up of enrollee premiums, general rev-

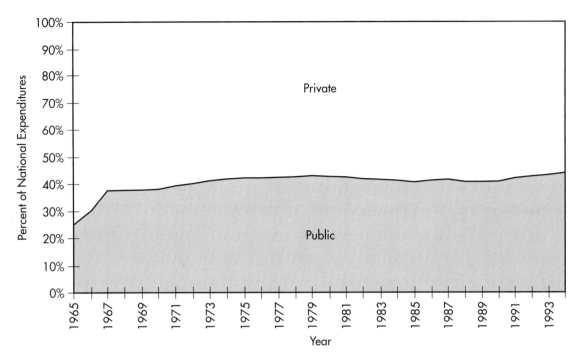

Figure 3-4 ■ Relative public and private health care expenditures. (From Health Care Financing Administration [1996]. *1996 Data compendium.* Baltimore: U.S. Department of Health and Human Services. Health Care Financing Administration.)

enue, and interest on investments (HCFA, 1997). Other cost-sharing strategies are used in the Medicare program, including enrollee deductibles and co-insurance payments. Medicare pays providers through a variety of strategies in addition to diagnosis-related groups (DRGs), such as fee-for-service and managed care, which are discussed in more detail later.

Medicaid, a health insurance program that provides coverage for more than 37 million poor people in the United States, is jointly sponsored by state and federal governments (HCFA, 1997) and administered by individual states. Full payment for services is also extended to aged individuals who meet eligibility requirements, individuals who are blind or disabled, and chil-

dren with absent parents. The proportion of Medicaid paid through state contributions ranges from 21% to 50%, and federal contributions range from approximately 50% to 79%, depending on a state's income level (HCFA, 1997; Standard & Poor's Industry Surveys, 1996). Eligibility is established by individual states, and coverage and services vary accordingly. Federal and state contributions to Medicaid come from federal, state, and local tax revenues.* Medicaid

---

* It should be noted that there are other sources of public funding not mentioned here; for example, the government also funds the cost of health care for veterans, active military personnel, and employees covered by workers' compensation. These sources of funding account for a relatively small portion of overall health care spending.

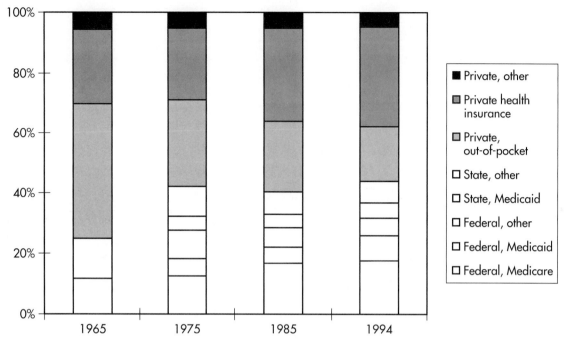

Figure 3-5 ■ Source of funds (1965, 1975, 1985, 1994). (From Health Care Financing Administration [1996]. *1996 Data compendium.* Baltimore: U.S. Department of Health and Human Services. Health Care Financing Administration.)

pays providers through a number of arrangements, such as DRGs, managed care, fee-for-service, and per-diem rates.

Private Health Care Funding

Five sources of private funding for health care are discussed here. The first of these, *private insurance,* is an arrangement between consumers and payers to cover the cost of medical care and to protect the consumer* against an unlikely health event (Folland et al., 1993). Health insurance is based on a pooling of money and risk,

and it operates under the law of large numbers; that is, although the likelihood of a certain health problem and its associated costs may be unpredictable for any one individual, that same health problem and its costs are much more predictable for a large group of people.

The oldest and largest health insurance company in the United States is Blue Cross/Blue Shield, founded in 1939.* The development of Blue Cross/Blue Shield inextricably linked health insurance to employment. Today, health insurance is obtained through employers, based on a mix of employer and employee contributions: employers may agree to pay the entire

---

* The term *consumer* is used loosely to mean the person who receives, or consumes, health care services. In a true economic sense, consumer implies that money is exchanged between the person who receives services and the entity who provides the service.

* Blue Cross provides hospital coverage, and Blue Shield provides physician coverage.

BOX 3-2

Sources of the U.S. Health Care Dollar (1995)

• Insurance	$0.31
• Medicare	$0.19
• Medicaid	$0.14
• Other government programs*	$0.13
• Out-of-pocket	$0.19
• Other private sources†	$0.04

From Vital statistics (1997, March 11). *The Washington Post,* p. 5 (Health Supplement).
*Includes the system for providing health care to veterans, current members of the military, and persons covered under workmen's compensation.
†Includes privately financed construction and foundations.

Key terms

Term	Definition
Medicare	Federally funded national health insurance program for all persons (1) age 65 years and older and/or (2) disabled (Standard & Poor's Industry Surveys, 1996)
Medicaid	Jointly funded federal and state program providing (1) health care services for low-income persons and (2) nursing home services for low-income persons age 65 years or older (Standard & Poor's Industry Surveys, 1996)
Managed care	System of financing and health care delivery that monitors and controls the types, utilization, quality, and cost of care for a defined population over a given period of time (Folland et al.,1993; Standard & Poor's Industry Surveys, 1996)
Retrospective payment	Hospital payment scheme whereby payment occurs after a service is rendered
Prospective payment	Inpatient hospital payment mechanism whereby payment is set for different patient groups before the delivery of a service

cost of health insurance, the employer and employee may share the cost of insurance, or the employee may be responsible for paying the entire cost of health insurance.

Insurers assume the financial risk for groups of individuals and often take steps to place certain limits or controls on those risks. For example, an insurance company may require second opinions for certain procedures, readmission certification, or inpatient length-of-stay reviews (Knickman & Thorpe, 1995). Insurance coverage can be based on any number of arrangements, including usual and customary charges, DRGs, a percentage of charges, a per-diem rate, or a capitated arrangement.

The increasing emphasis on cost containment in the late 1980s and 1990s has brought about the corporatization and privatization of health care known as *managed care.* Managed care is a system that monitors and controls the types, utilization, quality, and costs of health care (Folland et al., 1993). Although certain managed care arrangements have been around for some time, the number of people employed in the private sector who are enrolled in managed care plans through their employer has increased in recent years: from 40% in 1992 to 77% in 1996 (Hilzenrath, 1997). Two common types of managed care organizations (MCOs) (identified in Chapter 1) are HMOs and PPOs.

A key feature of managed care is capitation, whereby the MCO and provider agree on a pre-set, negotiated fee to provide care for a described group of patients during a certain period of time (often a monthly fee per enrollee). A premise of managed care is to shift the financial risk from the insurer to patients and providers through certain incentives and restrictions. For example, under some managed care plans, patients pay higher co-payments if they see physicians outside the plan, or physicians may need approval from the MCO before ordering certain tests, procedures, and medications.

Another feature of managed care is utilization management, which places certain controls on provider practice patterns (Folland et al., 1993). Again, all these efforts are aimed at controlling costs and achieving efficiencies; since MCOs represent such large numbers of individuals, they can dictate many of those cost-controlling strategies.

Employers are the largest purchaser of health care and, in fact, were the primary force behind recent changes in health care financing. Employers often represent large numbers of people and provide certain economies of scale to insurers. In return, employers can typically obtain better prices for health care coverage than can individuals. Because employers make decisions about specific benefits that will be purchased and set spending levels, they have to make certain trade-offs, recognizing that the money they spend on employee health care is money that could go toward other things, such as investments or profits. Moreover, there are tax incentives for businesses that provide health care benefits—they do not pay taxes on the money that goes toward employee health care. In short, employers and businesses have an enormous impact on health care financing (Folland, 1993; Knickman & Thorpe, 1995).

Some large businesses are bypassing insurance companies and MCOs altogether and are contracting directly with providers who agree to provide health services for employees. By cutting out the middle person and the associated administrative costs, employers can lower their costs of health benefits even more. Other businesses are offering wellness programs and other incentives to obtain, attract, and keep a healthy work force.

Finally, *individuals* may assume all or part of the costs of health care. For example, various insurance programs often require that individuals covered under the program pay premiums, co-insurance, co-payments, and/or deductibles (Folland et al., 1993). A premium is a set amount an individual pays for a certain level of health insurance coverage under a particular policy. For example, Medicare beneficiaries currently pay a premium of $42.50 per month for SMI coverage (HCFA, 1997). Co-insurance is the percentage an individual covered by a health program pays for charges associated with health services received. For example, Medicare SMI requires that covered individuals pay 20% co-insurance for physician services (HCFA, 1997). Co-payment is the actual dollar amount that an individual in a particular plan pays for services. For example, a Medicare beneficiary responsible for a 20% co-insurance payment for physician services that cost $40 would be responsible for a co-payment of $8. A deductible is a set amount that a person covered under a certain plan must assume responsibility for paying before receiving insurance coverage. For example, Medicare SMI requires individuals in the program to pay $100 deductible each year (HCFA, 1997). Frequently, insurance programs require some combination of these payment mechanisms for individuals covered under a plan. A good case in point is that of Medicare SMI cited above.

Other sources of private funding for health care include foundations, such as the Robert Wood Johnson Foundation and the Commonwealth Fund, and associations, such as the American Diabetes Association and the American Heart Association. The types of health care

Key terms	
Term	**Definition**
Health care premium	Set amount paid by an individual for health care insurance, based on the specifics of the policy (Folland et al., 1993)
Deductible	Set amount that an individual must pay before insurance payment takes effect, based on the specifics of the policy (Folland et al., 1993; HCFA, 1997)
Co-payment	Dollar amount paid by an individual to a provider at the time of service, based on the specifics of the policy (Folland et al., 1993; HCFA, 1997)
Risk plan	Type of managed care contract whereby individuals are required to receive all care through the plan or through plan referrals (HCFA, 1997)
Cost plan	Type of managed care contract whereby individuals are allowed to receive care within or outside the plan by assuming a portion of the cost for services received (HCFA, 1997)
Upcoding	Strategy used by HCOs aimed at maximizing Medicare reimbursement, whereby a DRG code is assigned that does not correspond to the actual care delivered (Lagnado, 1997)

funded by these groups vary, depending on their mission. For example, in keeping with the Robert Wood Johnson Foundation's mission of ensuring access to cost-effective health care for Americans, the foundation would likely provide funds to study innovative models of care delivery and innovative models of health care financing. Other private sources of health care funding include assets, such as stocks, bonds, cash, and equity, and loans that organizations might use to pay for health care or to invest in new health care programs.

Although funding for health care comes from the sources just mentioned, it is important to remember that the money channeled through these sources comes from ordinary citizens. For example, buying a car, groceries, clothes, and any other good or service pays for the cost of providing health care in that a portion of the money spent pays for health care benefits for employers and employees or goes to taxes that provide health care coverage for certain groups within society.

■ TYPES OF PAYMENT STRATEGIES IN HEALTH CARE

Several payment strategies are used by payers to compensate for health services delivered. These strategies, albeit complex and often overlapping, have developed over time and in response to changes in health care financing. Although each strategy will be presented individually, payers typically use a combination of strategies to pay for health services delivered, rather than a single strategy. Retrospective payment and prospective payment are common payment mechanisms for hospitals, whereas fee-for-service and capitation are common payment mechanisms for physician, outpatient, and other provider services (Knickman & Thorpe, 1995; Box 3-3).

Retrospective payment is often associated with Medicare, although it is more reflective of a time when payers had little or no incentive to control the costs of health care. Retrospective payment simply means that a payer provides compensation to a provider or hospital for a service after the service is delivered (Knickman & Thorpe, 1995). For example, before the mid-

Data from Knickman, J.R., & Thorpe, K.E. (1995). In A.R. Kovner (Ed.), *Jonas's health care delivery in the United States* (pp. 267-293). New York: Springer.

1980s, Medicare reimbursed hospitals on a retrospective basis; that is, the hospital determined the cost of providing services for patients after the services were delivered. Retrospective payment is typically based on one of two mechanisms: charges or costs (Knickman & Thorpe, 1995). Charge-based payment is set by the HCO and may not reflect the actual costs of providing a service. For example, a hospital might try to recoup the cost of providing "charity" care to an unusually high number of patients by charging a higher price for providing care to a Medicare patient with heart failure than it actually costs to deliver the care. A recent article noted that charges may exceed 40% of the actual costs of providing services to patients (Langley, 1997). Cost-based reimbursement reflects a price that is negotiated by the payer and hospital to provide care to patients: the payer reimburses the hospital a certain amount per patient per day for costs that the payer deems "allowable"(Knickman & Thorpe, 1995).

Prospective payment is a type of payment for inpatient hospital services that is based on a pre-established amount for providing care to a certain type of patient, with payments varying by some type of patient grouping (Knickman & Thorpe, 1995). The payment amount is established based on anticipated services and before the receipt of services. Again, prospective payment is associated with Medicare; in 1984, Medicare began reimbursing hospitals on a prospective basis through DRGs. Each DRG is clinically based and represents a group of patients considered to be similar with respect to the resources they are likely to consume (i.e., amount of care needed).

There are 25 major diagnostic categories, and each category contains several diagnostic subcategories that reflect resource consumption based on procedures, gender, and other clinical information (Adams, 1996; Knickman & Thorpe, 1995). In all, 429 DRGs are derived from the 25 major diagnostic categories (Adams, 1996). Patients are assigned a principal diagnosis from information abstracted from patient records (Knickman & Thorpe, 1995). Each DRG is assigned a relative weight, which is tied to the anticipated amount of resources that will be consumed to care for patients assigned to a given DRG; DRGs with higher relative weights are reimbursed at a higher rate (Adams, 1996).

Each hospital is assigned a hospital payment rate by HCFA, adjusted to account for differences in costs that might be associated with geography and demographics. Hospitals can determine their case mix index, which reflects the average relative weight for a specific group of patients or the overall hospital during a specific period of time (Adams, 1996). The case mix index can be used to determine total Medicare reimbursement received by a unit or hospital. For example, if a hospital, based on its case mix index, anticipates receiving a payment of $2000 from Medicare to provide care for a patient with a particular DRG coding and the hospital can provide care for less than that amount, the hospital will retain the difference. If, however, it costs the hospital more than $2000 to provide care for a patient in a particular DRG, the hospital must assume responsibility for that difference. Hence, the incentive is for hospitals to

Key terms	
Term	**Definition**
Diagnosis-related groups (DRGs)	Clinically based patient groupings for determining hospital payment (Adams, 1996; Knickman & Thorpe, 1995)
Hospital payment rates	HCFA-adjusted hospital payment for services rendered that takes into account differences in geography and community demographics (Adams, 1996)
Case mix index	Average relative weight for a specific group of patients (or the hospital overall) for a given period (Adams, 1996)
Fee-for-service (FFS)	Payment made to providers for services rendered, based on typical fees for a specific community (Folland et al., 1993; Knickman & Thorpe, 1995)
Resource-based relative values scale (RBRVS)	A measure of relative resource input levels required to produce services and procedures; categorizes physician "work" into four categories: time, mental effort and judgment, technical skill and physical effort, and psychologic stress (Hsiao et al., 1988)
Capitation	Payment method whereby providers are paid in advance of services rendered for a specific population over a defined period of time (Folland et al., 1993)

provide care that costs less than the amount of reimbursement.

Fee-for-service can be conceptualized as a type of retrospective payment for physicians and other health care providers. In this case, a physician or other health care provider is paid a fee for each health service rendered to individuals (Folland et al., 1993); the provider sets a price for the service, provides the service, submits a bill, and receives payment for the service from the payer (Knickman & Thorpe, 1995). Fee-for-service is the typical method used by Medicare and certain insurance companies for physician reimbursement and is based on physician fees within a given community. For example, Medicare fee-for-service payments to physicians must not exceed the 75th percentile of prevailing physician fees within the community (Knickman & Thorpe, 1995). In 1992, Medicare revised its fee-for-service reimbursement basis to a resource-based relative value scale (RBRVS) (Knickman & Thorpe, 1995). This scale

was developed to equalize payment across physician specialty groups and to recognize and compensate physicians who provide intense cognitive and diagnostic skills, as opposed to highly compensating physicians who perform primarily technical skills. Knickman and Thorpe (1995) note, however, that less change has been achieved with this system than was anticipated.

On the other hand, *capitation* can be thought of as a type of prospective payment made to physicians. Capitation is an arrangement between a physician or other provider and a payer whereby the provider agrees to render services to a group of individuals for a fixed amount charged to the payer (usually a monthly fee per member enrolled), regardless of the amount of services delivered (Folland et al., 1993). A cornerstone of managed care, capitation is an effort to set limits on costs before services are provided through a prearranged agreement. These limits provide a framework for resource consumption within which physicians and other providers must operate in providing care to individuals and groups. Like the discussion previously on prospective payment, if physicians and other providers consume resources in providing care to a particular patient that are above the capitated fee, the provider has to assume responsibility for the cost of those resources; if the provider delivers care that consumes a level of resources below the capitated fee, the provider keeps the difference.

Contracts establish a formal relationship between providers and payers. The agreement typically involves the negotiation of a lower rate of payment to providers for delivering care to well-defined patient populations. Medicare has recently partnered with MCOs to offer beneficiaries a choice of two managed care plans, each based on a different type of provider contract and each with a different emphasis on risk and risk sharing. *Risk plans* typically require that covered individuals receive all care through the plan or through referrals made by the plan; any care received outside the plan is typically the responsibility of the enrollee (HCFA, 1997). However, emergency care is typically covered under a risk plan, including emergency care that is received outside the plan's service area (HCFA, 1997). The agreement between Medicare and the MCO is outlined in a risk contract, whereby the MCO agrees to provide care to beneficiaries for a capitated fee, regardless of the services consumed by the beneficiary. Under this arrangement, the MCO assumes the financial risk for providing care to these Medicare enrollees (Health Care Financing Review, 1996). Some Medicare managed care risk plans offer a point-of-service (POS) option, which allows an enrollee to receive care from a provider outside the plan for certain services, and the plan and enrollee share responsibility for a percentage of the cost of care received (HCFA, 1997).

A Medicare *cost plan* provides enrollees with greater flexibility in the selection of a care provider (HCFA, 1997). Under this type of plan, en-rollees are allowed to choose a care provider from within or outside the MCO. If an enrollee selects a provider who is outside the plan, Medicare will cover a portion of approved charges and the beneficiary is responsible for co-insurance, deductible, and other fees (HCFA, 1997). A cost contract establishes the formal agreement between Medicare and the MCO, whereby Medicare agrees to pay the actual cost for delivering care to enrollees (Health Care Financing Review, 1996). Under this scenario, the risk is shared by Medicare and the Medicare beneficiary.

■ WHERE THE MONEY GOES IN HEALTH CARE

Up to this point, the discussion has focused on where the money comes from to pay for health care. The next obvious question is "Where does the money go?" In 1995, more than one third of the money went to hospitals and one fifth went to pay for physician services ("Vital statistics," 1997; Box 3-4).

A large portion of health care dollars goes into HCOs, whether those organizations are hospitals, skilled nursing facilities, home health care agencies, or physicians' offices. Once the

---

B   O   X   3   -   4

Recipients of the U.S. Health Care Dollar (1995)

• Hospital care	$0.36
• Other personal health care*	$0.25
• Physician services	$0.20
• Other spending†	$0.11
• Nursing home care	$0.08

Data from Vital statistics (1997, March 11). *The Washington Post*, p. 5 (Health Supplement).
*Includes dental, home health, drugs, medical supplies, and other miscellaneous health care services.
†Includes program administration, research, and construction.

money reaches an HCO, funds are further distributed to pay employees (in the form of salary and benefit compensation), to purchase equipment and new technologies, to buy supplies and pharmaceuticals, to pay consultants, to pay for overhead and maintenance, or to pay for *anything*—human, material, or capital resources—that is used to produce a particular organization's service.

■ MICROECONOMICS: BEHAVIOR WITHIN THE HEALTH CARE MARKETPLACE

The health care marketplace comprises providers, suppliers, consumers, regulators, payers, and HCOs (Finkler & Kovner, 1993). Microeconomic issues within the health care marketplace encompass the behaviors of units (organizations and individuals) within the health care sector. This section focuses on the behaviors and incentives of HCOs, professionals, and consumers to underscore driving and restraining forces within the environment.

Health Care Organizations

HCOs, like any other type of organization, strive to maximize profit.* Achieving this objective requires that HCOs focus on mission, structure, and service delivery while keeping their costs low, operating efficiently, and constantly comparing themselves with others in the industry and industry standards (i.e., benchmarking).

Thus HCOs have incentives related to cost containment and achieving operating efficiencies. First, HCOs obviously want to maximize reimbursement and minimize expenditures. Vigilant attention to documentation and coding allows organizations to receive appropriate and

---

* Many people erroneously believe that not-for-profit HCOs do not make or strive to make a profit. Not-for-profit HCOs do, in fact, strive to make a profit; unlike their for-profit counterparts who are concerned about paying stockholders, the "profits" of not-for-profit HCOs are reinvested in programs and services to serve the community, as dictated by their particular mission.

Key terms	
Term	**Definition**
Demand	Quantity of a good or service requested by buyers at a certain price (Folland et al, 1993)
Complement	Goods that must be consumed together; an increase in the price of one good will decrease demand for both goods (Folland et al., 1993)
Entrepreneurship	The identification of opportunities for change (Drucker, 1985)
Innovation	The creative application of knowledge and skill to bring about a change (Drucker, 1985)
Marginal	The incremental cost of producing and/or the incremental revenues generated from the sales of one additional unit (Wonnacott & Wonnacott, 1982)
Opportunity costs	The value of a foregone alternative (i.e., the next best choice) when an investment decision is made (Folland et al., 1993)
Substitute	Goods that satisfy the same need; an increase in the price of one will increase demand for the other (Folland et al., 1993)
Supply	Quantity of a good or service offered by a seller for a given price (Folland et al., 1993)

reasonable compensation for services delivered (Adams, 1996). An unfavorable outcome of coding has resulted in a practice known as *upcoding,* whereby HCOs assign a particular code for Medicare reimbursement to maximize billings within certain DRG categories, even if that code does not reflect the actual costs of delivering care for a particular patient or patient condition and/or resources consumed. In fact, organizations select a DRG code with a higher reimbursement (hence the term *upcoding*) than the DRG code associated with the actual patient condition. Although organizations certainly want to optimize billing codes to maximize reimbursement (Adams, 1996), the practice of upcoding may push the boundaries of optimization to deceit and fraud (Lagnado, 1997).

Second, HCOs strive to achieve operating efficiencies by focusing efforts on decreasing patients' length of stay (LOS) (e.g., through the use of critical pathways). In the same vein, HCOs strive to price themselves competitively within a given geographic region to attract patients and payers. They price themselves competitively by containing the use of expensive technologies, tests, and procedures; achieving staffing efficiencies by substituting lower-paid workers for higher-paid professionals and by changing the mix of staff used to provide the service; negotiating lower fees with payers and providers; and containing the use of referrals and consultations.

Finally, HCOs have an incentive to change their respective cultures from "best care regardless of cost" to "best care at the best cost." The culture within many HCOs today still remains consistent with the reimbursement system of the past—and many subcultures continue to value the inefficiencies of the retrospective payment system. To achieve the efficiencies that are possible, fundamental changes in the delivery of care can come about only when the culture and individuals within the

culture truly value the possibilities offered by those efficiencies.

Individuals

An often overlooked fact of microeconomics is that individuals, like organizations, have the same incentive for maximizing profits. Individuals and their behaviors, as units within health care, have a tremendous impact at the point of service, or the point of interface between the consumer and organization. Likewise, professional groups made up of individuals within the health care sector (nurses, physicians, dentists, physical therapists, and all other health care professionals) and their behaviors affect health care delivery at the organizational and system levels. All these groups are trying to maintain their position and role in the changing health care system. HCOs are pushing substitution with lower cost providers and other ways to achieve operating efficiencies, and as a result, these groups sometimes compete for power and jobs.

Nurses

Nurses, as the largest group of health care professionals, do and can have an enormous impact on health care organizations and, in turn, the health care system. The most recent National Sample Survey of Registered Nurses (Division of Nursing, 1997a), conducted in March 1996, estimates the current work force to be more than 2.5 million, with 82.7% of nurses employed in nursing. The average age of the working nurse is 42.3 years, up from 40 years in 1980 (Moses, 1982). The Division of Nursing (1997a, 1997b) also estimates that approximately 10% of the nursing work force represents an ethnic or racial category other than white and that roughly 5.4% is male. Approximately 40% of the nursing work force has a baccalaureate or higher degree in nursing, with approximately 32% possessing a baccalaureate as the highest nursing degree, 9% having a master's degree, and 0.6% of the nursing work force having a doctoral degree (Division of Nursing, 1997a). The average registered nurse's (RN's) salary in 1996 was $42,071, compared with $37,738 in 1992 (Division of Nursing, 1997a).

Given recent changes in health care delivery, the proportion of nurses working in various health care settings has changed. Approximately 60% of nurses work in hospitals, compared with 67% in 1992; 17% work in public health, compared with 15% in 1992; 8.5% work in ambulatory care settings, compared with 8% in 1992; and 8% work in long-term care facilities, compared with 7% in 1992 (Division of Nursing, 1997a; Moses, 1994). The actual numbers of nurses employed in various settings provide additional insight. For example, the number of nurses employed in hospitals actually increased between 1992 and 1996, from approximately 1,232,717 nurses employed in hospitals in 1992 to 1,270,870 in 1996 (Division of Nursing, 1997a). In addition, the number of nurses employed in public health more than doubled during the 4-year period (180,132 in 1992 versus 362,648 in 1996), while the number of nurses employed in ambulatory care settings and extended care facilities increased 24% and 32%, respectively. Approximately 59% of the nursing work force was employed full-time in 1996, compared with 57% in 1992 (Division of Nursing, 1997b).

This shift in nursing employment patterns clearly reflects recent changes in care delivery within the United States. As the demand for nursing services has changed, so too has the supply of nurses employed in various health care settings. HCOs' recent focus on cost containment has intensified efforts to look at alternative ways of enhancing flexibility and achieving efficiencies in service delivery. For example, hospitals may use substitutes for and complements to nursing care. In substitution, HCOs would replace RNs with unlicensed personnel in the overall mix of staff, whereas HCOs that employ unlicensed personnel as complements would do so to augment the care delivered by nurses.

An organization's choice of whether to use substitution or complementation reflects its mission and strategy. As noted in the Key Terms box on p. 79, the use of substitutes and complements is tied to price. When the cost of a certain group is perceived as high, an organization might consider substituting lower-paid personnel who can perform the same service. Although unlicensed personnel cannot perform the same services as nurses, they can perform certain tasks that are appropriately delegated by nurses and other health care professionals and that do not need to be performed by a nurse or other professional. The employment of unlicensed personnel as complements, on the other hand, would mean that an organization values the fact that RNs and unlicensed personnel must be employed together, and, for example, an increase in the price of RNs would bring about a concomitant decrease in the employment of both RNs and unlicensed personnel. Obviously, HCOs have employed unlicensed personnel as neither purely substitutes nor purely complements, but rather in ways that best meet organizational missions and the demand for services (Griffith, 1984).

Aiken et al. (1996) report that nursing personnel declined by 7.3% between 1981 and 1993 and nonclinical categories of hospital personnel, including administrators and other professionals, increased by almost 50%. Aiken and colleagues note that the staff mix in hospitals is "richer," because there has been an overall increase in RNs as a percentage of total nursing personnel, yet increasing acuity levels make it difficult to truly appreciate this richness. Moreover, Aiken et al. note that there has been a decline in non-RN nursing personnel during the period, leaving fewer overall nursing personnel to care for more acutely ill patients.

At the other end of the spectrum, nursing has advocated the substitution of nurse practitioners and other advanced practice nurses for other health care professionals. Under this scenario, nurses would be employed to provide many of the same services as other professionals at a lower cost. However, Griffith (1984) points out that some organizations may view nurse practitioners and other nurses with graduate education as complements to the care delivered by other groups of health professionals rather than substitutes for the care delivered by these other professionals. Again, how a particular HCO views nurses—as substitutes or complements—would likely be a function of its overall mission and direction, and HCOs are not likely to employ advanced practice nurses as either substitutes or complements in the purest economic sense (Griffith, 1984).

The government influences the supply of and demand for nursing services. For example, funding allocated through the federal budget to educate nurses with a special type of training sends a message to the nursing labor market and, in turn, increases the supply of a specifically educated category of nurse. The government influences the demand for nursing services at the policy level through the establishment of health care financing policies and by direct employment of nurses within federal programs. Once again, the impact of macrolevel decision making cannot be dismissed at the individual level.

Incentives That Drive Behavior

Nurses and other health care professionals may perceive that, in some cases, they have no choice in accepting the cost-cutting strategies employed by HCOs. For example, nurses may believe that other groups within health care are willing to step in and accept certain situations that may actually improve their economic well-being. In addition, within certain groups of health care professionals (e.g., certain specialty

physicians), a glut of providers has, in fact, left them with little bargaining power.

However, incentives within the current health care environment drive the behaviors of nurses and other health care professionals. First, there are clear incentives for health care employees to meet the demands of the market; these demands might include cross training and acquiring new knowledge and skills through advanced education. Second, there are incentives for risk taking, entrepreneurship, and innovation within health care service delivery. Those individuals and groups who think about and configure health care delivery in new ways will likely be rewarded. Third, there is a strong incentive for health care professionals to manage resources efficiently. Individual health care providers (physicians, nurse practitioners, and others) are being put at financial risk for the cost of patient care delivered. The day may soon come when HCOs will quantitatively evaluate each employee's ability to be productive and consume fewer resources in delivering care.

Consumers, not to be overlooked as important individuals within the health care system, also have certain incentives imposed by our evolving health care system. Consumers have incentives to stay healthy, become more knowledgeable, and take responsibility for their overall health, whenever possible, especially since insurance premiums are projected to rise 5% to 8% in the next few years (Hilzenrath, 1997).* Financial incentives, in the form of lower coinsurance and deductibles and increased coverage, are also provided to consumers covered under certain managed care arrangements who receive care from providers under contract with the organization. As individual consumers increasingly make trade-offs between purchasing

---

* Interestingly, Hilzenrath (1997) notes that insurance costs have increased twice as fast as the amount paid by employers.

health care or purchasing other goods and services, they will become more knowledgeable about their health and the health care system.

The incentives within the evolving health care system are numerous. However, there is the potential for conflict between individuals and organizations in health care as they each seek to maximize their profits. Therefore it is important to appreciate incentives within the system and recognize opportunities to work together in resolving those conflicts. Examining the costs of change and analyzing its effects on individuals and the organization can circumvent potential conflicts in the system. The following section discusses the cost of change and presents strategies for making informed decisions that minimize costs and maximize benefits.

■ THE COSTS OF CHANGE

In the current market environment of health care delivery, organizations must produce many services that make the most efficient and effective use of increasingly scarce human, material, and capital resources. As organizations adapt service and production processes to meet market demands, persons in decision-making roles must be able to analyze the economic costs and benefits of change proposals. Analysis of a proposal's direct and indirect effects on an organization and its members and constituents in terms of costs and benefits allows the organization to maximize its resources in the production of health care services.

Change has capital, material, and human costs. Weisbrod (1961) classified health care service costs and benefits in terms of direct, indirect, and intangible effects. Organizational costs associated with change include actual cash investments for equipment, personnel, and materials to bring a project into reality; personal stressors of matching the behaviors of individuals and groups to accept and carry out a new process or service; and commitments for the maintenance of organizational technology, whether in the form of employee training and skill development or durable equipment maintenance and upkeep.

The identification of a project's direct and indirect costs and benefits is an essential part of the resource distribution and investment process. The effects of change on consumers, employees, and ultimately the organization must be considered in short-range and long-range planning and goal-setting activities. Ideally, the identification of a project's effect on organizational functioning, consumer benefit, and investment return makes it possible for organizations to effectively manage and meet the demands of a turbulent market environment. In light of the cost-efficient nature of health care delivery, investment decisions an organization makes today will affect its ability to make investments in the future.

Examining the Costs of Change

Three methods to identify and select the best investment opportunity from a group of alternatives are benefit/cost analysis (BCA), cost-effectiveness analysis (CEA), and internal rate of return (IRR). These methods apply the concepts of efficiency, marginal analysis, and the time value of money to quantify a project's resource consumption and potential outcome for involved parties (Due, 1989; Folland et al., 1993; Klarman, 1982; Box 3-5).

BCA is a method used to evaluate and identify the least costly, most efficient project among a group of alternatives. The benefit/cost method considers a project's costs and benefits along with the direct and indirect effects of a project on constituent groups. The BCA method quantifies the human, capital, and material costs and benefits of a given project and is expressed as a ratio of benefits to costs. Ratios greater than one indicate the present value of a project's social

---

B O X   3 - 5

Tools to Aid Decision Making in the Current Environment

- Benefit/cost analysis (BCA): ranks programs based on direct and indirect costs and benefits
- Cost-effectiveness analysis (CEA): compares the costs of alternative programs with some predetermined objective or goal
- Internal rate of return (IRR): ranks investments based on expected return

---

Data from Brigham, E.F., & Gapenski, L.C. (1989). *Financial management: Theory and practice.* Chicago: Dryden Press; Folland, S., Goodman, A.C., & Stano, M. (1993). *The economics of health and health care.* New York: Macmillan Publishing; Klarman, H.E. (1982). In R.D. Luke & J.C. Bauer (Eds.). *Issues in health economics* (pp. 457-484). Rockville, Md.: Aspen.

benefits exceeds the costs and the project has a positive net benefit (Folland et al., 1993).

The application of BCA for health care investments is an underused analytic technique (Klarman, 1982). BCA assumes that the costs and benefits of a project can be expressed in monetary terms. Identifying relevant and meaningful direct and indirect costs and benefits, project life spans, and the appropriate interest rate for health care service investment is a challenging task. The precision of BCA can be enhanced through the use of sensitivity analysis. Sensitivity analysis is a technique in which benefit/cost ratios are calculated using different interest rates and project life spans to identify the scenario that yields the greatest net benefit (Jacobs, 1997).

The quantification of intangible characteristics (e.g., time, illness, life, health improvement, social welfare) as outputs of health care service delivery is a limitation of this analysis method (Klarman, 1982; Pruitt & Jacox, 1991). As the need for service efficiency grows, advances in defining, measuring, and analyzing the costs and

benefits of health care services will provide a foundation for the identification and development of improved service offerings (Grady & Weis, 1995).

CEA is a project evaluation method that compares alternative projects on the basis of cost only. CEA is used when the indirect effects of a project cannot be assigned a dollar value. Instead, a project's objectives are assumed to be socially desirable and the benefits of a given project outweigh the cost of production. This method compares projects of equal output or outcome to identify the project that uses human, capital, and material resources in the most efficient manner. The goal of CEA is to minimize the costs associated with producing a product or service of benefit to society.

Increasingly, the cost effectiveness of a variety of nursing practices has been demonstrated. In a comprehensive review of published nursing research, Fagin and Jacobsen (1985) evaluated the body of BCA and CEA studies specific to nursing practice. The benefit/cost ratio or cost effectiveness of nursing practices was segmented into four broad categories: (1) the organization of nursing services, (2) the testing of specific nursing interventions, (3) the substitution of nurses for other health care providers, and (4) the testing of alternative models of practice. Fagin and Jacobsen emphasize the importance of systematic and thorough analysis of the cost effectiveness and benefit/cost ratio of nursing practices and also call for the improvement of study designs by individuals engaged in research. As the need for cost-effective service delivery grows and analysis methods are refined, nurses practicing within organizations will have the ability to demonstrate the economic feasibility of new service offerings.

IRR is the third method useful in analyzing the cost of change. The IRR is a financial management technique necessary for capital budgeting decisions undertaken by organizations. Capital budgeting is the process of planning cash

B O X   3 - 6

Example Alternatives for Providing Services for Chronic Renal Patients

Alternative	Cost	Benefit	B/C Ratio	BCA Rank	IRR	CEA Rank
One	$25 M	$40 M	1.60	2	6%	2 (or 1)
Two	$12 M	$10 M	0.83	3	−2%	3
Three	$ 4 M	$7.5 M	1.88	1	0%	1 (or 2)

B/C ratio, Benefit/cost ratio; *BCA,* benefit/cost analysis; *IRR,* internal rate of return; *CEA,* cost-effectiveness analysis; *M,* million.

expenditures on assets (something of value) whose returns are expected to extend beyond 1 year (Brigham & Gapenski, 1989). Capital budgeting is one component of an organization's overall resource distribution process. IRR is a method of ranking investment proposals based on the amount of money that an investment will bring back into the organization.

The IRR method is based on the time value of money concept. This financial principle states that one dollar in the future is worth less than one dollar in hand today. This principle holds true because money can be invested at a certain interest rate and grows by that factor over time. The IRR method determines the interest rate that forces the present value of an investment's expected cash inflows to equal the present value of the project's expected costs (Brigham & Gapenski, 1989). To conduct an IRR analysis of an investment proposal, one must know the project's life span, usually expressed in years; the projected cash inflow for the project at each year; and the total investment costs for the project. An equation describing the relationship between these elements is solved, yielding the project's IRR. The widespread availability of financial calculators and spreadsheet programs makes the calculation of project IRR a simple task. Projects with an IRR more than the current interest rate at which the organization borrows money are typically considered for capi-

tal investment. In addition, projects are evaluated and ultimately selected based on their fit with the organization's overall mission, strategy, and service capabilities.

An Example

Consider a not-for-profit HCO that aims to provide outpatient care to patients with chronic renal disease—a service currently unavailable in the community—and, in turn, improve the quality of life for renal patients and the overall health and well-being of the community. To meet this goal, the HCO generates three alternative projects (Box 3-6).

Alternative one involves building and staffing a freestanding renal care facility in an area of the community with easy access by bus and free parking. Over 5 years, this alternative is projected to cost approximately $25 million (construction and operation), and benefits are projected at $40 million. The benefit/cost ratio is 1.6, and the IRR is estimated to be 6.0%.

Alternative two will expand an existing facility but will not be as convenient as alternative one for many of the community's patients. Under this scenario, the 5-year costs are projected to equal $12 million (renovation and operation), benefits are estimated to be $10 million, the benefit/cost ratio equals 0.83, and the IRR is calculated at −2.0%.

Alternative three will send advanced practice nurses into renal patients' homes for ongoing monitoring and treatment; close ties between the existing facility and an expanded patient population will be developed. This project is estimated to cost $4 million over 5 years, benefits are estimated at $7.5 million, and the benefit/cost ratio equals 1.88. The IRR under this scenario is 9.0%.

Using BCA, these three projects can be ranked as follows: alternative three is ranked first; alternative one is ranked second; and alternative two is ranked last. This ranking also is consistent with the IRR calculations for each project.

Consider, however, that the anticipated outcome of such a program—improved quality of life for patients with chronic renal disease—is a difficult objective to quantify in dollars and cents. Guided by a cost-effectiveness analysis, program planners should consider implementing the program with the lowest production costs that, in the long run, best meets the needs of community residents and provides the best improvement in the quality of life for patients with chronic renal disease. Because alternative three is the least costly and is anticipated to improve the quality of life for program participants, this selection would be ranked first. Alternative one, however, would reach and bring about an improved quality of life for a greater number of community renal patients, so this alternative should be considered. Again, choice of alternatives using CEA should reflect the organization's mission and project aims.

Although the discussion of these strategies has focused on organizational-level decision making, individuals can apply concepts from these analytic techniques to make personal decisions. For example, a nurse employed as a case manager in a hospital setting might weigh the quantifiable benefits and costs of accepting a position as an outcomes manager with a nearby HMO. If the personal goal is to achieve greater flexibility in work scheduling (a benefit that is difficult to calculate), the nurse might consider the costs of achieving this goal in the present position of case manager compared with accepting the position of outcomes manager. These decision-making tools provide a systematic means for thinking through alternatives and arriving at a conclusion that meets individual or organizational goals and objectives.

■ FUTURE DIRECTIONS FOR NURSING PRACTICE

Change is occurring in every facet of the health care industry. As the above discussion illustrates, cost savings, cost containment, and improved resource efficiency are shaping health care service delivery. Within this environment of change, nurses and other health care professionals need to understand where health care dollars come from and where they go to make more informed resource allocation decisions. Increased economic awareness of all health care practitioners is the key to creating a system of integrated, population-based, patient-centered, health-promoting service delivery for the twenty-first century.

The turbulence of the current practice environment can be daunting; however, professional nurses have the knowledge, skills, and tools to improve service delivery. Within organizational systems, nurses are the single largest group of health care professionals—at the interface of patients, organizations, and service delivery; they have the ability to question, envision, and create a cost-effective health care delivery system.

The first step in modifying professional nursing practice is a heightened awareness of the economic forces that drive health care delivery. Nursing practice has a profound effect on the cost of health care delivery, yet many nurses have relatively little appreciation of their role in organizational resource consumption (Caroselli, 1996). In the economic era of health care delivery, financial and economic knowledge is as much a part of professional nursing practice as pathophysiology, pharmacology, and patient care interventions (Box 3-7).

Keeping abreast of changes in the national economy, health care industry, delivery organizations, and population demographics influences practice and resource allocation behaviors. Financial and economic information about health care delivery is available from a variety of sources. Some of these are World Wide Web home pages maintained by the Department of Health and Human Services (DHHS, *http://www.os.dhhs.gov/*), Health Care Financing Administration (HCFA, *http://www.hcfa.gov/*), the National Institutes of Health (NIH, *http://www.nih.gov/*), the Centers for Disease Control and Prevention (CDC, *http://www.cdc.gov/*), and the Agency for Health Care Policy and Research (AHCPR, *http://www.ahcpr.gov/*); annual expenditure and utilization reports published by the Health Care Financing Administration; and professional journals and programs sponsored by professional organizations.

The second step in modifying professional nursing practice to meet the demands of a changing market environment is the application of economic knowledge to daily practice behaviors. A strong understanding of the macroeconomic and microeconomic forces shaping health care delivery makes it possible for nurses to act as effective change agents within organizational systems. Proficiency in financial and economic topics strengthens the ability of the advanced practitioner to communicate with members of multiple disciplines and constituent groups. In addition, the ability to communicate the economic feasibility of new service or care delivery processes supports the evolution of professional nursing practice.

The emerging model of seamless, patient-centered, community care networks parallels professional nursing's vision of health care service delivery (American Nurses Association, 1992). Professional nurses possess the knowledge and skills necessary for the creation of a new system of health care delivery. The professional nurse has the ability to identify and design new services; to coordinate, integrate, and manage patient care services; to facilitate service delivery among health care professionals; and to create an ethic of ongoing service delivery improvement. Contributions such as these enable organizations to develop services that meet changing market demands for health care service delivery.

There is speculation that, in the years since the introduction of capitated service reimbursement, the health care sector has "reaped the one-time windfall of savings" from managed

B O X   3 - 7

From the Field

Caroselli (1996) examined the relationship between the economic awareness of staff nurses, supply use, and the budgetary responsibility of unit-level nurse managers. Overall, she found that the economic awareness of participating staff nurses and unit managers was relatively low. Economic awareness of the nurses did not increase with age, experience, gender, marital status, education, or management experience but did increase with professional certification. Additionally, 41% of the sample believed that an understanding of finance and budgeting was not applicable to their clinical practice. Caroselli advocates budget-neutral strategies that provide staff nurses with financial information, such as the cost of frequently used items, the amount of items consumed on a monthly basis, and the amount of linen used per patient day. Strategies such as these demonstrate the important relationship between staff nurse clinical practice behavior and unit resource consumption. Ultimately, practice information of this type could have a major impact on the cost savings and overall financial health of unit operating budgets.

care (Hilzenrath, 1997, p. H9). Cost savings have been achieved through decreases in staffing costs, patient length of stay, or service rationing. However, analysts predict that cost savings by these means may be at a maximum. Greater efficiencies within the health care industry will be achieved through fundamental changes in care delivery as opposed to further cuts in staffing and other areas (Hilzenrath, 1997).

The creation of a heath care system focused on disease prevention, health promotion, and primary care depends on organizational structures, systems, and cultures that allow evolutionary change to occur (Shortell et al., 1995). At the heart of the change process is the need for innovation and entrepreneurship within organizations.

Typically, innovation takes one of two basic forms. Product or revolutionary innovation introduces a new product of service that is unrelated to an organization's current or core technology (Dewar & Dutton, 1986). In hospitals the production of health promotion services can be viewed as a revolutionary innovation because the core service of hospitals traditionally has been illness treatment. Process or evolutionary innovation refines or enhances current organizational technology to capitalize on organizational capabilities (Dewar & Dutton, 1986). The adoption of clinical guidelines or critical pathways for the care of specific patient groups is an example of process innovation (Box 3-8).

Within health care delivery organizations the cycle of service development and process improvement occurs with the integration of information about population health needs, current clinical practices, and service technology capabilities. Underlying the innovation dynamic is the systematic examination of current practices to identify areas of productivity gain in conjunction with the application of specialized knowl-

B O X   3 - 8

Types of Innovation Within Organizations

- Product, or revolutionary, by introducing a new product or service that is unrelated to an organization's core technology
- Process, or evolutionary, by refining and enhancing current organizational technology to capitalize on organizational capabilities

From Dewar, R.D., & Dutton, J.E. (1986). *Management Science 32*, 1422-1433.

edge leading to the development of new services. In the new era of health care, innovations will emerge from an empiric base that describes outcomes of services delivery in terms of resource efficiency and relative effectiveness leading to the attainment of improved health status in served populations (Standard & Poor's Industry Surveys, 1996).

The nursing profession is presented with a variety of opportunities to contribute a unique disciplinary knowledge ultimately leading to the creation of an efficient and effective health care delivery system. Nurses must cultivate a spirit of entrepreneurship leading to innovations in patient care service delivery. Now, more than ever, nurses must be aware of opportunities; communicate the feasibility of proposed service changes in terms of human, capital, and material resources; and be willing to envision a new reality of health care service delivery for the twenty-first century.

■ KEY POINTS

- The escalating costs of health care have brought about an increasing emphasis on the economic and financial side of the health care system.
- Changes in the demographics of the U.S. population, the behaviors of health care pro-

viders, the mechanisms of health care payment, consumer expectations, the provision of care to the indigent population, the provision of care to uninsured individuals, and technology are reasons offered for the increase in health care costs.

- The federal government exerts a tremendous macroeconomic influence on the health care system through policymaking.
- Health care is paid for through public, private, and individual sources.
- Managed care was introduced in the 1980s as a financing and health care delivery system aimed at curbing excess health care spending.
- Health care dollars go to organizations and individuals who provide health care services.
- Analytic techniques for evaluating the cost of change are benefit/cost analysis, cost-effectiveness analysis, and internal rate of return.
- Nursing, as the largest health care profession, has the potential to effect change in the manner in which health care is delivered and resources are allocated.
- Nurses can effect change by increasing awareness of economic issues, maintaining an up-to-date knowledge base, and translating and applying this knowledge in nursing practice and health care delivery.

■ CRITICAL THINKING QUESTIONS

1. Differentiate and describe sources of health care funding. Identify strategies commonly used by each source to pay for health care services.
2. What incentives exist within the health care system to influence the choices and behaviors of individuals and organizations?
3. Describe a change scenario in which it would be appropriate to apply the benefit/cost analysis technique. Could cost-effectiveness analysis also be used to evaluate this same situation? Why or why not? Would

it be appropriate to evaluate this same scenario using the internal rate-of-return technique? Why or why not?

4. Why is it important for nurses to have specific knowledge about the costs associated with care delivery? How would nurses go about acquiring this knowledge?
5. What is the relationship between innovation and the economics of health care delivery? Identify a recent nursing innovation, and evaluate the effects of that innovation on the cost of care delivery.

■ REFERENCES

Abraham, I.L. (1997). *Will an aging population break the health care bank?* Unpublished manuscript.

Adams, T.P. (1996). Case mix index: Nursing's new management tool. *Nursing Management, 27*(9), 31-32.

Aiken, L.H., Sochalski, J., & Anderson, G.F. (1996). Downsizing the hospital nursing workforce. *Health Affairs, 15*(4), 88-92.

American Nurses Association (1992). *Nursing's agenda for health reform.* Washington, D.C. : The Association.

Boyes, W.J. (1991). *Macroeconomics: Intermediate theory and policy* (3rd ed.). Cincinnati: South-Western Publishing.

Brigham, E.F., & Gapenski, L.C. (1989). *Financial management: Theory and practice.* Chicago: Dryden.

Caroselli, C. (1996). Economic awareness of nurses: Relationship to budgetary control. *Nursing Economic$, 14*(5), 292-298.

Cleland, V. (1990). *The economics of nursing.* Norwalk, Conn.: Appleton & Lange.

Dewar, R.D., & Dutton, J.E. (1986). The adoption of radical and incremental innovations: An empirical analysis. *Management Science, 32,* 1422-1433.

Division of Nursing (1997a). Advance notes I from the National Sample Survey of Registered Nurses, March 1996. Available at *http:www.hrsa.dhhs.gov/bhpr/DN/advnote1.htm/ (Dec. 16, 1997).*

Division of Nursing (1997b). Advance notes II from the National Sample Survey of Registered Nurses, March 1996. Available at *http:www.hrsa.dhhs.gov/bhpr/DN/advnote2.htm/ (Dec. 16, 1997).*

Drucker, P.F. (1985). *Innovation and entrepreneurship: Principles and practice.* New York: Harper & Row.

Due, R.T. (1989). Determining economic feasibility: Four cost/benefit analysis methods. *Journal of Information Systems Management, 6*(4), 14-19.

Fagin, C.M., & Jacobson, B.J. (1985). Cost-effectiveness analysis in nursing research. In H.H. Werley & J.J. Fitzpatrick (Eds.). *Annual review of nursing research* (vol. 3, pp. 215-238). New York: Springer.

Finkler, S.A., & Kovner, C.T. (1993). *Financial management for nurse managers and executives.* Philadelphia: W.B. Saunders.

Folland, S., Goodman, A.C., & Stano, M. (1993). *The economics of health and health care.* New York: Macmillan.

Grady, M.L., & Weis, K.A. (1995). *Cost analysis methodology for clinical practice guidelines.* Baltimore: U.S. Department of Health and Human Services, Agency for Health Care Policy and Research.

Griffith, H. (1984). Nursing practice: Substitute or complement according to economic theory. *Nursing Economics, 2*(2), 16-23.

Health Canada (1997). National health expenditures in Canada, 1975-1996. Available at *http:www.hwc.ca/ (Dec. 16, 1997).*

Health Care Financing Administration (1996). *1996 Data compendium.* Baltimore: U.S. Department of Health and Human Services, Health Care Financing Administration.

Health Care Financing Administration (1997). Overview of the Medicare program & HCFA statistics [on-line]. Available at *http://www.hcfa.gov.*

Health Care Financing Review (1996). *Medicare and Medicaid statistical supplement.* Baltimore: U.S. Department of Health and Human Services, Health Care Financing Administration.

Hilzenrath, D.S. (1997, July 6). What's left to squeeze? Managed care firms find health costs rising—and cuts harder to come by. *The Washington Post,* pp. H1, H9.

Hsiao, W.C., Braun, P., Yntema, D., & Becker, E.R. (1988). Estimating physicians' work for a resource-based relative value scale. *New England Journal of Medicine, 319*(13), 835-841.

Jacobs, P. (1997). *The economics of health and medical care.* Gaithersburg, Md.: Aspen.

Jones, C.B. (1996). Issues in health care delivery and nursing. In J.L. Creasia & B. Parker (Eds.). *Conceptual foundations of professional nursing practice* (2nd ed., pp. 168-190). St. Louis: Mosby.

Kalish, P.A., & Kalish, B.J. (1995). *The advance of American nursing* (3rd ed.). Philadelphia: J.B. Lippincott.

Klarman, H.E. (1982). Application of cost-benefit analysis to the health services and the special case of technological innovation. In R.D. Luke & J.C. Bauer (Eds.). *Issues in health economics* (pp. 457-484). Rockville, Md.: Aspen.

Knickman, J.R., & Thorpe, K.E. (1995). Financing for health care. In A.R. Kovner (Ed.). *Jonas's health care delivery in the United States* (5th ed.) (pp. 267-293). New York: Springer.

Kovner, A.R. (1990). *Jonas's health care delivery in the United States* (4th ed.). New York: Springer.

Lagnado, L. (1997, April 17). Hospitals profit by "upcoding" illnesses. *The Wall Street Journal,* pp. B1, B12.

Langley, M. (1997, July 14). Nonprofit hospitals sometimes are that in little but name. *The Wall Street Journal,* pp. A1, A6.

Levit, K.R., Lazenby, H.C., Sivarajan, L., Stewart, M.W., Braden, B.R., Cowan, C.A., Donham, C.S., Long, A.M., McDonnell, P.A., Sensenig, A.L., Stiller, J.M., & Won, D.K. (1996). National health care expenditures, 1994. *Health Care Financing Review, 17*(3), 205-242.

Mansfield, E. (1988). *Microeconomics: Theory, applications* (6th ed.). New York: Norton.

Moses, E.B. (1982). *National sample survey of registered nurses. II. Status of nurses, November 1980* (HRP-0904375). Rockville, Md.: Health Resources and Services Administration, Bureau of Health Professions.

Moses, E.B. (1994). *The registered nurse population: Findings from the National Sample Survey of Registered Nurses, March 1992.* U.S. Department of Health and Human Services, Public Health Service. Health Resources and Services Administration (ISBN: 0-16-042616-2). Washington, D.C.: U.S. Government Printing Office.

National Center for Health Statistics. (1982). *Health in the United States.* Department of Health and Human Services publication no. (PHS) 83-1232, Public Health Service. Washington, D.C. : U.S. Government Printing Office.

Newhouse, J.P. (1993). An iconoclastic view of health cost containment. *Health Affairs, 12*(supplement), 152-171.

Pruitt, R.H., & Jacox, A.K. (1991). Looking above the bottom line: Decisions in economic evaluation. *Nursing Economics, 9*(2), 87-91.

Shortell, S.M., Gilles, R.R., & Devers, K.J. (1995). Reinventing the American hospital. *Milbank Quarterly, 73*(2), 131-160.

Standard & Poor's Industry Surveys. (1996). Proposed Medicare/Medicaid cutbacks: Winners & losers. *Healthcare, Hospitals, Drugs, and Services: Current Analysis, 164*(2), H1-H51.

Stevens, R. (1989). *In sickness and in wealth: American hospitals in the twentieth century.* New York: Basic Books.

Thomas, L. (1974). *The lives of a cell: Notes of a biology watcher.* New York: Bantam Books.

Vital statistics (1997, March 11). *The Washington Post,* p. 5 (Health Supplement).

Weisbrod, B.A. (1961). *Economics of public health.* Philadelphia: University of Pennsylvania Press.

Wonnacott, P., & Wonnacott, R. (1982). *Economics* (2nd ed.). New York: McGraw-Hill.

Organizational Theory and the Change Process

Juliann G. Sebastian

INTRODUCTION

The organization of health care is changing rapidly and profoundly, and these changes in the structure, financing, and administration of health services create the environment within which clinicians provide health care and patients receive health services. Health care agencies are merging, acquiring other health care agencies, and joining together in partnerships and alliances. Agencies are also making significant internal changes by eliminating some departments and adding others, redesigning jobs, and creating new services. Terms such as *downsizing, right sizing,* and *reengineering* (Hammer & Champey, 1994) are being used to describe changes in personnel and work processes.

Organizational changes influence caregiving in fundamental ways. Organizational changes influence the type of care that can be delivered, how it is delivered, what it costs, and consumer satisfaction with the care. Further, the ways in which health care is organized influence how changes in care delivery (e.g., new models of care delivery and clinical innovations) are implemented, evaluated, and improved. This reciprocal relationship is shown in Figure 4-1 and is the basis for this chapter.

This chapter uses organizational theories to explain why structural changes are occurring both within agencies and across agencies in communities. Different types of organizational structures are described, and the potential relationship of organizational design to health outcomes is discussed. The impact of the way health care is organized on the spread of clinical innovations and implementation of new care delivery models is discussed. Finally, the concept of integrated delivery systems is explained, and the impact of changing organizational arrangements on vulnerable populations is analyzed.

Figure 4-1 ■ Relationship between organization of care and change.

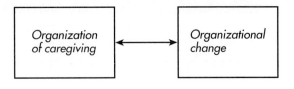

Figure 4-1 ■ Relationship between organization of care and change.

OBJECTIVES

After reading this chapter, you will be able to:

1. Evaluate the contributions organizational theory can make to the design and function of health care delivery systems
2. Explain the key concepts and propositions from selected organizational theories and their relevance for care delivery systems
3. Analyze the advantages and disadvantages of various forms of intraorganizational and interorganizational structure
4. Describe the link between organizational structure, population needs, outcomes of care, and issues related to cost effectiveness
5. Analyze the contributions of change theory to processes of organizational change
6. Evaluate the contributions of organizational theory to processes of change
7. Examine the impact of organizational structure and function on vulnerable populations

■ WHAT IS ORGANIZATIONAL THEORY?

Organizational theory is the science of understanding why and how people organize into work groups and how such work groups function. It has roots in sociology and social psychology and focuses on aggregate-level issues. Organizational theory differs from theories of organizational behavior, despite sounding similar, because organizational theory is concerned with the behavior of entire organizations and groups of organizations. Organizational behavior, on the other hand, focuses on the behavior of individuals and small work groups and has its roots in psychology (Sebastian & Stanhope, 1996).

What Is an Organization?

An organization is a group of people who have joined together to accomplish goals they cannot achieve alone (March & Simon, 1958). Employees are those people who enter into a contract with an existing organization to help achieve those goals in exchange for compensation. Basically, then, organizations help people aspire to shared visions.

Work has not always been done in organizations. Before the twentieth century, most work was done in small shops, in guilds, or on farms (Morgan, 1986). Industrialization changed the way people work by making it possible to achieve previously unimagined outcomes by combining the work of groups of people with technology. This led to migration into cities so people could live closer to large workplaces and to the formalization of employee/employer relationships in legally defined organizations.

Organizations have become an accepted part of daily life within industrialized countries in the twentieth century. They form a deep part of social culture, creating daily routines around "going to work" and accommodating the demands of work on family and social life. Organizations influence individuals' sense of self, because careers are often closely connected with organizational life, and both intrinsic and extrinsic rewards influence job satisfaction and self-esteem.

With the move away from industrialization and toward a service- and information-based economy, the organization of work is changing as well. Information technology has reduced the need for employees to work at central locations. For example, home health nurses with access to computers have little need to be based at a single agency location. The term *virtual organization* has real meaning as people in geographically diverse areas have opportunities to work together through electronic mail, Web-based chat rooms, and teleconferencing.

What Does Organizational Theory Contribute to Health Care?

Health care in the United States has been characterized as fragmented, with duplication of services and costly inefficiencies (Iglehart, 1992). This is a public problem, because an increasingly large proportion of the gross domestic product (GDP) is spent on health care in the United States, leaving fewer dollars for other goods and services. It is a problem also because health statistics indicate that the population is not as healthy as it could be, and inefficiencies within the health care system are thought to contribute to these less than optimal outcomes (U.S. Public Health Service, 1991). Finally, health services are often difficult to access, confusing, and frustrating. Patients do not always know which agencies provide the services they need, and they may not know if they are eligible for such services or how to obtain them. Obtaining help with health care needs from multiple agencies poses tremendous demands on patients in terms of (1) the time and energy required to keep multiple appointments with different providers, (2) frustration over answering the same question repeatedly, and (3) the feeling that providers are intruding into patients'

Key terms	
Term	**Definition**
Downsizing	Reducing the number of positions within an organization; normally done to reduce organizational costs and often accompanied by changes in job design to enhance the productivity of the remaining staff
Organizational theory	Science of understanding why and how people organize into work groups and how these work groups function
Virtual organization	A group of people working together to accomplish shared goals but without coming together in the same physical location; most often done through electronic linkages, such as electronic mail, participation in a single computer local or wide area network, Web sites, and teleconferencing

personal lives. These problems have led to discussions by clinicians and policymakers about ways to promote seamless care and integrate services. Organizational theory explains why some strategies for service integration work better than others and under what circumstances they are likely to work best.

Another trend that has developed as one way of containing costs is organizational restructuring. This may involve downsizing, or reducing the size of the work force. Sometimes restructuring involves eliminating a formal department, such as the department of nursing. Organizational theory helps predict what type of structures will be most effective in different situations.

Organizational theory helps to explain not only which lines of communication might be most effective, but also how decision making might be handled, how formal rules for working together should be (e.g., the extent to which people should rely on written policies and procedures), and what the relationships are between the ways groups are organized (structure) and the ways people work together (process) with organizational outcomes. Organizational outcomes are broader than individual patient outcomes and include those things that

are important to stakeholders in an organization (Yuchtman & Seashore, 1967).

Health, social service, and financial organizations work together in a variety of ways. Sometimes they simply refer patients to each other and pay bills submitted on patients' behalf. Sometimes organizations enter into formal agreements to co-sponsor various types of programs, and other times they enter into contracts to provide certain services or personnel to one another in exchange for compensation. An example of this occurs when a temporary personnel agency supplies personnel for a hospital. Increasingly, hospitals and physicians are entering into contractual agreements that make it possible for them to jointly control insurance payments (Riley, 1994). This creates a situation advantageous in local markets heavily saturated by managed care organizations (MCOs) for two reasons. First, it gives these two large provider groups more control over financial and administrative decisions. Second, integration between clinical and administrative structures is thought to foster alignment between providers and payers, leading to increased efficiency and effectiveness. These kinds of arrangements are called *physician-hospital organizations (PHOs)* (Riley, 1994).

Key terms	
Term	**Definition**
Restructuring	Making decisions about new ways in which people will work together to accomplish organizational goals; one of the early outcomes of restructuring is development of a new organizational chart; however, this is not as important as the new working relationships themselves; the organizational chart is simply a drawing that represents the final decisions about new patterns of working relationships
Stakeholders	Persons who stand to gain or lose from organizational activities; may include patients, employees, stockholders in for-profit organizations, community members, and payers

At the community level, some organizations join together to provide more seamless care for patients. This may be done by one organization acquiring others or by contractual arrangements in which all parties agree to work together. Finally, the way work is organized within single agencies and across multiple agencies influences how changes are implemented and how successful changes spread from one place to another. This has come to be known as *diffusion of innovation* (Rogers, 1983) and can be helped or hindered by organizational arrangements.

Organizational theories help explain the working relationships within and between orga-

nizations. Organizational theories help predict which relational patterns will lead to certain outcomes under particular circumstances. Organizational design, functioning, and management are important because they either facilitate or impede caregiving.

■ ORGANIZATIONAL THEORIES AND CORE CONCEPTS

Organizational theory can be analyzed at four levels (Figure 4-2). First, work is organized at the individual level by both the way a job is designed and the way that individual sequences tasks and manages time. Second, groups of indi-

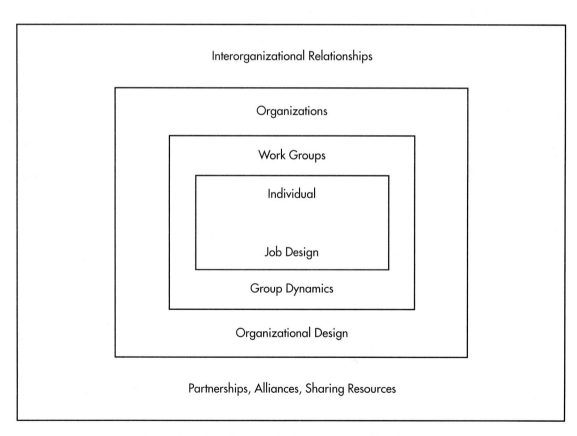

Figure 4-2 ■ Levels of analysis in organizational theory.

viduals organize their work together, either on a relatively long-term basis, such as on a nursing unit, or on a temporary basis, such as a community coalition established to work on a specific problem. Third, organizations are arranged, or designed, in terms of reporting relationships, policies, and procedures. Reporting relationships are formalized, or written, as organizational charts, which are drawings that depict reporting relationships. Policies represent decisions about the nature of work (i.e., what is appropriate, when it will be done, and by whom). Procedures are step-by-step instructions for accomplishing tasks.

Although organizational design refers to formal decisions about how organizations will function, every organization has a parallel informal organizational structure that is very real. The informal structure includes the actual communication patterns and the day-to-day ways of working. Finally, at a broader level, groups of organizations within a single community may work together, such as when health and social service agencies refer patients to one another.

Key terms

Term	Definition
Policies	Decisions about what kinds of activities are appropriate and when, how, and by whom those activities will be done; may be formal (written) or informal (unwritten), although those that are written have more legitimacy
Procedures	Specific written instructions about the manner in which particular tasks are to be accomplished

Organizations spread across a wide geographic area also may work together, such as when hospitals join together in purchasing consortia to enable them to negotiate favorable prices with suppliers of medical equipment or pharmaceuticals.

Prominent Organizational Theories

The primary organizational theories under discussion by scholars in the field today that are related to organizational structure, functioning, and outcomes are (1) structural contingency theory, (2) resource dependence theory, (3) institutional theory, (4) population ecology, and (5) transaction cost economics. These theories, the scholars originally most responsible for their development, the areas emphasized by the theories, and the major propositions of each theory are outlined in Table 4-1. Each theory offers a different perspective on organizational life and differing recommendations for action.

One of the oldest organizational theories is structural contingency theory. This theory was originally proposed by Burns and Stalker (1961), who noted that organizations seemed to be structured in distinct ways and the outcomes of these structures varied by the nature of the work people were doing. They observed that some organizations were very bureaucratic. Bureaucracy simply means that an organization has many rules and procedures, clear lines of authority, and specialized jobs and departments. Although bureaucracies are often criticized for creating barriers to work, Burns and Stalker suggested that bureaucratic structures were effective in situations where the work was routine and jobs were designed in a way that workers had little need to make multiple, complex decisions. These types of structures (called *mechanistic*) seemed to work well when workers were not highly skilled and did not have a high level of education.

Burns and Stalker noted that other organizations operated in more fluid ways, with few

T A B L E 4 - 1

Overview of Organizational Theories

Theory	Primary Authors	Area of Emphasis	Major Propositions
Structural contingency theory	Thompson (1967)	Organizational structure	There is no "best" organizational structure. The situation itself helps determine whether more or less centralized decision making will work best. Factors such as the type of work, the level of worker preparation, the size of the organization, and the nature of the environment all interact to determine which type of structure will be optimal. This theory emphasizes the impact of the external environment on how organizations are set up and how they should function. It also emphasizes the nature of the people working in the organization and the work in which they are engaged.
Resource dependence theory	Pfeffer and Salancik (1978)	Relationships between organizations	Organizations gain or lose power in relation to other organizations based on the resources they have and those they need. If an organization needs resources that another organization has, the first has less power and will behave in ways that will enable it to gain power. This theory emphasizes political processes and focuses attention on the impact that political processes have on organizational decision making.
Transaction cost economics	Williamson (1975, 1986)	Relationship between parties involved in an exchange of valued resources	Organizational life is essentially a series of transactions between parties exchanging valued resources. A variety of factors influence the motivations that underlie the ways in which the parties behave. This theory emphasizes the exchanges that occur between parties, so it focuses not only on the interrelationships, but also on the goals and motivations of each actor. It helps to explain why aligning incentives with goals is so important, since the theory proposes that organizations act based on their own self-interest.

Continued

T A B L E 4 - 1

Overview of Organizational Theories—cont'd

Theory	Primary Authors	Area of Emphasis	Major Propositions
Institutional theory	DiMaggio and Powell (1983); Scott (1987)	Prevailing norms, values, and beliefs	Organizational structure, functioning, and preferred outcomes are more heavily influenced by prevailing norms, values, and beliefs than by perfectly rational processes. Factors such as desires to imitate other organizations believed to be good ones, to be seen as legitimate by more powerful actors, and to adhere to regulations and avoid sanctions all determine how organizations will actually behave. This theory emphasizes social and psychologic processes.
Population ecology	Hannan and Freeman (1977, 1984)	Systems (populations) of organizations	This theory proposes that organizational systems behave much like living systems, with those that are most well suited to the environment surviving. The theory focuses on the behavior of entire populations or organizations and how segments of an industry adapt to changing environmental demands. It has been criticized for suggesting that actions of individual managers and leaders matter little in the long-term survival of a population of organizations. Population ecology emphasizes an examination of change at the systems level and encourages "big picture" thinking.

written policies and procedures. Professionals, researchers, and artists seemed to work best in these situations. The work in these environments was not routine and demanded ongoing decision making and a certain amount of background education for workers to be both comfortable with and effective in making decisions about novel and individualized situations. Burns and Stalker referred to this type of structure as *organic.* The important feature of their work was their observation that the "best" organizational structure was one that took into account certain features of the situation, such as the nature of the work and the level and type of preparation people had for that work.

Thompson (1967) expanded this idea and theorized that the best structure depended on the situation. This came to be known formally as *structural contingency theory.* Although frustrating for managers, since it offered no advice for any one best way to organize, it did focus attention on analyzing the nature of the situation and led to further understanding of the factors that needed to be taken into account when reorganizing. For example, both the size of the organization and the nature of the external environment are critical factors in determining an optimal structure. Larger organizations often must rely on formalized policies and procedures, as well as clearly delineated lines of authority, to avoid chaos. Organizations in rapidly changing industries function more effectively with more fluid, loosely structured arrangements because they need to be able to respond to changes in the environment rapidly and decisively. This presents a paradox in health care, because the pace of mergers and acquisitions has led to larger organizations, while the sociopolitical and economic environment is extremely dynamic (hyperturbulent).

Resource dependence theory is a political theory that helps explain power relationships within and between organizations (Pfeffer &

Key terms	
Term	**Definition**
Mergers	Two or more organizations joining together in a single new organization
Acquisitions	One organization buying another, with the acquired organization no longer carrying its original identity
Bureaucracy	Organization with rules, procedures, clear lines of authority, specialized jobs, and defined units (e.g., departments)

Salancik, 1978). According to this theory, much of human behavior in organizations can be explained by the motivation to acquire those resources necessary to achieve the organization's goals. Those organizations or departments that have resources desired by others (e.g., money, personnel, space, equipment, prestige) have more power than others because they can give or withhold their resources from others. This theory explains the source of some administrative power, because organizational administrators typically make final budgetary decisions. It helps explain why third-party payers in health care have gained so much decision-making power in recent years, since those groups are the largest source of reimbursement for health care providers. Resource dependence theory focuses on the relationships among departments and organizations and not simply on how a single entity is structured.

Another theory that focuses on relationships is *transaction cost economics,* or *organizational economics* (Williamson, 1975, 1986). According to this theory, organizations arise based on characteristics of the exchange relationships between two parties. The key characteristics that determine organizational form are (1) uncertainty of the extent of future demand for a service, 2) the expected frequency of future transactions, and (3) interchangeability of suppliers of needed services (Renshaw et al., 1990). If future demand for a service is not expected to be high, the exchange is expected to occur only once or sporadically, and the service can be purchased from one of many different suppliers, it is likely to be most efficient to buy that service. This is referred to as the *market form of governance* (or *organization*) (Williamson, 1975, 1986). On the other hand, if future demand for a service is expected to be relatively high, the need to buy the service will occur frequently, and it matters a great deal that the service be purchased from a party with considerable specialized knowledge and skills, the most efficient form of organization is to own the service. These choices are often referred to as *make-or-buy decisions* or *outsourcing*.

Many organizations have made decisions to buy, or contract for, services that in the past were provided by the organization itself. For example, it is not uncommon for a hospital to contract with vendors to operate the hospital food service rather than the hospital employing its own dietary department. It is also becoming common for home health agencies to employ nurses on a contractual basis, in which the nurses are essentially independent contractors with access to the agency's patients, records, and administrative support. Sometimes make-or-buy decisions lead to creative forms of providing service, but in other instances, they may lead to unexpected and unwanted outcomes. For example, if home health nurses on contract are paid on a per-visit basis, they may have incentives to make high numbers of visits, potentially leading to a reduction in quality of care.

However, make-or-buy decisions do raise interesting questions about new ways of providing service. Would it be advantageous for an independent nursing group to contract with a hospital or nursing home to staff the agency, rather than the nursing staff being employees of the agency? These types of decisions also create new ways of thinking about careers. Nurses may increasingly become entrepreneurs responsible for marketing their own skills and moving from one professional opportunity to another, as opposed to being employees of a single large organization for many years.

Institutional theory emphasizes the role that values, beliefs, and norms play in organizational life. This theory has it roots in sociology and has been widely used in helping understand organizational life in health care agencies (Scott & Backman, 1990). Because professionals adhere to standards of practice that are broader than just those requirements of the agencies with whom they work and because they have ethical codes of conduct that again transcend any single health care agency, the behaviors of groups of professionals within organizations do not reflect the policies and procedures of just those organizations. Professionals' behavior is heavily influenced by the norms, values, and belief systems of their own professions and is also likely to be influenced by the organizational cultures within which the professionals work. Thus it is necessary to understand these conflicting pressures to have a more complete picture of why health care organizations (HCOs) function as they do.

For example, the growth of managed care led to the institution of "gag rules" in some HCOs, which prohibited health care professionals (primarily physicians) from telling patients about all possible options for treatment. This occurred because not all MCOs cover payment for all forms of care. However, this posed a serious ethical problem for health care professionals because it conflicted with standards of practice that provide for fully informed decision making by patients. Ultimately, the courts decided this was not a legal practice, but not until after great organizational turmoil occurred.

Institutional theory also explains that organizational choices are responses to several different types of pressures: coercive pressures, mimetic pressures, and normative pressures. Coercive pressures are manifested by the need to conform to externally imposed rules and regulations. Examples include accreditation and certification requirements and legal requirements. Adhering to these pressures seems perfectly rational, but they often cause frustration within organizations.

Mimetic pressures originate when organizations imitate other organizations. Especially during times of uncertainty, organizations often adopt successful practices of others (DiMaggio & Powell, 1983). Adoption of what are thought to be best practices is efficient and enhances the perceived legitimacy, or appropriateness, of the organizations (Meyer & Rowan, 1977). Being viewed as legitimate by others is a helpful strategy for organizations that may have some difficulty clearly demonstrating goal attainment or in situations where goals are multidimensional, such as in health care (Provan & Milward, 1991). Mimetic pressures lead to what is referred to as *institutional isomorphism* (DiMaggio & Powell, 1983), in which organizations within a particular service sector come to look increasingly alike. Isomorphic tendencies create stability within a hyperturbulent environment, but they also create inertia and can interfere with making needed changes (Jepperson, 1991). Understanding the impact of mimetic pressures can help nurses know when to question certain taken-for-granted ways of working and propose innovative approaches to health care.

Normative pressures arise from professional standards of practice, codes of conduct, and belief systems. Norms are transmitted through professional education and professional organizations and are enforced through licensing and certification policies. Norms and professional belief systems transcend the values and culture of individual organizations themselves. The pervasive influence of professional norms creates interesting challenges for HCOs because of the impact of many different professional groups being involved in providing care. Although all health care professionals share certain values, differences in world views can influence how each defines problems, priorities, and appropri-

Key terms	
Term	**Definition**
Coercive pressures	The need to conform to a specific way of doing things is imposed by external rules and regulations
Mimetic pressures	Occur when an organization tries to be like or mimic some other organization
Normative pressures	Exerted on an organization by professional standards of practice, codes of conduct, or professional belief systems
Hyperturbulent environment	One in which the rate of change is exceedingly fast
Environmental munificence	The extent to which the environment contains the resources necessary for organizational survival and the amount of demand for the products or services of the organizations within a particular niche

ate interventions. For example, physicians may define problems in terms of curing patients' illnesses, whereas nurses may define problems in terms of helping patients promote health and manage health problems. These seemingly subtle variations can lead to conflicts within HCOs, or if the caregivers work collaboratively, their unique focus can provide a more comprehensive picture of health services.

Population ecology is a theory about organizational change and survival within a population of similar organizations. According to population ecologists (Hannan & Freeman, 1977, 1984), all organizations exist within a niche, or a segment of a market. The environment holds a finite number of resources for all organizations within a particular niche. The challenge for each organization is to compete successfully for a share of the resources that it needs to survive. Examples of important resources include funding streams, patients, and talented personnel.

Population ecology theorists state that environmental characteristics are the most important variables determining organizational survival; that is, organizations that effectively adapt to environmental constraints and demands are the most likely to survive. Characteristics of the environment that influence organizational choices and survival are munificence, uncertainty, and competition.

Environmental munificence is the extent to which the environment contains the resources necessary for organizational survival and the amount of demand for the products or services of those organizations within a particular niche (Renshaw et al., 1990). Uncertainty refers to the ability to forecast changes in resource availability and demand, as well as the amount of control organizations have over the environment. Finally, competition describes the behavior of organizations within a particular niche as they attempt to gain the share of environmental resources they believe to be necessary for survival.

Organizational behavior can focus on either gaining first-mover advantages or winning patients through low prices (Renshaw et al., 1990). Those organizations that adopt a first-mover strategy choose to compete by being the originators or early adopters of innovations. By comparison, those who compete based on low price tend to wait until innovations have become well established and then modify services to be as efficient as possible.

Adaptation suggests that organizations must change over time. However, inertial forces counteract organizations' efforts to change. Examples of these inertial forces include the institutional pressures previously described and, ultimately, the policies and procedures within organizations themselves. Another important inertial force is what is referred to as *bounded rationality* (March & Simon, 1958), which is the difficulty people have in comprehending all the demands in a complex, hyperturbulent, and information-rich environment. Population ecology helps explain and predict the circumstances under which organizations are likely to change successfully. The two important aspects of this theory are the emphases it places on organizational change (including entry into a new market niche, transformation over time, and exit from a particular niche) and on entire systems of organizations. Professional nurses should consider these factors when developing clinical innovations.

Key Organizational Concepts

Certain concepts are basic to an understanding of organizational theories. Table 4-2 outlines these. The first task is to distinguish *differentiation* and *integration*. Differentiation refers to the extent to which an organization specializes in some way, whether in terms of the market it serves (i.e., target population) or the product or service it provides. For example, an HCO that specializes in home infusion therapy for a five-

TABLE 4 - 2

Key Concepts in Organizational Theories

Concept	Primary Authors	What It Means	Relevance in Health Care Today
Differentiation versus integration	Lawrence and Lorsch (1967)	Organizations have to manage needs to both specialize (or differentiate) and coordinate (or integrate) their activities. These needs are somewhat conflicting, so organizations face special challenges with managing to accomplish both differentiation and integration effectively.	One of the biggest challenges in health care today is determining when and how specialized care should be delivered and when and how health care delivery should be coordinated.
Tight versus loose coupling	Weick (1976)	Tight coupling occurs when coordination and communication are very closely connected across organizational units or across organizations themselves. Loose coupling indicates that fewer checks and balances exist, and fewer required communications must occur. This is similar to the differences between efficiency and redundancy. In a very efficient situation, little duplication of services will exist. Patients will be referred to services from a single provider who specializes in that service.	When care is "managed," the implication is that the system is tightly coupled. More parties must agree to the care that is planned, and information must flow across more parties. Loose coupling gives more decision-making autonomy to patients, families, and providers. Very tightly coupled health care markets can be difficult for vulnerable populations to navigate. It may be simpler for people with complex health and socioeconomic problems to have multiple entry points into care.
Monopolies, oligopolies, monopsonies	Economic theory	Monopolies occur when there is only one viable supplier of a particular good or service in a local market. Oligopolies refer to situations in which two or three suppliers exist within a particular market. Consumers lose decision-making power in monopolistic and oligopolistic markets. Monopsonies are situations in which a single buyer dominates the marketplace. This places pressure on suppliers of goods and services to comply with the wishes of the buyer.	The more a single provider of services acquires other providers, the more a local market will tend toward monopolistic or oligopolistic features. Also, when employers offer only one or two health plan choices within their benefit packages, the more the consumer will experience the market as monopolistic or oligopolistic. Large managed care organizations and large employer groups can create situations that function like monopsonies and place pressure on clinicians to practice in ways desired by the purchaser.

county area is highly differentiated in terms of both market and service. Integration refers to the degree to which specialized services or functions are coordinated across specialty lines. An example of a highly integrated health care agency is a community health center that provides a broad array of services on-site and coordinates those services through interdisciplinary planning.

Lawrence and Lorsch (1967) were the first organizational scientists to say that achieving the right balance between differentiation and integration was a key challenge for organizations. Differentiation and integration require different and sometimes conflicting skills. Integration is more easily achieved with the mindset of a generalist, whereas differentiation benefits from an emphasis on specialization. Primary health care takes a more integrated approach and works well for people with common health problems. However, people with complex, less common problems are thought to have better outcomes when cared for by specialists. Disabled and some chronically ill individuals often require specialty care, although they frequently need care provided by many different agencies and

specialists. Their care needs to be both differentiated and integrated at the same time.

A national study of integrated delivery systems (Shortell et al., 1994) determined that achieving the appropriate blend of differentiation and integration is the key challenge in today's health care environment. Shortell and his colleagues (1994, p. 49) say the following:

> The differentiation challenge involves being able to offer or arrange to offer the full continuum of care at geographically accessible locations throughout a given market to capture a sufficient number of enrollees to make the system viable. The integration challenge lies in coordinating the continuum of care across the relevant market area of interest. At the heart of this process is the ability to clinically integrate services in local markets. Providers acting alone or in loose affiliation will have great difficulty providing and coordinating the full continuum of care to compete effectively in the new world of managed care economics. This need to simultaneously differentiate and integrate represents the internal logic of system development in the new managed care economy.

Simultaneously differentiating and integrating services requires decisions about how tightly connected services should be. This is referred to in the organizational literature as *tight versus loose coupling* (Weick, 1976). An example of tightly coupled services occurs in a large organization that owns primary care, acute care, and home health care services. If such an organization develops policies and procedures that make it possible for a nurse to see his or her patients in each of those areas, have access to patient charts, make referrals, and coordinate services, the organization is tightly coupled. If the organization has uniform patient records and particularly if those records are electronic, it is even more tightly coupled.

Tight coupling potentially can create a stronger sense of seamlessness for patients.

Key terms	
Term	**Definition**
Differentiation	The extent to which an organization specializes in some way, whether in terms of the market it serves (i.e., target population) or the product or service it provides
Integration	The degree to which specialized services or functions are coordinated across specialty lines

However, very tightly coupled organizations also have high potential for serious problems, because a problem in one part of the system is likely to influence other parts of the system with which it is tightly linked. For example, if a health care agency uses computerized patient records and the computer malfunctions, no one in the system will have access to patient information unless a backup plan is in place.

Loose coupling refers to a situation in which individual parts of a system function more independently. Although the autonomy available in such a situation may be appealing to staff, it may not leave patients with a sense of coordination. Benefits of loose coupling, however, are not only that individual system components can continue functioning when problems arise in other components, but also that decisions can be made more quickly and innovations developed and implemented more quickly. The challenge today is to determine the right blend of tight versus loose coupling in different situations.

As discussed in Chapter 3, several key economic concepts are important to understanding how health care is organized. Those HCOs that vertically integrate by merging with or acquiring other HCOs create market consolidation by reducing the numbers of separately owned organizations within a local area. Complete market consolidation (i.e., where one entity owns all HCOs within an area) represents a *monopoly* market. It is unlikely that many, if any, actual monopolies exist within the United States because of constraints imposed by antitrust law. The Sherman Antitrust Act prohibits development of monopolies because of the adverse impact monopolies can have on consumers and other suppliers of a particular good or service.

Problems associated with monopolies include limitations on consumer choice of providers and services, the potential for higher prices

than would be found in a competitive market, and the potential for lower levels of service and clinical quality because of the lack of choice for another provider. As the health care system changes, nurses should be aware of the problems that can result from development of monopoly markets. Although antitrust law offers some protection, ongoing development of integrated delivery systems has led to some reinterpretation of antitrust law in some areas and to exemptions from certain provisions in others. This can have beneficial effects in terms of creating more seamless experience for health care for consumers, but nurses engaged in local or state level policy debates should always be aware of the disadvantages associated with complete market consolidation.

Oligopolies are more common in local health care markets. An *oligopoly* is present when only a few major providers exist within a local area. Oligopolies represent heavy market consolidation but not the complete consolidation of a monopolistic situation. Oligopolistic markets can result in the same problems as with monopolistic markets, although this is less likely. More likely is the generation of efficiencies, such as economies of scale and development of clinical and service delivery expertise.

The term *economies of scale* means that organizations are large enough that they can negotiate favorable discounts with suppliers (e.g., of durable medical equipment) and that the average cost of providing services is lower than for smaller providers. For example, if it costs $1,000,000 to open a new health care facility, providing service to 1000 patients results in an average cost per patient of $1000. On the other hand, if that same facility serves 10,000 patients, the average cost per patient decreases to $100. Assuming that adequate staff and facilities are available, serving 10,000 patients rather than 1000 will also give clinical and administrative staff more experience and presum-

Key terms	
Term	**Definition**
Monopoly	Complete market con-solidation where one vendor has all stores or organizations in an area
Oligopoly	A limited number of providers in an area offer products or services
Monopsony	A single purchaser of goods or services exists within a market
Economics of scale	An organization is suffi-ciently large to nego-tiate favorable prices or contracts

ably will result in greater expertise and efficiency in operations.

Finally, *monopsony* refers to a situation in which a single purchaser of goods or services exists within a market. Large MCOs, other private and public third-party payers (e.g., Medicare, Medicaid, large commercial insurance companies), and large employers can function like monopsonies. In a monopsony, buyers of services are so large that they have increased bargaining power over prices and can effectively determine what they will and will not pay for. Monopsony power is becoming increasingly evident in health care as third-party payers insist on certain limits on charges and as they establish precertification and utilization review processes for their enrollees. An example of insisting on limits on charges occurs when a public payer, such as Medicare or Medicaid, regulates payment of no more than 80% of prior rates. This forces HCOs to do one of two things. Organizations can accept a lower excess of revenues

over expenses, which means fewer dollars will be available for ongoing clinical and organizational improvements, such as developing new services, upgrading buildings, or raising staff salaries. The other response is to reduce expenses. Because the majority of expenses in HCOs are in staff salaries, this often means redesigning jobs, offering early retirement options, layoffs, or limiting new hiring.

What do these macrolevel economic influences on organizational design have to do with clinical nursing? These economic pressures are important for nurses to understand because the "trickle down" effect occurs in the delivery of clinical services. Nurses need to understand the problems so they can help propose viable solutions. It is not enough to argue that reduction of nursing positions in hospitals has a negative impact on patient care. If the hospital goes bankrupt and closes, the impact on patient care is devastating. It is critical for nurses to understand the pressures and propose feasible alternatives to manage the impact of economic changes on organizations. To do so, nurses should understand how health care is currently organized.

■ HOW IS HEALTH CARE ORGANIZED TODAY?

Most organized health care in the United States in the past has been provided by single agencies, typically structured to provide a particular set of health services, such as by a community hospital with the mission to provide acute care services or a primary care clinic designed to provide strictly primary care services with referrals for secondary or tertiary care. These single mission agencies worked with other agencies, either by making referrals or by sitting on joint health planning bodies. However, these relationships were typically voluntary in nature and comprised what has been called a *service implementation network* (Provan & Milward, 1995). More frequently now, small agencies are either merging with others or being acquired by larger agencies, or working together in a myriad of formal and informal ways. What follows is a description of how single agencies are organized internally followed by an explanation of how current interorganizational relationships are configured.

Forms of Internal Organizational Structure

Functional Structure Functional structure refers to organizing around clinical departmental lines. This way of thinking about structure originated in businesses organized around various professional functions, such as marketing, accounting, and human resources. In health care, organizations with functional structures are likely to have departments of nursing, physical therapy, respiratory therapy, and other disciplines focused on the professionals themselves. Figure 4-3 illustrates a simple functional structure in a hospital.

These structures have the advantage of giving professionals a clear voice in the delivery of services through their department heads. This can add strength to clinical service delivery, since the departments have a straightforward way of contributing their knowledge about best practices in their fields to program and service decisions. The disadvantage is a tendency to become embroiled in "turf" issues, limited interdisciplinary decision making, and reduced programmatic flexibility. Chapter 8 describes typical lines of communication among staff on the same unit and also between units.

Product Line Structure Product line structures refer to organizing around specific products. In some cases, such structures are called *service line structures* to better reflect the fact that HCOs most often focus on providing services rather than products. Of course, pharmaceutical and biotechnology companies are exceptions, since they do produce goods. Product

line structures are often organized around sets of similar diagnosis-related groups (DRGs) and focus on provision of care throughout a continuum for those groups of patients. Figure 4-4 depicts a product line structure.

One example of this type of product line is cardiovascular services, linking all clinicians involved in providing care for patients with cardiac diagnoses. Such a structure incorporates outpatient, inpatient, and rehabilitative care for people with cardiac problems. Another example, organized around gender rather than diagnosis, is a womens' health product line. This type of product line might include all clinical services provided to women older than 18 years, such as reproductive services, perimenopausal services, cardiovascular services focusing on womens' unique needs (e.g., clinical decisions about the physiologic and emotional aspects of hormone replacement therapy after menopause), and caregiver issues for young adult, middle-age, and older women.

Product line structures have the advantage of focusing attention on the needs and outcomes of a particular target population. The manager of a product line can be any type of clinician or a health administrator. The disadvantage of such systems is that clinical specialty expertise may be lost with the dissolution of clinical departments, such as nursing, physical therapy, and pharmacy.

Matrix Structure A matrix structure combines the clinical expertise facilitated by the functional structure with the patient-centered coordination fostered by product line structures. With this arrangement, employees report both to a director in the area of their professional education (e.g., the director of nursing services) and to the manager of the product line within which they work. Such a structure is depicted in Figure 4-5. Matrix structures require a great deal of communication to be effective, and they require that employees report to dual lines

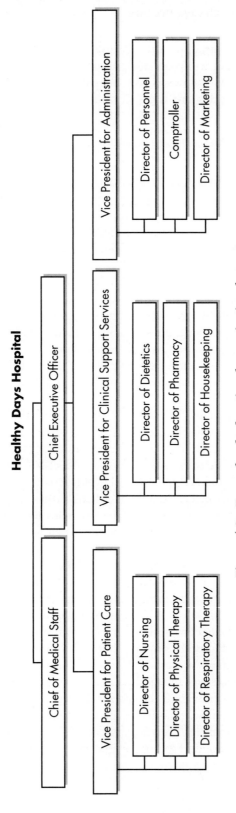

Figure 4-3 ■ Example of a functional organizational structure.

Healthy Days Health System

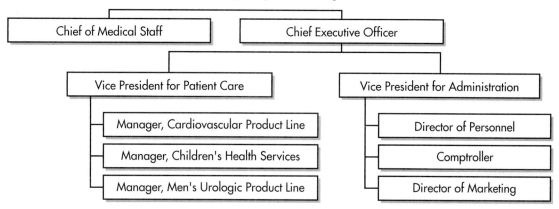

Figure 4-4 ■ **Example of a product line organizational structure.**

Healthy Days Hospital and Health Care Systems

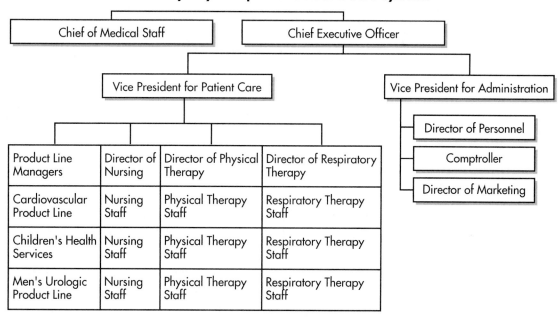

Figure 4-5 ■ **Example of a matrix organizational structure.**

of authority. The time involved in communication makes matrix structures costly, and they are normally adopted only in large, complex organizations.

Professional Practice Models Professional practice models are participatory structures in which clinicians share governance responsibilities with administrators. This approach to organizational structure is increasing in popularity because it builds on the accountability that clinicians are prepared to assume for their practices. Professionals prefer a large amount of decision-making autonomy and often resent being required to go through multiple lines of authority to initiate new ideas.

Professional practice models that formalize shared governance reduce these requirements but demand that professionals take time for issues they may not have had to deal with. Self-scheduling is one example of a task that employees often take on in shared governance systems that they may not have dealt with in other systems. Sometimes employees are not prepared for, or comfortable with, the time involved and the difficulties inherent in making decisions such as these.

Four common shared governance models are the congressional, unit-based, administrative, and councilor models (Yanko et al., 1995; Figure 4-6). These models vary in terms of whether they are used throughout the organization or within single departments and the nature of the coordinating mechanisms that are present.

Forms of Interorganizational Relationships

Vertical Integration In the United States, vertical integration refers to a single organization owning all types of health services necessary along a continuum. Patients of such organizations should then have access to services from primary care to hospital care to nursing home and home health care. The key is a single owner of all such services. Large, vertically integrated organizations enjoy "economies of scope," which means that such organizations can offer a wide range of different types of health services. The larger they are, the more likely they are to also enjoy "economies of scale," which means they can accomplish certain activities less expensively than smaller organizations.

CONGRESSIONAL	ADMINISTRATIVE
• All staff belong to congress. • Structure is similar to federal government. • Committees submit work to cabinet for action.	• Practice and management structures exist. • Forum integrates work of councils. • Councils submit work to executive council for decisions.
UNIT-BASED	COUNCILOR
• Each unit establishes its own system. • Multiple models may exist within one institution. • There are no department-wide coordinating activities.	• Coordinating council coordinates activities on departmental level. • Unit councils reflect department councils. • Staff nurses are accountable for clinical decision making.

Figure 4-6 ■ **Types of shared governance models.** (From Rowland, H.S., & Rowland, B.L. [1997]. *Nursing administration handbook* [4th ed., p. 121]. Gaithersburg, Md.: Aspen.)

For example, large organizations can negotiate for better prices from vendors of durable medical equipment and pharmaceuticals. A disadvantage to vertical integration occurs when such organizations become so large that smaller organizations find it difficult to compete in a local market. This can lead to monopoly or oligopoly conditions and reduce the level of consumer choice with respect to service type and quality and health care providers.

There is more than one way to conceptualize vertical integration. A recent World Health Organization (WHO) report (1996) defined vertical integration as programs designed around single disease categories. Similarly, the public health system in the United States has been and still is organized around categoric health programs in some areas.

Horizontal Integration   Horizontal integration refers to clusters of the same types of organizations being owned by a single entity. A hospital company that owns multiple hospitals in one or more regions of the United States is an example of horizontal integration. Similarly, a company that owns nursing homes is horizontally integrated. These types of companies have the advantage of developing expertise with a particular health service, such as acute or long-term care. They can develop efficiencies because they specialize in delivering certain services. Horizontally integrated companies always have the potential for economies of scale, because they use many of the same raw materials repeatedly and can negotiate for discounts from suppliers as a result. Again, the larger the organization, the more likely it is to create monopoly or oligopoly conditions.

Strategic Alliances   Strategic alliances give organizations greater economies of scale, or the ability to negotiate for lower prices because of the buying power of the purchasing organization. Alliances make it possible for individual organizations to retain their autonomy and indi-vidual ownership. Purchasing alliances or consortia (Brown, 1996) allow many organizations to come together under one umbrella group for the purpose of making bulk purchases. As members of a purchasing group, participants can often negotiate lower prices for health care equipment and supplies and can then pass these savings on to purchasers of health care, such as insurance companies, self-insured employer groups, and Medicare and Medicaid.

Strategic alliances are linkages between autonomous organizations that foster achievement of critical organizational goals (Lazo-Miller & D'Andrea, 1996). These alliances give participating organizations opportunities to garner additional resources, reduce costs, and increase their political and economic power. Although the exact nature of strategic alliances can vary from subcontracting for services or staff, to joint programs and services, to more formal partnerships, and ultimately to mergers or acquisitions, they can be characterized in terms of seven dimensions (Leatt & Barnsley, 1994):

1. They vary in the extent of coordination required by the connection between the organizations.
2. They may be quite formal, requiring written contracts, or quite informal, based on trust.
3. These interorganizational relationships differ in the amount of risk assumed by the parties. Risk may be financial, political, and reputational.
4. They involve varying levels of commitment by the participating organizations, including commitment of "money, personnel, space, and time" (Leatt & Barnsley, 1994, p. 764). These alliances are more likely to be successful when complementary resources are committed by participating groups.
5. Comparability of commitments makes a difference in the interorganizational dynamics. Those situations in which one partner in-

vests significantly more than others can lead to imbalances of power and expectations.

6. They vary in the extent to which they are central to the participating organizations' missions.

7. Alliances vary in the degree of uncertainty of the anticipated outcomes, with greater uncertainty associated with greater risk (Leatt & Barnsley, 1994).

Integrated Delivery Systems Integrated delivery systems are those local sets of organizations that choose to work together in systematic ways to ensure that patients receive a full continuum of services and that patients experience service delivery as seamless. This refers not only to system integration, but also to clinical integration. Integrated delivery systems represent different strategies for overcoming the fragmentation that is occurring in the U.S. health care system without resorting to single ownership of all health services by one organization. Integrated delivery systems at their best align financial and administrative incentives with clinical care delivery goals. For example, rewarding cli-nicians for seeing as many patients as possible within a given time period while saying that individualized patient-centered care is the goal of the organization does not represent alignment (i.e., consistency).

A recent report of WHO (1996) argued that integration of social, economic, and health services is necessary to achieve a goal of health for all people. Achievement of this goal will facilitate a higher quality of life through enhanced economic productivity and improved functional status of individuals, families, and communities.

According to this report, integration can be defined in either functional or organizational terms. Defining integration in functional terms refers to "a series of operations concerned in essence with the bringing together of otherwise independent administrative structures, functions, and mental attitudes in such a way as to combine these into a whole" (WHO, 1996, p. 4; WHO, 1965). An organizational definition of integrated health services is "those services necessary for the health protection of a given area and provided under a single administrative unit, or

Key terms	
Term	**Definition**
Strategic alliances	Linkages between autonomous organizations that foster achievement of critical organizational goals (Lazo-Miller & D'Andrea, 1996)
Integrated delivery systems	Local sets of organizations that choose to work together in systematic ways to ensure that patients receive a full continuum of services and that patients experience service delivery as seamless; include both system and clinical integration
Alignment	Making things consistent with one another; when used to describe incentives, it means that the incentives that are present in a system match the requirements of the system
Partnership	One or more organizations working together to achieve a common purpose; that purpose may not necessarily be directly linked to a strategic goal of each partner individually (as with a strategic alliance) but is linked to shared goals.

under several agencies, with proper provision for their coordination" (WHO, 1996, p. 4; WHO, 1954). This definition is one that allows for either vertical or horizontal integration. The key is having some form of coordinating structure in place. A WHO study group defined integration of health services as follows:

> . . . the process of bringing together common functions within and between organizations to solve common problems, developing a commitment to shared vision and goals, and using common technologies and resources to achieve these goals. The aim is to promote primary health care services which are fully integrated under the management of a district health team, led by a district health manager, in order to make the most efficient use of scarce resources (WHO, 1996, p. 4).

The report notes that "integration is not a panacea . . . [but] . . . is a way of optimizing the use of scarce resources and responding more effectively to people's needs. By improving efficiency and effectiveness and with the involvement of education and other social services, integration aims to increase consumer satisfaction with the health services" (p. 4).

Finally, WHO recommends the district health system as the optimal form of integration in most areas. District health systems are focused on local needs and depend on local community members for participation in planning. This is in contrast to "top down" planning methods that rely on administrators, policymakers, and clinicians to determine what is best for a commu-

nity. The concept of district health systems is similar to the local health department in the United States. Because health care in the United States is provided by both public and private agencies, the important part of the WHO recommendation is the concept of local planning that involves partnerships with local agencies, clinicians, and community members.

Community Partnerships Porter-O'Grady (1995) argues that partnership is the key principle for the contemporary health care environment. With organizational structures moving more decision-making authority to the point of service and encouraging more interdisciplinary collaboration, clinicians must work together effectively. As health care moves from institutional facilities, in which health care professionals had a certain amount of authority, to homes, schools, workplaces, and places of worship, where health care professionals have limited (less) authority, stronger partnerships with community members are essential. Further, few organizations currently function independently; most work with others as partners in alliances, joint ventures, and networks. These interorganizational arrangements require stronger collaborative and partnering skills.

At the organizational level, four primary forms of partnership are seen, ranging along a continuum based on the degree of organizational control over administrative decisions (Figure 4-7). At the left side of the continuum, no one organization has complete control over ad-

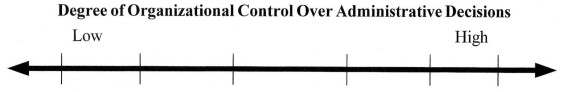

Degree of Organizational Control Over Administrative Decisions

Low   High

Consortia   Shared staff   Joint programs   Strategic alliances   Mergers   Acquisitions

Figure 4-7 ■ Interorganizational relationships and degree of organizational authority.

ministrative decisions, whereas at the right side of the continuum, a single organization has actually purchased another and as a result now has complete authority for administrative decisions. The less authority any one organization has over decision making, the more negotiation and conflict resolution skills become critical to the success of the partnership relationship. For example, in situations in which two or more organizations work together to operate joint programs, negotiations must occur over decisions about the goals of the program, where it will be located, how it will be staffed, how the administrative functions supporting the program will occur, how billing and reimbursement will be handled, and how conflicts will be resolved. These decisions must be made before the program begins and throughout the life of the program as situations change.

■ KEY AREAS OF EMPHASIS IN ORGANIZING NURSING CARE DELIVERY

Population-Based Approaches and Care Management

Traditional methods of organizing nursing care delivery have focused on the site of care rather than on linking systems of care on behalf of patients and families. Team nursing, primary nursing, functional nursing, and modular approaches have all been used within both inpatient and community-based sites. Increasingly, nurses are focusing on population-based approaches to organizing care across a continuum of time and place. They are emphasizing the shared needs of populations of patients while continuing to tailor care to the unique needs of individuals. Organizations form the context for delivery of clinical care but are less likely to be the fulcrum around which nurses organize. Instead, the patient and family are the nexus around which care is organized and the focus is on managing care across sites and over time. This is a more distributive approach,

although it incorporates nursing care of patients during episodes of illness (Walker & Sebastian, 1997). For example, nursing care in an MCO might be focused on the needs of frail, elderly individuals and their families. The nurses involved in such an approach may provide home-based health assessment of the frail, older person and his or her caregiver, support for the family, education about therapeutic and health promotion measures for the older individual and family, and consultation with acute care clinicians when the older individual is hospitalized. In this example, the nurse emphasizes managing care across time and space rather than managing people.

Accountability for Clinical and Fiscal Outcomes

Nurses are held accountable for outcomes of care, including both clinical and fiscal outcomes. Standard nomenclatures are available that describe the problems with which nursing care is designed to deal, interventions, and outcomes (McCloskey & Bulechek, 1994). Organizing care and documenting care using standard nomenclature make it more likely that nurses can determine when their care is cost effective and when alternative approaches might more effectively achieve the same outcomes. It is important for nurses to develop innovative strategies for care delivery that focus on integration and demonstrate the impact new care delivery models have on quality of care, service utilization, and costs.

Nursing care can be organized so it helps patients and families maximize health and experience their care as seamless, with good continuity, comprehensiveness, and minimal duplication of services or information. Integrated community nursing services have been shown to help reduce hospital utilization and costs for high-risk elderly patients (Burns et al., 1996).

■ HOW DOES CHANGE THEORY FACILITATE SMOOTH TRANSITIONS IN HEALTH CARE ORGANIZATION?

Change theory helps explain why and how organizational changes unfold. Theories of organizational change can help to develop strategies to implement changes as effectively as possible with fewer unanticipated results. Unexpected events always occur, of course, but understanding how people respond to change helps plan for smooth organizational transitions. For example, changes in organizational structure should involve much communication throughout the process to minimize anxiety, morale problems, and subtle obstruction of the process. More important, actively soliciting input from organizational participants throughout the process can yield helpful suggestions and insights that may lead to improvements in the original ideas.

The outcomes of organizational changes can include enhanced organizational flexibility and responsiveness to the environment, decisions about programs that should be expanded, reduced, or eliminated to meet current needs, and better match between the organizational mission and capacity with appropriate programming. However, restructuring is sometimes accompanied by psychologic effects on all participants. Survivors of downsizing experience a range of emotions, including guilt, anxiety, and depression. It is important to acknowledge these normal reactions early in the process and plan ways for those remaining on staff to share their feelings and use those emotions to improve the working environment.

The same principles of inclusiveness and broad-based communication and participation apply at the system level. The five-stage model of change shown in Figure 4-8 is one approach for building coalitions of families, educators, and clinicians focused on improving systems of care for children (Melaville et al., 1993). Key el-

ements of this process involve mutual goal setting, building and nurturing trust, and joint evaluation and monitoring. Note that all participants are involved in some way in planning for and managing critical resources, including hiring people and developing the budget.

■ ORGANIZATIONAL INTEGRATION AND VULNERABLE POPULATIONS
Conceptual Model of Interorganizational Collaboration

Polivka (1995) developed a conceptual model of interorganizational collaboration that incorporates elements from structural contingency, resource dependence, transaction cost economics, and institutional theory (Figure 4-9). The model is designed to help community health nurses understand how and why such collaborative relationships function as they do and to help predict strategies that will foster more effective collaboration.

To understand the nature and function of relationships that develop across organizations, the nurse must analyze three sets of characteristics. First, it is important to analyze those environmental factors that create political, social, demographic, and economic pressures for organizations to function in particular ways. Second, the nurse should evaluate situational factors that are related to the organizations themselves, such as their awareness of particular problems and opportunities, their dependence on others for resources such as patients and funding, the extent to which they serve similar patients and have goals similar to those of others, and the extent of agreement across organizations on areas such as goals, tasks, and issues (Polivka, 1995). Finally, it is important to consider the nature of the clinical work being done, such as the breadth of services provided by each agency in the relationship, the complexity of those clinical services, and the degree of unpredictability about the course or outcomes of services. For

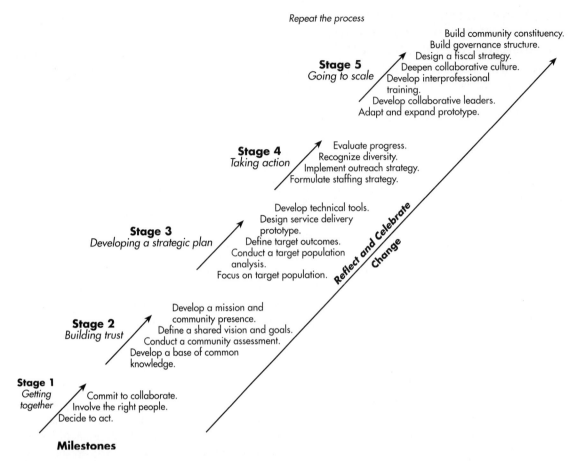

Repeat the process

Stage 5
Going to scale

Build community constituency.
Build governance structure.
Design a fiscal strategy.
Deepen collaborative culture.
Develop interprofessional
    training.
Develop collaborative leaders.
Adapt and expand prototype.

Stage 4
Taking action

Evaluate progress.
Recognize diversity.
Implement outreach strategy.
Formulate staffing strategy.

Stage 3
Developing a strategic plan

Develop technical tools.
Design service delivery
    prototype.
Define target outcomes.
Conduct a target population
    analysis.
Focus on target population.

Reflect and Celebrate Change

Stage 2
Building trust

Develop a mission and
    community presence.
Define a shared vision and goals.
Conduct a community assessment.
Develop a base of common
    knowledge.

Stage 1
*Getting
together*

Commit to collaborate.
Involve the right people.
Decide to act.

Milestones

Figure 4-8 ■ Five-stage process for change. (From Melaville, A.L. et al. [1993]. *Together we can: A guide for crafting a pro-family system of education and human services.* Washington, D.C.: U.S. Government Printing Office.)

many vulnerable patients (those with multiple health and social problems), the complexity of their health and social situations leads to a high level of unpredictability about how their courses of treatment will progress and the level of outcomes they will achieve.

The interorganizational relationships themselves can be characterized in terms of their intensity, degree of formalization (written policies and procedures), the extent and nature of joint decision making, and the structure of the network in which the relationships are embedded. Describing a network of interorganizational relationships is a bit like describing the structure of a single organization. Single organizations have both formal structures, which are written and consciously planned descriptions of decision-making authority, and informal structures, which are the unwritten, but quite real patterns of how decisions are actually made.

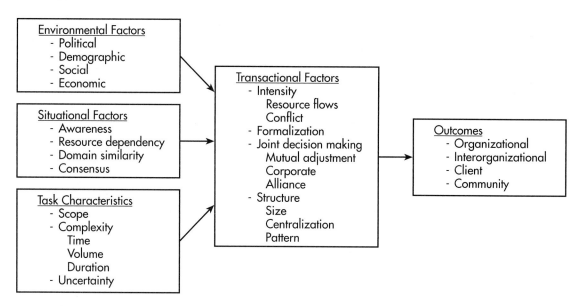

Figure 4-9 ■ **Conceptual framework for community interagency collaboration.** (From Polivka, B.J. [1995]. A conceptual model for community interagency collaboration. *IMAGE: Journal of Nursing Scholarship, 27*[2], 110-115.)

Interorganizational relationships are much the same. Some of these are written and planned, such as collaborative agreements for health programs, whereas others develop informally. For example, if a nurse at the local health department makes referrals to the same person at a community medication program and finds that individual serves the patients well and provides thorough follow-up, those two individuals have effectively developed an interorganizational linkage that is not written anywhere but is nonetheless real and has a positive impact on patient outcomes.

One can often identify which individuals work together regularly and draw a modified sociogram to reflect the structure of the network. Figure 4-10 shows three types of structural arrangements for interorganizational relationships. Dyadic relationships occur between two parties only. The dyadic relationship in Figure

4-10 is undirected. This means that the relationship does not involve one party sending resources or information to the other. For example, two nurses who interact because they are both members of a staff development committee have an undirected relationship. The triadic structure depicted in Figure 4-10 shows three parties, with two of those directing some resource to the third. An example of this type of network structure would be two primary care clinics that direct patient referrals to the same specialty physician group. Note that in this case, the nodes represent organizational groups rather than individuals.

Cliques are special network structures in which each party is linked with every other party in the group. This type of highly integrated structure is likely to lead to a strong sense of shared values, norms, and ways of working together since all parties are connected with all

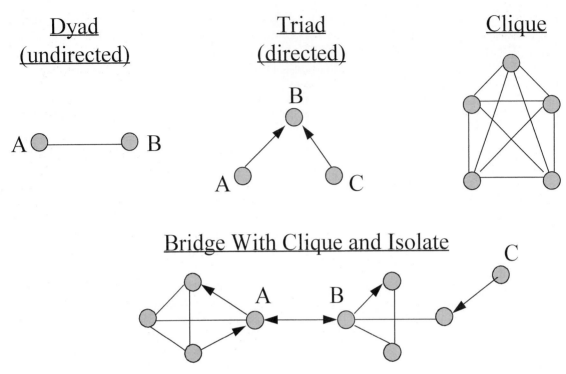

Figure 4-10 ■ Examples of interorganizational network structures. (Data from Scott, J. (1991). *Social network analysis: A handbook.* London: Sage.)

others. Finally, Figure 4-10 also shows a bridging structure with a clique connected with point A and a set of partially connected nodes and one isolated node connected to point B. An example of this type of situation might occur if point A represents a nurse case manager in an MCO who is linking information from his or her organization to the referral source represented by point B. The person represented by point B may be in a social service agency, with point C representing a therapist who provides information to one of the other members of the organization. Figure 4-10 shows how varied interorganizational networks can be and leads the nurse to ask questions about how to most effectively facilitate organizational linkages to help enhance patient and family outcomes.

The last component of Polivka's model is that of the outcomes of interorganizational collaboration. Outcomes occur within four levels: within the organization itself, within the interorganizational network, at the patient level, and at the community level. One important organizational outcome is the impact that such relationships have on the cost of providing care. Interorganizational collaboration has the potential to reduce costs within the organization because it is easier for the organization to focus its efforts on only those services with which it has the greatest expertise and refer patients to organizations with complementary services. However, maintaining interorganizational relationships is time consuming and may actually cost the organization more if attention is not paid to this aspect. Potential outcomes within the network itself include the ability to reduce system-wide costs by a reduction in duplication of services and the potential for more rapid and profound system changes. When organizations collaborate, they are more likely to ask different questions and develop original solutions to problems as multiple perspectives are brought to bear on the issues (Bolland & Wilson, 1994). Patients are more likely to have improved clinical outcomes in situations in which care is coordinated through one central agency (Provan, 1996). Finally, at the community level, well-planned interorganizational cooperation has the potential to lead to improved community health as multiple groups come together to set goals and determine implementation strategies.

Organizational Integrations That Meet the Needs of Vulnerable Populations

Vulnerable populations, such as those with multiple health, economic, or social problems (Aday, 1993; Sebastian, 1996), have a particular stake in the ways in which organizations are configured. The complex health, social, and economic needs of vulnerable groups make it particularly important that services are either provided within a single, comprehensive organization or carefully coordinated across agencies (Provan, 1996). Although providing all services within a single organization may seem like the ideal way to structure services for vulnerable populations, it is both impractical and politically unrealistic in many situations. Further, centralization of services can lead to monopolistic situations with the disadvantages associated with any monopoly. However, patient outcomes do seem to be better when services are coordinated and administered through one lead organization (Provan & Milward, 1995).

Coordination and cooperation between agencies has both benefits and costs (Bolland & Wilson, 1994; Polivka, 1995). These reflect the benefits and costs of tight coupling versus planned redundancy. Deliberate, thoughtful coordination and collaboration generate benefits for patients in terms of a perception of greater seamlessness and reduced service acquisition burden. It is easier for patients with multiple, complex problems to benefit from health and human services if they can devote all their energies to working with health professionals in treating current problems and preventing future ones, rather than having to self-manage multiple agency requirements, payment requirements, and issues such as transportation and multiple clinic appointments. On the other hand, to coordinate services and collaborate effectively, organizations must give up a certain degree of decision-making autonomy and must commit to some level of shared goals. Thus organizations suffer a loss of scarce resources. At a minimum, coordination and collaboration require additional time, and time costs money in staff salaries. More likely, coordination and collaboration also require that organizations give up a certain amount of decision-making flexibility (Morrissey et al., 1985).

At the community level, the most important type of coordination appears to be that which is related directly to the needs of the patient. This has been referred to as *service delivery coordination* (Bolland & Wilson, 1994) and as *clinical integration* (Shortell et al., 1994). Agencies can work together in administrative matters; for example, in health-planning groups and in developing rules and procedures for reimbursement, prior authorization, and joint programs. Such strategies are important but seem to have less impact on patient outcomes than cooperative relationships most directly related to the patients themselves, such as making referrals and sharing clinical information necessary to referral success (Provan & Sebastian, 1998). This underscores the important role nurses play in making service delivery networks truly feel seamless to patients and families and in achieving the best possible clinical outcomes in these networks.

Nurses can manage the health care system in a way that most directly benefits patients themselves through case management. Nursing case management has both patient- and system-oriented goals (Stahl, 1997). Patient-oriented goals relate to meeting patient health needs, ensuring access to appropriate services, and supporting caregivers. System goals relate to coordinating services, ensuring appropriate service utilization, and controlling costs (Stahl, 1997).

Shortell et al. (1994) argue that community assessment and planning health promotion, wellness, and illness prevention programs are critical skills that must be incorporated into integrated delivery systems. Focusing on the health of a local community and not just the enrollees of a particular system better ensures that vulnerable populations will receive the care needed to facilitate good health. However, these areas have traditionally been the responsibility of public health systems. Whether integrated delivery systems adopt a community-focused approach or public health systems are strengthened to focus on core public health functions (i.e., assessment, policy development, assurance; Turnock, 1997) may be a matter of local competence and preference. Regardless, both systems should work together to ensure that care is well coordinated for vulnerable populations while remaining fiscally responsible.

Organizational theory helps explain and predict the patterns of human relationships that will best enable groups of people to work together to accomplish health care goals. Although organizational structure is often thought of simply in terms of an organizational chart, it is far more than that, involving collective decisions about how people will work together, both inside single organizations and in partnership across organizations. Understanding organizational theory can help nurses set a context for clinical services that facilitates the delivery of high-quality services in a fiscally responsible manner and makes it possible to develop and implement clinical innovations in a way that promotes quality of care and job satisfaction.

■ KEY POINTS

- Organizational theories help explain the working relationships within and between organizations. Organizational theories help predict which relational patterns will lead to certain outcomes under particular circumstances. Organizational design, functioning, and management are important because they either facilitate or impede caregiving.

- The most widely used organizational theories are structural contingency theory, resource dependence theory, institutional theory, population ecology, and transaction cost economics. Structural contingency theory emphasizes the impact of the situation on the choice of organizational design. Resource dependence theory focuses on power relationships among organizational participants, on the way organizations are designed, and on the way they behave. Institutional theory emphasizes the important role of values and norms in organizational decisions. Population ecology focuses on the behavior of entire systems of organizations as they change. Transaction cost economics explains how organizations determine whether to "make" or "buy" services.

- Health services are organized within individual organizations and between organizations at the system level. Internal forms of organization include functional structures, product line structures, matrix structures, and professional practice models. External forms of organization at the system level include vertical integration, horizontal integration, strategic alliances, integrated delivery systems, and community partnerships.

- Organization of professional nursing care is increasingly focusing on application of population-based approaches and management of care delivery. Nurses increasingly are recognizing their accountability for clinical and fiscal outcomes and are developing innovative models of care delivery that will promote optimum clinical and fiscal outcomes. Although attention to fiscal outcomes has not always been emphasized, nurses recognize that organizations that are not fiscally sound eventually close, with the potential for negatively affecting the health status of local communities.

- Organizational structures and cultures influence the extent to which clinical innovations and other changes are adopted and the speed with which they are adopted. Change theory offers insights into strategies for implementing changes in organizational design, clinical delivery processes, and administrative changes. Change theory also suggests strategies for developing and implementing community-wide innovations in health care delivery.

- The complex health, social, and economic needs of vulnerable groups make it particularly important that services are either provided within a single, comprehensive organization or carefully coordinated across agencies. Nursing case managers can ensure such coordination by focusing on patient goals and system goals. Nurses and other health care professionals should work with other community members to determine the health needs and strengths of the community and to develop plans that best meet the needs while building on community resources.

■ CRITICAL THINKING QUESTIONS

1. Imagine you are a nurse in a hospital that is planning to develop a mobile clinic to serve disadvantaged populations within your community. Which organizational theory would you use to help you develop collaborative relationships with other agencies within the community in order to make referrals and develop joint programming? Explain how the theory you selected will influence your course of action.

2. The urgent care clinic in which you work has just contracted with two large employer groups to provide employee health screenings and occupational injury services for those employers. Your clinic is part of a large chain of clinics throughout the state, all with a single owner. Six urgent care clinics within the chain are located in your community. The clinics employ nurses, nurse practitioners, physicians, radiology technicians, laboratory technicians, and clerical staff. How would you recommend that the new employee health services be organized within your city and why? Take into account demographic and economic factors, as well as determinations about which types of staff are best prepared to provide specific types of services.

3. Imagine that your state has just enrolled all Medicaid recipients into mandatory managed care plans. Providers are worried about the cost of caring for high-risk populations, such as those Medicaid recipients in the aged, blind, and disabled categories. Consumers are worried about losing the access to health care professionals with whom they have long-standing relationships.

   Look up the Medicaid home page on the World Wide Web, and determine what proportion of Medicaid recipients nationally and in your state are in these categories. Then determine what proportion of expenditures result from their care. Work with a group of classmates to develop a plan to provide professional nursing care to a target population within the overall Medicaid population in your state, using as much data from your state as possible. Include data on morbidity and mortality related to the target population you have selected. How would organizational theory help you implement the innovation you propose within your state?

4. The chapter points out how important it is for professional nurses to propose viable solutions to the problems resulting from the economic pressures facing HCOs today. Simply saying that administration is not doing the right thing is not enough for a professional. Describe what you think would be a viable solution to the reduction of professional nursing care in acute care facilities today. Focus your answer on what patients need and who is best prepared to meet those needs, rather than on saving nursing jobs.

■ REFERENCES

Aday, L.A. (1993). *At risk in America: The health and health care needs of vulnerable populations in the United States.* San Francisco: Jossey-Bass.

Bolland, J.M., & Wilson, J.V. (1994). Three faces of integrative coordination: A model of interorganizational relationships in community-based health and human services. *Health Services Research, 29*(3), 341-366.

Brown, M. (1996). Mergers, networking, and vertical integration: Managed care and investor-owned hospitals. *Health Care Management Review, 21*(1), 29-37.

Burns, L.R., Lamb, G.S., & Wholey, D.R. (1996). Impact of integrated community nursing services on hospital utilization and costs in a Medicare risk plan. *Inquiry, 33*, 30-41.

Burns, T., & Stalker, G.M. (1961). *The management of innovation.* London: Tavistock.

DiMaggio, P.J., & Powell, W.W. (1983). The iron cage revisited: Institutional isomorphism and collective rationality in organizational fields. *American Sociological Review, 48*, 147-160.

Hammer, M., & Champey, J. (1994). *Reengineering the corporation: A manifesto for business revolution.* New York: Harper.

Hannan, M.T., & Freeman, J. (1977). The population ecology of organizations. *American Journal of Sociology, 82*, 929-964.

Hannan, M.T., & Freeman, J. (1984). Structural inertia and organizational change. *American Sociological Review, 49*, 149-164.

Iglehart, J.K. (1992). The American health care system: Introduction. *New England Journal of Medicine, 326*(14), 962-967.

Jepperson, R.L. (1991). Institutions, institutional effects, and institutionalism. In W.W. Powell & P.J. DiMaggio (Eds.). *The new institutionalism in organizational analysis.* Chicago: The University of Chicago Press.

Lawrence, P.R., & Lorsch, J.W. (1967). *Organization and environment.* Boston: Harvard Business School.

Lazo-Miller, C., & D'Andrea, D. (1996). Strategic alliances: The wave of the future. *National Medical-Legal Journal, 7*(3), 3, 7.

Leatt, P., & Barnsley, J. (1994). Physicians in health care management. 9. Strategic alliances and relationships between organizations. *Canadian Medical Association Journal, 151*(6), 763-767.

March, J.G., & Simon, H.A. (1958). *Organizations.* New York: Wiley.

McCloskey, J.C., & Bulechek, G.M. (1994). Standardizing the language for nursing: An overview of the issues. *Nursing Outlook, 42*(2), 56-63.

Melaville, A.L., Blank, M.J., & Asayesh, G. (1993). *Together we can: A guide for crafting a pro-family system of education and human services.* Washington, D.C.: U.S. Government Printing Office.

Meyer, J.W., & Rowan, B. (1977). Institutionalized organizations: Formal structure as myth and ceremony. *American Journal of Sociology, 83*, 340-363.

Morgan, G. (1986). *Images of organizations.* Newbury Park, Calif.: Sage.

Morrissey, J.P., Tausig, M., & Lindsey, M.L. (1985). *Network analysis methods for mental health service system research: A comparison of two community support systems.* Pub. no. ADM 85-1383. Washington, D.C.: U.S. Government Printing Office.

Pfeffer, J., & Salancik, G.R. (1978). *The external control of organizations: A resource dependence perspective.* New York: Harper & Row.

Polivka, B.J. (1995). A conceptual model for community interagency collaboration. *IMAGE: Journal of Nursing Scholarship, 27*(2), 110-115.

Porter-O'Grady, T. (1995). Managing along the continuum: A new paradigm for the clinical manager. *Nursing Administration Quarterly, 19*, 3.

Provan, K.G. (1996). Services integration for vulnerable populations: Lessons from community mental health. *Family and Community Health, 19*(4), 19-30.

Provan, K.G., & Milward, H.B. (1991). Institutional-level norms and organizational involvement in a service-implementation network. *Journal of Public Administration Research and Theory, 1*(4), 391-417.

Provan, K.G., & Milward, H.B. (1995). A preliminary theory of interorganizational network effectiveness: A comparative study of four community mental health systems. *Administrative Science Quarterly, 40*, 1-33.

Provan, K.G., & Sebastian, J.G. (1998). Networks within networks: Service link overlap, organizational cliques, and network effectiveness. *Academy of Management Journal, 41*(4), 453-463.

Renshaw, L.R., Kimberly, J.R., & Schwartz, J.S. (1990). Technology diffusion and ecological analysis: The case of magnetic resonance imaging. In S.S. Mick. *Innovations in health care delivery: Insights for organization theory.* San Francisco: Jossey-Bass.

Riley, D.W. (1994). Integrated health care systems: Emerging models. *Nursing Economic$, 12*(4), 201-206.

Rogers, E. (1983). *Diffusion of innovation* (3rd ed.). New York: Free Press.

Rogers, E.W., & Kincaid, D.L. (1981). *Communication networks.* New York: Free Press.

Scott, W.R. (1987). The adolescence of institutional theory. *Administrative Science Quarterly, 32,* 493-511.

Scott, W.R., & Backman, E.V. (1990). Institutional theory and the medical care sector. In S.S. Mick. *Innovations in health care delivery: Insights for organization theory* (pp. 20-52). San Francisco: Jossey-Bass.

Sebastian, J.G. (1996). Vulnerability and vulnerable populations: An introduction. In M. Stanhope & J. Lancaster (Eds.). *Community health nursing: Promoting health of aggregates, families, and individuals* (pp. 623-646). St. Louis: Mosby.

Sebastian, J.G., & Stanhope, M. (1996). Community health nurse managers and consultants. In M. Stanhope & J. Lancaster (Eds.). *Community health nursing: Promoting health of aggregates, families, and individuals* (pp. 849-877). St. Louis: Mosby.

Shortell, S.M., Gillies, R.R., & Anderson, D.A. (1994, Winter). The new world of managed care: Creating organized delivery systems. *Health Affairs,* pp. 46-64.

Stahl, D.A. (1997). The hub of integrated health care delivery systems: Case management. In S.S. Blancett & D.L. Flarey. *Case studies in nursing case management: Health care delivery in a world of managed care* (pp. 12-29). Gaithersburg, MD: Aspen.

Thompson, J.D. (1967). *Organizations in action.* New York: McGraw-Hill.

Turnock, B. J. (1997). *Public health: What it is and how it works.* Gaithersburg, Md.: Aspen.

U.S. Dept. of Health & Human Services, Public Health Services (USDHHS/PHS). (1991). *Healthy People 2000: National Health Promotion and Disease Prevention Objectives.* (DHHS Publication No. [phs] 91-50213). Washington, D.C.: U.S. Government Printing Office.

Walker, M.K., & Sebastian, J.G. (1997). Complementarity of advanced practice nursing roles in enhancing health outcomes of the chronically ill: Acute care nurse practitioners and nurse case managers. In S. Moorhead & D.G. Huber (Eds.). Nursing roles: Evolving or recycled? *Series on Nursing Administration, 9,* 170-190.

Weick, K. (1976). Educational organizations as loosely coupled systems. *Administrative Science Quarterly, 21,* 1-19.

Williamson, O.E. (1975). *Markets and hierarchies: Analysis and antitrust implications.* New York: The Free Press.

Williamson, O.E. (1986). *Economic organization: Firms, markets, and policy control.* New York: New York University Press.

World Health Organization (1954). *Methodology of planning an integrated health programme for rural areas: Second report of the Expert Committee on Public-Health Administration.* WHO Technical Report Series, no. 83. Geneva, Switzerland: The Organization.

World Health Organization (1965). *Integration of mass campaigns against specific diseases into general health services: Report of a WHO Study Group.* WHO Technical Report Series, no. 294. Geneva, Switzerland: The Organization.

World Health Organization (1996). *Integration of health care delivery: Report of a WHO Study Group.* WHO Technical Report Series, no. 861. Geneva, Switzerland: The Organization.

Yanko, J.R., Hardt, M., & Bradstock, J. (1995). The clinical nurse specialist role in shared governance. *Critical Care Nursing Quarterly, 18,* 3.

Yuchtman, E., & Seashore, S.E. (1967). A system resource approach to organizational effectiveness. *American Sociological Review, 32,* 891-903.

Organizational Dynamics

Jean Sorrells-Jones

INTRODUCTION

This chapter focuses on some of the important dynamics of organizations: what they are; how they work; what is known about changes to and within organizations; and what is projected for the organization of the future. It is important for nurses and other clinicians to understand organizational dynamics. For at least the past 50 years, most nurses have worked and practiced nursing within an organization of some type. At least two thirds of nurses traditionally have practiced within hospitals; many others have practiced in community health or home health agencies, schools, or business or industrial organizations. A recent shift has occurred in the number of nurses practicing in hospitals as many hospitals have downsized, merged, or even closed; however, more than half of active professional nurses still practice in hospitals today.

Organizations of all types are undergoing radical and rapid change. The scope of the changes has created new vocabulary. Terms not even coined a decade ago, such as *downsizing,* *seamless, re-engineering,* and *strategic alliances,* have become commonplace in the discussion of organizational change. Health care organizations (HCOs) are not immune to these radical changes. Indeed, many HCOs are now experiencing fundamental changes in structure, operations, and mission.

The changes occurring in organizations are deeply embedded in broader societal changes. Much has been written in books, journals, and scholarly papers to address the turbulent changes of the late twentieth-century industrialized world. When trying to understand a complex phenomenon, it is often helpful to step back and attempt to place that phenomenon within a larger context—to "see the bigger picture." The next section describes this bigger picture as currently posited by leading scientists, writers, and philosophers. This description provides a broader context and helps to make sense of some changes occurring to and within organizations that may seem irrational when viewed in isolation.

After reading this chapter, you will be able to:

1. Compare and contrast the "Industrial Age" organization and its views and expectations of workers with the emerging "Information Age" organization and its views and relationships with workers
2. Discuss the concepts of "knowledge workers" and "intellectual capital" and how you as a professional nurse will be affected by these developing concepts

3. Discuss the successful development and use of teams within organizations and the implications for interdisciplinary practice in nursing and health care
4. Analyze the importance of organizational culture and its impact on an organization's ability to change and adapt
5. Evaluate how the changes in organizational structure, function, and definition are changing traditional management and managers

■ A CHANGE IN WORLD VIEW

In history class, students learn about the major "Ages" into which human history can be divided and what happened during each Age. For example, after the Middle Ages, Western civilization moved into an era known as the Renaissance. Likewise, students have learned about the dawning of the Industrial Age during the eighteenth century. Movement from one Age to another is not an abrupt or rapid occurrence but happens over many transitional years. Those years of transition may be characterized by turmoil and instability as basic understandings, beliefs, and structures of the "old" Age are re-

Key terms	
Term	**Definition**
Industrial Age	The period from approximately 1750 AD until the mid-1950s, during which a large part of the world moved from an agrarian society, economically and socially centered on farming, to an industrial society, economically and socially centered on factories and manufacturing; the industrial age is believed to be waning now
Information Age	The popular title given to the current period, beginning in the mid-1950s with the rapid development of the computer, and the evolving transition from a manufacturing economy to a service- and information/knowledge-based economy
Intellectual capital	The intangible assets of knowledge, skill, and information
Knowledge work	Nonrepetitive, nonroutine work that entails substantial levels of cognitive activity; it includes professional and specialists' work
Knowledge workers	Persons who work both with their hands and with theoretic knowledge

placed or modified by new scientific and economic understandings and changed social and economic structures.

Philosophers, scientists, and economists say that just such a transition is occurring now and that when people in 2100 look back at the last half of the twentieth century, it will be apparent that the years from 1950 to 2020 were transitional years between the Industrial Age and the Information Age. Although any detailed discussion of this topic is beyond the scope of this chapter, a brief explanation is important because this is part of the big picture that helps to explain some of the changes in organizations and roles that are now occurring, which will affect the working lives of current and future workers.

The major change occurring in this transition to the Information Age is movement from an economy and a work force based primarily on the manufacture of material products to an economy and a work force based on the production of services and the use of information and knowledge.

When the agrarian economy gave way to an industrial economy, there was a great shift in the work force. The percentage of workers who were farmers dropped dramatically, and the percentage of factory and industrial workers ballooned. Another shift is occurring now. In 1950, industrial workers who made or moved things were the single largest group in every developed country in the world; by 1990, industrial workers who made or moved things accounted for less than one fifth of the American work force. By the year 2000, it is estimated that no developed country in the world will have more than one sixth to one eighth of its workers in industrial roles of making and moving goods (Drucker, 1994). Already, nearly two thirds of Americans work in the service sector. In economics, this is described as the movement from a manufacturing base to a service base.

As industrial jobs and opportunities decline, a new group of workers is gaining dominance. These workers are referred to as *knowledge workers,* a term coined by Peter Drucker. Drucker (1994, p. 56) defines knowledge work as "nonrepetitive, nonroutine work that entails substantial levels of cognitive activity." Knowledge workers are described as people who work both with their hands and with theoretic knowledge (Drucker, 1992, 1994). Drucker is specific in his descriptions. He stresses that the education required for knowledge workers can be gained only through formal schooling and cannot be gained through apprenticeship or on-the-job training. Knowledge workers must be able to acquire and apply theoretic and analytic knowledge as well as significant manual/physical skills. Given the rapid changes in knowledge and information, the knowledge worker must also be committed to and skilled in the habit of continuous learning.

In this new era, knowledge is the primary ingredient in what is done, made, bought, and sold. Knowledge assets, rather than land, buildings, machines, or factories, are the capital assets needed to create wealth. *Fortune* magazine declared in 1994: "Intellectual assets undoubtedly far outweigh the material assets which appear on balance sheets" (*Fortune,* April 3, 1994, p. 71). Knowledge workers use their combination of theoretic knowledge and related physical skills to produce new knowledge, information, and services, as well as new products. Engineers, information and computing specialists, and new product designers are all knowledge workers. Physicians, nurses, and other health care professionals (occupational and physical therapists, pharmacists, certain technicians) are knowledge workers.

In the industrial era, workers (labor) were seen as a necessary cost of doing business—a means to an end. The majority of employees were considered "hands" or "muscle" needed to

---

Key terms

Term	Definition
Team	A small number of people with complementary knowledge and skills who are committed to a common purpose, performance goals, and approach for which they hold themselves mutually accountable
Accountable	Being responsible for the performance or completion of some obligation, duty, or trust
Shared or aggregate accountability	The promise or commitment of each individual to be responsible for his or her own performance and for the performance and results of the group in its pursuit of mutual goals
Performance goal	Specific and measurable objective(s)
Cross-functional team	A group of individuals from different departments or professions, or with different knowledge, skills, or functions, who are committed to a common goal or purpose
Team building	Educational or experiential exercises or opportunities for individuals to learn or develop skills as team members; the intent of team-building efforts is to help teams develop trust and commitment as a basis for effectiveness
Teamwork	A set of values that encourage behaviors such as active listening, responding constructively, providing support when needed, and recognizing and respecting the interests and achievements of others; these values promote team performance
Team learning	The process of aligning and developing the capacity of a team to create the results its members desire; involves learning how to tap the potential for many minds to be more intelligent than any one mind

---

produce things; as such, most were considered largely interchangeable and easily replaceable. Many organizations are beginning to understand that in this emerging Information Age, knowledge workers are their most important asset and knowledge workers are neither interchangeable nor easily (or cheaply) replaced. In *Intellectual Capital: The New Wealth of Organizations,* Stewart (1997) writes that a company's knowledge workers and their ability to use that knowledge in the vigorous pursuit of the goals of the company are the company's keys to competitive advantage.

Traditional organizations with their hierarchies, single function departments, and close supervision of workers were designed to fit the Industrial Age's definition of work, workers, and production tasks. Much of the current turmoil within organizations is the result of the need to redesign the organization to meet the challenges of a knowledge-based world and to optimize the work of the knowledge workers.

■ TEAMS WITHIN ORGANIZATIONS

The use of teams has been and continues to be an important topic in management and leadership literature. Many different organizations have found that teams can outperform individuals, even extremely knowledgeable, skillful individuals, in accomplishing complex work. As organizations continue evolving to function more effectively in the Information Age, the team is being recognized widely as the primary work unit, rather than the individuals within functional departments of the old-style organizations. "We believe that teams—real teams, not just groups that management calls 'teams'—should be the basic unit of performance for most organizations, regardless of size," say Katzenbach and Smith, authors of *The Wisdom of Teams* (Katzenbach & Smith, 1993, p. 15). Peter Senge, of MIT's prestigious Center for Organizational Learning, says, "Teams, not individuals, are the fundamental learning unit of an organization. This is where 'the rubber meets the road'; unless teams can learn, the organization cannot learn" (Senge, 1990, p. 10). The organization that can learn, he says, will have the critical, competitive edge in times of turbulent change. Drucker says flatly that the only way for knowledge workers to be truly productive is for them to work in teams, and health care researchers Schweikhart and Smith-Daniels report that teams are now considered the basic unit of work performance in hospitals undergoing reengineering (Schweikhart & Smith-Daniels, 1996).

Teams are hardly new. Almost everyone has been a part of some team at some time and believes that he or she understands what a team is, how teams work, and how to be a team player. In their years of research into teams, however, Katzenbach and Smith (1993) found that opinions differed widely about what a team is, can and should do, and needs in order to be successful. For example, some people think only of sports, with its focus on coaching, individual best records, stars, practice, and winning. Others emphasize teamwork and the values they believe define teamwork, such as cooperation, equality, trust, and confidence. Many, especially managers with experience in traditional organizations, believe teams are a fad and that teams waste time, squander re-

sources, and interfere with decisive individual action and performance.

Why is there so much emphasis on teams in organizations now? Why is there so much research going on and so many reports and books being written on the topic? Katzenbach and Smith (1993) believe that the urgency stems from the growing link between teams and the high levels of performance needed for organizations to remain competitive. Literally every organization is faced with the challenges of improving performance, decreasing costs, and speeding up processes. These are formidable challenges. A *high-performance organization* is defined as an organization that has consistently outperformed its competitors for an extended period (10 years or more) (Katzenbach & Smith, 1993). In this era of turbulent change, becoming high performance is seen as the key to success and possibly even survival. Few organizations have achieved the designation, although many are aggressively seeking to become high performers. However, of those organizations recognized as being high performers, most have credited the effective use of teams as key to creating and sustaining their high performance.

Thus one of the reasons for the emphasis on teams is the growing perception that teams that work are the key to a higher performing, more successful organization, but not all teams are effective performers or even reasonably productive performers. Some "teams" never become more than "a mob of people . . ." sinking in seas of contention or working at cross purposes (Robbins & Finley, 1995). Some organizational leaders, reading about the extraordinary successes accomplished through teams at companies such as Motorola, Westinghouse, General Electric, and Texas Instruments, have launched teams and "waited for the magic," only to experience serious, expensive problems and grave disappointment.

Basics About Teams

Webster's Third International Dictionary gives several definitions of *team,* including "two or more horses, oxen, or other draft animals harnessed to the same vehicle (as a coach, wagon, or sled) or to the same plow or other work implement" and "a number of persons associated in work or activity." About all these two definitions have in common is the concept of two or more entities working together toward the achievement of some joint effort or work.

More helpful is the definition from Katzenbach and Smith. They define a team as "a small number of people with complementary skills who are committed to a common purpose, performance goals, and approach for which they hold themselves mutually accountable" (Katzenbach & Smith, 1993, p. 43).

There are different kinds of teams, such as teams that recommend things (task forces or planning teams), run things (management teams), and make or do things.

Research into teams, both successful productive teams and teams that just never made it, can now provide some clearer understanding of teams. In compiling the key findings of several researchers, the following themes emerge:

- The size and composition of the group are important.
- A clear and commonly understood goal is critical.
- Commitment to achieving the goal is essential.
- There are key skills and values that team members must have to be successful.
- There are stages in the development of teams, and teams can "get stuck" and fail to progress.

Size and Composition

Effective teams range in size from 2 to 25 people, although the average size is 10 or fewer people. Size may differ according to the job of the team, but groups larger than 25 have trouble interacting constructively or agreeing on key issues and plans. In theory, a group as large as 50 could be a team, but groups of that size are generally forced to break into smaller working groups rather than function as a single team.

The composition of the team is important. To be successful, a team must have people with the right mix of knowledge and skills to accomplish the goal. When deciding on team membership, therefore, it is important to consider what theoretic, functional, or technical expertise will be needed to achieve this goal. Drucker's definition of the knowledge worker is particularly clear and helpful here, because the question becomes "What combination of knowledge workers is appropriate for this team to ensure that the knowledge and technical expertise that need to be applied will be available within the team?"

A narrower, more circumscribed goal may need a team whose members are much alike, whereas broader or more complex goals often need members with clearly different knowledge and skills. Teams requiring a mixture of people from different functions or disciplines are called *multidisciplinary teams,* or *cross-functional teams.* Cross-functional teams are effective and productive when they function well, but they often experience difficulties becoming successful. Examples of cross-functional teams include (1) a product design team composed of several varieties of engineers, marketers, and even customers and (2) a health care team made up of physicians, nurses, a pharmacist, and a physical therapist. The composition depends on the goal of the team and the characteristics of the patients being cared for by the team.

Clear and Commonly Understood Purpose and Goals

To work successfully together, teams need to understand clearly what they are trying to accomplish. Research shows that a common barrier to good team performance is the lack of a commonly held, clearly understood purpose and goals. Robbins and Finley (1995), describing why teams so often "don't work," found that confused goals are common. Team members would admit that they didn't know where the team was going or supposed to go (goals) or even why it was put together in the first place (purpose).

Much has been written, some of it contradictory, about the development of the team's purpose and goals. Some of the concern from managers about teams wasting time stems from misunderstanding the process of developing a commonly held team purpose. The process often goes something like this. A team is brought together and presented, often by senior management, with a general demand, problem, or opportunity, such as launching a new product or reducing the cycle time and unnecessary steps of a major process. One health care example is improving the process and decreasing delays and the cost of providing care for a woman with a breast lump that might be malignant. Another example is improving the clinical outcomes and patient satisfaction while significantly decreasing the cost of a hip or knee replacement procedure.

In the best scenarios, direction from management broadly frames the issue or problem, the rationale and supporting information, and the performance challenge but leaves plenty of solution space for the team to set specific goals, decide the timing, and agree on the approach. Research has shown that the most successful teams then spend considerable time and effort together exploring, shaping, and agreeing on a purpose that really belongs to them, both collectively and individually (Fisher & Fisher, 1998; Mohrman et al., 1995). Transforming broad directives into specific steps and measurable performance goals that require contributions from all team members is the surest first step to a successful team. In doing this, team members define a teamwork product that is different from their individual jobs or functions and more specific than the organization's overall mission. Setting specific, measurable objectives also facili-

tates clear communication and collective responsibility, both of which are key to team success.

Commitment to Achieving the Goal

Even when the purpose is clearly and commonly understood and the goals clearly articulated, it all must be seen as important and of value to the organization and team members. Katzenbach and Smith (1993, p. 12) found that the purpose and goals must be seen as both meaningful and challenging: "No team arises without a performance challenge that is meaningful to those involved. . . . A common set of demanding performance goals that a group considers important to achieve will lead, most of the time, to both performance and a team." They go on to say that it is important to remember that the team is the means to achieving an end (a goal), not the end itself.

Teams and individuals can understand clearly what the goal is and still not believe in it or fully commit to achieving it. They may not believe that the goal, once reached, will be of any value to the organization. They may not believe that the goal is reachable. Perhaps they believe that the basic premise is flawed because it is based on inaccurate figures or that achieving the goal would require too much time or effort.

Failure by team members to commit to a goal may be related to the organization's overall performance ethic. Organizations with weak performance ethics consistently have difficulty fielding successful teams. Leaders who fail to make clear and meaningful performance demands of their people and, more important, of themselves contribute to an organizational culture that does not support team success. (Organizational culture is discussed in more detail on pp. 140-146; Chapter 9 discusses the responsibilities of leaders.)

There are several levels of involvement with a purpose or a goal. Senge (1990) discusses the difference between *compliance* and *commit-*

ment. Although Senge is talking about involvement with the greater vision of the organization, these descriptions can be applied equally well to the attitude of team members to the purpose and goals of the team (Box 5-1).

Senge believes, and research on teams agrees, that many people in organizations are in states of formal or genuine compliance. They "go along," sincerely trying to contribute. They

Modified from Senge, P.M. (1990). *The fifth discipline: The art and practice of the learning organization* (p. 219). New York: Doubleday Publishers.

B O X   5 - 1

Possible Attitudes of Team Members

Commitment: Really wants to achieve goals. Will make it happen. Brings energy, passion, and creativity to work. Is absolutely and completely "on board."

Genuine compliance: Genuinely sees the benefit and wants to accomplish the goal. Does everything expected and sometimes more. Is diligent; follows the "letter of the law" and is a "good soldier."

Formal compliance: On the whole, sees the benefits and would like the goal accomplished. Does what is expected but no more. Is "on board" unless or until controversy or difficulties arise.

Grudging compliance: Does not see the benefit and has no stake in delivering the goal but does not want to lose job. Does enough of what is expected because he or she has to but makes it known in various ways that he or she is not really "on board."

Noncompliance: Does not see the benefit nor want the goal accomplished. Will not do what is expected. "I won't do it, and you can't make me do it."

Apathy: Has no opinion; is neither for nor against the goal. Unengaged. No interest. No energy.

---

try to play by the rules. They are upbeat and generally positive. In short, they live up (or down) to the general expectations of the organization (see discussion of organizational culture on pp. 140-146). When placed on teams, they are acceptable team players, especially in the earlier stages of team formation.

What is the difference, then, between compliance and commitment, and why is it important to team effectiveness? The truly committed person brings an energy, passion, and excitement to his or her performance that is not found in the compliant worker. Senge (1990, p. 221) says that ". . . the committed person doesn't [just] play by the rules of the game, he is responsible for the game. . . . A group of people truly committed to a common [goal] is an awesome force. They can accomplish the seemingly impossible."

DePree (1989, p. 56) also speaks of commitment when talking about an individual's relationship with work: "When one thinks carefully about why certain people who are competent, well-educated, energetic, and well supported with good tools fail, it is often the red thread of superficiality that does them in. They never get seriously and accountably involved in their own work."

Research shows that commitment to—not compliance with—the purpose and goals by all or most of the members of a team is an important condition for the team to be successful. "Groups that fail to become teams rarely develop a common purpose that they own and can translate into specific and actionable goals. For whatever reason—an insufficient focus on performance, lack of effort, poor leadership—they do not coalesce around a challenging aspiration" (Katzenbach & Smith, 1993, p. 52).

Specific skills and values are essential to team effectiveness. In spite of resounding agreement on this point, however, organization after organization attempts to launch teams without sufficient attention to the important skills and values needed by team members.

Key Skills and Values

The skills needed by team members fall roughly into two categories: knowledge and functional skills and problem-solving and interpersonal skills. The knowledge and functional skills needed for the team are usually addressed during decisions about the team composition. However, there can be problems within organizations with varying levels of competence of individuals with given credentials. A team may require an engineer: which engineer with what kinds of knowledge and experience? A team may require a nurse: which nurse with what level of knowledge and experience? Careful selection of team members with demonstrated knowledge and competency is important. One cannot use knowledge one does not have, and no amount of enthusiasm can substitute for sophisticated knowledge.

A paradox of teams and team research concerns the assessment of problem-solving and interpersonal skills of potential team members. Some sources advocate that careful attention be paid to personal compatibility or formal positions in the organization as prerequisites for team membership. On the other extreme, some authors extol the power of the team as a vehicle for personal growth and development and suggest that limited attention should be paid to the interpersonal skills of potential members. These latter sources seem to suggest that the technical knowledge and skills are the key consideration and that sufficient team-building exercises and the team process itself will develop the interpersonal and problem-solving capabilities of the team members. Still other sources advise that team members need to possess only basic skills and values and the potential to learn.

Evidence suggests that there is accuracy in all these suggestions. Certain basic interpersonal and problem-solving skills are important to team success, whether they are present in full measure at the onset or develop as the team coalesces. Effective communication skills are critical, and the need for active listening skills is important. Conflict resolution skills are of great importance, since lack of constructive conflict within a team is a key indicator of an unsuccessful team. Certain underlying values (e.g., respect, trust) are generally reflected in such behaviors as recognizing and appreciating the achievements and talents of other team members, risk taking, and refraining from personal attacks or ridicule of others' ideas. Last, much evidence suggests that effective teams can and usually do learn and refine their interpersonal skills and problem-solving skills individually and as a group.

Some basic level of all these skills, or the clear potential for developing them, seems, then, to be a prerequisite for anyone expected to function well on a team. Although it would clearly be inappropriate to select team members solely on their personalities, it would be wise to consider whether their interpersonal and problem-solving skills, or lack of them, would actively impede the work of the group.

Providing formal support and assistance for specific team-building activities is recommended by many organizational development experts, although these activities are not always held in high esteem by organizations or some team members themselves. With or without formal team-building activities, most successful teams set ground rules of behavior for the group and hold themselves and each other accountable for observing their own ground rules (Katzenbach & Smith, 1993).

Stages of Development of Teams

The development of a group of individuals into a team follows some predictable patterns. B.W. Tuckman, a psychologist, identified and named these stages of group process/team development: forming, storming, norming, and performing. This model has been used often by organizational development trainers and in nursing school curricula. It has been featured in several books on groups or teams, including Robbins and Finley's *Why Teams Don't Work* (1995). Therefore it is not at all unusual to hear people within organizations using the names of these stages as a brief description or explanation. For example, one might hear someone dismiss the report of a conflictive team meeting with the comment, "Oh that is just the necessary 'storming' that has to go on in a team. . . ."

Forming is the first stage of a team or group. It begins when the different parts of the team are brought together and given a charge or task. Typically, people are unsure of their roles and the roles of others. There is a wariness about team members, and frequently there are questions about why certain team members are included. For those who may not have worked in groups or teams before, there may be prejudices or misconceptions about how teams work and who has the power. People cast about for alliances. Formal or informal team leaders may be selected or elected. If a formal team leader has been appointed as part of the team formation, he or she needs to clarify why people were asked to be a part of the team and explain individual responsibilities. The team begins to learn to deal with each other, but little work toward the goal gets accomplished.

Storming is the name given to the second formative phase of teams or groups. During this phase, which is often marked by conflict and struggle, the team works out its goals, its specific plans, the relationships among team members, and the roles of each person. Conflicts arising from different personalities, different agendas, and different backgrounds surface and have to be resolved before the team can move on. Tuckman, as described by Robbins and Fin-

ley (1995) sometimes referred to this stage as a group's *trial by fire*—a period of significant risk for the team. Many teams fail to make it through this stage and dissolve in conflict. The role of the team leader during this phase is one of guidance and limit setting to try to keep the disagreements from shattering the team. Team-building efforts to teach effective conflict resolution skills may be helpful.

Norming is the stage that occurs after team members have resolved most conflicts regarding their identities, their roles on the team, and their shared commitment to the goals of the team. Team members are less defensive, and a team identity begins to develop. The group begins to gain focus and unanimity and works together to find solutions.

Performing is the stage at which the team "comes of age" and reaches the optimum stage of performance together. The team is united, and synergy develops as the members work together as a group. Although there may be conflict during this stage, it is conflict about ways to meet the goal, not about destructive turf issues of previous stages.

Robbins and Finley (1995), who use the Tuckman model in their discussion of effective and noneffective teams, describe the first two stages of this model as struggles to develop trust and cooperation in place of mistrust and defensiveness. They point out that teamwork is impossible without trust among the members and that trust must be earned by and among team members.

Another model of team development is the team performance curve (Figure 5-1) featured in the best-selling book *The Wisdom of Teams* (Katzenbach & Smith, 1993). This model is used frequently in business school classes so it is familiar to many people within organizations. The underlying assumption is that any small group's performance depends on the basic approach it takes and how well the approach is imple-

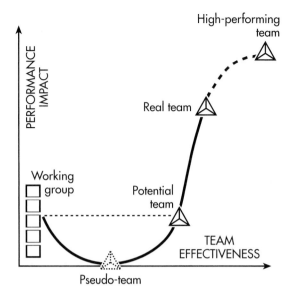

Figure 5-1 ■ **The team performance curve.** (From Katzenbach, J.R., & Smith, D. [1993]. *The wisdom of teams: Creating the high-performance organization.* Boston: Harvard Business School Press, p. 84.)

mented. This model describes several levels of small group performance, from the working group to a high performance team.

In their introduction to the team performance curve model, Katzenbach and Smith stress that an organization needs to make clear decisions about when a team is needed to obtain a particular goal and when it is not. In many situations, using a structured working group makes more sense and incurs less risk than opting for a real team. Too often, organizational leaders do not recognize that they have a viable choice or how to make a good decision.

> The basic distinction here turns on performance. A working group relies primarily on the individual contributions of its members for group performance, whereas a team strives for a magnified impact that is incremental to what its members could achieve in their individual roles. The choice depends largely on whether individual achievements

can deliver the group's performance aspirations, or whether collective work-products [an outcome that is more than the sum of the individuals' efforts], skills, and mutual accountability are needed (Katzenbach & Smith, p. 89).

Katzenbach and Smith go on to describe the operational dynamics of a working group, a pseudoteam, a potential team, a real team, and a high performance team.

A *working group* is not a team at all. Working groups are prevalent and often quite effective in large organizations, particularly in traditional hierarchies where individual accountability and individual performance are most valued. A working group relies on the sum of "individual bests" for its performance. There is no collective work product that requires joint effort or a merging of individual performances. There is no incremental performance goal that requires that the total performance equals more than the sum of the individual parts.

The most effective working groups come together often to share information and insights, to make decisions that help each person do his or her job better, and to clarify and reinforce the individual's role and performance standards. The focus is on individual accountability. Each person is accountable for the quality of his or her own work, but the working group members do not take responsibility for results other than their own. The roles assigned to each individual often match that person's organizational position. There is frequently a type of constructive competition among the small group members in pursuit of their individual performance targets.

A *pseudoteam* is a group for which there *could* be a significant, incremental performance need, but the group has not focused or agreed to collective performance and is not really trying to achieve it. Although pseudoteams often call themselves teams, they have not shaped either a common purpose or a set of performance goals. Members of the pseudoteam may be "faking it" by espousing a willingness or desire to work together as a team while remaining unwilling to trust or accept mutual accountability. It requires a leap of faith to work as a team. People cannot contribute to real team performance without taking responsibility for their peers and letting their peers assume responsibility. This is very difficult for rugged individualists who believe that the only way to ensure a job is done right is to do it themselves. It is also difficult for the individuals who believe, openly or covertly, that their own work is the only really important work needed to achieve the outcome.

Senge sums up the problem of the pseudoteam (or the immature potential team) succinctly: "How can a team of committed [people] with individual IQs above 120 have a collective IQ of 63?" (Senge, 1990, p. 9).

The pseudoteam can be a significant drain for an organization. Members may get diverted from doing their individual best yet achieve little as a group. Work does not get done, costs outweigh benefits, and people resent the imposition on their time and priorities. It is possible that much of the distrust of teams voiced by managers in organizations stems from experience with nonproductive pseudoteams instead of real teams.

The *potential team* is a group for which there is a significant, incremental performance need that the group is trying to achieve. The team members are sincere in their commitment, but they have not yet become a team. Most generally at this stage, the group has not yet established collective accountability and has not yet achieved necessary clarity about purpose, goals, or a common working approach. As a team, this group is definitely a work in progress.

Potential teams abound in organizations. Because they are at a stage of struggle to come together around mutual performance goals and shared accountability, potential teams are marked by conflict and varying levels of frustration. Some teams overcome the obstacles and move on to become real teams, but other teams get stuck. It is often at this stage that a team seeks assistance via "team-building" efforts. It is important that teams maintain their focus on performance, not on team building for the sake of becoming a team. If team members need to improve their skills, it is most effectively accomplished within the context of performance. Too many team-building activities focus on becoming a team, almost as an end in itself, instead of focusing on learning to achieve the work together. "The worst thing a stuck team can do is to abandon the discipline of the team basics " (Katzenbach & Smith, 1993, p. 87). Team basics include size, purpose, goals, skills, approach, and accountability.

A *real team* is a small number of people with complementary skills who are equally committed to a common purpose, goals, and working approach for which they hold themselves mutually accountable. This is the team that was described earlier. Not only does the team achieve more than any single individual could achieve, but also their group outcome is more than the sum of the individual parts.

The real team demonstrates both individual and group accountability, and the group goal transcends individual goals. Senge used a quote from basketball player Bill Russell of the Boston Celtics: "[We] were a team of specialists, and like a team of specialists in any field, our performance depended both on individual excellence and on how well we worked together. None of us had to strain to understand that we had to complement each others' specialties; it was simply a fact, and we all tried to figure out ways to make our combination more effective" (Senge, 1990, p. 232). The Celtics were a high-performance organization, winning 11 world championships in 13 years.

Key terms

Term	Definition
Mental models	Deeply ingrained assumptions, generalizations, or even pictures or images that influence individuals' understanding of the world and their actions
Multidisciplinary team	A team composed of members from different disciplines or professions
Multidisciplinary practice	A team process in which members of different disciplines assess and treat patients (usually independently) and then share information
Interdisciplinary practice	A deeper level of collaboration than multidisciplinary practice, in which certain processes, such as evaluation and development of plans of care, are done or created jointly by a team of professionals working together
Professional identity	A sense of belonging to or being part of a particular profession, which includes being entitled to the rights accorded the profession and committed to the values, responsibilities, and obligations of the profession

Teams in Health Care

The use of teams in health care is expanding rapidly. HCOs, challenged by intense pressure to improve quality and reduce costs, are beginning to recognize the significant potential of effective interdisciplinary teams. Nurses and other health care providers need to understand team functioning and learn to function as effective members of sophisticated intradisciplinary and interdisciplinary teams.

The use of teams in HCOs is a complex and compelling topic. All of what has been said about teams in other settings is equally true of teams in health care. Some additional issues and conditions in health care, however, make the development of teams even more challenging—and possibly more necessary—than in some other organizations.

All types of teams are used in HCOs, sometimes effectively, often not very effectively. Teams that recommend things (task forces or planning teams) have been almost ubiquitous, tackling both large policy issues and small operational problems. Teams that run things, such as management teams, exist at least in name and structure, from the executive management teams to unit-based management teams. The most intense focus in the past decade has been on teams that make or do things, specifically teams that plan and deliver care to patients (i.e., teams of care providers).

Caregiver teams may be composed of like professionals, as in a nursing team, a pharmacy team, or an occupational therapy team. Multidisciplinary teams, as the name implies, are composed of different kinds of professionals. Multidisciplinary teams may also be called cross-professional teams, and both are analogous to the cross-functional teams of the business world.

Teams composed of like professionals, or professionals and nonprofessional assistants, are quite familiar, particularly in nursing, where such teams have been used for decades. Most generally, these teams consist of at least one registered nurse (RN) and one or more licensed practical nurse/licensed vocational nurse (LPN/LVN) or unlicensed assistants. Using the new definitions, this would be a team consisting of knowledge worker(s)—the RN(s)—and non-knowledge worker assistants. The roles in this type of team are clear. The RNs are the team leaders and carry the ultimate authority and responsibility. They make the decisions and delegate the work that does not require their knowledge and judgment. There are clear limits on the possibility of shared accountability because of the differences in knowledge and skill and because of legal responsibilities. RNs retain the responsibility and accountability although they may delegate specific tasks. Nurses tend to be rather comfortable with this type of team and its designated roles, perhaps because of its familiarity.

Cross-professional or multidisciplinary teams are a much more recent phenomenon and present both greater challenges and greater opportunities for improving care. Rather than a team of knowledge workers and assistants, the multidisciplinary team is composed of several different types of knowledge workers, each with his or her own area of knowledge and skills. Presumably the team has been assembled and the membership determined because the goal requires this particular combination of knowledge and skills or because the process being examined includes segments or activities performed by the different professionals. Multidisciplinary teams have most often been brought together to improve complex patient care processes in which they have all participated. Usually the goal is to integrate the process, and possibly the care itself, into a seamless whole.

Multidisciplinary and Interdisciplinary Practice

The words *multidisciplinary* and *interdisciplinary* often are used interchangeably, even though their actual definitions differ. Multidisciplinary means many disciplines and is correctly used to describe a team composed of professionals of different disciplines. *Multidisciplinary practice* has come to mean a team process in which members of many disciplines assess and treat patients (usually independently) and then share information. The intent of the sharing is to streamline the process and enable each professional to accomplish his or her part of the process or care more effectively.

When examined within the context of the team performance curve, a multidisciplinary team doing multidisciplinary work such as that just described is not a real team but a work group. Work groups can be very effective, and they can greatly improve the process by improving each piece or segment of the process, as well as achieving better alignment and sequencing of the segments. Certainly the earliest clinical pathways were examples of work groups improving a multidisciplinary process.

Interdisciplinary refers to a deeper level of collaboration, where certain processes, such as evaluation and development of plans of care, are done or created jointly by a team of professionals working together. Interdisciplinary practice involves a merging of knowledge and sometimes of functions and processes. Role boundaries of the various professionals are more blurred and may be determined by patient needs rather than being rigidly prescribed (Hedelt & Holden, 1995). When examined within the context of the team performance curve, the mature interdisciplinary team involved in interdisciplinary practice is a real team. The developing interdisciplinary team fits the description of a potential team.

These differences between multidisciplinary practice and interdisciplinary practice are not universally held. However, as health care teams gain more experience and skill in becoming real teams, the differences are becoming more clearly defined and understood. Schweikhart and Smith-Daniels (1996) talk about functional teams, coordinated teams, and focused teams. Although they are speaking primarily of team structure, it is clear that the designations also describe different levels of integration of care functions and processes.

Professionals and Teams

Bringing cross-professional teams together and making them effective have proven to be especially difficult. They require professionals to learn new ways of working together. Tjosvold and Tjosvold (1995, p. 3) have studied cross-professional teams, and they are blunt in their evaluative comment: "Specialists who try to do it all are not specialists. They must apply their specific [knowledge and] skills in conjunction with other professionals and employees. They can only be successful together." They go on to say that professionals are often more responsive to the ideas and contributions of like professionals than to "outsiders" and that professionals may tend to be parochial in their conceptualization of the issues. "Professionals are thought to be too narrow-minded and high-handed, perhaps more committed to maintaining their own professional identity and goals than to achieving the goals of the organization."

There have been successes, however, and the Tjosvolds cite their own work and that of others in describing ways for professionals to learn to work cooperatively and constructively across professional boundaries. "Studies demonstrate that professionals who develop strongly cooperative goals and discuss their opposing [or nonaligned] views constructively combine their expertise to solve [complex problems and utilize emerging knowledge and technology]" (Tjosvold & Tjosvold, 1995, p. 3).

One of the unique and potentially complicating characteristics of the cross-professional or multidisciplinary team in health care is that most or all members of the team have a professional identity that transcends their organizational position. Further, each professional is licensed, registered, or certified to practice his or her profession within certain parameters defined and monitored by legal statute or the operating rules of a regulatory board. Thus some actions and decisions can be done only by a particular professional, and the responsibility for those actions cannot be delegated.

Health care professionals themselves often assume that these legal definitions and responsibilities prevent the multidisciplinary or cross-professional team from developing the mutual or shared accountability described as key to real team functioning. In fact, although team functioning may be more complex than in some other settings, real cross-professional teams can and do find ways to develop mutual goals and shared accountability. The real team, as described previously, develops specific performance goals and plans. These plans incorporate the contributions and responsibility of each professional. Real teams, whether cross-functional or cross-professional teams, develop a rich and interesting mix of individual and team performance, with strong commitment to hold each other and themselves accountable for performance.

One perceptive researcher wrote that "as organizations become more flexible, the boundaries that matter are in the minds of managers and employees" (Hirschhorn & Gilmore, 1992, p. 105). The most powerful barrier to developing real teams, engaged in true interdisciplinary practice and shared accountability, is in the

Key terms	
Term	**Definition**
Organizational culture	The values, assumptions, beliefs, and behavior patterns that are shared by people in the group (organization) and that tend to persist over time even when group membership changes
Work group rules	The behaviors (verbal and nonverbal) that group members consider to be appropriate responses to given situations, or typical ways of acting; seldom, if ever, written down
Entitlement	The attitude or belief that one gets something because one is owed it, because one is entitled to it
Extracontractual behavior	Working at a level above the minimum required for job maintenance
Trust	A willingness to place oneself in a position of vulnerability with reliance on someone or something to perform as expected

minds of the various practitioners. They have developed mental models that influence or frame the way they see the world, themselves, and other professionals. Sometimes those mental models contribute to a parochialism that prevents them from seeing new possibilities.

Health care professionals, whether physicians, nurses, pharmacists, occupational therapists, or physical therapists, tend to have very strong professional identities. They describe themselves clearly as nurses, or as physicians, or as pharmacists, with a clear understanding of what that means and of their rights and responsibilities as members of that profession. They have a strong sense of belonging to that profession and a deep commitment to the individual responsibility that is inherent in the practice of that profession. Schools for health care professionals work hard to acculturate their members into the culture and identity of the profession. However, health care professional curricula, for the most part, prepare the professional to see himself or herself and to practice as an individual practitioner, placing high value on professional autonomy. Until recently, there has been little opportunity for health care profes-

sionals to learn as students how to work as part of an interdisciplinary team. Schools, urged onward by learned commissions, such as the Pew Health Professions Commission, and oversight groups, such as the Joint Commission for Accreditation of Healthcare Organizations, are now exploring ways to educate health care professional students for effective interdisciplinary practice.

There is no question that interdisciplinary teams will become more important in the coming years. Even the prestigious Institute of Medicine recommends that interdisciplinary teams of physicians and other health care professionals are the best answer to many of the United States' challenging health care needs. Health care professionals will have to learn how to work effectively as knowledge workers on interdisciplinary teams. Launching and supporting such teams will also require changes in organizational cultures and management practices.

■ ORGANIZATIONAL CULTURE

Organizational culture is difficult to define concisely. The concept has its roots in anthropol-

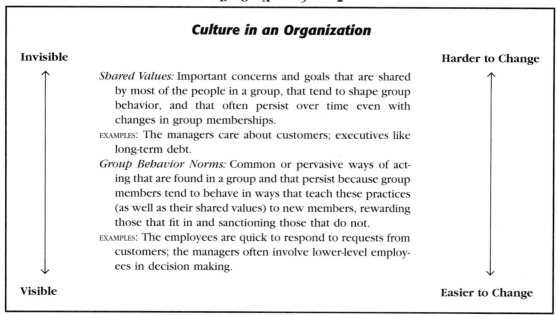

BOX 5-2

Culture in an Organization

Invisible

Harder to Change

Shared Values: Important concerns and goals that are shared by most of the people in a group, that tend to shape group behavior, and that often persist over time even with changes in group memberships.

EXAMPLES: The managers care about customers; executives like long-term debt.

Group Behavior Norms: Common or pervasive ways of acting that are found in a group and that persist because group members tend to behave in ways that teach these practices (as well as their shared values) to new members, rewarding those that fit in and sanctioning those that do not.

EXAMPLES: The employees are quick to respond to requests from customers; the managers often involve lower-level employees in decision making.

Visible

Easier to Change

From Kotter, J.P., & Heskett, J.L. (1992). *Corporate culture and performance* (p. 5). New York: The Free Press.

ogy, sociology, psychology, and management theory, and there are numerous, sometimes conflicting, approaches to describing and dealing with it. There is widespread agreement, however, that organizational cultures do exist, are very important, are often complex, and can have tremendous effects on the performance of the organization. One reasonably complete definition of organizational culture is that it is the values, assumptions, beliefs, and behavior patterns that are shared by people in the group (organization) and that tend to persist over time even when group membership changes.

Kotter and Heskett (1992) find it helpful to think of organizational culture as having two levels that differ in their visibility and their resistance to change (Box 5-2). At the deeper, less visible level are values, including beliefs and thoughts about what is important in life, in this work, and in this organization. At this level, culture can be extremely difficult to change, partly because members of the group are often unaware of many values that they share and that bind them together (Kotter & Heskett, 1992).

At the more visible level, culture involves behavior patterns and norms. Coeling and Wilcox (1988) use the term *work group rules* to describe this level of organizational culture. Work group rules are the behaviors (verbal and nonverbal) that group members consider to be appropriate responses to given situations, or typical ways of acting. These rules are developed over time by the group members themselves, usually growing out of the group's perception of what works or what have been successful solutions to work problems or situations. They are seldom, if ever, written down (Coeling & Wilcox, 1988).

Each level of culture influences the other, although it is widely believed that the deeper level—values and beliefs—more often affects behaviors. For example, the underlying belief that patients are entitled to courteous, rapid response from caregivers is likely to influence how quickly caregivers respond to patient requests or needs. However, Kotter and Haskett emphasize that causality can flow in the other direction, too, with behavior and practices affecting values. Box 5-2 depicts Kotter and Heskett's two-level model of culture in an organization.

There is no culture unless there is a group, because culture is embedded in and owned by the group. Cultures are formed, over time, by groups that share problems and solutions, interpret the effects of solutions or actions, and see people come and go from the group. Culture is used by the group in many ways. Shared beliefs, thoughts, and behaviors make groups more efficient (not necessarily more effective) because they produce a consistency of expectation about how work is done and about priorities. Culture is used to orient newcomers to conform and thus to perpetuate cultural norms. Depending on the strength of the culture, this can contribute to stability of the group and its work.

It is simplistic to speak of an organizational culture as a single entity. Although an organization consists of a group of people, most organizations have multiple subunits or subgroups within them. These subgroups are likely to have their own subcultures, varying to greater or lesser extent from the overarching large organizational culture. Whether the subculture varies greatly or is consistent with the larger culture, at least at the values level, depends on the strength of the larger organizational culture.

Coeling and Wilcox (1988) suggest that understanding the culture at the work group level, rather than the larger organizational level, is easier because it is at the work group or work unit level that people discover, create, and use culture. They go on to report an interesting analysis of the differing cultures of two patient care units within the same hospital. There were differences between the units on nurses' pref-

erences and practices regarding the following areas:

- Working together: unit A preferred a group approach, with everyone helping each other until the work was done; unit B had a more independent ethic, expecting everyone to accomplish his or her own load.
- Competition: unit A avoided competition, describing themselves as a "family" and being unwilling to vote an award for "best" nurse; unit B allowed, even promoted, competition among themselves about who was the best nurse.
- Authority: unit A nurses avoided telling each other what to do, relying more on the manager to do that; unit B nurses used their personal authority to persuade others and recognized an internal staff hierarchy based on skills, knowledge, and assertiveness.
- Organization and use of time: unit A valued efficiency and organizational skills, identified priorities, and got people out on time; unit B placed a limited emphasis on efficiency and accepted that they might not get out on time because "we stay and do it all, and don't skip any patient needs."
- Following established standards: nurses on unit A preferred standardized guidelines and procedures to ensure consistency and quality; unit B nurses desired to use their own judgment regarding procedures and preferred individual decision making.
- Change: unit A nurses preferred stability to change and made use of certain kinds of classes but assumed no need of others; unit B nurses preferred changing situations and attended as many classes as possible "to avoid tunnel vision."

It is important to stress that although the cultures were observably different, and recognized as different by the nurses on the unit, one was not better or worse than the other; neither was right or wrong. Both units achieved similar high-quality patient care and patient satisfaction outcomes; they just did it differently in terms of working practices, beliefs, and norms. Further, the managers of both units had learned how to interview, select, and hire new nurses who would be comfortable and "fit" within the unit's specific culture, thus perpetuating the unique characteristics of each culture (Coeling & Wilcox, 1988).

Culture can prove to be both beneficial and detrimental. The very stability, consistency, and predictability accomplished via a strong organizational culture can be counterproductive when the strategic achievement needs of the organization are not met or supported by the organizational culture. In times of great change and turbulence, the "old" culture may make it difficult for an organization to be adaptive and creative.

Can Corporate Cultures Be Changed?

In the 1970s and 1980s, many American companies discovered, quite painfully, that they were no longer competitive in the world's marketplaces. Companies in the Asian rim, particularly Japan, were outproducing, outclassing, and outselling many American companies. As American companies began to scramble to recover and survive, many found that the very corporate cultures that had served them well were now contributing to their maladaptiveness.

The business literature described and then recommended multiple approaches to achieving rapid change in corporate culture. Organizations redefined their missions and developed value statements. Major programs and culture change efforts were rolled out, hoping to encourage employees to accept a new set of values and behaviors. Few of the efforts succeeded, which caused considerable disillusionment to corporate trainers and leaders.

Several researchers since have noted that the early corporate culture studies had culture control as the goal, seeing culture change as the "quick fix" to cure the ailing American corporation. Researchers discovered the power and tenacity of the organizational culture and the importance of attempting to understand it and its impact on organizational change. Now, rather than describing the change in corporate culture and values as something done to an organization, it is seen as something that must arise from within the organization. Accomplishing a deliberate change in corporate culture requires strong and visionary leadership from the top of the organization and is likely to take years. (For more on visionary leadership, see Chapter 9.)

HCOs, especially hospitals, are experiencing rapid, radical change as managed care and other reforms evolve (Nordstrom & Allen, 1987). Like other American corporations, many hospitals are finding that their "old" entrenched cultures impede their efforts to adapt to new challenges. "Hospitals are among the most discipline-fragmented of all organizations," report Tjosvold and Tjosvold (1995, p. 5). The various subcultures of professional groups, functional departments, and hospital units create multiple barriers to collaborative integration of care and services. The status of nurses and other health care providers as hospital employees and the designation of physicians as independent contractors have contributed to the traditional culture. The changing relationship between employers and knowledge workers gives promise of significant change in this traditional paradigm.

The Changing Employer/Employee Relationship

One of the powerful but not very visible values that has underpinned traditional corporate culture is the implied "contract" between the organization and its employees. Although rarely put into explicit words, millions of employees and thousands of organizations understood the implicit promise in place since the 1940s: lifetime job security in return for loyalty and hard work (Handy, 1990). The restructurings, downsizings, and other turbulent changes of the 1980s and early 1990s seemingly have ended that expectation. Philosophers discussing the change from the industrial age to the information age would say that such a contract would have to end, indeed could not survive, in a knowledge-based, performance-focused world. Yet the radical disruption of the "old" value has generated much distress, anger, and cynicism among American workers, including nurses and other health care professionals.

A "new" implied contract between organizations and employees is evolving. According to *Fortune* magazine (June, 1994, p. 44), it goes something like this:

> There will never be [guaranteed] job security. You will be employed by us as long as you add value to the organization, and you are continuously responsible for finding ways to add value. In return, you have the right to demand interesting and important work, the freedom and resources to perform it well, pay that reflects your contribution, and the experience and training needed to be employable here or elsewhere.

The authors go on to explain that this new approach requires companies to relinquish much of the control they have held over employees and give genuine authority to work teams. Companies must work hard to make themselves attractive places to work, because their most productive knowledge worker employees are mobile and in high demand. Employees become far more responsible for their work and their own careers. "No more paternalism," they say; "this is an adult-to-adult business deal."

Some sources see this change in the employment arrangement as part of a much larger evolution of corporate design, structure, and culture. They compare the large, traditional, slow-moving hierarchies with thousands of full-time employees to ocean liners: hard to steer, hard to turn, impossible to make nimble and quick. Moreover, they say, the old paradigm led to some serious entitlement mindsets in employees, in the corporate world, and in health care.

Entitlement is the attitude or belief that one gets something because one is owed it, because one is entitled to it. Bardwick (1991, p. 9), a psychologist, says, "When this rich nation stopped requiring performance as a condition for keeping a job or getting a raise, it created a widespread attitude of entitlement. Entitlement destroys motivation. It lowers productivity. In the long run, it crushes self-esteem." She goes on to describe many workers doing mediocre work but still expecting to get their regular raise and their next scheduled promotion. This corporate failure to hold people accountable for performance, for quality, has fostered a standard of "good enough," as in "this is good enough to get by."

Although agreeing that the standards and levels of performance are inadequate to achieve excellence in most organizations, Senge (1990) sees this as a failure of the corporation—not the worker. Traditional organizations with the command and control hierarchy have not asked for anything more, he says. Most have settled for compliance and never built the kind of organization, with the kind of corporate culture, that could elicit true commitment and full engagement of their work force.

Others agree with this assessment (Johns, 1996, p. 15):

> Behavior of employees in traditional organizations often reflects the characteristics assumed by management. Managers traditionally have regarded employees as reluctant to work. Because of this, they believe that employees must be closely controlled through immediate supervision and, if necessary, coerced because employees have little ambition, prefer to be directed, and want to avoid responsibility.

The Information Age organization will have to build a different kind of corporate culture, with different values. The structure of the new organization is smaller, with fewer full-time personnel, more contracted or outsourced specialized services, few departments, and more cross-functional or cross-professional work teams. These new companies (and many already exist) tend to invest more than average in research and development, training, education, and human resources. Ferocious competition forces them to innovate continuously, and they are engaged in providing a dazzling, ever-changing array of services (Toffler & Toffler, 1994). With the focus on innovation, greatly improved services, and enhanced achievement, there will be little room for "good enough" performance by workers. Extracontractual behavior, or working at a level above the minimum required for job maintenance, is becoming the norm.

More important than the structure are the values of the new organization. Innovation and transformational improvements require risk-taking behavior and new levels of commitment—not compliance. Organizational culture strongly affects the willingness of employees to engage in risk-taking behavior, which is the key to innovation. Finding and trying new ideas are full of risk, because not all new ideas or innovations are successful. How organizations regard persons who fail may be the most significant determinant of whether employees will take the risk of innovation. Some organizations regard the failure of seemingly good ideas as an inevitable cost of doing business and use failures as learning experiences. The innovator is regarded positively in spite of the lack of success. Other organizations, although claiming to be innovative, regard failed efforts as disasters and the would-be innovators as failures.

Trust is the cornerstone to build both commitment and risk-taking behavior, and sustained trust is closely linked with organizational performance. Johns (1996, p. 14) defines trust as "a

willingness to place oneself in a position of vulnerability with reliance upon someone or something to perform as expected." Trust, or the lack of trust, is an inherent element in the culture of any organization. An organization's character is determined, in great part, by the degree to which trust exists between leaders and employees. Trust appears as attitudes, beliefs, and behaviors. Trust, says Johns, is the glue that holds an organization together.

Organizations recognized as high trust organizations usually share some other characteristics. These include patterns of consistent, effective, and open communication; cooperation; accountability; and effective leadership.

A Change in Management Practice

The role of the manager or administrator is changing. In the Industrial Age organization, the primary role of the manager was control. Johns (1996) described the philosophy quite clearly in the last section: workers were believed to need close supervision, much direction, and tightly developed work rules and job descriptions. The manager supervised the work. Most managers were selected for their positions because they were the best, most skilled, or most knowledgeable at the work and could provide direction for the workers.

In a knowledge-based world, the workers often have more knowledge in a given field or area than the manager. Attempts to control or coerce not only are ineffective, but also often are counterproductive. Knowledge workers cannot be forced to think or create; caregivers cannot be forced to be compassionate. Further, knowledge workers tend to be in high demand and mobile. They have many options and feel little loyalty to a manager or organization that fails to recognize their contributions. When knowledge workers leave, they take their knowledge with them (Stewart, 1997). Somehow, then, the organization must find ways to persuade knowledge workers to use and share their knowledge voluntarily and in ways that serve the mission of the organization. The manager is key in these efforts.

Drucker succinctly sums up the evolution of the management role. After World War II, a manager was "someone who is responsible for the work of subordinates." Management was about rank, power, and bosses. For some, this definition is still cherished. However, the definition began to change to "one who is responsible for the performance of people." This is the usual current definition, but Drucker says this, also, is too narrow. The evolving definition, he says, is "one who is responsible for the application and performance of knowledge" (Drucker, 1993, p. 44). The manager accomplishes this by bringing people with varying knowledge together for joint performance.

Management, like any work, has its own tools and techniques: analytic tools, such as budgets and projections, and people-management skills, such as coaching, setting expectations, and encouragement; but the essence of management is to ensure performance, and the tools and techniques to accomplish this work are changing as the work world is changing. (For more on management and leadership, see Chapter 9.)

■ SUMMARY

Thinking about the emerging role of nurses as knowledge professionals working in sophisticated interdisciplinary teams can be exciting and challenging; it can also be somewhat intimidating, because these changes force rethinking long-held beliefs and assumptions. As Peter Senge would put it, this requires examining some powerful and entrenched mental models. It is probable that most nurses and other health care knowledge professionals will continue to be employed by or at least closely affiliated with an organization. The evolving employment "contract" discussed in this chapter can work well for health care knowledge workers.

They must be clear about what they have to "sell" in the more corporation-like health care marketplace: their knowledge, skill, judgment, and time. Both they and the HCO that employs them must learn not to waste any of these assets. Being successful will require commitment and self-discipline, because the knowledge professional is responsible for the quality of his or her own knowledge and skills. The habit of continual learning must be cultivated, because it is the nature of knowledge to change rapidly.

In addition to knowledge, skill, judgment, and time, the knowledge worker must have what DePree (1989) calls "a relationship" with his or her work. This means he or she must be willing to risk full commitment (not compliance) and must be accountable. It also means that he or she works with integrity and compassion. It means that he or she *cares.* Workers report that it is easier to stay committed, accountable, and caring when they can readily see the value of their work and recognize that their hard work makes a difference. Health care professionals have an advantage here, because the work they do every day makes an obvious impact on the lives and well-being of their patients.

The movement toward interdisciplinary practice will require that nurses, physicians, and other health care professionals expand their understanding and respect for each other's competence and potential contributions. The interdependency of real team members is one key to the effectiveness of the team itself. It is hard to trust and depend on a colleague if one's knowledge of that person's capability is limited.

Much of the literature on organizational change emphasizes renewing and reenergizing the core values of trust, integrity, and respect. This emphasis does not grow from altruism alone. Research has shown that organizations characterized by high trust and a focus on effectiveness, people, vision, and a long-term perspective on profit are more successful. Whereas leaders set the tone and direction for an organization, employees are key in developing and maintaining organizational cultures that are value centered and productive. That is true now, and it is likely to be true in the future.

The Information Age, with its emphasis on knowledge work, interdisciplinary collaboration, and accountability, holds great promise for nurses and other health care professionals. Success will require new levels of commitment, personal responsibility, and team skills. It will also require the ability to change. As DePree (1989, p. 100) points out, "In the end, it is important to remember that we cannot become what we need to be by remaining who we are."

■ KEY POINTS

- The emerging role of nurses as knowledge workers will require that they increasingly work as part of an interdisciplinary team.
- Working effectively in a team requires a change in some powerful and entrenched mental models and in some firmly held and often long-held beliefs.
- The contract between employee and employer has changed in recent years; this necessitates that nurses must be clear about what they have to "sell" in the more corporatized health care marketplace (e.g., their knowledge, skill, judgment, time). In addition, knowledge workers must have a "relationship" with their work, must be willing to risk full commitment, must be accountable, and must work with integrity and compassion.
- The movement toward interdisciplinary practice will require that nurses, physicians, and other health care professionals expand their understanding and respect for each other's competence and potential contributions.
- Organizations that are characterized by the core values of trust, integrity, and respect and have a focus on effectiveness, people, vision,

and a long-term perspective on profit are more successful than their counterparts that do not demonstrate these core values.

- The Information Age, with its emphasis on knowledge work, interdisciplinary collaboration, and accountability, holds considerable promise for those nurses who change, grow, continue learning, and are able to meet the challenge of the new workplace.

■ CRITICAL THINKING QUESTIONS

1. Pay careful attention to your environment, and describe at least 10 factors that support the thesis in this chapter that we are moving rapidly into an Information Age.

2. Think about the last job that you had. Were you a knowledge worker? If yes, in what ways was this true? If no, what would have needed to change for you to be a knowledge worker in that role?

3. Consider the teams that you observe in the clinical area in which you practice. Think of both a successful team and an unsuccessful team, using the characteristics presented in the chapter. Describe the successful team. What do you attribute to its success? Describe the unsuccessful team. What hindered its success? What would need to be changed to transform the unsuccessful team into one that is visibly successful? Is this possible?

4. Review the chapter in terms of what makes a team successful both in general and in health care. Describe the qualities that the person who leads the team would need to have. Is it likely the team leader would remain the same over time or change? If the team leader would change, at what intervals would this happen? What might lead to a change in team leadership?

5. Debate this statement: Nursing as a profession is diluted as a unique group when nurses function as part of an interdisciplinary team. Give the pros and cons.

■ REFERENCES

Bardwick, J.M. (1991). *Danger in the comfort zone.* New York: American Management Association.

Coeling, H.V.E., & Wilcox, J.R. (1988). Understanding organization culture: A key to management decision-making. *JONA, 19*(11), 16-23.

DePree, M. (1989). *Leadership is an art.* New York: Dell Publishing.

Drucker, P.F. (1992, September-October). The new society of organizations. *Harvard Business Review.*

Drucker, P.F. (1993). *Post capitalist society.* New York: Harper Business Publishers.

Drucker, P.F. (1994, November). The age of social transformation. *Atlantic Monthly.*

Fisher, K., & Fisher, M.D. (1998). The distributed mind: Achieving high performance through the collective intelligence of knowledge work teams. New York: AMACOM (American Management Association).

Handy, C. (1990). *The age of unreason.* Boston: Harvard Business School Press.

Hedelt, A., & Holden, M. (Eds.). (1995). *Guide for interdisciplinary practice: A report of the interdisciplinary practice task force.* Charlottesville, Va.: University of Virginia Division of Patient Care Services.

Hirshhorn, L., & Gilmore, T. (1992, May-June). The new boundaries of the "boundaryless" company. *Harvard Business Review,* pp. 104-115.

Johns, J. (1996). Trust: Key to acculturation in corporatized health care environments. *Nursing Administration Quarterly, 20*(2), 13-24.

Katzenbach, J.R., & Smith, D. (1993). *The wisdom of teams: Creating the high-performance organization.* Boston: Harvard Business School Press.

Kotter, J.P., & Heskett, J.L. (1992). *Corporate culture and performance.* New York: The Free Press.

Mohrman, S.A., Cohen S.G., & Mohrman, A.M. (1995). *Designing team-based organizations: New forms for knowledge work.* San Francisco: Jossey-Bass Publishers.

The new deal: What companies and employees owe one another (1994, June 13). *Fortune.*

Nordstrom, R.D., & Allen, B.H. (1987). Cultural change versus behavioral change. *Health Care Manage Review, 12*(2), 43-49.

Robbins, H., & Finley, M. (1995). *Why teams don't work: What goes wrong and how to make it right.* Princeton, N.J.: Petersons/Pacesetter Books.

Schweikhart, S.B., & Smith-Daniels, V. (1996). Reengineering the work of caregivers: Role redefinition, team structures, and organizational redesign. *Hospital & Health Services Administration, 41*(1), 19-36.

Senge, P.M. (1990). *The fifth discipline: The art and practice of the learning organization.* New York: Doubleday Publishers.

Sorrells-Jones, J. (1997). The challenge of making it real: Interdisciplinary practice in a "seamless" organization. *Nursing Administration Quarterly, 21*(2), 20-30.

Stewart, T.A. (1997). *Intellectual capital: The new wealth of organizations.* New York: Bantam Doubleday Dell Publishing Group.

Toffler, A., & Toffler, H. (1994). *Creating a new civilization: The politics of the third wave.* Atlanta: Turner Publishing Co.

Tjosvold, D., & Tjosvold, M. (1995). Cross-functional teamwork: The challenge of involving professionals. In Beyerlein, M., Johnson, D., & Beyerlein, S.T. (Eds.). *Advances in interdisciplinary studies of work teams.* Greenwich, Conn.: JAI Press.

Managing Change

Jeanette Lancaster

INTRODUCTION

Managing change is crucial to the survival of every staff nurse, manager, teacher, and administrator in health care today. Many people say the profession of nursing is changing, and the changes are not for the best. However, the reality is that change is occurring rapidly in health care; organizations are being restructured, purchased or sold, reengineered, and re-formed. Nurses must learn about change and be able to lead, manage, and participate in the process of change (Zukowski, 1995).

The drivers or influencers of change in health care are multiple and complex; a primary driver is the imperative to reduce costs. Qualifications are being set for what will be reimbursed, and limits are being set on the actual level of reimbursement. Other change drivers are the availability of sophisticated technology and the need for large amounts of information. In the changing reimbursement system, the time used by all health care providers, including nurses, in delivering care has become crucial because "time is money" and it costs to pay skilled people to provide effective care. Technology is often seen as a way to expand the talent and time of nurses, physicians, and other skilled professionals. However, new, expanded, and upgraded tech-

nology requires users to learn, practice, and become proficient in its use even though they may have limited time to spend on practicing and mastering the technology.

Information and the need for more of it, to have it faster, and to have it in any location also have accelerated the rate of change. There are almost no places today where people can be free from receiving and sending information. With the use of beepers, cellular telephones, voice mail, satellite and fiber-optic broadcasting, electronic mail, faxes, and overnight mail delivery, the "ends of the earth" are reachable. Better and more rapidly informed people accelerate the anticipation that change can occur quickly.

Major change efforts have enabled some organizations to adapt effectively to shifting conditions, thereby improving their competitive standing and positioning them for a much better future. In contrast, other organizations have been unable to respond in a timely, thoughtful, market-driven way, and they have wasted resources, disrupted the lives of their employees, and seen a decrease or demise of their usefulness.

Health care organizations (HCOs) today have two choices in relation to change. They can in-

149

organizations that are more nimble and able to change. However, successful innovation or change is not a random, haphazard effort. Instead, innovation must be managed through a systematic, organized process called *planned change* (Manion, 1993).

Nurses are challenged to respond to change in a thoughtful, proactive, interactive, and collaborative way. Nurses have some useful skills for the process of planned change. First, the nursing process is a systematic problem-solving approach that is consistent with the planning of change. Second, nurses are taught in school and experience in practice the need to work effectively with others (i.e., to be inclusive and bring others in rather than exclusive and try to work alone). People who must now be included in this changing health care environment include other members of the multidisciplinary health care team, payers (i.e., those who fund health care such as insurers or managed care companies), families, the people being served, as well as groups such as philanthropic organizations, health care associations, and regulators. During times of rapid change, roles, relationships, processes, and partnerships change.

Some of the most effective change efforts in nursing were developed by nurses who under-

ganization. In HCOs, nurses often realize that quality care is central to the organization's effectiveness. Nurses are at the point of patient care that is the business of health care; they are also generalists with a good, broad knowledge of the needs of patients, families, organizations, and communities. They may, however, not know how to manage change. This chapter provides information to assist the nurse serving in the role of change leader or change manager.

Change stimulates a range of responses in people, and these responses may be proactive or reactive, stimulating or frightening, creative or confining. Rarely are people neutral to change. Change can provide opportunities for growth, survival, extinction, or retrenchment. The environment for change can be exciting and energizing, encouraging risk taking and calling for creativity and innovation. Effective nurse leaders promote successful change processes that enable their organizations to grow and their employees to feel valued and able to influence the change process. They do this by understanding the change process; by helping others see change as an exciting opportunity; and by communicating effectively throughout the process (Kerfoot, 1996).

OBJECTIVES

After reading this chapter, you will be able to:

1. Define at least five types of change
2. Design a systematic process of planned change
3. Evaluate a situation that requires change and develop a plan for managing the change
4. Consider an individual whom you have known to be charged with making a signifi-

cant change and evaluate the effectiveness of the change agent's skills
5. Analyze the role that communication plays in a systematic change process
6. Analyze at least seven typical responses to change, and describe effective ways of dealing with the negatively perceived responses

■ TYPES OF CHANGE

Change can be described in a variety of ways, including the use of polarities such as haphazard versus planned. *Haphazard* change is often random with no advance preparation, in contrast to *planned* change, which results from deliberate and conscious actions taken to adjust the way a system functions (Bennis et al., 1976). Similarly, change can be seen as being on a continuum ranging from developmental through spontaneous and on to planned change. *Coercive* change is characterized by nonmutual goal setting, unbalanced distribution of power, and deliberate intention on one side only. *Developmental* change occurs through the natural growth of people, groups, or organizations. In general, developmental changes tend to be sequential, with one phase naturally leading into another in a more or less orderly fashion. *Spontaneous* or *natural* change occurs in response to natural, uncontrollable events outside the system being affected. This type of change is unpredictable and often unexpected; thus planning is typically not possible.

Planned change is intentional and thought out, occurs over time, and includes mutual goal setting, an equal power distribution, and deliberation. It is easier to manage and positively use planned change rather than change that happens in the course of human development (developmental) or without warning (haphazard or spontaneous) or change that is coercive and in which power is unequally divided among participants. For this reason, nurses are well served when they understand the process of planned change and become skilled in managing the change process.

■ PROCESS OF PLANNED CHANGE

The process of planned change is complex because of the many interacting people, factors, and forces involved. In general, planned change is a process whereby new ideas are created or developed (invention), communicated to all participants (diffusion), and either adopted or rejected (consequences). Planned change, like the nursing process, requires a carefully thought-out effort on the part of an individual or group. Problem solving, decision making, critical thinking, astute assessment, and the effective use of interpersonal skills, including communication, collaboration, negotiation, and persuasion, are key in planning change. Before looking at the strategies for making change, it is useful to summarize selected change theories. The works of Lewin, Lippitt, and Rogers continue to influence current views of change and the process of making change.

Key terms	
Term	**Definition**
Haphazard change	Random, with no advance preparation (i.e., "things just happen")
Developmental change	Natural growth of people, groups, organizations (i.e., as children grow and develop)
Spontaneous change	A response to natural, uncontrollable external events (e.g., a fire)
Coercive change	Nonmutal goal setting, unbalanced power (i.e., a person is told to do something)
Planned change	Intentional, thought-out, deliberate process with equal power distribution among participants

Lewin's Theory

The origin of classic change theory is credited to Lewin (1951), who described three steps in the change process: unfreezing, moving to a new level, and refreezing. *Unfreezing* is recognizing that a problem exists; it is the "thawing out" of the old way of looking at and doing things. During this phase, participants see the need for change. This may be a time of considerable stress, especially if change managers or facilitators use techniques such as threats and coercion, since they increase fear and uncertainty. The aim of planned change is to motivate participants to become engaged in the process of change because they see the need rather than because they are afraid not to participate.

In the second phase of Lewin's change cycle, participants *move to a new level* of behavior. They gather sufficient information to know that change is needed and begin to diagnose the problem and generate a solution by examining a variety of options. The change manager needs to gain the confidence of the participants so they will listen, offer ideas, examine options, and agree that change is needed. Considerable information is usually gathered at this time so many options can be examined. This is the restructuring stage of change that many organizations go through.

Refreezing is the stage in the change cycle when the newly acquired behavior is integrated into the participants' personal ties and way of doing things. The new behaviors should be supported and nurtured through continuous or intermittent reinforcement. That is, the behavior is either rewarded every time it occurs (continuous reinforcement) or periodically reinforced (intermittent reinforcement); the latter is generally more realistic given the demands on people's time and attention.

Lewin also proposed a force-field analysis framework for looking at problem solving and change. He described driving and restraining forces that either support or interfere with the process of change. *Driving forces* move people in the direction desired by the change agent. In contrast, *restraining forces* hamper the change cycle. When the driving and restraining forces are equal, the status quo is maintained. Change occurs when one set of forces outweighs the other. In making change, it is important to identify the driving and restraining forces, which may be people (who oppose or support), time, financial constraints, knowledge, habits, or traditions. Some of the current driving or motivating factors in health care changes are capitation, changes in the amount and types of reimbursement, increasing patient acuity, shorter hospital

Key terms	
Term	**Definition**
Unfreezing	"Thawing out"; awareness that a problem exists
Move to new level	Gather information, diagnose problem, examine options, and begin to move from status quo
Refreezing	Incorporation of new behavior into actions
Continuous reinforcement	Rewarding behavior every time it occurs
Intermittent reinforcement	Periodic reinforcement of behavior
Driving forces	Those that move people toward the change
Restraining forces	Those that hamper the change process

stays, managed care, and the changing staffing mixes found in some agencies.

Rogers' Theory

Planned-change theory has been discussed by many writers using Lewin's theory as a foundation. Rogers (1962) expanded on Lewin's three phases of change by emphasizing both the background of the people participating in the change process and the environment in which the change takes place. Rogers described five phases in the change cycle: awareness, interest, evaluation, trial, and adoption.

Essentially Rogers believed that the process of adopting any change was more complex than the three steps discussed by Lewin. Specifically, each participant in the change process could initially accept the change or reject it. In addition, although the change might initially be accepted, it could later be discontinued; or it could initially be rejected and later adopted. Rogers called attention to the fluid and sometimes reversible characteristics involved in change. The relationship between Rogers' five phases and Lewin's three phases is depicted in Figure 6-1.

Rogers said that the effectiveness of change depended on whether the participants were keenly interested in the innovation (the change) and had a commitment to work toward implementing it. Five factors were cited by Rogers and Shoemaker (1971) as determinants of successful planned change. These factors—relative advantage, compatibility, complexity, divisibility (trial-ability), and communicability (observability)—have stood the test of time and are still considered useful. They are discussed later when the essential elements in the diffusion of a new idea are presented.

Lippitt's Theory

Lippitt (1973, p. 37) defined change as "any planned or unplanned alteration of the status quo in an organism, situation, or process" and planned change as "an intended, designed, or purposive attempt by an individual, group, organization, or larger social system to influence directly the status quo or itself, another organism, or a situation." Lippitt contended that no one can escape change: the question is "How do people handle change?" The key to dealing with change is to develop a thorough and carefully thought-out strategy for intervention. To do this, Lippitt (1973, p. 52) identified seven stages in the change process: diagnosis of the problem, assessment of the motivation and capacity for change, assessment of the change agent's motivation and resources, the selection of progressive change objectives, choosing an appropriate

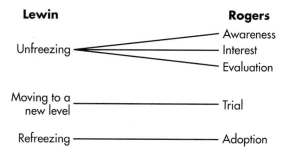

Figure 6-1 ■ **Comparison between Rogers' and Lewin's phases of change.** (Data from Rogers, E. [1962]. *Diffusion of innovations.* New York: Free Press of Glencoe; Lewin, K. [1951]. *Field theory in social science.* New York: Harper & Row.)

role for the change agent, maintenance of the change once it has been started, and termination of a helping relationship. Figure 6-2 compares Lippitt's phases of change and those of Lewin. Lippitt's stages are consistent with the steps in the nursing process.

Stage 1: Diagnosis of the Problem Diagnosis of the problem requires that participants keep an open mind and avoid jumping to conclusions before considering all possible causes. Frequently participants think they know what is wrong and thus omit the critical first step of data collection and problem identification. Ideally all who will be involved in the change process or affected by the change should be included at this time, kept informed, and encouraged to raise questions and make suggestions. The more information the change manager has, the more likely an accurate assessment and problem identification will be made. Key people, especially those with considerable power and authority in the organization, need to be involved in the change process as early as possible. Each participant is responsible for being informed about the issues, such as learning why capitation and managed care are being used.

Stage 2: Assessment of the Motivation and Capacity for Change Change seldom comes easily; on the contrary, successful planned change generally involves considerable

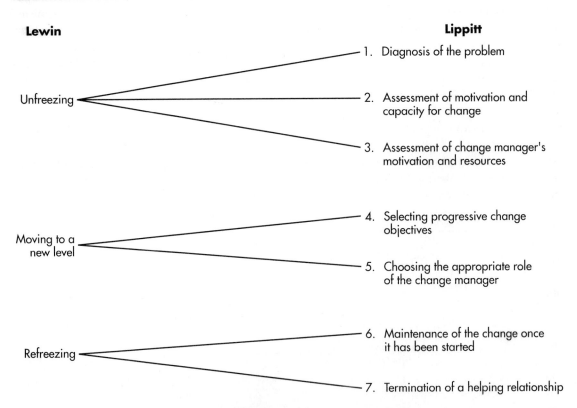

Figure 6-2 ■ Comparison between Lewin's and Lippitt's change cycles. (From Lewin, K. [1951]. *Field theory in social science.* New York: Harper & Row; Lippitt, G.L. [1973]. *Visualizing change: Model building and the change process.* La Jolla, Calif.: University Associates.)

hard work and commitment to the project. During this stage, both the people involved and the environment need to be assessed to identify the resources, constraints, and change facilitators and supporters. Because the majority of nursing practice takes place in some type of agency or institution, the organizational structure should be examined to determine whether the rules, policies, norms, and people involved will help or hinder the change process. The availability or limitations of financial resources are considered. Can the institution afford to became involved in the project? Are those who control policies, budget, and personnel well informed and supportive of the change? During stage 2, possible solutions are identified and prioritized by listing the pros and cons of each one.

Stage 3: Assessment of the Change Manager's Motivation and Resources This stage requires a great deal of honest and critical self-assessment on the part of the change manager. The degree to which the change manager is trusted and respected within the organization will influence acceptance of the idea. For example, if many of the change manager's ideas are viewed as radical, proposals for change are likely to be viewed with skepticism, especially by more conservative members of the establishment. If more than one person is responsible for introducing the change, they need to have similar goals, objectives, and styles of leadership so that all involved receive consistent messages about the project.

Stage 4: Selection of Progressive Change Objectives Once the problem is diagnosed and the resources and constraints are listed, a step-by-step strategy is developed for implementing the change. This planning stage must be specific as to the steps to be taken, by whom, and when.. Deadlines are essential, and a trial period can be instituted at this time. If a trial period is used, careful and critical evaluation is necessary to determine the effectiveness of the change strategy. Goals can be reevaluated based on the

trial experience, and alterations in the plan can be devised.

Stage 5: Choosing the Appropriate Change Manager Role The change manager may choose to be an expert role model, catalyst, teacher, or group leader. He or she may actively gather information and demonstrate new procedures or may serve more as a motivator for others who will actually implement the project. The change process is more effective if both the participants and the change manager have similar conceptions of the change manager's role. Lack of congruence between role perceptions breeds discontent and uncertainty, in that few people's expectations of one another are met.

Stage 6: Maintenance of the Change Once a change has been instituted, the interest and enthusiasm seen during the developmental phase may wane, and old behaviors may emerge. Once the change is implemented, communication should be kept open so that questions, concerns, and ideas can be addressed to provide frequent reports about the change to managerial personnel as well as participants. When the change has been successfully instituted, plans must be made for diffusion of information, since other people in the organization may want to become involved in a similar project. Members of the original change group may serve as resource people to other work units, keeping in mind that the actual design of a change project may require modification to meet the unique needs of a different setting. Also, each setting has its own personality and structure that may necessitate modification of the original plan.

Stage 7: Termination of the Helping Relationship During the termination stage the change manager, following a prescribed plan, withdraws from the situation. This should be accomplished gradually so that participants can increasingly assume more responsibility for the maintenance functions. The change manager may continue to serve as a consultant or resource person but should actively encourage autonomy on the part of the change implementers.

· · ·

Lippitt's model for planned change is a problem-solving approach that is consistent with the components of the nursing process. This model points out that successful change efforts take thoughtful planning. Time spent on this planning generally pays off in that the outcome is more likely to be positive if many variables are considered early in the process. The success of planned change depends not only on the steps used, but also on how clearly and in what manner the ideas are explained to the involved parties. There is a systematic process for diffusing new ideas that can be used by change managers to move the process forward.

Diffusion of New Ideas

The main elements in the diffusion of new ideas include the *innovation* itself, which is communicated through a variety of *channels* over *time* and among designated *participants* (adopters or rejecters). Simply stated, an innovation is brought to a receptive social (patient) system by a change agent or manager. Participants tend to evaluate an innovation according to five characteristics: relative advantage, compatibility, complexity, trialability, and observability (Rogers & Shoemaker, 1971, p. 22).

Characteristics of Innovation

1. *Relative advantage* is the degree to which the new idea is considered superior to the old one. Although the degree of relative advantage may be measured in economic terms, it is often judged by social factors, convenience, time involvement, and general satisfaction with the idea. The participants' perception of the advantage is more critical to its adoption than the actual, objective advantage. The greater the perceived relative advantage, the more rapid the adoption.

2. *Compatibility* refers to the degree of congruence between the innovation and existing values, habits, past experiences, and needs of the participants. The adoption of an incompatible innovation is slow because it often requires the prior adoption of a new set of values and attitudes. Because compatible ideas are more familiar, they tend to be less threatening and thus more readily accepted.

3. *Complexity* describes the amount of difficulty that participants have in understanding and subsequently using the innovation. Complexity of the innovation and adoption vary inversely. Often participants are embarrassed to acknowledge that they do not understand the process so they refuse to participate lest their lack of understanding becomes widely known. Astute observation by the change manager is important to assess receptivity to ideas on a continuing basis.

4. *Trialability* is the degree to which the new idea can be pretested or tried on a limited basis. New ideas that can be tried on a small-scale basis are less frightening than massive changes and are more likely to be accepted. An innovation that can be pretested generally presents less risk, since failure or difficulties are less obvious.

5. *Observability* refers to how visible the innovation is to participants and onlookers. The easier it is for an individual to see the results of an innovation, the more likely its adoption will be.

Communication Channels　Communication is the process by which messages are sent from a source to a receiver. Speaking from the perspective of change, *source* refers to the person initiating change who introduces the new idea, approach, or procedure and communicates it in the form of a message through a predetermined channel to the intended participants in the process (Figure 6-3).

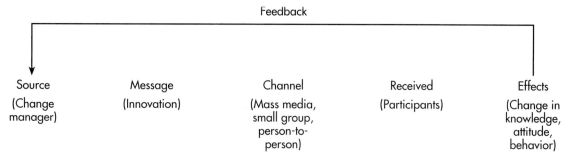

Feedback

Source	Message	Channel	Received	Effects
(Change manager)	(Innovation)	(Mass media, small group, person-to-person)	(Participants)	(Change in knowledge, attitude, behavior)

Figure 6-3 ▪ Communication process for change.

The communication channel chosen influences whether the innovation or change will be accepted. The following factors influence the selection of a channel for the communication:

1. The purpose of the message
2. The characteristics of the audience to whom the message is being sent
   • The flexibility and general receptiveness of the group
   • The size of the audience: that is, if the audience is large and the goal is to inform them, the mass media are effective and rapid; if the audience is small and the objective is to persuade them, an interpersonal or small-group approach can be used
3. The degree of ambiguity and controversy surrounding the innovation
4. The degree of institutional support for the innovation: if the change will be mandated regardless of participant response, an announcement can be used, assuming acceptance by participants; however, if the change is mandated and negative feelings abound, small-group discussion works best
5. The degree of urgency for the change
6. The personality of the organization, including what usually works best and what the established lines and channels of communication are

Timing Timing is critical in the successful introduction of change. A good idea at the wrong time (e.g., when participants are tired, upset, angry, or thinking about other more pressing ideas) is generally greeted with little enthusiasm. An effective change facilitator critically assesses whether A or B is the best solution at a given time and in a particular environment. It is important to remember that change happens slowly and innovations take time for their introduction, acceptance, and implementation. Generally, the more people involved, the more complex the innovation; and the greater the incompatibility with past procedures, the more time that will be needed for successful change to occur.

The process of change, then, includes a problem-solving process as well as attention to the method of communication used and the timing. The person introducing change needs also to recognize general patterns of people responding to the change and appreciate that responses to innovations can vary from enthusiastic acceptance to active rejection. It is important to recognize how people typically react to change in terms of their participation or adoption of the change.

Categories of Adopters Individual responses to change are described according to six categories of adopters that form a continuum from eager participation (innovators) to rejection (Rogers & Shoemaker, 1971, p. 357):

1. *Innovators.* These people are the pacesetters. They are venturesome, curious, eager for new experiences, and enthusiastic. They are often considered radical and disruptive by colleagues but frequently bring great change, albeit often amid controversy, to an organization.

2. *Early adopters.* This group moderates their enthusiasm and vigor in introducing an idea according to the readiness of the organization. These individuals tend to be well-established members of the group who are often sought out as advisors. Because the early adopters prefer to maintain esteem within the group, they usually do not introduce highly radical or controversial ideas.

3. *Early-majority adopters.* Accepting innovation just before the mass of participants do so, the early-majority adopters are followers with deliberate willingness and dedication to the innovation, but they rarely lead. This group generally constitutes an effective support system for change.

4. *Late-majority adopters.* For this group adoption is an economic necessity. They view the change with skepticism and, although they may not be active dissidents, they cannot be counted on for support.

5. *Laggards.* Members of this category tend to be socially isolated within the organization. Suspicious of change, they may discourage others from participating by their attitude of general negativism.

6. *Rejecters.* Members of this group openly reject the innovation and actively encourage others to do so.

Groups typically will have a mixture of people who respond to change in these six ways. The balance is important, and it is helpful to have several early and early-majority adopters who will promote the change.

Change rarely occurs in isolation; it has multiple effects on the individuals and organizations involved. There is often a "domino effect," with one change leading to other, and at times unexpected, outcomes. To deal with potential "ripplelike" or "snowball" effects of change, it is important to know what strategies are effective when making change.

■ **STRATEGIES FOR MAKING CHANGE**

Changes in organizations can occur at three different levels: changing the individuals working in the organization, changing the organizational structure and systems, and changing the interpersonal style of the organization (Goodstein & Burke, 1991). Regardless of the level of the organization in which the change occurs, the strategies used have common characteristics.

The first requirement for successful change is to have a clear *vision* of what the change will look like. This vision should be one that can be stated simply and will evoke a mental image for the listener. For example, two classic examples are John F. Kennedy's vision of "putting a man on the moon before the end of this decade" and Bill Gate's statement of a "computer in every home" as the mission statement for Microsoft. Unless there is a clear, short, easy-to-comprehend, and inspiring vision, the change will get off course as people set off on different paths depending on their interpretation of the goal (Cauthorne-Lindstrom & Tracy, 1992). Moreover, the person with the vision must be able to sell it to others.

Creating a culture that supports trust is crucial. Specifically, change is typically better accepted when people value and trust one another and feel that they themselves have value. People are more willing to take risks in a trusting environment than if the setting is characterized by anger, mistrust, and bitterness. Whatever the atmosphere is when the change is planned, it must be addressed openly and in an honest, straightforward manner.

B O X   6 - 1

Requirements for Successful Change

- Vision of what the change will look like
- An organizational culture in which people value and trust one another
- Communication system that is clear, concise, and frequent and that uses appropriate mechanisms
- Involvement of the right people

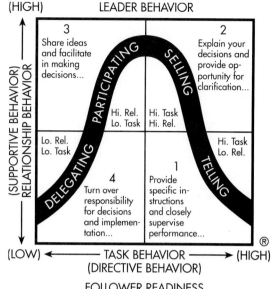

Figure 6-4 ■ Situational leadership model. (From Hersey, P. [1996]. *The management of organizational behavior utilizing human resources* [7th ed.]. Escondido, Calif.: Center for Leadership Studies.)

Communication is the backbone of effective change. Everyone must be kept informed to decrease the potential for rumor and misinformation. The more people know about a situation, the better able they are to visualize the future, which reduces anxiety and fear (Kerfoot, 1996). Failure to communicate clearly and adequately what changes are to be made and the effects they will have on people will intensify fear. According to Silber (1993, p. 61), one-way (top-down) communication is insufficient and produces ambiguity because people do not know what is going on so they tend to "fill in the blanks" (Box 6-1).

Questions to ask early in the change process to improve communication while also involving more people in the process and building the vision for change are as follows (Doerge & Hagenow, 1995, p. 32):

1. What is going right?
2. What could be better?
3. If you were in charge, what would you do?

People must be kept *involved* in the process. The change may be designed in part by a steering group, but as soon as possible the group must involve people at all levels of the organization. Involvement leads to support and advocacy. Planned change is systematic and requires that its management be carefully designed, implemented, and evaluated (Figure 6-4).

Managing Change

Managing change has become a core competence that today's nursing managers must have. Ineffectively implementing change is expensive in the time involved and the emotions expended as people try to deal with the process and its consequences. Too often in HCOs, participants are informed of the change that will occur and affect them after plans have been made and the changes are ready to be implemented. People want to learn about possible change from their frontline supervisors, who often serve as opinion leaders for the group (Kerfoot, 1996). Bolton et al. (1992) described 10 steps for managing organizational change based

B O X   6 - 2

Steps for Managing Organizational Change

STEP 1: Define the Project Goals. Conduct a needs assessment by interviewing key people; examine documents and written materials already developed; and consistently keep an eye on the shared vision for the future.

STEP 2: Make Sure Project Goal(s) Are Congruent with the Organization's Strategic Plan. When the fit is good, participants will be more willing to join in.

STEP 3: Decide Who Will Lead the Project. The leader must communicate the vision effectively to people at all levels of the organization and coach, mentor, listen, and support work groups and their leaders.

STEP 4: Obtain Commitment From Key Stakeholders who come from all levels of the organization.

STEP 5: Identify Specific Measurable Objectives that provide a ready description of the effects of the change.

STEP 6: Establish Work Groups to Address Objectives. These groups must fit the tasks at hand and be able to communicate with one another and also negotiate and resolve their differences.

STEP 7: Use a Patient Care Focus to Involve Individuals From All Levels of the Organization. The world of health care is a world of teams, partnerships, and collaboration; thus the involvement should be both from all levels of the organization and from the various groups of key people at each level. These groups should reflect the stakeholders, be flexible, and able to deal with new issues and needs as they emerge.

STEP 8: Build on Past Efforts to Avoid "Reinventing the Wheel." Draw upon the past work of group members; don't redo what has already been done in a different setting, time, or context.

STEP 9: Educate Work Groups to the "Interactive Planning" Process. Work group leaders need ongoing training in change management.

STEP 10: Develop a Comprehensive, Ongoing Communication Plan. Think ahead about what people need to know; how, when, and who should convey the information; and what reactions might be.

From Bolton, L.B., Aydin, C., Popolow, G., & Ramseyer, J. (1992, June). *Journal of Nursing Administration, 22,* 14-20.

on their work at Cedars-Sinai Medical Center in Los Angeles (Box 6-2).

Before change can take place, members of the organization must become dissatisfied (the unfreezing) with how things are going. The person managing the change must have a vision of where the process needs to go and the best options for getting there. As stated, planned change is not instantaneous and cannot simply be announced. The process for change requires an orderly sequence of events in which people are engaged in the change process and commit to both the process and the direction in which the change is going. Coalitions must be formed to support change, and this may be through task

forces, key committees, or other groups that bond people to the process and make them feel that they are creating the change.

Kotter (1995) talks about leading change from the perspective of understanding why transformation efforts fail. He contends that the "change process goes through a series of phases that, in total, usually require a considerable length of time" (Kotter, 1995, p. 59). Box 6-3 identifies the eight steps to transforming an organization.

Kotter (1995) also points out that most people underestimate the amount of effort required for large-scale change. It is important to energize people and create excitement for the

B O X 6 - 3

Steps to Transforming Your Organization

1. *Establish a sense of urgency:* avoid high complacency levels.
2. *Form a powerful guiding coalition:* teams transform organizations.
3. *Create a vision:* direct, align, and inspire the people.
4. *Communicate the vision:* use every communication tool available.
5. *Empowers others to act:* use a team effort.
6. *Plan for and create short-term wins:* plan for, create, and recognize the wins.
7. *Consolidate improvements and produce more change:* hire, promote, and develop people to implement the vision.
8. *Institutionalize new approaches:* develop ways to ensure succession.

Data from Kotter, J.P. (1995, March-April). *Harvard Business Review,* pp. 60-67; Kotter, J.P. (1996). *Leading change.* Boston: Harvard Business School Press.

change or the participants become complacent. Without a sense of urgency, people will not make needed sacrifices; instead, they will hold onto the status quo. It takes a team to make change happen. No matter how much enthusiasm there is for change in the beginning, countervailing forces emerge and without a guiding coalition or team, the project is in trouble. Making effective change happen and last is not the work of a soloist but rather an orchestra or at least a quartet!

The team, of course, must have a guiding vision to succeed at getting others to join in, stay on, and become some of the "movers for change." The vision must be clear, crisp, and understandable. As Kotter (1995, p. 8) says, "A useful rule of thumb: Whenever you cannot describe the vision driving a change initiative in 5 minutes or less and get a reaction that signifies

both understanding and interest, you are in for trouble." A successful team has four qualities: open and effective communication; involvement of members; clearly defined goals; and trust among members (Antai-Otong, 1997, p. 48). These qualities affect how teams and their members manage and respond to change.

■ RESPONSES TO CHANGE

Human forces operate to either support or resist change. People try to maintain their equilibrium or balance by resisting new things and ways of behaving. The changes currently affecting the health care system seem to come from one of two categories: those that are imposed and are not a matter of choice and those that are initiated through a matter of choice (Miller, 1988, p. 37). To understand how people respond to change and why they might resist, it is useful to cite several characteristics of people. First, people will stay with an organization and be productive as long as the organization meets most or all their real or perceived needs. Second, people do things for only one of two reasons—to gain something or to keep from losing something. Third, a person is motivated first to take care of that which hurts the most. Fourth, the single most significant person in people's lives is the person who affirms them the most. And last, a person will accept change from someone seen as significant much more often than from one seen as indifferent to him or her (Miller, 1988, p. 38).

Connor (1992) says there are three fundamental aspects to a structured approach to change. First is *pain management* or "the concentrated orchestration of information to lead people to believe that the price for the status quo is significantly higher than the price for transition" (Connor, 1992, p. 34). The second element is called *remedy selling* and is the process of suggesting remedies that can pull people toward a desired state. Pain management precedes putting remedies into effect. The third element is an *implementation plan,* and this plan should include four key factors:

- Develop commitment among those sponsoring the change.
- Identify and deal with resistance.
- Orchestrate a fit between the organization's culture and the change.
- Adequately prepare the change managers for the task of leading the change process.

Change may threaten a person's status in the organization as well as his or her power, opportunities to pursue future goals, level of security, and comfort. Major change involves a shift in power, and this type of shift is never automatic or greeted with enthusiasm by all involved. Also, changing to a new way of working or a new structure within the organization means that some competencies that have served people well in the past may become obsolete and new ones will be necessary. Major organizational change typically requires some reassignments of people, changes in titles, and changes in reporting relationships and may involve alterations in compensation and other forms of reward. People may experience an alteration or loss of identify that is frightening and typically something they will try hard to avoid. For these reasons, virtually all change meets some degree of resistance.

Resistance to Change

Resistance is often one of two types: resistance because of the nature of the proposed change and resistance resulting from misconceptions and inaccurate information about what the change will mean. The human side of change is not logical, rational, or reasonable. It involves people's feelings, including fear, uncertainty, doubt, threat, comfort with the ways things are, and insecurity. As Iacovini (1993, p. 66) says, "For many, the experience [of change] is like standing at the edge of a chasm and being challenged to jump to the other side—with nothing in between but fog." People do not ask how far it is to the other side; instead, they feel trapped.

It is essential to remember that fear of moving out of one's comfort zone and readily embracing the change is hard for many. People do not resist merely to be obstructive and difficult. Managers and change agents can employ some useful strategies to enable participants to "let go" (Box 6-4).

Sometimes people get stuck in the middle of the change. They reach an impasse, and this can be frustrating to their colleagues and the organization. When an impasse is reached, the following actions can be taken to help the person or group move beyond this:

- Take time to think about where things stand.
- Encourage creative thinking, and tolerate diversity of people and ideas.
- Encourage reminiscing about the past and thinking about the future.

B O X   6 - 4

Strategies to Assist People to Engage in Change

- Give visible support.
- Look for those stable areas that are not changing.
- Provide opportunities for people to interact informally.
- Build on the past instead of discounting the past.
- Be sensitive to people at different stages in making change.
- Help people identify what they are holding onto and why.
- Support people in letting go.
- Give information constantly.
- Provide a safety net when people make mistakes.

From Iacovini, J. (1993, January). *Training & Development,* pp. 65-68.

- Let people express their feelings.
- Encourage exploration of new ideas.

An impasse presents an opportunity for all participants to look at their roles, where they have been, where they are going, and if they should still be going down that path.

It is important that nurses who function as change agents recognize that the degree of resistance will typically depend on the answers to the following questions:

1. How great is the change? How much does it deviate from the current norm of expectations?
2. How much emotional investment by the participants is there in the "old way"?
3. To what degree and in what manner are the people involved threatened? Most people when confronted with change ask themselves either consciously or subconsciously the following set of questions (Stevens, 1975, p. 24):
   - Will the change alter my role by either increasing or decreasing my power or status?
   - Will this change affect the activities or content of my job?
   - Will my freedom to perform my job be altered? How will my range of choices be affected?
   - Can I expect to be inconvenienced by this innovation?
   - How will my financial status be affected?
   - Exactly what advantages or disadvantages can I expect from this change?
4. How reasonable or profitable is this change?
5. Will new skills and procedures be executed? If so, how complex are they?
6. How much involvement at each level of the implementation can be encouraged?
7. How do participants feel toward the change agent?
8. How clear and well informed are the expected participants about the total change project and about what is expected of them?
9. How effective is the communication network surrounding the change process? Is two-way communication adequate?
10. What financial resources will be required?

On the other hand, resistance can be minimized when the following conditions are met:
1. All involved parties, including members of the administration, are kept well informed.
2. The change is possible from a budgetary viewpoint.
3. The proposal is reasonably in line with established norms, procedures, and beliefs within the organization.
4. Communication is open and readily used for suggestions, questions, and feedback.
5. The project has been carefully thought out, potential problems have been identified and handled, and alternatives have been considered.

Certainly not all resistance is bad; it may in fact be a warning to assess the idea carefully before implementing it further. Resistance can call attention to the lack of effective communication about the proposed change: people may resist simply because they do not know what is going on; they feel left out, angry, or poorly prepared for future expectations of them. In truth, it is usually wise to listen carefully to dissenters; their hesitancy to participate may save the change manager and the organization the embarrassment of embarking on an impossible or poorly thought-out strategy. What is often seen as irrational resistance to change may in the long run help to maintain organizational integrity. Hence, resistance to change and the people who quietly attempt to defend the status quo should be taken seriously.

No matter how irrational, hostile, or disruptive the resister or defender may be, this type of behavior communicates a great deal about the nature of the system. The change manager needs to determine what the resister is trying to protect and why such resistance is being evidenced. It may be helpful to modify the change strategy to gain the support of nonparticipants.

■ EMBRACING INSTEAD OF FEARING CHANGE

Many people go through life thinking that their "glass is half full." No matter what happens, they see the potential for good, for growth, and for new opportunities. In contrast, others go through life with their "glass half empty." Regardless of what happens, they place a negative "spin" on it. Those with a positive attitude and a willingness to see the possible value in change will generally have many more interesting adventures during the change process and will eventually benefit from the rigors demanded of the change process. Some tips for dealing positively with one's own change experiences are described by a variety of writers.

First, when you are the change manager, remember that "No one really likes a change agent, especially during the change" (Cauthorne-Lindstrom, 1993, p. 72). It is human nature for people to grieve for the old ways and resent the new, and they will naturally look for a recipient or "lightning rod" for their frustrations. Give people the space, acceptance, and time to express these frustrations without responding angrily or defensively. Remember, it is about the process, not you.

Second, listen carefully. In those times when there is just nothing you can do, listen! Some problems with the change will remedy themselves over time. Some things that are criticized do not reflect problems or flaws in the change design or implementation. Be able to assess which concerns, actions, and needs truly require discussion and which people with concerns need to be provided with support (Cauthorne-Lindstrom, l993, p. 72).

Third, stay flexible and adaptable, knowing that more changes may need to be planned as the process is implemented. It is not possible to design the perfect change plan. There will always be a need to rethink and modify. While adhering to the key values and goals of the plan, modifications may alter some of the methods.

Fourth, change is filled with uncertainty, ambiguity, mistrust, grief, and fear. There will be emotional reactions. A useful strategy is to focus on the long-term goal rather than stay absorbed in the discomfort of the moment.

Vicenzi et al. (1997) offer suggestions for nurses to cope more effectively with the "chaos" in nursing and the health care system. They base their recommendations on chaos theory and the concept of complexity. Dealing with the current situations in health care requires that nurses abandon false notions of control and recognize that there may be more haphazard and spontaneous change than is desired and that the goals of planned change may not be achieved in the turbulence. They agree that nurses may need to take time to accept the reality of the change, grieve for what is thought of (often erroneously) as the good old days, and move on to the new days.

Their third recommendation, to "accept the unpredictability of the future, including the uncertainty of your own job," is difficult (Vicenzi et al., 1997, p. 28). Jobs are not an entitlement, and change in the system often shifts the need for certain skills and people. The recommendation to keep learning logically follows from thinking about the lack of permanence in the job. Nurses need to continue learning and growing so they can increase their value to current and future employers. They need also to build and strengthen relationships with nurses and other professionals—to learn from them.

■ CHANGE MANAGER

The *change manager* or *agent* is the catalyst who initiates the change process and sees it through to completion. This person generates ideas, introduces the innovation, develops a positive climate for planned change by identifying potential sources of resistance, developing strategies to overcome them, and marshaling forces for acceptance of the change. The change manager is also responsible for implementing and evaluating the change. Nurses, by the very definition of their role, are change managers. That is, "a nurse is brought into a situation precisely because the patient's status quo is not acceptable" (Curtin, 1995, p. 8). The patient can be an individual, a family, a group, or a community. The role of the nurse is to bring about a desired change, and this is done through astute observation and analysis. The individual serving as the change agent should recognize that a person's ability to cope with change depends on (1) his or her flexibility, (2) his or her evaluation of the current situation, (3) expected consequences both if things stay the same and if they change, and (4) his or her view of what would be gained or lost if the individual did or did not engage in the change.

Observation, communication, group process skills, and political astuteness are key to effective change managers. These people must listen carefully to what is said as well as what is not said. Attention is paid to who says what. How much power and respect or fear does the person expressing the idea or opinion have? The change manager must also be decisive and able to gather information quickly and then move on it. Communication is critical to effective change. It must be direct, honest, complete, and factual. Communication must also flow both up and down the organization.

Howell and Higgins (1990) refer to what this text calls change managers or agents as *change champions.* These people are supportive of change and know how to implement change and how to overcome adversity to ensure completion of the project. They see four qualities as essential in the change champion: self-confidence, persistence, high energy, and the willingness and ability to take risks. These champions must be able to work the political system to get needed resources, information, and support (Cauthorne-Lindstrom & Tracy, 1992). They also need to be civil to others (i.e., they should respect people and work to build a sense of community among the change participants) (Doerge & Hagenow, 1995).

Cauthorne-Lindstrom (1993) provides some advice to the person in charge of change. First, she says that forces that demand change all share one characteristic: dissatisfaction with the status quo. She calls this stage a period where change agents help people "smell the smoke and feel the fire" (Cauthorne-Lindstrom, 1993, p. 70). Now people see the need to change because they have become uncomfortable with the old way (unfreezing as Lewin would say). Soon, however, they begin to explore their options and may at this time become ambivalent about their own discomfort. Maybe the change will not really help; maybe it is just a leap of faith.

Next, change participants begin to screen information and pay attention to that which supports their decision to change. They then eliminate or ignore information that supports the status quo. Lewin (1951) calls this "moving to the new level." Part of letting go is grieving for the old way. People need support, encouragement, and to be heard when they express feelings, reservations, and fears.

To help participants deal with these responses to change, four techniques are helpful: (1) create the "smoke and fire" early in the process by asking people to describe a perfect situation and differentiate between perfection and the status quo; (2) ensure a strong support system; (3) involve all participants in the change's design, since those who participate in creating and controlling the change will have the most buy-in; and (4) support the self-esteem of all people involved.

Change agents need also to assess whether they are functioning as insiders or outsiders. The diagnosed problem, the environment, and the characteristics of the participants determine whether it is better for a change agent to be an insider or an outsider. External change agents are often better able to view the situation clearly in that they are less affected by vested interests and biases. Also, the outsider is independent of the organizational power structure and cliques. The external change agent comes to the situation as a stranger, which may be a disadvantage until participants gain trust and confidence in this person's ability. It helps if the change agent has impressive credentials, is well informed about both the organization and the proposed change, and can communicate effectively with involved individuals and groups.

The internal change agent has the advantages of knowing the system, being able "both literally and figuratively to speak the language" of the participants, and being familiar to the organization (Olson, 1979, p. 325). The insider, however, may be influenced by vested interests and biases that impede clear examination of the situation. Internal change agents may also be handicapped by group impressions of their ability, by their past failures, and by jealousies within the group. There is no simple solution regarding which is consistently best: an internal or an external change agent. The needs and resources of each situation are unique. Although choice may not be possible because of administrative decisions, availability of competent people, or finances, the change agent needs to recognize the advantages and disadvantages of each option.

The change agent assists the group to (1) define the problem; (2) list all possible alternatives and the positive or negative consequences of each; (3) determine the most suitable alternative

at this time and for this setting; (4) organize an implementation plan; (5) provide ongoing supervision, direction, and support; and (6) work toward developing an evaluation format. The following guidelines for implementing change are offered to nurses in change agent roles.

In some instances the change agent is the designated manager or leader for a group. Sometimes the change agent comes from outside the organization to manage the change process. Regardless of whether the change agent is from within and has position authority or comes from without, leadership qualities are essential and the person should be able to express a captivating vision that inspires others; pursue unconventional and perhaps un-thought-of and untried action plans; bring out the best talents possible in those involved in the process; and frequently give positive feedback and recognition to others (Kawamoto, 1994, p. 4). The following nine guidelines will be useful in managing change.

Guide to Implementing Change

1. *Involvement.* No one person knows everything. Therefore respect the knowledge and wisdom of others, and involve all who will be affected by the change in its development from the beginning. Listen carefully. People will usually cooperate and accept innovations that they perceive as nonthreatening and beneficial.

2. *Motivation.* People participate in activities when they are motivated, and they are generally motivated when they feel that their contributions are valuable for the outcome of the project, that they are listened to, and that they are respected.

3. *Planning.* This includes considering where the system is inflexible as well as what, how, and when change can be brought about.

4. *Legitimization.* Any change, to be accepted, must be sanctioned by the participants in the

project and ultimately by those who will be affected.

5. *Education.* Change typically implies reeducation or the switch from one way of thinking to another.

6. *Management.* The change agent finds a balance between leading and developing the leadership capacities of participants. It is helpful to manage by delegation of responsibility so that others may develop their talents.

7. *Expectations.* A variety of expectations should be held by change agents: expect the outcome to be somewhat different from what was originally planned; expect resistance and unforeseen problems; also expect unbelievable reactions from participants.

8. *Nurturance.* Recognition and support for participants are imperative. People need to be acknowledged for what they do right, and they also need to discuss in private how their actions interfered with the project.

9. *Trust.* The key element in implementing change is developing trust. Participants must trust the change agent to think carefully before involving them in projects, and the change agent should trust the participants to do a good job.

• • •

The change agent serves as a vital communication link between each of the interacting parts of subsystems in the change project. To be effective, the change agent must do the following:

1. Be accessible to all who are involved in the change process.

2. Develop trust among participants.

3. Be honest and straightforward about goals, plans, priorities, and problems.

4. Keep the goals clearly in mind, and assist others to do so and not get diverted by side issues or activities.

5. Define the responsibilities of others; allow participants the freedom to do their part.

6. Listen.

The process of planned change is essentially a problem-solving process like the nursing process. Change is a complex, continuous process that can rarely be rushed or imposed on unwilling participants. Before the onset of any change process, a careful assessment must be performed as to the readiness to participate and support for the project of those who will invariably be involved. Each situation and organization have unique features that influence the response to innovation. Change is essentially goal-seeking behavior, and one key to success lies in careful delineation of the project goals. What is the need as defined by the change agent? Do others who will be involved perceive the need in a similar way? Once the goals of the change project are established, clarified, agreed on, and prioritized, it is essential to determine what forces, internal or external, will direct the project toward its goal. Not only helping forces but also hindering factors must be identified so that the detrimental influences can be neutralized before the initiation of the change activity. Once the goals are established and resources and hindrances are identified, the change agent can begin to delegate and assign responsibility to participants.

The change agent will spend considerable time conveying information. All relevant information must first be sought and then clarified and synthesized into a logical format as a guide to action. The ideas and suggestions of a wide range of people must be listened to, elaborated on, and synthesized into a plan that allows all involved to feel that their ideas were heard. The wise change agent tests information against reality to determine whether proposed plans seem realistic, workable, and economically feasible. Often the overexpenditure of human, economic, and technical resources in the implementation of change can be directly attributed to poor or incomplete planning.

If at all possible, it is helpful to try to implement a change strategy on a limited basis so that weak points can be assessed early and remedied before the complete process commences. Evaluation at each stage is crucial. Few projects cannot be improved.

■ SUMMARY

The following model for change is offered:
1. Stimulation of idea: diagnosis of need or problem
2. Assessment of motivation and resources for change
3. Assessment of resources and capability of change agent
4. Diagnosis of the type of change strategy needed
5. Development of the implementation strategy
6. Pretesting (trial) of the implementation strategy
7. Revision of strategy as needed
8. Implementation of the change project
9. Observation, handling, avoidance, or overcoming of resistance to the project
10. Evaluation of the effectiveness of the change
11. Formulation of recommendations for future actions or modifications

■ KEY POINTS

- There are a variety of ways in which change can be made; however, in nursing it is generally thought that planned change is the most effective method.
- The process of planned change is a systematic, problem-solving process that has many similarities to the nursing process.
- People respond to new ideas and the anticipation of change in a variety of ways, and for this reason it is useful to understand the unique ways in which individuals approach innovation and change.
- The way in which the change is communicated will influence how effectively it is adopted. Communication includes the channel for conveying the message, the timing, and an understanding of the way in which persons adopt change.
- The process for managing change has several steps and requires that the leader of the change have a vision for the change as well as a clear understanding of the culture of the organization and the people who will be involved.
- A common reaction to change is resistance. The change manager needs to be prepared for this response and have a plan for dealing effectively with those who resist. It is important to realize that people resist change for a variety of reasons, including fear of what effect the change will have on them; lack of clear understanding; or a sense of threat that the status quo, including the power relationships, will be changed.
- The effective change manager needs to work with the resistance and change it from a negative and impeding force to a force that is positive, is thoughtful, and helps to identify potential areas in the change process that require further examination.
- Change managers are often called *change champions,* and they have these four qualities: self-confidence, persistence, high energy, and the willingness and ability to take risks.

■ CRITICAL THINKING QUESTIONS

1. Think about a situation in the clinical area in which either the manager or another member of the staff attempted to introduce a change. Did the person who tried to introduce the change follow the steps recommended for planned change? What was the reaction of the majority of those involved?

Was there a minority group? If so, how did they respond? What do you think caused them to react both positively and negatively?

2. Given the change process analyzed above, what would you have done differently? What would your rationale be for handling things differently?

3. Design a strategy for change at work, at school, or in a social group. Identify the categories of adopters. How will you change the resisters into supporters? What skills do you have that will serve you well as a change manager? What skills will you need that are not a natural part of your behavior?

4. In the change process that you are planning, what specifically is your vision for this change?

5. Consider the clinical population with whom you are working, and design a change process that will positively affect the health of that group. Be specific about the process. Identify potential resisters. Design a plan to alleviate the resistance.

■ REFERENCES

Antai-Otong, O. (1997). Team building in a health care setting. *American Journal of Nursing, 97*(7), 48-51.

Bennis, W.G., Benne, K.D., & Corey, K.E. (1976). *The planning of change* (4th ed.). New York: Holt, Rinehart & Winston.

Bolton, L.B., Aydin, C., Popolow, G., & Ramseyer, J. (1992, June). Ten steps for managing organizational change. *Journal of Nursing Administration, 22,* 14-20.

Cauthorne-Lindstrom, C. (1993). Change: The chain of events. *Nursing Management, 24*(6), 70-71.

Cauthorne-Lindstrom, C., & Tracy, T. (1992, July/August). Organizational change from the "mom and pop" perspective. *Journal of Nursing Administration, 22,* 61-63.

Connor, D. (1992, March). Five views of change. *Training & Development,* pp. 34-37.

Curtin, L.L. (1995, March). Blessed are the flexible . . . *Nursing Management, 26,* 7-8.

Doerge, J., & Hagenow, N. (1995, December). Management restructuring: Toward a leaner organization. *Nursing Management, 26,* 32-38.

Goodstein, L.D., & Burke, W.W. (1991). Creating successful organization change. *Organizational Dynamics, 19,* 5-17.

Howell, J.M., & Higgins, C.A. (1990). Champions of change: Identifying and understanding and supporting champions of technological innovations. *Organizational Dynamics, 19,* 40-55.

Iacovini, J. (1993, January).The human side of organization change. *Training & Development,* pp. 65-68.

Kawamoto, K. (1994). Nursing leadership: To thrive in a world of change. *Nursing Administration Quarterly, 18*(3), 1-6.

Kerfoot, K. (1996). On leadership: The change leader. *Medical Surgical Nursing, 5*(5), 384-385.

Kotter, J.P. (1995, March-April). Leading change: Why transformation efforts fail. *Harvard Business Review,* pp. 60-67.

Kotter, J.P. (1996). *Leading change.* Boston: Harvard Business School Press.

Lewin, K. (1951). *Field theory in social science.* New York: Harper & Row Publishers.

Lippitt, G.L. (1973). *Visualizing change: Model building and the change process.* La Jolla, Calif.: University Associates.

Manion, J. (1993, May). Chaos or transformation? Managing innovation. *Journal of Nursing Administration, 23,* 41-48.

Miller, J.T. (1988, July). Change: Getting them to meet you half way. *Management Solutions, 33,* 37-41.

Olson, E.M. (1979). Strategies and techniques for the nurse change agent. *Nursing Clinics of North America, 14*(June), 323-336.

Rogers, E. (1962). *Diffusion of innovations.* New York: Free Press of Glencoe.

Rogers, E., & Shoemaker, F. (1971). *Communication of innovations: A crosscultural approach.* New York: Free Press of Glencoe.

Silber, M.B. (1993, September). The "C"s in excellence: Choice and change. *Nursing Management, 24,* 60-62.

Stevens, B.J. (1975, February). Effecting change. *Journal of Nursing Administration, 5,* 23-26.

Vicenzi, A.E., White, K.R., & Begun, J.W. (1997). Chaos in nursing: Make it work for you. *American Journal of Nursing, 97*(10), 27-31.

Zukowski, B. (1995, August). Managing change—before it manages you. *Medical Surgical Nursing. 4*(4), 325-326, 330.

Role Theory and Effective Role Acquisition in the Health Care System

Vickie A. Lambert and Clinton E. Lambert, Jr.

INTRODUCTION

Over the past decade, the health care system has undergone massive change and restructuring. Such events as cross training, downsizing, rightsizing, and the blurring of role boundaries have occurred. To deal with these changes, nurses need appropriate skills to negotiate a variety of roles within their specific health care organization. This chapter discusses theoretic approaches to the study of roles, socialization for effective role acquisition, changes occurring in the newly emerging health care system, ways to deal with role changes in that system, and ways to achieve effective role acquisition. The information presented is drawn from the works of contemporary theorists, current experts in role development, and organizational visionaries.

OBJECTIVES

After reading this chapter, you will be able to:

1. Compare and contrast the two leading approaches to role theory
2. Discuss the socialization process for effective role acquisition
3. Analyze changes occurring in the emerging health care system
4. Examine ways to deal with role changes in the emerging health care system
5. Analyze ways to achieve effective role acquisition in the emerging health care system

■ THEORETIC APPROACHES
TO THE STUDY OF ROLE

According to Conway (1988, p. 63) role theory "represents a collection of concepts and a variety of hypothetical formulations that predict how actors will perform in a given role, or under what circumstances certain types of behaviors can be expected." The term *role* has its roots in theatrical usage and denotes the part an individual plays or is assigned in a dramatic production. It was not until the early 1920s that the term *role* appeared in scientific literature (Thomas & Biddle, 1979). It was at this time in the history of the United States that changes in job activities occurred as a result of major movement from the agricultural to the industrial setting.

In the 1930s several social theoreticians formally created the basic knowledge area of role theory (Mead, 1934; Thomas & Biddle, 1979). As role theory developed, two main complementary bodies of knowledge emerged: the structural-functionalist view and the symbolic interactionists' view. Much of the work on symbolic interaction occurred from 1920 to 1935, whereas the majority of the development of structural role theory took place in the 1950s and 1960s. In the late 1960s, when there was a heightened awareness of the nature of social theory, structural role theory was dislodged from its place of dominance and symbolic interaction, because of its humanistic perspective, became the theoretic approach of choice.

In the 1970s, nurses became increasingly interested in role theory as a result of the role dissatisfaction experienced by nurses in acute care settings (Lambert & Lambert, 1988). Thus a movement to conduct research on such topics as role conflict, role dissatisfaction and role strain occurred. Nursing's interest in role theory has continued as reflected by the type of research in the area that has been and continues

to be carried out (Meleis, 1975; Mineham, 1977; Keteran, 1985; Lambert & Lambert, 1993).

Both structural-functionalists and symbolic interactionists have had as their goal the understanding and explanation of social order. However, structural-functionist role theory focuses more on society, social systems, and social structure. Social structures are seen to shape and determine individuals' behavior. In comparison, symbolic interactionist role theory focuses on individuals who actively create their environment through a process of self-reflexive social interaction. Although the theories differ in level of analysis and theory development strategies, they have in common such concepts as role, role behavior, and sanction.

To better understand both the structural-functionalist and the symbolic interactionist approach to role theory, it is helpful to compare and contrast their theoretic underpinnings (Box 7-1). The structural-functionalist view has linked role theory with such terms as *status, position,* or *office*. This approach has emphasized systems of interrelated roles (Linton, 1936; Merton, 1957; Nadel, 1957). Rules and norms governing these roles indicate that there are specific norms that dictate appropriate role behavior. Roles are treated as "social facts": facts that are passed on to succeeding generations as objective, real entities. In other words, the behavior of the individuals assuming a given role is determined by the social forces dominant in a society at any point in time (Brim, 1966).

The assumption exists that the division of labor within a given society is an expression of its state of development. In other words, the more developed a society, the more complex are its structures and, thus, the more differentiated are the components of its labor force. Durkheim (1964), one of the early proponents of structural-functionalism, indicated that as social form evolves and changes over time, the di-

Theoretic Approaches to the Study of Roles

Structural-Functionalist View

1. Environmental forces act to produce behavior.

2. Prescriptions for actions dictate appropriate behaviors.

3. An act will take place with or without any interpretation taking place on the part of another.

4. Group action is the expression of society's demands and shared values.

Symbolic Interactionist View

1. An individual accepts, rejects, or transforms the meaning of environmental forces by way of self-indication.

2. Others' attitudes are the basis for an individual's actions.

3. An act is validated by the response of another.

4. Group action is the expression of individuals confronting life situations.

vision of labor will adjust or reconstruct itself to reflect these changes. A very recent example of this change is the evolution of roles for unique professionals, technologists, and skilled laborers as a result of computerization.

In the structural-functionalist view, roles are perceived as primary mechanisms that serve essential functional prerequisites of the social system (Parsons, 1951). A relationship exists between roles and the social structure that is comparable to the relationship that exists between organs and functions in a biologic system. Even though roles, in the structural-functionalist schema, are conceptualized as fixed or stable in character, they can be seen to change as the institutions of society evolve. Buckley (1967) contends that each institution undergoes a developmental process, over time, that leads to a re-creation of the institution.

A recent example of this process is the developmental change that has occurred in the health care system in response to managed care. Managed care has altered the way in which health care providers are allowed to deliver patients care based on a prescribed reimbursement system. Providers now are required to obtain per-

mission from a patient's managed care corporation for the right to deliver certain health care services. If approval is not obtained, service rendered will not be reimbursed. As a result, the quality and timeliness of care delivered to a patient can be compromised.

The symbolic interactionist view of role theory advocates a reciprocal interrelationship of roles (Blumer, 1962; Turner, 1962). Each actor regulates behavior and responses to what is expected from the other individual(s). The symbolic interactionist approach does not construct individual roles as being controlled by a set of rules. Roles are perceived as relationships between what an individual does and what others do (Lambert & Lambert, 1981). In other words, a role is an internally consistent series of responses by a member of a social situation, whereby the individual enacts his or her behavior based on the responses of others.

To understand a role from the symbolic interactionist perspective, the counter-role must be understood. Every role is oriented toward one or more existing other roles. For example, the role of mother makes no sense without the role of child. The role of health care provider makes no sense without the role of patient. For either the mother or the health care provider to appropriately carry out their respective roles, they must comprehend what constitutes the role of child or the role of patient. Inappropriate role enactment occurs when an individual interprets the counter-role(s) incorrectly. If the nurse interprets the counter-role of the patient incorrectly, he or she will take on inappropriate behaviors when enacting the role of health care provider. This, in turn, may cause the nurse to expect responses from the patient that are incompatible with or inappropriate for the role.

Role enactment becomes incomplete when role behavior is not continually evaluated by the individual or by members of the counter-role. Evaluation can lead to maintaining existing behavior or to changing the behavior of the role. A change in one's role often reflects a change in perception because of assessment by the individual or members of the counter-role. Thus it becomes apparent that the symbolic interactionist approach involves learning, reciprocal interaction, change, and growth. The newly appointed charge nurse who seeks and evaluates feedback from members of the nursing staff and subsequently changes professional leadership

Key terms	
Term	**Definition**
Counter-role	Acts by others that serve as cues to guide specific role performance
Role acquisition	The act of acquiring new role behaviors
Role enactment	The manner in which an individual carries out the behaviors of a role

behavior is an example of one who is working toward complete role enactment.

According to Thornton and Nardi (1975), an individual progresses through four stages when taking on a new role: anticipatory, formal, informal, and personal. These stages reflect the change and growth that occur in new role acquisition. The *anticipatory stage* involves the period of time before taking on a new role. During this time the individual is exposed to a very general and stereotyped view of the role. The person may fantasize about the role, and thus the perception of the role may be incongruent with what the role actually entails. An example of the anticipatory stage is the senior nursing student, in the final semester of school, who has an unrealistic and stereotyped view of the role of the nurse in a home health care setting. Ultimately this inaccurate anticipation of the role could impede adjustment to the role.

The *formal stage* takes place when the individual's perception of the role changes from "outside" viewing to "inside" viewing. During the formal stage a focus on expected behaviors and abilities, not attitudes, occurs. This is when the individual begins to assimilate what is expected in the performance of the role. For the recently graduated nurse working in a home health care setting, it is during the formal stage that the nurse realizes the importance of being able to organize a workload of more than one or two patients efficiently.

The *informal stage* occurs when the individual's personal reactions become involved. Expectations are communicated to the individual by members of society who already assume the particular role. In other words, the "mays" that can be done in the enactment of the role are brought to the individual's attention. It is at this point that the person begins to formulate personal meaning for the role and for the performance of the role. It is during the informal stage that the recently graduated home health care nurse learns from peers what is acceptable in enacting the professional role of the nurse in a home setting.

The *personal stage,* the final stage of role acquisition, occurs when the individual imposes the "self" upon the role. The person's conceptions and needs become part of the role. This is also the time when the individual reconciles the situational demands of the role. For the recently graduated nurse, it is during the formal stage of role acquisition that one comes to terms with the physical and emotional demands of the work setting. It is also during this stage that the nurse assimilates personal professional needs into the newly acquired nursing role.

An individual fully acquires a new role when he or she anticipates the role, learns others' expectations of the role, formulates personal expectations of the role, and reconciles these expectations. Successful completion of each of these stages leads to successful role acquisition. If, however, a person fails to meet each of these challenges, he or she will enact the role unsuccessfully.

A great deal of literature attempts to support the usefulness of both the structural-functionalist view and the symbolic interactionist view. The major difference between the two approaches is that the structural-functionalist view conceives an action as a learned response that is communicated during the process of socialization and reinforced in the person by approval or disapproval by significant others (Goslin, 1969). In contrast, the symbolic interactionist view suggests that the individual engages in interactions with others and selects certain cues for action that, for him or her, have more relevance than others. Thus the behavior enacted is not simply a learned response, but an interpretation of cues in one's environment.

Both theoretic perspectives have merit. Neither perspective alone can account for the wide variety of human responses possible in the multiple scenarios where individuals confront each other. However, the symbolic interactionist approach to role has taken precedence, in the health care environment, over the structural-functionalist approach. This is because the structural-functionalist view does not account for the wide variations in behavior that take place within complex social structures, such as the health care system. In addition, the structural-functionalist view fails to account for the numerous social and psychologic characteristics of human beings. Instead, this view perceives the human as an object in the environment that does not have any intrapsychic meaning attached to its behavior.

■ SOCIALIZATION FOR ROLES

For an individual to effectively take on a specific role within a society, he or she must be appropriately socialized for the role. The role socialization process involves learning to meet, for a variety of situations, the behavior requirements that are delineated by other members of society. This process requires the acquisition of knowledge, skills, and dispositions that lead to the individual becoming a more or less able member of society. Members of society develop both prescriptive and performance aspects of a specific role in an attempt to regulate the behavior of societal members so that the function of society will be successfully carried forward (Brim, 1957).

Socialization into a role is perceived as successful if the process prepares a person to respond to a variety of situational demands with the appropriate amount of a given role characteristic. Socialization accomplishes this process by enhancing the person's repertoire of behavior through the range and complexity of responses that can be enacted, by freeing the person from a learned series of stereotyped responses, and by providing the person with the ability to discriminate among social situations.

According to Brim (1960), successful role acquisition involves *awareness* and *knowledge* of the demands of the role, the *ability* to fulfill the demands of the role, and *motivation* to meet the demands of the role. Socialization is not successful if the person cannot call forth appropriate responses in a variety of social situations that rely on role awareness and knowledge, role ability, and role motivation.

Socialization for a given role is a continuous and cumulative process that begins in infancy and evolves throughout one's life. Thus any role that a person assumes is continually evolving with each new life experience related to that role. As a result of this continuous evolution, the average person tends to move from a status of lower role responsibility to a status of higher role responsibility. This increase in responsibility is accompanied by an increase in net social gains, increased rewards, a larger sphere of decision making, a larger number of people over whom one has authority, a smaller number of persons who have superior authority, and a sense of greater social recognition. Thus it becomes apparent that as one obtains more mastery in the socialization of a given role, one obtains more positive social outcomes.

Mastery of the socialization of a given role can be enhanced in a number of ways. According to Roscow (1974), socialization mastery of a given role within an organization can be fostered when supervisors or administrators work to do the following:

- Decrease rewards for conformity to previous role performance
- Reinforce expectations associated with a newly acquired level of role responsibility
- Clarify the responsibilities associated with the new role
- Provide opportunities for rehearsing a future role and thus cultivating skills, techniques, and insights associated with the new role
- Increase the individual's commitments to new role behavior
- Change the self-image of the person associated with the new role
- Provide opportunities for successful role performance

Conformity to previous role performance involves continuing to carry out the "old" ways of doing the job even though the job responsibilities and expectations have changed. In other words, it is maintaining the status quo. For example, for the individual who has just changed from the student nurse role to the professional nurse role, the supervisor may decrease rewards for conformity to previous student role performance by denying merit increases, delaying promotions, not providing improved office space, or not enhancing the job perks if the new graduate continues to behave like a student.

Key terms	
Term	Definition
Role awareness	Perception of what constitutes the responsibilities of a given role
Role knowledge	Possession of information related to a specific role
Role ability	Possession of skills needed to carry out the responsibilities of a given role
Role motivation	Incentive or drive to carry out the responsibilities of a given role
Role rehearsal	Practicing the new role with the guidance of a supervisor or mentor

A newly acquired level of role responsibility involves the acquisition of a wider and more comprehensive range of skills. To reinforce the expectations associated with a new level of role responsibility, the skills and job responsibilities required must be clearly delineated in a job description. When an individual, such as a nurse who was recently assigned to the emergency room, performs at the expected level, both verbal and written positive reinforcement need to be provided.

Clarifying the responsibilities associated with a new role involves providing both a clearly written job description and verbal reinforcement of the tasks to be accomplished. When the responsibilities of a new role are unclear, the individual is likely to engage in inappropriate and/or inadequate role enactment. For example, if a newly assigned charge nurse is not made aware of the administrative responsibilities of the role, inappropriate role performance is likely to occur.

Cultivating appropriate skills, techniques, and insights into a new role can be accomplished by allowing time for role rehearsal. Role rehearsal can provide the individual with the opportunity for carrying out the responsibilities of the new role under supervision with feedback. For example, allowing a nursing anesthesia student to perform anesthesia skills in a human simulation laboratory under the direction of a faculty member provides the opportunity for learning the aspects of the new role within the context of a controlled and/or protected environment (Box 7-2).

Increasing an individual's commitment to new role behavior involves providing meaning and value for acquisition of the skills and techniques for the new role. It is only when an individual, such as a new advanced practice nurse, perceives the significance of a new role that he or she gains a sense of ownership for assuming the new role.

Changing the self-image of the person associated with the new role involves enhancing how the person views himself or herself in the role. This can be accomplished by providing frequent positive feedback for appropriate role performance. For example, when the new staff nurse in the operating room thinks that there is a "goodness of fit" with the role, he or she will manifest positive self-image within the role.

Providing opportunities for successful role performance involves designing sequential, graduated situations in which the person can accomplish various components of the new role. For example, the graduate student in mental health nursing who over time is taught the interviewing and counseling skills required to engage in independent private practice with patients will have an increasing sense of achievement. A person who develops a sense of achievement with each sequential, graduated situation is likely to feel a sense of positive role performance.

Although these strategies cannot guarantee successful role socialization, they certainly can

---

B O X   7 - 2

Fostering Role Socialization

1. Decrease rewards for conformity to previous role performance.
2. Reinforce expectations associated with a newly acquired level of role responsibility.
3. Clarify the responsibilities associated with the new role.
4. Provide opportunities for rehearsing a future role, and thus cultivate skill, techniques, and insights.
5. Increase the individual's commitment to new role behavior.
6. Change the self-image of the person associated with the new role.
7. Provide opportunities for successful role performance.

From Roscow, I. (1974). *Socialization to old age.* Berkeley: University of California Press.

enhance the likelihood of success. The more opportunities for successful role performance that a supervisor or administrator can provide, the more likely it is that an individual will be appropriately socialized into his or her new role.

■ CHANGES OCCURRING IN THE EMERGING HEALTH CARE SYSTEM

Over the past decade, the health care system has undergone massive change and evolution. According to the Pew Commission (1995), these changes are a result of five major forces:

- The need to contain the nation's health care costs
- An aging population
- Expansion of science and technology
- Consumer empowerment
- A greater degree of tension between the two core values of the rights of the individual and the importance of the common good.

Each of these forces has had and will continue to have an impact, now and on into the next century, on the roles that health care providers assume.

The need to contain the nation's health care costs, the first major force influencing the direction of the future health care system, has had a dynamic and powerful influence on how health care providers *carry out* their professional roles. The health care system has been pushed toward an increasingly complex array of management and incentive structures. As a result, there has been an increase in the diversification of the mix of providers, as well as in the roles that these providers play. This diversification has led to a dramatic alteration in who delivers care to whom, when, and where (O'Malley et al., 1996). Less often does the physician serve as the point of patients' entry into the health care system. As a result, advanced practice nurses are playing a pivotal role in this arena. No doubt this is because the focus in the health care system is now on population health rather than on the provision of individual care.

For decades nurses have served as the champions of health promotion and disease prevention and as proponents of "community" health. This shift in the overall health care system has created an increased demand for ambulatory and community-based care alternatives rather than the acute care pattern of hospitalization. According to Mundinger (1994), research has shown that nurse practitioners can provide 80% of the health care needs of adult patients and 90% of the health care needs of pediatric patients in a primary care setting. The cost of an advanced practice nurse to the public is less than that of a physician. According to Lamm (1996), it costs between one-fourth and one-eighth as much to educate an advanced practice nurse (i.e. nurse practitioner) as it does to educate a primary-care physician.

As a result of the push for cost containment in health care, the diversification in the mix of providers also has led to an increase in the delivery of certain aspects of care by *nonlicensed* health care providers such as "patient care assistants" or "nursing assistants." This trend has created an increased awareness of both legal and professional issues related to the regulation and supervision of these health care providers. Some state regulatory bodies are grappling with what type of tasks can be delegated to unlicensed personnel and what level of direct or indirect supervision these individuals require from the professional nurse. Many of the questions related to these specific areas of concern have not yet been completely answered.

The aging of the population is the second major force directing the future of the health care system. The rapid increase in the number of elderly individuals is creating a movement from an acute to a chronic disease burden for the nation that will become even more evident in the early part of the next century. Thus the health care system is moving away from being a system that largely treats acute disorders and acute manifestations of chronic illness to a system that delays the onset of chronic disorder through health promotion and disease prevention. The health care system is shifting from a cure to a care mode.

The ever-growing number of elderly people has placed an increased responsibility on the younger segment of the population to provide and pay for the expanding services needed by this group. In addition to an aging population, there is also a smaller pool of young people to pursue health care careers and to replace health care providers who are retiring. In addition, with expanded career roles for women, a professional life in health care is no longer seen as one of the few major job opportunities. Thus there are fewer and fewer health care providers available to care for the burgeoning number of elderly people. This fact has created more reliance on the delivery of care by nonlicensed personnel who are directed or supervised by licensed health care providers. As mentioned, the regulatory and supervisory issues of this group remain to be resolved. Without question, nurses are and will need to continue to play a major role in these regulatory and supervisory issues.

Over the past three decades, the expansion of science and technology, the third major force identified by the Pew Commission, has greatly influenced health care. The public has benefited greatly from these recent technologic advances. However, there is a need to balance the use of technology with the values of quality of life, consumer choice, risk-benefit, and the integrity of human life. Without question, a health care system driven by technology can lead to a depersonalization or dehumanization of patient care delivery. Nurses need to be sensitive to this factor as patient contacts become shorter and more fragmented.

Advances in technology have created a new way of recording and retrieving information (Simpson, 1996). Nursing informatics, a fairly new specialty in nursing, has facilitated nurses in ways of collecting and analyzing large data sets to better understand and evaluate clinical practice from the perspective of population health and welfare. Through nursing informatics nurses are now able to communicate world wide, and to disseminate new knowledge and the latest research findings more quickly.

Over the past 20 years, the relationship between the consumer and the health care provider has changed. This relationship, the fourth factor identified by the Pew Commission (1995) as a factor influencing the evolution of the health care system, has caused the consumer and the health care provider to view each other in a new light. As a result, there is an increased emergence of expectations and obligations between the consumer and the provider because of more emphasis on health promotion and consumer cost sharing. The consumer and health care provider are required to be partners in managing each consumer's agenda for health promotion and disease prevention. The result is more empowerment on the part of the consumer.

Key terms	
Term	**Definition**
Nursing informatics	A combination of computer science, information science, and nursing science that is designed to assist in the management and processing of nursing data, knowledge, and information for the purpose of supporting the practice of nursing and the delivery of care

A better-educated population also has led to the consumer demanding more from the knowledge base of the health care provider. Mass media have provided a wealth of information on health care, which has led to the consumer not accepting his or her "lot" in the health care system without a fight.

Consumers are bearing a greater share of their health care costs. This increased cost sharing has led to more active involvement in decision making about health care. Consumers are beginning to exercise greater discretion in selecting providers and in purchasing health care services. A greater expectation for accountability, effectiveness, and efficiency from the provider is occurring. In addition, consumers are starting to make decisions about their health care based on issues of convenience, quality, and cost. Health care is being perceived as a commodity to be purchased, much in the same way as a home or a car.

The fifth and final trend that the Pew Commission (1995) suggests is driving changes in the health care system is tension between the right of the individual and the importance of the common good. Many of these tensions are fueled by issues of access to care, equitable use of health care by consumers, quality of life, and extension of life. The United States is one of only two industrialized countries in the world that does not guarantee financial access to health care for all citizens. Citizens in nonurban areas are dealing with limited access to physicians and closure of hospitals. Such areas are ripe for the picking for advanced practice nurses.

The issues of quality of life, extension of life, and death are becoming increasingly complicated. In the past, the decision to extend life using all measures was the rule of thumb. This rule no longer applies in all settings for all patients. Resources eventually do have a limit, and there must be some form of equitable distribution of services to all members of the public. Thus nurses and other health care providers are being forced to confront difficult decisions for dealing with these concerns.

In summary, the Pew Commission (1995) has indicated that health care costs, an aging population, advances in science and technology, consumer empowerment, and tension between the rights of the individual and the importance of the common good have contributed to the rapid changes that are occurring in the health care system. To confront the results of these factors (i.e., hospital downsizing or rightsizing, the hiring of fewer professionals, the hiring of more unlicensed personnel, the growth of more ambulatory/community based health care facilities, and the blurring of health care role boundaries), the nurse needs to develop new skills for the development of the roles that he or she will be expected to play in the newly emerging health care system. How to develop these new role skills is discussed below.

■ WAYS TO DEAL WITH ROLE CHANGES IN THE EMERGING HEALTH CARE SYSTEM
Guidelines for Dealing With Changes in Role Responsibilities

If nurses are to meet the challenge of the constantly evolving health care system, they must acquire new skills to meet the many opportunities that lie ahead. To maintain the status quo and to assume that current skills will be sufficient for role survival is a mistake. Health care careers have already stopped working as they used to work (Davidson, 1996). No longer is the corporate structure sensitive to personal opinions or to "old" assumptions and expectations of how careers *should* operate. According to Pritchett (1994), thirteen guidelines can be initiated to facilitate one's management of his or her role in the job market.

The first guideline is to become a quick-change artist (i.e., be able to manage perpetual motion). Expect job responsibilities to constantly be realigned and possibly to be short-lived. Not every organizational change in a health care system will be to the liking of those in that system. Those who do not learn to adapt quickly may become work casualties of the past. Change can be painful. However, resistance to change in the health care work environment is almost certain to lead down a dead-end street. Taking personal responsibility for adapting to the work environment changes that are occurring is a must.

Committing fully to your work role is the second guideline proposed by Pritchett (1994). Nurses should anticipate that the health care system will expect more from them. The marketplace is more demanding than ever, and patients want more services for less cost. Each nurse needs to buy into the philosophy of the work setting in which he or she functions. Survival in today's marketplace requires a high level of job commitment. This commitment often makes job responsibilities more satisfying and fulfilling.

Speeding up your level of performance is the third guideline. Health care organizations that do not accelerate will become extinct. The emphasis on *action* is a must. Organizations can no longer wait for employees to work through a lengthy adjustment process to change. To be successful, a nurse needs to develop a reputation as one who facilitates the change taking place in the health care system.

Accepting ambiguity and uncertainty is the fourth guideline for role success in the evolving health care system. As aptly put by Pritchett (1994, p. 14), "pinning down your job during change can be like trying to nail Jell-O to the wall." Nurses need to come to terms with the fact that the blur of ambiguity can be in the best interest of their career. Ambiguity can create multiple role opportunities. Nurses need to learn to create role clarity for themselves. Taking personal responsibility for determining the

top priority and then moving in that direction is a key to success. Nurses need to develop the ability to improvise and come to terms with the fact that the parameters of their role are going to be a bit fuzzy around the edge (Box 7-3).

Behaving as though you are in business for yourself self is the next guiding principle. In today's market, everyone—including nurses—needs to think and behave as though they are in business for themselves (even if they are not). Organizations are reshaping themselves in an attempt to become more entrepreneurial. When the nurse begins to act like an owner of the organization, he or she becomes more empowered and more visionary. Becoming empowered provides the opportunity and the freedom to excel. By so doing, the nurse has assumed the personal responsibility for career mobility and, in turn, has enhanced the likelihood for self-marketability.

B O X 7 - 3

Guidelines for Success in Dealing With Changes in Role Responsibilities

1. Become a quick-change artist.
2. Commit fully to your job.
3. Speed up your level of performance.
4. Accept ambiguity and uncertainty.
5. Behave as though you are in business for yourself.
6. Be a lifelong learner.
7. Hold yourself accountable for outcomes.
8. Add value.
9. See yourself as a service center.
10. Manage your own morale.
11. Practice *kaizen.*
12. Be a fixer, not a finger pointer.
13. Alter your expectations.

From Pritchett, P. (1994). *The employee handbook of new work habits for a radically changing world.* Dallas: Pritchett & Associates.

There have been careers that have never had the chance to change and thus have disappeared (i.e., gas station attendants, certain types of assembly line workers). Lifelong learning is the only way to remain competitive in the job market. Nurses need to constantly learn new information in their chosen field. This information can be obtained through formal education, by attending workshops, and/or by reading professional journals. Nurses should never assume that they have "completed" their education. This is the age of the knowledgeable worker (Drucker, 1994), who possesses highly developed capabilities and skills. An educated individual is someone who has learned how to learn and who continues to learn throughout his or her lifetime.

Holding yourself accountable for outcomes constitutes the seventh guideline for successful role acquisition. Responsibility and authority are being placed in the lowest levels of organizations and, for this, one has to be accountable for the results. Being accountable requires thinking broadly, looking beyond the specifics of the individual job, learning to work across departmental boundaries, avoiding turf issues, and combining efforts to complete the task at hand. Being accountable requires streamlining the approach to what needs to be done. Thus nurses are going to have to put to rest many of the "sacred cows" of practice (eliminate steps and tasks that no one can justify). Now, more than ever, health care providers are going to be questioned about whether the approach is interfering with the expected and desirable outcome. The goals in today's market are to direct your energies toward the outcomes that count the most.

Making certain that you contribute more than you cost is how the nurse adds value, the eighth guideline, to his or her existence within an organization. It is a person's contributions that count—not the hours or years "put in." Experience does count; however, it counts only if it makes the nurse a worthy investment to the or-

ganization. Nurses need to think in terms of being paid for performance and for the value they add to the health care system. No longer will nurses be paid for tenure within the organization, for good intentions, or for a high "activity" level. To be successful in today's health care system, nurses need to add enough value to the organization so that if they left, others would see that something very important and valuable would be missing.

Managing your own morale constitutes guideline number ten. Over the years we have come to believe that higher administration/management was accountable for employee morale. Not so! We have to be personally accountable for our own attitudes and feelings. Putting others in charge of our morale disempowers us. To regain a sense of empowerment, nurses need to take charge of their own emotions. Wallowing in negative emotions such as anger, depression, or conceit requires an overwhelming and unnecessary expenditure of energy. Rather than focusing on negative aspects of the workplace, the nurse needs to think positively, act upbeat, and feel good about the smallest accomplishment. Everyone in the health care system carries some battle scars from the rapid changes that are occurring. Rather than being bitter about what is happening, it is more productive for the nurse to demonstrate what he or she can contribute. Such behavior displays the characteristics one needs to be a viable candidate for a role in the job market of the future.

Pritchett's eleventh principle for dealing with changes in role responsibilities is practicing *kaizen*. In today's market, what counts is being able to improve the quality of your product at a more rapid rate than your competitor. Thus no health care organization can rest on a past reputation. Circumstances in the health care industry are changing constantly, and what was considered outstanding yesterday is only acceptable today. Nurses who practice *kaizen* assume a personal responsibility for continually upgrading their professional skills. Continuous improvement may come one small step at a time, but over time these small incremental gains will constitute a valuable competitive edge in the workplace.

Being a fixer and not a finger pointer, the twelfth guideline, leads to becoming a valuable problem solver. Unfortunately, it has become easy to be involved in the "blame game." Dodging personal accountability and responsibility carries with it terrible costs to the health care system and ultimately to society. Rather than finger-pointing, nurses need to assume ownership of problems and proceed accordingly.

Altering your expectations, the final guideline proposed by Pritchett (1994), means that nurses should do their best to stay flexible, upgrade their skills, and never convince themselves that the employer is supposed to protect their future. The age of entitlement is over. Nurses need to take responsibility for their own career growth and development. Change should be embraced and work habits need to be developed that keep one marketable in this age of information. It should be remembered that organizations cannot stop the world from changing. Thus the only guarantee that nurses have in today's health care market is change. Reframing one's relationship with the health care system by addressing all thirteen of Pritchett's guidelines is a good foundation for successful survival in today's world.

Key terms	
Term	**Definition**
Kaizen:	Quest for a better way to accomplish a task; in other words, continuous improvement

An Action Plan for Addressing Changes in Role Responsibilities

Continuing change in the health care system is inevitable and so is the role expansion that nurses are facing and will face in the future. Nurses need to develop an action plan to actualize the guidelines for success in dealing with changes in role responsibilities, as delineated by Pritchett (1994). Professional behavior needs to be driven by design, rather than by accident or by fate. As agents of action, nurses are responsible for the design of their own behavior. To assist in the design of an action plan, Johnson (1995) has described several helpful steps.

The first step is to acknowledge and resolve personal conflicts about role expansion in the changing health care system. For example, if the nurse believes that it is appropriate for him or her to supervise numerous nonlicensed personnel in a number of geographically distant sites (such as in a school system) but *truly* does not believe these responsibilities are appropriate, he or she will have a sense of insecurity, as well as difficulty in carrying out the responsibilities. As a result, the nurse may resort to what Argyris (1985) calls "defensive routines," or acts that protect a person from threat or embarrassment. For example, instead of confronting issues of concern directly, the nurse will smooth over differences, intellectualize, and speak in abstract terms. Such behavior prevents the nurse from learning the components of the new role responsibilities and leads to the creation of a reputation of being incompetent. To assist in working through personal conflicts about role expansion, the nurse is encouraged to establish a network of trusted colleagues with whom he or she can confidentially discuss and process concerns.

Refining skills in balancing inquiry and advocacy, the second component of the action plan, involves examining the insights of many people with diverse points of view. In the past, nurses were educated to identify a problem and then to quickly move on and "fix" the problem. This is not a bad trait to have, but in today's health care market, solving and confronting the ever-increasing complex problems requires more than the standard problem-solving skills. Once nurses learn about others' views, they need to learn how to advocate or put ideas forth in a way that explains what they think should be done and why it should be done. Combining inquiry and advocacy assists individuals in seeing each other's points of view and has the potential for developing new and creative ideas. Because there is no single blueprint for charting the course of the evolving health care system, inquiry and advocacy are means of using the brightest minds in the organization to identify and create solutions to difficult problems.

Realistically assessing one's mental model of nursing in today's market constitutes the third step in Johnson's (1995) action plan. This aspect and all of the remaining steps described by Johnson are taken from the work of Senge (1990). Senge states that the only organizations that will flourish in the future are those that can overcome learning disabilities for the purpose of clearly understanding threats and recognizing opportunities. Mental models are assumptions that are deeply integrated into our being. These models have significant influence over how we perceive the world and thus how we act upon the world. For example, if we see a male nurse with a pierced ear, we may make certain assumptions about his life-style. If we see a female nurse who is untidily dressed, we may assume that she does not care what others think about her. It is quite likely that neither of these assumptions is correct. (See Box 7-4.)

Mental models are difficult barriers to change. Senge (1990) suggests that when one realistically assesses his or her mental model, the individual starts by turning the mirror inward—learning to unearth internal images of the world and bringing these images to the fore-

BOX 7 - 4

Action Plan for Addressing Changes in Role Responsibilities

1. Acknowledge and resolve conflicts about role expansion.
2. Refine skills in balancing inquiry and advocacy.
3. Realistically assess your mental model of nursing in today's market.
4. Develop a plan to achieve personal mastery in your role.
5. Build a shared vision of patients and their care.
6. Promote team learning as a norm.
7. Become a systems thinker.

front for rigorous scrutiny. For example, the nurse in today's market needs to ask whether his or her mental model of health care delivery is small and limited or large and diverse. To survive in today's health care arena, nurses need to create a mental model of care delivery that addresses patients who are in all settings and who are of all ages. In addition, this mental model needs to include the delivery of health care by the right type of health care provider, at the right time, and for the right cost. For example, excellent mental health counseling at a reasonable price to all age-groups can be provided by an advanced practice nurse (who is a psychiatric/mental health clinical nurse specialist) in an outpatient setting.

Developing a plan to achieve personal mastery is the fourth step in the action plan. Personal mastery, according to Senge et al. (1994, pp. 6-7), is "the discipline of continually clarifying and deepening our personal vision, of focusing our energies, of developing patience and of seeing reality objectively." Personal mastery is not the gaining of dominance over others; rather it involves gaining a special level of proficiency in one's work responsibilities. Individu-

---

C A S E   S T U D Y

Case Example: Steps to Successful Change in Clinical Role and Responsibilities

Mr. Beck is a masters-prepared psychiatric/mental health clinical nurse specialist who is currently working in an acute care psychiatric facility. He has been informed by administration in his health care organization that he and six other nurses will be assuming new job responsibilities. The new responsibilities will entail working as a mental health counselor in a community-based outpatient clinic that is owned by the health care organization but housed in the basement of a local church. Mr. Beck's immediate response to this job reassignment was one of anger and dismay. However, he soon realized that he needed to acknowledge and resolve his conflicts about his new role responsibilities. Wallowing in his negative emotions would not benefit his career mobility nor his professional growth and development.

To appropriately deal with his new role responsibilities, Mr. Beck developed a plan of action. First he set up an appointment for himself and the six other nurses to meet with administration. The purpose of the meeting was to inquire about how administration perceived the role of the nurses in the outpatient clinic and to share with administration their views on what issues might foster successful acquisition of the new role responsibilities. Such an action is an example of Mr. Beck refining his skills in balancing inquiry and advocacy.

Next, Mr. Beck assessed his mental model of nursing. He realized that his perception of nursing practice did not incorporate a continuum of psychiatric/mental health care that was delivered in a community-based, nontraditional setting. Once he recognized that he had a limited view of the world of mental health nursing, Mr. Beck worked to accept a more expansive view of his nursing practice. Such an action is an example of

Mr. Beck's assessment of his mental model of nursing in today's market.

The two aspects of Mr. Beck's plan of action were to work to achieve personal mastery and to promote team learning. Thus arrangements were made for him and his colleagues to form a journal club. They met twice a month to discuss specific journal articles that dealt with the latest developments in outpatient psychiatric/mental health care. In addition, Mr. Beck arranged for himself and his six colleagues to attend, together, a series of continuing education workshops on outpatient mental health therapies.

While attending the series of workshops, Mr. Beck and his colleagues again met with their supervisors to discuss the vision that the health care organization had for the growth and development of the community-based clinic. Dialogue ensued among Mr. Beck, his colleagues, and administration that facilitated the nurses' understanding of the mission of the clinic. This action helped foster the nurses' belief in what was intended to be accomplished. This action is an example of building a shared vision of patient care.

The final aspect of Mr. Beck's action plan for addressing changes in his role responsibilities was to develop himself as a systems thinker. Mr. Beck worked to move away from thinking as an individual entity in the organization. Instead, he focused on understanding and thinking about the interrelationships that shaped the health care organization that employed him. As Mr. Beck developed his skills as a systems thinker, all of the other components of his actions to address changes in his role responsibilities were brought together as one functioning entity. As a result, he was highly successful in taking on the responsibilities of his new role.

---

als who possess a high level of personal mastery are capable of consistently realizing the results that, to them, matter the most. They approach life as an artist approaches a work of art. Personal mastery is fostered by lifelong learning. It

starts with clarifying the things that really are of importance to us and of living our lives in the service of our highest aspirations.

Building a shared vision of patient care constitutes the next step in the action plan. A shared vision is something that is not seen, but rather is felt and believed (Moore et al., 1996). It is the binding together of people within an organization around a common identity and sense of destiny (Senge, 1990). When there is genuine vision, individuals excel and learn because they want to. To practice a shared vision of patient/ patient care, nurses need to create within the organization a common picture of the future for nursing that fosters commitment rather than just compliance.

Promoting team learning as a norm, the sixth step in the action plan, exists when the intelligence of the team exceeds the intelligence of the individuals on the team (Senge, 1990). To create team learning, one has to start with dialogue. The dialogue requires team members to be objective, to suspend judgment, and to begin thinking as one. In ancient Greece the term *dialogos* meant a free-flowing of meaning through a group, thus allowing the group to discover insights that were not attainable individually. The ability to dialogue involves learning to recognize interaction patterns of teams that might undermine learning. For example, if patterns of defensiveness exist, they can undermine the learning of the team. If defensiveness is recognized and brought to the surface, it can actually enhance team learning.

In team learning, the team is the unit of analysis, not the individuals. *Working* in teams is a familiar concept for nurses; however, *learning* as a team will require new skills. According to Moore et al. (1996, p. 58), "team learning requires that team members change behaviors, give up control, become objective, learn to trust enough to 'create out loud' and feel secure enough to challenge the current reality."

Becoming a systems thinker constitutes the final step in the action plan for addressing changes in role responsibility. For many individuals, this component is probably the most difficult aspect of the action plan. Systems think-

ing is "the way of thinking about, and a language for describing and understanding, the forces and interrelationships that shape the behavior of systems" (Senge et al., 1994, pp. 6-7). It is the glue that connects shared vision, mental models, personal mastery, and team learning. Moving people from rampant individualism to a certain connectedness where they are a part of the greater whole is accomplished by systems thinking. It is systems thinking that brings all the steps of the action plan together to make them work. Systems thinking is necessary for an organization to survive into the next century.

In summary, these seven steps of an action plan for addressing changes in role responsibilities can prove helpful for nurses as they face the ever-evolving role expansions and role changes that are occurring in the health care system. Senge and associates (1994) propose three guiding principles, along with steps three through seven of the aforementioned action plan, that are likely to assist in producing a more integrated organization. Understanding how to foster a more integrated organization also facilitates one's ability to be more successful in appropriate role acquisition. These principles are primacy of the whole, community nature of self, and generative power of language.

The principle of *primacy of the whole* facilitates an understanding that the whole is greater than the sum of its parts. Thus a well-integrated health care system is greater than the individual components of that system. According to Moore et al. (1996), a seamless continuum of care for an individual that is managed across the lifespan is an excellent example of primacy of the whole. Seamless managed care is the whole, and it is greater than the sum of its parts (Box 7-5).

Individual patient advocacy on the part of the nurse is another example of primacy of the whole. The nurse who advocates for improved policies guiding care will have a major impact

Guiding Principles for Creating an Integrated Organization

- Primacy of the whole suggests that relationships are more fundamental than things, and that wholes are primordial (first created or developed) to parts.
- Community nature of self is a perspective that provides an individual with the opportunity to see himself or herself as a part of the community in which he or she is embedded.
- The generative power of language is the tool used to emphasize the interdependency that operates whenever individuals interact with their external reality.

From Senge, P., Kleiner, A., Roberts, C., Ross, R., & Smith, B. (1994). *The fifth discipline fieldbook: Strategies and tools for building a learning organization.* New York: Doubleday.

on the outcomes of the *whole* policy system of the organization.

Unfortunately, in the realm of leadership and management, people are conditioned to perceive organizations as things instead of patterns of interaction. When problems arise in the health care system, we tend to look for solutions to fix the problems, as if the problems were external and could be fixed without correcting that within us that leads to the creation of the problems. As a result, we are drawn into an ongoing process of "quick fixes" that, in the long run, only intensify a sense of powerlessness in regard to our role responsibilities. Fostering the primacy of the whole helps individuals break this vicious and nonproductive cycle.

The principle of the *community nature of self* facilitates an individual's understanding of relationship to the community. In other words, the concept recognizes the integrated delivery network (such as the evolving health care system) as an integral part of the community. This

perception fosters the network's assessment of the community's needs and the development of strategies to meet those needs. When the network (such as the health care system) does not perceive itself as a necessary part of the community, evaluation of need will be based on the internal needs of the network rather than on the needs of the community. The community nature of self opens the doors to powerful and beneficial changes in our underlying values. As Senge et al. (1994, p. 26) point out, "when we do not take other people as objects for our use, but see them as fellow human beings with whom we can learn and change, we open new possibilities for being ourselves more fully." Thus relationships among health care organizations, nurses, and the community are fundamental to the strategic objective of an integrated delivery network.

The *generative power of language,* the third and final principle, brings together multiple realities into a meaningful language. Language provides us with the opportunity to freshly interpret our experiences and thus enables us to bring forth new realities from our environment. Perceptions of the world vary among individuals and can create conflict. The generative power of language provides us with the ability to use these perceptual differences to bring forth new realities rather than to create barriers to change. Think about the new realities of computer technology and the new language and ideas that have grown from this field of science. Envision a new language for nursing within the structure of the continuum of health care. A new common language is more than a list of terms. A new language establishes common meanings and values—a must for survival of the health care system in the next century.

In summary, addressing the use of primacy of the whole, community nature of self, and generative power of language brings into question some of the organizational tactics of the past.

These principles are much easier to articulate than they are to practice. However, they serve as a guide in assisting the nurse in successful role acquisition in an evolving and ever-changing health care system.

■ ROLE ACQUISITION IN THE EMERGING HEALTH CARE SYSTEM

A new framework for building and acquiring roles must be adopted to transform nursing into a profession that continues to serve the needs of society in the ever-changing health care system. The ways of the past will no longer work. Nursing needs to transform its strategies if it is to survive in the next century.

According to White & Begun (1996), history has shown that nursing's professional strategies have been focused on inward-directed sets of activities to build the strength of the profession. The profession has tried to create a "closed" system in an attempt to foster strength to deal with the external environment. These strategies are no longer effective for nurses in today's health care market.

White & Begun (1996) propose 12 factors that can assist nurses in successful role acquisition in today's contemporary health care system (Box 7-6). The first factor, *developing interdependence,* speaks to the fact that nurses no longer can focus only on independent and dependent nursing functions. Nursing needs to place its emphasis on working collaboratively with other members of the health care team. Working collaboratively places emphasis on teamwork. With nursing's broad-based primary care approach to patient care, nurses are in an excellent position to serve as leaders in the evolving health care system.

Being accountable to stakeholders, the second factor, indicates that nurses need to be responsible to the purchasers of nursing services. Patients, managed care corporations, third party reimbursement agencies, and health mainte-

---

B O X   7 - 6

Successful Role Acquisition in Today's Contemporary Health Care System

1. Develop interdependence.
2. Be accountable to stakeholders.
3. Create flexible boundaries.
4. Develop a focus on nursing as possessing skills and knowledge.
5. Be a partner in prevention and treatment.
6. Seek more professional diversity.
7. Establish job security through contributions to the organization.
8. Develop multidisciplinary theories.
9. Increase corporatization.
10. Diversify settings of nursing care.
11. Create multiple entry pathways to nursing.
12. Decentralize professional organizations.

Data from White, K., & Begun, J. (1996). *Nursing Administration Quarterly, 20*(3), 79-85.

---

nance organizations are just a few examples of entities who are purchasing nursing services. They are demanding more input into the quality and quantity of services that are being requested and received. Nurses are no longer in a position to consider themselves outside the loop of accountability for market performance. Entrusting accountability solely to one's employer will not enhance one's successful role acquisition in today's health care system.

Creating flexible boundaries involves continual redesign and reengineering of the profession. In other words, role responsibilities should constantly be reexamined for appropriateness in the ever-evolving health care market. This will result in an increased diversification of the new type of nurse that must emerge from educational programs. For example, nursing education programs are and will continue to be redesigned to address such issues as managed care, private practice, integrated health care systems, and delivery of care in nonhospital settings/nontraditional settings.

Developing a focus on nursing as a profession that possesses health care skills and knowledge for the next century implies that nurses need to take their knowledge, skills, and talents to the marketplace with a price tag. Nurses need to market the fact that they can add value to health care by contributing improved quality of care at a reduced cost. This will, as already demonstrated, lead to less of a demand for nurses at the bedside in the hospital and a greater demand for nurses in advanced practice roles, such as nurse practitioners, nurse midwives, certified registered nurse anesthetists, and psychiatric/mental health clinical nurse specialists (Lamm, 1996). Research has already begun to examine the impact that advanced practice nurses have on quality outcomes in patient care (Mundinger, 1994; Safriet, 1992).

Being a partner in prevention and treatment places advanced practice nurses in a role of primary caregiver. Historically, nurses have been involved in prevention and treatment, but in the evolving health care system, they will be more in positions of decision-making and accountability for outcomes and effectiveness of practice. Direct involvement in prevention and treatment provides an open playing field for nurses who desire to engage in private practice, such as nurse practitioners or clinical nurse specialists.

Seeking more diversity in the professional membership of nursing will lead to increased creativity and innovation for problem solving. More cultural and gender heterogeneity will provide for better insights into the multiplicity of society's health care needs. This, in turn, will contribute to better outcomes of the health care services rendered by nurses.

Establishing job security through contributions to the organization requires the nurse to keep pace with new knowledge and changing technology in the discipline. Education to address new knowledge and changing technology can occur through formal degree-granting programs, through continuing education programs, by reading professional journals on a regular basis, and by attending workshops and seminars. Health care organizations that wish to survive into the next century can no longer provide job security based on longevity. The quality of one's contributions to the organization is the bottom line.

Developing multidisciplinary theories requires health care disciplines to work together in the creation of theories that guide practitioners in producing healthy patients in the most cost-effective and efficient way. According to Meleis (1993), nursing theory development in the next century will be less concerned with nursing's domain and more concerned with health care theories that address the needs of populations. Being involved in such theory development gives nursing an invested interest in multidisciplinary collaboration. To prepare nurses to develop multidisciplinary theories may require an increased emphasis on interdisciplinary education in schools of nursing. Understanding and respecting the knowledge and skills of other disciplines can foster nursing's ability to develop valid and useful multidisciplinary theories.

Increasing corporatization means becoming actively involved in decision making at the executive level. Decisions affecting nurses who are at the bedside in hospitals or with patients in clinics or extended care facilities will no longer be made locally. Rather, most of the decisions influencing patient care will be made at the top administrative level of an organization. As hospitals, HMOs, and other health care agencies become part of regional or national chains, decisions may be made by individuals who are located in a different city or in a different part of the country. To be prepared to be involved in such decision making, an increased number of nurses will find it necessary to receive formal education in business, finance, marketing, and health administration.

Diversifying settings of nursing care means that no longer are acute care settings, such as hospitals, the focus of nursing practice. Care is now and will continue to be delivered in outpatient settings, in the home, in day care settings, in schools, at work sites, and in churches, to name a few. Understanding the continuum of care is a necessary asset. Nurses are in an excellent position to assume leadership roles in case management, advanced practice, private practice, and population-based primary care.

Creating multiple entry pathways to nursing involves creating nursing curricula that address the needs of the nontraditional student. Articulation models among schools of nursing have become a reality. For example, in Georgia, schools of nursing across the state have worked collaboratively to develop an articulation model that is acceptable to all schools for whom it is applicable (Kisch et al., 1997). Such a model expedites students' ability to move from an associate degree program into a baccalaureate program without having to jump through additional and unnecessary hoops before being admitted. Other examples of multiple entry pathways include such programs as LPN to BSN, RN to BSN, RN to MSN/MN, nonnursing baccalaureate degree to MN/MSN, nonnursing baccalaureate degree to ND (nursing doctorate), and BSN to PhD.

The final factor in addressing successful role acquisition in today's health care system is *decentralizing professional organizations.* As the health care system becomes increasingly more complex, so will the various specialty segments of nursing become more complex. New segments of nursing will arise and join the existing ranks of nurse midwives, nurse anesthetists, nurse practitioners of various types, nurse executives, and clinical nurse specialists of various types. These specialties will be in touch with their respective stakeholders and thus more likely understand the stakeholders' specific health care concerns. Therefore one *major* professional organization, such as the American Nurses Association (ANA) or the National League for Nursing (NLN), will become increasingly inadequate to address all of the issues related to either practice or education. Nursing will need to work to effectively decentralize the major professional organizational structures.

Although White and Begun's factors may not guarantee a nurse's successful role acquisition within today's health care system, they certainly will foster and facilitate acquisition as the system constantly undergoes change. With promotions, job security, income, and rewards based on more definitive measurable outcomes, it behooves the nurse who intends to move forward in his or her career to be flexible and to stop relying on how things used to be done.

■ KEY POINTS

- Two ways to consider role theory are to use the structural-functionalist view or the symbolic interactionist view.
- People progress through four stages when taking on a new role: anticipatory, formal, informal, and personal.
- People must be socialized into a role if they are to be effective in assuming the role. There is a defined process for role socialization.
- Multiple and significant changes in the health care system require that successful participants reevaluate and when needed modify their roles to meet the new needs and expectations.
- Dealing with role changes may not be easy and will require that participants learn new skills and ways of working and interacting with others.
- Nurses who lead or participate in contemporary and changing organizations must acquire

the role behaviors that will be most valued by the organization.

■ CRITICAL THINKING QUESTIONS

1. Compare and contrast the structural-functionalist view of role theory and the symbolic interactionist view of role theory.
2. Discuss what steps a nursing supervisor can take to enhance a staff nurse's ability to master the responsibilities of a new role within the health care system.
3. Identify two major changes that have occurred in the health care system over the past decade, and discuss what impact these changes have had on the delivery of nursing services.
4. Because of the restructuring that has occurred in the health care system over the past decade, nurses are confronted with addressing changes in their role responsibilities. Identify and discuss four actions that nurses can take to effectively deal with role changes within the emerging health care system.
5. Identify and analyze five factors that can assist nurses in successful role acquisition within the health care system.

■ REFERENCES

Argyris, C. (1985). *Strategy, change and defensive routines.* Boston: Pitman.

Blumer, H. (1962). Society as symbolic interaction. In A. Rose (Ed.). *Human behavior and social processes* (pp. 179-192). Boston: Houghton & Mifflin.

Brim, O. (1957). The parent-child relation as a social system: I. Parent and child roles. *Child Development, 28*(3), 345.

Brim, O. (1960). Personality development as role-learning. In H. Iscoe & W. Stevenson (Eds.). *Personality development in children* (pp. 127-160). Austin: University of Texas Press.

Brim, O. (1966). Socialization through the life cycle. In O. Brim, Jr. & S. Wheeler (Eds.). *Socialization after childhood: Two essays* (pp. 1-50). New York: Wiley.

Buckley, W. (1967). *Sociology and modern systems theory.* Englewood Cliffs, N.J.: Prentice-Hall.

Conway, M. (1988). Theoretical approaches to the study of roles. In M. Conway & M. Hardy (Eds). *Role theory: Perspectives for health professionals* (pp. 63-72). Norwalk, Conn.: Appleton-Lange.

Davidson, D. (1996). The role of the nurse executive: In the corporatization of health care. *Nursing Administration Quarterly, 20*(2), 49-53.

Drucker, P. (1994). *The age of social transformation. The Atlantic Monthly,* November, 53-80.

Durkheim, E. (1964). *The division of labor in society.* New York: Free Press.

Goslin, D. (1969). Introduction. In D. Goslin (Ed.). *Handbook of socialization theory and research* (pp. 1-21). Chicago: Rand McNally.

Johnson, J. (1995). An expanded role for nurses: Point, counterpoint, and an action plan for success. *Nursing Administration Quarterly, 19*(4), 36-43.

Keteran, S. (1985). Professional and bureaucratic role conceptions and moral behavior among nurses. *Nursing Research, 34*(4), 248-253.

Kisch, C., Newsome, G., Dattilo, J., & Roberts, L. (1997). Georgia's RN-BSN Articulation Model. *Nursing & Health Care: Perspectives on Community, 18*(1), 26-30.

Lambert, C., & Lambert, V. (1988). A review and synthesis of the research on role conflict and its impact on nurses involved in faculty practice programs. *Journal of Nursing Education, 27*(2), 54-60.

Lambert, C., & Lambert, V. (1993). Relationships among faculty practice involvement perception of role stress and psychological hardiness of nurse educators. *Journal of Nursing Education, 32*(4), 171-179.

Lambert, V., & Lambert, C. (1981). Role theory and the concept of powerlessness. *Journal of Psychosocial Nursing and Mental Health Services, 19*(9), 11-14.

Lamm, R. (1996). The coming dislocation in the health professions. *Health Care Forum Journal,* January/February, 58-62.

Linton, R. (1936). *The study of man.* New York: Appleton-Century.

Mead, G. (1934). *Mind, self and society.* Chicago: University of Chicago Press.

Meleis, A. (1975). Role insufficiency and role supplementation: A conceptual framework. *Nursing Research, 24*(4), 264-271.

Meleis, A. (1993). Directions for nursing theory development in the twenty-first century. *Nursing Science Quarterly, 5*(3), 112-117.

Merton, R. (1957). The role set: Problems in sociological theory. *British Journal of Sociology, 8,* 106-120.

Minehan, P. (1977). Nurse role conception. *Nursing Research, 26*(5), 374-379.

Moore, B., Smith, S., Schumacher, L., & Papke, R. (1996). Client care leadership within an emerging integrated delivery network. *Nursing Administration Quarterly, 20*(2), 54-64.

Mundinger, M. (1994). Advanced-practice nursing: Good medicine for physicians? *New England Journal of Medicine, 330*(3), 211-214.

Nadel, S. (1957). *The theory of social structure.* London: Cohen & West.

O'Malley, J., Cummings, S., & King, C. (1996). The politics of advanced practice. *Nursing Administration Quarterly, 20*(3), 62-72.

Parsons, T. (1951). *The social system.* New York: Free Press.

Pew Health Professions Commission (1995). *Critical challenges: Revitalizing the Health Professions for the twenty-first century.* San Francisco: UCSF Center for Health Professions.

Pritchett, P. (1994). *The employee handbook of new work habits for a radically changing world.* Dallas: Pritchett & Associates.

Roscow, I. (1974). *Socialization to old age.* Berkeley: University of California Press.

Safriet, B. (1992). Health care dollars and regulatory sense: The role of advanced practice nursing. *Yale Journal on Regulation, 9*(2), 417-487.

Senge, P. (1990). *The fifth discipline.* New York: Doubleday.

Senge, P., Kleiner, A., Roberts, C., Ross, R., & Smith, B. (1994). *The fifth discipline fieldbook: Strategies and tools for building a learning organization.* New York: Doubleday.

Simpson, R. (1996). The twenty-first century nurse executive. *Nursing Administration Quarterly, 20*(2), 85-88.

Thomas, E., & Biddle, B. (1979). Basic concept for classifying the phenomena of role. In B. Biddle & E. Thomas (Eds.). *Role theory: Concepts and research* (pp. 23-45). New York: Wiley.

Thornton, R., & Nardi, P. (1975). The dynamic of role acquisition. *American Journal of Sociology, 80*(4), 870-885.

Turner, R. (1962). Role-taking: Process versus conformity. In A. Rose (Ed.). *Human behavior and social processes* (pp. 20-40). Boston: Houghton & Mifflin.

White, K., & Begun, J. (1996). Profession building in the new health care system. *Nursing Administration Quarterly, 20*(3), 79-85.

Communicating to Manage Change

Jeanette Lancaster and Melinda Lancaster

INTRODUCTION

Communication is a "complex, ongoing dynamic process in which the participants simultaneously create shared meaning in an interaction." (Sullivan & Decker, 1997, p. 172). For communication to be effective, a common understanding of the message sent and the one received must be achieved. Communication may be viewed in several ways, one of which is that of a pathway between two people. Far too often, although both parties are talking, neither is actually communicating. "Both are intent upon making a point, getting their way, or hurrying through the conversation." (Cornell, 1993, p. 42). For example, one person (manager, charge nurse, physician) may talk "down" to the other party (staff nurse) and effective communication is not achieved because little communication goes back "up" the pathway. Effective communication occurs when two people are talking and these same two people are listening.

A person seeking to influence change must recognize and understand the factors that facilitate the communication process, as well as the commonly occurring obstacles. This chapter describes how effective communication is an essential tool for making change. Both verbal and nonverbal communication are discussed, as well as barriers to effective communication and factors, including the climate of the environment, that influence communication. Suggestions are provided for dealing with these barriers to minimize their disruptiveness and to bring about effective communication. Particular attention is given to organizational communication, since so much work is done within the context of organizations.

OBJECTIVES

After reading this chapter, you will be able to:

1. Describe the communication process
2. Explain at least five factors that influence communication
3. Evaluate factors that contribute to creating a positive climate for change

4. Analyze the ways in which both verbal and nonverbal communication affect how information is heard
5. Differentiate the channels for communications in organization
6. Demonstrate a process for effectively managing conflict

■ PROCESS OF COMMUNICATION

Communication includes conscious and unconscious behavior; spoken and written words, and a wide range of body gestures, movements, expressions, and symbols. Often an individual's nonverbal communication is more informative than what is actually said.

Various models can be used to illustrate the communication process. Commonalties in each model include a sender, a receiver, a message, an environment, signals, and feedback. The communication process in a systems theory perspective is shown in Figure 8-1. In the system perspective, either verbal or nonverbal information enters the system as input that is then processed according to the receiver's perceptual abilities, biases, and cognitive processes and subsequently expelled back into the environment of the system as output. The output of *B* is then fed back to *A* and has an additional effect on the communication. For example, individual *A* is a nursing manager who receives a new policy regarding the institutional procedure for

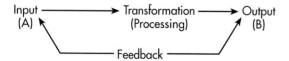

Figure 8-1 ■ Systems theory view of communication.

administration of intravenous fluids. The manager studies the procedure *(transformation)* and asks six charge nurses to explain the new technique *(output)*. After carefully going over the procedure with the charge nurses, manager *A* asks if there are any questions. No one says anything so the manager asks if everyone clearly understands how to implement the procedure on their respective units; all nod in agreement, but the manager notices frowns on the faces of three of the nurses *(feedback)*. After a few carefully worded questions, the manager learns that one part of the explanation was somewhat unclear, yet no one was willing to say this aloud in front of a group of peers. This feedback not only indicated a lack of clarity in the explanation of the procedure, but also called attention to group feelings of insecurity and a hesitancy to be open and honest.

A more comprehensive model of communication is shown in Figure 8-2. In this model, an idea is generated either by an individual or by a group and encoded or organized into a series of symbols that are designed to convey meaning clearly to recipients of the message. These symbols can be spoken, written, or shown as pictures. The sender of the message cannot give meaning to the receiver; instead, the sender transmits a set of symbols to the receiver, who then interprets and processes this information in a unique and subjective fashion *(decoding)* and takes action according to how the message was interpreted.

■ FACTORS THAT INFLUENCE COMMUNICATION

Of the many factors that influence communication, three—gender, cultural background, and organizational culture or climate—are discussed.

Gender

"Gender is a social construction that varies across cultures, over time within a given culture, and in relation to the other gender" (Zak-Dance, 1996, p. 18). People are born as either males or females; they learn to be masculine or feminine. Thus many communication differences are learned through socialization and enculturation. Although men tend to be masculine in their manner of communication and women tend to be feminine, this is not absolute; that is, some females communicate consistently or on occasion in a masculine form, and some males use what are typically considered feminine styles. For instance, feminine communication is characterized by attempts to connect with others, whereas masculine communication is characterized by attempts to compete with others (Zak-Dance, 1996, p. 18). For men, communication is a means by which to gain and maintain the upper hand, whereas

for women, communication is viewed as a tool for negotiation to facilitate confirmation and support. Considering recent statistics that 96% of hospital administrators are men and 97% of nurses are women, it is not surprising that communication may not always be effective (Heim, 1995).

It is important to remember that just because men and women communicate differently, neither one is "right" or "wrong." People have an innate ability to continually evaluate (or reevaluate) behavior and discard or modify what is not working and enhance those skills that are productive. In this respect, when the negative associations are removed from what is considered "masculine" or "feminine," a wide repertoire of behaviors remains from which to choose (Zak-Dance, 1996, p.18). For people who typically use feminine communicators the following strategies may be used to improve communication:

- Get right to the point; women often provide excessive details.
- Speak in a firm, moderately loud, confident voice; women often use a soft, tentative voice.
- Do not allow yourself to be interrupted by men; keep talking in a firm, slightly louder voice.
- Avoid ending statements with a questioning tone; be clear and firm. Men are more action-oriented in their speech.

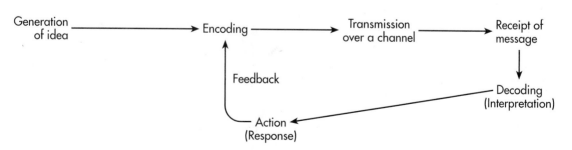

Figure 8-2 ■ Composite model of communication.

- Never apologize or discount what you say, such as by saying, "I'm not an expert in this but . . ."

Box 8-1 outlines some common differences in masculine and feminine communication styles.

Historically, women were at a disadvantage if they communicated according to tradition; however, they are also at a disadvantage if their behavior conflicts with gender expectations. Current research does not support the theory that masculine behaviors are more effective in motivating and getting results (Zak-Dance, 1996, p. 19). The most effective communication style is *androgynous:* embodying characteristics from both male and female, masculine and feminine communication styles.

Cultural Background

Cultural attitudes, behaviors, and beliefs all affect communication. Such elements as "body movement, gestures, tone, and spatial orientation are culturally defined" (Sullivan & Decker, 1997, p. 176). To achieve and maintain effective communication, cultural differences not only

B O X   8 - 1

Common Differences in Communication Styles

Masculine	Feminine
Assertive	Turn-taking (no one dominates)
Stick to the facts	Explain, analyze, justify
Hierarchic structure	Network of connections
Outcome	How it was reached

Data from Heim, P. (1995). Getting beyond "she said, he said." *Nursing Administration Quarterly, 19*(2), 6-18; Zak-Dance, C. (1996). The ties that bind leadership, communication, and gender. *Surgical Services Management, 2*(6), 18-20.

must be acknowledged, but must be understood. Cultural diversity workshops and training are effective tools for overcoming barriers that may be easily understood with proper guidance. Understanding cultural messages is essential for effective communication at all levels of the organization. Chapter 11 discusses social and culture issues in depth.

Organizational Culture and Climate

Organizational customs, norms, and expectations are powerful forces that shape communication. It is important to pay attention to the company culture to facilitate effective communication throughout the organization. Some organizations value and reward direct, straightforward communication. In contrast, other organizations develop more indirect patterns of communication. For example, in some organizations only positive topics are discussed in a large group. Negative or sensitive topics may be discussed only in small groups. It is crucial to recognize the dynamics of an organization to know what to say in what context and also to be vigilant about what message may not be conveyed directly or to everyone.

Few people always say the right thing at the right time. In a fast-paced society where change is continuous, communication is often rushed and little attention is directed either to what is said or to what is heard. Frequently, both time and energy can be saved in the long run if communication is viewed as a critical part of any relationship. A recognition of the significance of communication begins by establishing a climate that fosters clear, straightforward message transmission. This means that the message sender feels sufficiently secure in the relationship with the message receiver to say what he or she truly means. Further, to maintain clear communication, those who receive the information (both verbal and nonverbal) must feel free to respond as they see fit as well as to raise questions between the verbal and nonverbal messages. Creating such a climate requires that concepts such as trust, respect, and empathy be a part of the communication process.

Trust

Trust is key to effective communication; without such feelings, neither the sender nor the receiver will risk the transmission of an honest message. Trust is learned early in life in the parent-child relationship and is reinforced by all future involvements with people. Some people, because of earlier experiences, have concluded that "You can't trust anyone" or that "Everyone is out to get me." These individuals have generally experienced relationships in which they felt taken advantage of or discounted as a valuable person. People who lack trust, either in general or with selected people, are guarded in the information they choose to share, tend to be extremely private about their own lives, and spend considerable energy testing the reliability of others.

To gain the trust of co-workers, it is important to be careful about what is said, to whom it is said, and where the conversation is carried on. Often people inadvertently pass on information that was given to them in confidence. Trust is reduced when information is handled carelessly. For example, important and at times confidential information may be conveyed in a setting that does not provide privacy, such as in an office with the door ajar or in the hall, restroom, or elevator.

Be careful to protect the identity of the people concerned when giving real-life examples to illustrate a point. Although it is helpful to share examples both with patients and colleagues, it is thoughtless to be so explicit that the listener can guess who is being described. Likewise, information about staff or patients, although it may not necessarily be confidential,

should not be discussed in public areas when anyone in the vicinity can hear and possibly repeat the message.

Respect

Each individual is a blend of heredity and experiences, which means that each person is unique. Often we criticize or evaluate others in terms of how much they are like us. If communication is to be effective, each participant must feel accepted and respected as a unique and valuable person. Respect is a nonjudgmental acceptance of other people that implies "although we are different, we each have good qualities." It is generally easy to respect people who are like us or who have ideas and values consistent with ours. Yet respect means positive regard for people who are different—whose values, beliefs, and opinions are unlike our own To respect people who are different, we each need a clear idea of what we value or hold in high regard. Although it tends to be easier to talk with people who have similar ideas and values, the importance of new approaches and different ways of thinking should not be underestimated.

Respect does not mean that people must like or choose to spend time with everyone they meet. It does mean really listening to what people say to really hear their good ideas. Respecting a person whom you basically dislike requires that you honestly accept your negative reaction to the person. Too often we think we ought to like everyone. Then someone comes into our life who is offensive, yet we want to like him or her. It is not possible for most of us to like everyone, but be honest with yourself about whom you dislike. For example, a manager who has many good ideas might yet alienate you with her condescending attitude. Rather than avoid her, be honest and admit, perhaps, that her attitude is offensive and you would rather not spend much time with her; but also admit that she does have some useful ideas. Listen to her ideas, and avoid personalizing her provocative comments.

Respect also includes sharing negative comments with another person in private. If a co-worker has made an error, show that person the courtesy of a private audience for this discussion. Reprimands or other negative sanctions can be viewed as a form of two-way communication. People generally do not like to make mistakes; thus the error may reflect good intentions even though poor judgment may have been used. It is useful to help the person who made the error to look at other ways of handling similar situations in the future. Also, a reprimand should take place as soon after the event occurred as possible, while circumstances are fresh in people's minds. In any discussion of negative content, keep to the topic. This means dealing with one issue at a time and avoiding bringing up everything the other person did that was annoying. Remember that the other person also has a perspective on the situation; no one is always accurate. The information may have been inaccurate, or there may have been situations that were not obvious that prompted the person's behavior. During a period of change, the need for trust and respect is particularly great.

Empathy

Empathy is the ability to assess another person's feelings to view things from that person's perspective. Try to see the world through the other person's eyes to maintain objectivity and increase understanding. *Empathy* means "feeling with" the other person—in contrast to *sympathy,* which implies feeling (sorry) for the other person. In empathy the other person retains responsibility for personal feelings, whereas in sympathy it is tempting to assume some of the other person's responsibility.

To convey empathy you must be attentive to both the verbal and nonverbal messages. Listening is not enough; it is essential to hear and see the carefully disguised meanings and messages as well as the words. Empathy conveys acceptance of the other person's point of view or feelings, yet it does not mean that the listener must agree with the other person. The feelings one person perceives may be totally different from what was intended or what another listener might feel.

■ FACTORS INFLUENCING VERBAL AND NONVERBAL COMMUNICATION

As mentioned, communication takes place on two levels: verbal and nonverbal. Verbal communication includes the spoken word, whereas nonverbal communication includes the signals and cues conveyed by a person's actions, expressions, gestures, and tone of voice. It is estimated that, in an average conversation, less than 10% of the message actually comes from the words. The meaning of any message is not as much in the words used as in the interpretation, which is influenced by vocal tone and body language. Also, people interpret both the verbal and nonverbal aspects of communication based on experiences, needs, desires, and frame of reference (Davis, 1994).

Verbal Communication

The world is full of symbols, and people use words to express thoughts, needs, desires, attitudes, and feelings to others. Through the use of words or verbal symbols, individuals form images of people, places, things, and processes. Communication is a complex process, since words have different meanings for different people depending on their age, level of education, background, experiences, attitudes, biases, and frame of reference. For example, to a child the meaning of the phrase "a lot of money" may differ from the meaning an adult places on it. Likewise, in nursing a teacher or manager may ask students or staff members to do something "as soon as you can." In truth the person may want the item now, but the person being spoken to may interpret the words as "please do this when you have finished all your other assignments." Communication can be clarified by being as specific as possible in the words used; that is, if a person needs something "as soon as possible," it is important to tell the listener exactly when the work must be done. It also helps to avoid global pronouns such as *they, he,* or *we* unless the listener knows without a doubt whom is meant.

Words are used to express as well as to disguise feelings. When people say they are fine, they may mean that they are functioning quite well or they may feel terrible yet be unwilling actually to say how they are. People often use cliches as social amenities, and this discourages real communication. Seldom when someone asks, "How are you?" does he or she get a response other than "Fine," since the opening phrase is often a substitute for "Hi" or "Hello," rather than a sincere inquiry about the other person's well-being.

Nonverbal Communication

Nonverbal communication occurs whenever two people meet; each one sizes up the other and comes to some conclusions about the person. Nonverbal communication takes place continuously, and frequently it is not accompanied by verbal communication. Feelings, attitudes, and thoughts that people are hesitant to share aloud are often conveyed to observers by nonverbal cues. A grimace, twitching mouth, tapping fingers, or shaking of the foot frequently indicates that feelings are attached to what is being said to a greater extent than the words indicate.

The adage "actions speak louder than words" is true. People can try hard to make a good appearance by dressing appropriately, being punctual, and using the correct words; yet their image can be dramatically affected by their nonverbal reactions. For example, a calm tone of voice and well-planned speech cannot disguise the anxiety evidenced by tapping fingers or a twitching eye.

The eyes are particularly important as a medium for conveying nonverbal messages. It is hard to keep the truth and honesty out of one's eyes. Many people are described as "smiling from the eyes down"; that is, while they appear friendly and cheerful, if their eyes are not reflecting the same feeling, a different nonverbal message is conveyed. In American culture it is considered polite to look directly at someone when you are speaking to him or her. This projects honesty and trustworthiness when talking to one another. Avoiding eye contact can denote shiftiness, guilt, fear, or lack of self-confidence. However, in some other cultures

Key terms	
Term	**Definition**
Communication	Complex, ongoing process in which a message is sent and accurately received
Verbal communication	The spoken part of a message
Nonverbal communication	That part of a message that includes signals, cues conveyed by a person's tone of voice, gestures, actions, and facial expression

making direct eye contact is considered rude or invasive and should be avoided.

The eyes are also one of the most readily available avenues for quick communication. A glance can alert someone to the approach of another person. A wink can indicate that two people are coconspirators, or it may be a flirtatious gesture. Similarly, a frown can express disagreement with what is being said or it can mean that the listener did not clearly hear or understand what was said. Closed eyes may mean that the person is bored, sleepy, or has burning eyes or that he or she is trying to think about something and has closed the eyes to decrease distractions. When a person conveys a definite message with the eyes, yet the listener is uncertain what is really being communicated, clarify the message. For example, if the person is frowning, inquire whether the message sent was clearly heard. Remember, people frequently say with their eyes what they will hesitate to write or speak.

In any person-to-person exchange, it is important to listen carefully to what is being said to determine whether it matches the nonverbal message. For example, does the emotion in the speaker's tone of voice match the words? Are the words friendly while the person's eyes or the expression around the mouth is cold or tense? Where does the speaker direct his or her eyes? Whenever the nonverbal and verbal messages are contradictory, further dialogue and exploration are indicated.

The clear receipt of any message depends on the degree of congruence between the message sent and the nonverbal message that was simultaneously conveyed. If a manager, Ms. Jones, frowning or in an irritated tone of voice, says to staff nurse Ms. Smith, "You are doing a fine job," Ms. Smith will no doubt receive an incongruent message. Such messages establish barriers to effective communication in that the respondent may not know which level of communication to

address in the reply. The only way to determine what the speaker actually means is to mention tactfully the incongruence between what was said and the simultaneously conveyed unspoken message. For instance, in this example, Nurse Smith might ask her manager, Ms. Jones, whether she had any reservations about her performance, since Nurse Smith noticed a frown. The manager may be quite satisfied with the staff nurse's progress, and by inquiring about the incongruence, Nurse Smith may learn that the frown is in response to a fleeting thought about another responsibility.

■ BARRIERS TO EFFECTIVE COMMUNICATION

The work environment is improved when communication is effective. In fact, stress can occur when communication is repeatedly ineffective. Nurses may become moody, withdrawn, or irritable when there is an inability to communicate effectively. For this reason, it is useful to learn ways in which effective communications can be fostered (Hanlon, 1996). The communication process breaks down when the environment is distracting: either the sender's ability to present the information clearly is impaired; the receiver cannot clearly present or hear the information; or the approach used thwarts the conveyance of the message. Distractions in the environment such as noise, other people trying to gain the attention of either the sender or receiver, or visual stimuli can impair the process of message transmission and reception. If something is worth saying, the environment should be carefully selected. This means that important issues should not be discussed in a hallway, elevator, or restroom; they deserve the privacy of a meeting or a telephone call. Electronic mail is not generally a good medium to use when one or both participants are angry.

Some people have impaired abilities either to speak clearly or to hear all that is said. Impaired speech is generally obvious, but hearing defects may go unnoticed. For this reason, it is helpful for people with hearing impairments to make this known so that the speaker can direct comments to the unimpaired ear, increase the volume of the voice, or look directly at the listener. Many people can hear better out of one ear than another; others have trouble hearing what is being said if there is background noise such as machinery, the voices of other people, or music. Also, rapid speech may interfere with a receiver's ability to comprehend accurately the intended message. The listener may simply not hear every word.

An additional communication barrier may arise when participants have differing frames of reference about the topic. Because of experience, cultural influences, age, or race, two individuals may interpret the same message differently. Communication may also be ineffective when one or more participants listen only partially to what is being said. People have a tendency to "block out" what is being said if they are otherwise preoccupied, if they are disinterested, or if the new information conflicts with their beliefs or desires.

Source and Manner of Communication as Barriers

Both the source and manner of communication affect its receipt. If the speaker is not deemed trustworthy or competent, or if the message is not clearly conveyed in language appropriate both to the situation and to the receiver's level of understanding, the likelihood of an accurate message being received is decreased. Also, communication can be hampered when the speaker expresses value judgments that may not be held by all participants, as well as when time pressures limit thorough discussion. In addition, when messages are hurriedly sent, someone or some part may be left out, thereby confusing the listener. Biased messages also may get in the

way of effective communication. Some people ask for the opinion of others by first inflicting their own opinion. "Questions" such as, "Don't you want to go to lunch now?" or "Don't you think that was a useless meeting?" often discourage the expression of a different opinion. The speaker's message is clear, and unless the receiver feels comfortable and confident, it is easier just to agree than to state a disagreeing opinion. The speaker could gain more information by phrasing the above questions as, "When do you want to go to lunch?" or "What do you think about that meeting?"

Communication is often affected when one of the participants uses jargon or an acronym that is unfamiliar to others. Listeners may not wish to appear ignorant or ill prepared, so they do not ask what the jargon or acronym really means; they merely nod appropriately and try to end the conversation. This occurs also when speakers and writers use acronyms, abbreviations, or words that are more sophisticated or complex than the listeners understand and know.

Also, frequently giving advice can block communication by antagonizing the listener. The implication behind unsolicited advice is "My way is the best way." Thus the words "If I were you . . ." often serve as communication interrupters because the receiver simply smiles and quits listening. Not only does frequent advice giving tend to be offensive, it also encourages dependency. The receiver may think, "Why bother working out a solution? Joe will tell me what to do" or "Here goes little Miss (or Mr.) bossy."

Defensive Communication

Defensive communication can also be a barrier to effective transmission of messages. This form of communication is an ego-protective mechanism. It is natural for individuals to protect themselves from either real or perceived threats. The most common reactions to threat are fight or flight. Defensive communication refers to a reaction to a perceived psychologic threat and can be found in the sender, the receiver, or the actual message being sent. The following sections provide examples of defensive communication on the part of the speaker, receiver (listener), or the message itself.

Speaker Everyone knows at least one person whom they simply do not trust. Experience may show that this person is self-serving and will do almost anything to gain recognition. This person may be a notorious "brownnoser" who praises superiors frequently and in general spends a great deal of energy trying to look good. Let's call this distrusted colleague Joe. One day Joe comes up and tries to be warm and friendly while discussing a current work project. How do you react? Should you cooperate with him as he is requesting, or should you maintain your usual on-guard position and secretly question, "What's in it for ole Joe?" You have considerable historical information that would interfere with a cooperative venture, but do you give Joe one more chance? The defensive reaction is to hesitate and remain wary of Joe's motives.

Listener Under any circumstance, communication is a give-and-take process between sender and receiver. Some people have difficulty accepting what is said in a straightforward fashion. They hear every message from a defensive, doubtful perspective and are consistently suspicious of the sender's motives. These people are "prickly" and look for ways to hear messages as insults or attacks. Such defensive listening interrupts effective communication, in that a clear message is never received. For example, Sue always responds to statements of praise and encouragement defensively. One day Jane said to Sue, "You look so nice today. That hairdo is very flattering." Sue's defensive comment was "I guess you mean that I usually

don't look good." Such a response by Sue would certainly thwart future attempts by Jane to praise her.

Frequently, no matter what you say, defensive listeners cause the speaker to leave the interchange feeling guilty. The speaker often wonders, "Why did I say that?" A typical reaction by the speaker is to avoid, whenever possible, any future discussions with the defensive listener. Although a variety of ways are available for dealing with the defensive listener, perhaps the simplest and most effective way is to limit communication to essential job-related topics, thereby minimizing the opportunity for hurt feelings and defensiveness.

It is difficult to communicate with some people because of their communication styles. They may be generally aggressive, complainers, passive, and unresponsive, or they appear overly nice, which disguises other often-negative feelings. Aggressive communicators tend to keep people at a distance by their abrupt, intimidating, and often angry-sounding tones. People tend to back away from these communicators. The strategies for improving communication used throughout this chapter are especially helpful with aggressive communicators. Specifically react to the message, not the person; don't take it personally; clarify that you heard the message that was being sent; and be patient. People often avoid communicating freely with complainers because these communicators tend to cast a negative tone and perspective over the topic. Listeners walk away discouraged, which ultimately is time consuming and nonproductive. Likewise, listeners may find that it simply takes too much energy to carry on an extended conversation with a passive listener. They may perceive that getting feedback from the passive listener is like "pulling teeth." The communicator who appears excessively nice and polite and yet conveys a different message either by tone of voice, facial expression, or body language may make the listener uncomfortable because of the ambiguity of the message.

Message Defense-arousing messages may be sent when the content contains a challenge to the other person's competence; a threat; or a disregard for the listener's worth, value, or feelings. Several clues can be used to assess whether defense-arousing messages are being sent inadvertently. For example, when listeners ask, "How are you really doing?" or "What's the problem?" you may find that your messages are conveying incongruency and are heard as defensive arousing.

Other communication barriers in the message itself include poorly chosen or highly emotional words, jargon or terms not familiar to the listener, poor organization of ideas, or talking too fast or too slow, as well as rambling, slurring words, or mumbling.

Avoiding Defensive Communication Several strategies are available for avoiding defensive communication. Language, tone of voice, and nonverbal messages should be assessed for defensiveness. Some people say words that seem like a positive message, but the angry tone of voice or the frown conveys an entirely different message than the words alone imply. Defensive communication can be avoided by the following methods:

1. *Discuss the problem, not the person.* This means sticking to the issue and avoiding any reference to the other person's ability, appearance, intelligence, or other personal factors. A problem is rarely solved by casting blame. Instead, time can be more profitably spent in talking about new alternatives to solving the problem.
2. *When something is wrong or a person's behavior seems troublesome, deal with how it affects you.* Avoid talking about the other person's involvement. This can be done by using "I" more often than "you." For ex-

ample, "I am having trouble understanding the directions for this project," instead of, "You are not making the instructions clear."

3. *Avoid judgmental statements.* A sure way to activate defensiveness is to offer a judgmental reaction to another person's ability, statements, or projects. From early childhood, each of us has judged other people and things in terms of how we think and act. It is important to remember that there are always many ways to say and do things. Because others approach a task differently does not indicate that they are wrong. Also, our way may not be the best way for someone else.
4. *Listen.* Defensive communication can be decreased by listening carefully to what the other person is saying. Often people respond to a partially heard message in such a way as to offend the speaker, who then has to clarify what was really said or has to repeat the message in hopes that the person will listen this time.
5. *Clarify.* Before responding, be sure to check the sender's meaning by clarifying what you heard.

Responding to Defensive Communication

If channels of communication are to be kept open and information freely transmitted, it is necessary to learn how to respond to defensive communication in a way that curtails this form of interaction. Some people feel defensive much of the time, and all people feel defensive at least part of the time. How, then, can people respond to defensive communication? Several approaches are discussed for handling defensive communication, each of which is based on the assumption that words alone have no meaning. People give meaning to words by the way they speak, as well as by their expressions and gestures.

1. *Paraphrasing.* This technique is used to repeat to the speaker what *you* heard. In para-

phrasing, restate in your own words the message you received. Such an approach provides immediate feedback to the speaker about the message that was actually heard. For example:

Charge Nurse Agitation: "Where is that IV bottle that you were supposed to hang at 1 PM? Is it hung yet? Can't you ever get your work done on time?"

Staff Nurse Calm: "You think I have trouble getting my work done on time?"

Actually, the charge nurse may think that the staff nurse is quite efficient, but on this particular day nothing is going right on the entire unit. By paraphrasing, the staff nurse can avoid hurt feelings, and this also provides feedback to the charge nurse that the message sent is not really what was meant.

2. *Perception checking or validation.* This form of communication is similar to paraphrasing in that it describes what is perceived as the other person's message or psychologic state. For example, the charge nurse at change of shift says to the oncoming evening charge nurse, who ordinarily arrives early for work, "Why are you always 5 minutes late for report?" Instead of answering defensively, the evening charge nurse could respond with, "I am sorry, sounds like this has been a long day." Such a response avoids getting hooked on either the "Why?" or the blaming tone of the message and keeps communication open. Perception checking or validation is also useful when the verbal and nonverbal messages are incongruent. Because nonverbal cues are indirect expressions of feelings, it is important that they be put into words and handled.

3. *Voicing the implied.* Like paraphrasing and perception checking, voicing the implied allows the listener an opportunity to call attention verbally to the underlying message. Perhaps a negative evaluation is couched behind a smile and joking comment. It would be helpful to call attention to the negative implication, which may be a major issue that a person is reluctant to handle.

4. *Asking for clarification.* Too often people fail to ask for clarification—either because they are in a hurry, feel intimidated by the other person, or hesitate to acknowledge that they did not truly understand what was said. A person's self-evaluation is sometimes so fragile that the fear of exposing lack of understanding or knowledge deficits is entirely too threatening to risk. In effective communication, clarification is a continuous process.

Defensive communication impairs the productivity of any work group because people respond to one another more often with their feelings rather than with their thoughts. If a problem exists, it is important to deal with possible feelings of anger or hurt so that participants can deal as objectively as possible with the actual or perceived problem. Also, remember that effective communication requires careful planning. It is not uncommon to hear people say, "It wasn't what he said, but how he said it," or, "I can't stand for people to talk to me in that tone of voice." To a large extent the climate, efficiency, and overall functioning of any organization depends on the quality of the communication.

■ COMMUNICATION WITHIN THE ORGANIZATION
Directions for the Flow of Communication

Every organization should provide for communication in four directions: upward, downward, horizontal or lateral, and diagonal. *Upward communication* is essential if those in charge are to make decisions based on valid and accurate information. Also, upward communication gives employees a feeling of belonging and being part of the organization—when they know that what they think is important to the effective functioning of the work group as well as the total organization. Upward communication is of prime benefit to the administrator, who needs extensive and varied sources of information to make effective decisions. Communication modes such as group meetings, conferences with individuals or with small groups, suggestion boxes, and responses to memoranda tend to encourage upward communication. When employees think that they will receive a fair audience from members of the administration, they are more likely to be open in their messages and avoid "underground" channels such as gossip, anonymous letters, or the media.

The most frequent forms of *downward communication* are instructions, rules, policies, procedures, performance appraisals, letters, memos, electronic mail, newsletters, and annual reports (Marriner-Tomey, 1996). The effectiveness of downward channels of communication can be measured by how frequently employees complain that they never know what is going on. Certain behaviors increase the effectiveness of downward communication. First, the person who has a message to communicate should be well prepared and clearly understand the infor-

mation to be conveyed. This may mean doing a considerable amount of homework before embarking on the communication process. It is also important, once the information is assembled, to plan carefully for the actual communication activity. Some people need to be told about changes that will affect them before there is massive dissemination of information. The effectiveness of downward communication often depends on the confidence in which the communicator is held. Mutual respect and trust are integral aspects of effective organizational communication.

Horizontal communication between disciplines or departments is necessary for the organization and coordination of activities. Time and energy are saved when co-workers readily discuss projects, make plans together, and provide one another with evaluation of ideas and plans. Considerable peer support and a "team spirit" atmosphere can be generated through active, open, and honest horizontal communication. For horizontal communication to be effective, participants must trust one another and respect each other's opinions. Also, horizontal or lateral communication is enhanced when participants maintain a nondefensive attitude toward suggestions and critiques of their work. The need for

Key terms	
Term	**Definition**
Upward communication	That which moves up the organizational hierarchy and generally goes from staff to management
Downward communication	That which is often directive and is sent by an authority figure to people in staff roles
Horizontal (lateral) communication	That which is among people who are at the same level in the organizational hierarchy
Diagonal communication	That which occurs between individuals or work groups who are on different levels of the organization's hierarchy; one person typically has more authority than others

lateral communication increases when people work in teams.

Diagonal communication occurs between individuals or work groups that are not on the same level in the organization's hierarchy. The need for diagonal communication increases as interdependence grows. For example, a nursing manager may communicate directly with the medical chief-of-staff or the chief information officer to provide needed information quickly, instead of having to go through chains of command in order for the parallel nursing chief to provide information to his or her peers on the organizational chart, that is, to the chief-of-staff or chief information officer.

Formal and Informal Channels of Communication

Organizational communication occurs along formal and informal channels, as well as in upward, downward, horizontal, and diagonal directions. It is usually much easier to monitor formal communication, in that the organizational channels are easily identified. Each organization has procedures for formal dissemination of information. In some instances, all communication along formal channels is conveyed in a written format, whereas other organizations handle even formal communication in the organization in an oral tradition. The important thing to learn is the expected route for formal communication in the organization and how to use it, A great deal of confusion and misunderstanding can be avoided when everyone understands and uses the established formal communication channels.

Although it is generally easier to monitor formal communication channels, the informal medium may have the greatest impact on organizational functioning. Being part of the informal communication network is important for the nurse who wishes to introduce a change. Such inclusion does not generally happen by chance; the nurse must cultivate a role as a participant in the informal communication network by virtue of being trusted, respected, and valued by other group members. Good interpersonal relationships, both within and outside the nursing group, provide an opportunity to become privy to informal channels of communication. Inclusion in this network depends to some extent on the individual being willing to be friendly and responsive, to be respectful of the merits of the "grapevine," and to share information when appropriate. This means that information is always shared both formally and informally with discretion; that is, confidential information is never shared, and that which is passed on is carefully screened to avoid harming or embarrassing individuals, groups, or projects.

The informal communication medium, or grapevine, generally conveys information more rapidly than established channels. According to Keith Davis (1977, p. 349), the "grapevine moves with impunity across departmental lines and easily bypasses superiors in chains of command. It flows around 'water coolers,' down hallways, through lunchrooms and wherever people get together in groups." If the information carried via the grapevine is reasonably consistent with that which is disseminated across formal channels, the two modes of communication complement one another.

Rumors

Occasionally the information carried on the grapevine is a poor representation of reality. When rumors on the grapevine threaten the effectiveness of the organization, action is indicated. Rumors are not haphazard occurrences but instead arise from a variety of causes (Davis, 1975). A major cause of rumors is a feeling that participants lack information. When people do not know exactly what is going on around them, they begin to speculate, and speculation breeds rumors. In addition to lack of information, rumors are caused by insecurity and emo-

ultimately saves time because the information gained is generally accurate. Also, good listeners learn how well their messages were received by the quality of the reactions and responses they hear or observe.

Listening is rarely an innate characteristic; rather, it is a skill learned through practice. Listening is more than hearing; it is an active process that demands the person's entire attention and considerable psychologic energy. The ability to listen carefully requires the time needed to complete the communication without feeling rushed. Listening implies trying to hear what is being said from the other person's frame of reference; this cannot be done if the listener is in a hurry, is disinterested, is thinking about what he wants to say next, or is otherwise preoccupied. To hear a message from the other person's perspective, empathy is necessary. Empathy or listening to feelings as well as words means that the covert or subtle as well as the overt or obvious messages are addressed. For example, you might ask Ms. Wills, a new nurse on the unit, how her orientation is going. Although she answers "Fine," you notice that her tone of voice is low and that she avoids eye contact. The message you "hear" may be that she is a shy and hesitant person who is easily embarrassed by direct questions or that things are really not going particularly well. Ms. Wills may be reluctant to say how things are really going until she finds out whether you want to hear the truth or whether you are just making conversation by using "How are things going?" as a social phrase rather than a sincerely directed question. If you follow up the lack of consistency between the words and the nonverbal message by saying something like "Tell me about your orientation," "What is working well in your orientation?" or "What changes would you make in the orientation if you had planned it?" you may learn that Ms. Wills is intimidated by the charge nurse who speaks loudly and

is free with criticism. Listening for feelings means being willing to hear and, perhaps ultimately, to handle the ramifications of an honest message.

Listening also implies being nonjudgmental. Often when people truly listen to messages, they "hear" attitudes, feelings, and beliefs that are different from their own strongly held views. Specifically, in this example, the listener may encourage Ms. Wills to speak with the charge nurse and explain how she feels when criticized in front of a group. Ms. Wills may refuse even to consider this alternative, saying, "She is just like my mother—I could never talk to her about anything that really mattered." The listener, on the other hand, may perceive the charge nurse to be approachable. Although it is helpful to point out such a difference of perception, it would not be useful to argue with Ms. Wills about her perception or to deflate her self-image further by saying, "You are clearly mistaken about Ms. Jones; she is quite easy to talk with." Listening, then, often means hearing more than a person might like to know. The Ten Commandments for Effective Listening seen in Box 8-2 may be useful. The effectiveness of communication can be increased if some or all of the steps shown in Box 8-3 are taken (Davis, 1972; Gibson et al., 1976).

■ THREE C's OF ORGANIZATIONAL COMMUNICATION

Three C's are often found in organizational communication: collaboration, conflict management, and confrontation. Each communication mode has the capacity to be a positive or negative force in the communication process, depending largely on the participants, the setting, and the way in which the communication is handled. The nurse who is involved in change must be a master at handling each of these communication modalities, especially during times of rapid change and turbulence.

Ten Commandments for Good Listening

1. *Stop talking!*
   You cannot listen if you are talking.
2. *Put the talker at ease.*
   Help listener feel free to talk; create a permissive environment.
3. *Show listener that you want to listen.*
   Look and act interested. Do not read your mail or answer the telephone while the person talks.
   Listen to understand rather than to reply.
4. *Remove distractions.*
   Don't doodle, tap, or shuffle papers; perhaps close the door.
5. *Empathize with the person.*
   Try to put yourself in the other's place so that you can see his point of view.
6. *Be patient.*
   Allow plenty of time. Do not interrupt him.
7. *Hold your temper.*
   An angry person gets the wrong meaning from words.
8. *Go easy on argument and criticism.*
   They put people on the defensive and they may "clam up" or get angry.
9. *Ask questions.*
   This encourages communication and shows you are listening.
10. *Stop talking!*
    This is first and last, because all other commandments depend on it. You just can't do a good listening job while you are talking.

Nature gave man two ears but only one tongue, which is a gentle hint that he should listen more than he talks.

From Davis, K. (1972). *Human relations at work* (p. 360). New York: McGraw-Hill.

Collaboration

Prerequisite to effective collaboration is a basic understanding among individuals or groups as to each other's functions and abilities. Nursing as well as many other health professions is changing rapidly and substantially. Nurses who are graduates from one type of program cannot assume that they know about graduates from other types of nursing programs. Nor can nurses presume to know about the role, competencies, and skill sets of social workers, psychologists, physicians, or health technicians. There are areas of overlap as well as unique features in the roles of health professionals; thus a first step in collaboration is to learn about the role compe-tencies of other members of the team or work group. Each participant in a collaborative activity has a set of perceptions about the role of the other participants. It is helpful to validate these perceptions with each other to determine what set of tools each person brings to the project or group. Effective collaboration also implies that participants must be skilled communicators who are adept at responding both to verbal and to nonverbal cues and who understand and can use group-process skills. It is important for participants to recognize hindrances or stumbling blocks to group process and to take responsibility for moving the collaboration forward by clarifying issues or misperceptions, keeping the

B O X 8 - 3

Steps for Improving Communication

1. Use simple words and phrases that are chosen according to the vocabulary and understanding level of the listeners.
2. Convey empathy by being receiver oriented and consider how the message may be received. When possible, use the name of the person to whom you are talking.
3. Use charts, graphs, and illustrations to convey information in a succinct manner.
4. When writing, use short sentences and paragraphs and active verbs, and avoid excessive adjectives.
5. Use feedback; for example, a downward memorandum about a new policy does not always afford much opportunity for back-and-forth communication. In general, face-to-face communication provides greater amounts of feedback than messages sent in written format.
6. Repetition ensures that if one part of the message is not heard, repeating it is likely to provide the necessary information.
7. Timing is crucial to effective communication. People hear messages accurately only when they are psychologically ready to do so. Hence monitoring the emotional tone of the recipients of information is helpful to determine the level of anxiety, comfort, fear, or security.
8. Effective listening means giving full attention to the person(s) speaking in an environment that is as free as possible from distractions. When possible, use the grapevine, since it is inevitable in an organization and can be used to facilitate change.

Data from Davis, K. (1972). *Human relations at work.* New York: McGraw-Hill; Gibson, J.L., Ivancevish, J.M., & Donnelly, J.H. (1976). *Organizations: Behavior, structure, processes* (rev. ed.). Dallas: Business Publications.

group on the topic, and respecting one another's opinions and differences. In collaboration it is useful to realize that there is generally more than one way to attain the goals; the way chosen by the participants will not always satisfy everyone.

Effective collaboration is more likely to occur when participants feel confident about their skills and contributions and when they are willing to negotiate, disagree, and compromise when necessary. There may be considerable role overlap, and members may find it helpful if they can comfortably relinquish tasks and perhaps try new approaches. Collaboration is a "process of joint decision making among interdependent parties, involving joint ownership of decisions and collective responsibility for outcomes" (Liedtka & Whitten, 1996, p. 3). Collaboration does not occur unless two or more parties exchange messages in a process over

time—a process contributed to by both parties, involving attention to the communication content, the communication relationship, and the time needed to enact the process. (Coeling & Wilcox, 1994). Collaboration is an essential component of effective communication and is emerging as an ideal state for the nurse-physician relationship. In hospitals, decreased length of stay and increased severity of illness intensify the need for effective collaboration among physicians and nurses as well as among other team members.

Collaboration also offers potential reductions in both cycle time and number of contacts, each of which has the potential to increase patient satisfaction as well as to improve the satisfaction that caregivers receive from their work (Liedtka & Whitten, 1996, p. 4). By eliminating redundancy and enabling departments to work together, health professionals are creating new systems and processes to facilitate collaboration. However, these new methods require new ways of thinking, and in some cases the behaviors are not supported in traditional hospital structures. Effective collaboration requires health care providers to use skills rarely rewarded by health care organizations. Today it is essential to listen with an open mind; acknowledge and productively utilize conflict; and lead by supporting others and facilitating their work.

Organizational Conflict

Conflict is an inevitable component of the organizational communication process. Few decisions can be made and implemented without encountering conflicting viewpoints, differing action strategies, and opposing expectations. Because conflict is inevitable in interactions between two or more people, the change agent's goal is to use differing opinions and plans in a constructive way rather than to allow inherent differences to disrupt goal attainment. Often, conflict is viewed as a negative, disruptive force

to be avoided at all costs. To gloss over, ignore, or stifle organizational conflict may lead to later problems; open communication is a forerunner to organizational efficiency and change. To use conflict as a tool for making or responding to change, several factors need to be considered. First, the nature of conflict must be explained to differentiate positive and negative aspects as well as common sources of conflict. Next, the management of conflict is considered by looking at the reactions of participants and by describing a variety of strategies for conflict resolution.

Nature of Conflict   Conflict results from "real or perceived differences in mutually exclusive goals, values, ideas, attitudes, beliefs, feelings or actions" (Sullivan & Decker, 1997, p. 186). Conflict is generally seen in one of four forms: *intrapersonal,* which is within the person; *interpersonal,* which is between two or more people; *intragroup,* which is within the group; and *intergroup,* which occurs between two or more groups.

Although conflict within a group may seem painful and disruptive at the time it erupts, it is

Key terms	
Term	**Definition**
Conflict	A clash, disagreement, or different perspective that occurs when people have differing goals, ideas, values, beliefs, needs, or feelings; can be useful or a hindrance
Collaboration	Mutual sharing and joint work toward either achieving a common understanding or reaching a common goal
Confrontation	A problem-solving approach to conflict management
Avoidance	Not directly acknowledging or dealing with conflict; a passive form of conflict management
Accommodating	A passive form of conflict management where one or more participants put aside their own concerns to support the group
Compromising	When two or more people have a different goal that can be met only if each participant modifies his or her position; implies a "give and take" or "finding a middle ground"

important to recognize that conflict can be useful when it points out differences that would emerge later and possibly be even more disruptive. The expression of conflict prevents stagnation and often is a healthy prelude to change. In any successful change activity, it is essential that all participants agree on their goal. Consensus on both a goal and an action plan is basic to the change process. Reaching consensus generally means that a wide range of often different opinions and approaches are considered. Consensus is essential when the change will affect each of the participants. Before a group can achieve consensus, however, the views of different members must be heard, given fair consideration, and critically evaluated.

Conflict can be either constructive or destructive for organizational effectiveness. When it is used for personal gain—to achieve vested interests and hidden goals—or when it is expressed to hurt someone or some project, it is a destructive force. There seems to be an optimal level of conflict within an organization; an excessive amount of conflict typically threatens the group and has negative consequences. Too much and too frequent conflict that is poorly managed and never resolved keeps the organization in turmoil and severely works against goal attainment and progress. For example, overt, angry disagreement tends to squelch communication, so relief of the feeling tone or velocity may be needed. Conflict is a signal that something is amiss and, as such, generates the need for further dialogue and idea generation.

Sources of Conflict Conflict often results from *faulty communication,* and it is inevitable when all participants do not have the same information. Thus any effective change process requires clear, consistent communication to all participants and influential parties. It is not enough just to discuss the proposed plan with the anticipated participants. Everyone who is likely to be affected, from the administrator to the cleaning personnel, needs to be informed if conflict, confusion, and angry feelings are to be decreased.

Another source of conflict arises from *incompatible goals* among participants. People tend to be motivated and to become involved in projects according to their own personal goals and vested interests. The expression of conflict can be a useful barometer for measuring clashing goals and personal need-attainment strategies.

Differing opinions about a project or plan may be a further source of conflict. This type of conflict is easier to address than when divergent personal goals and needs constitute the roadblock to the communication process. In hierarchic form, it is easiest to handle conflict that arises from lack of information. Once this gap is noted, an action plan can be formulated to provide effective communication to all who are or will be affected by the decision or project.

Conflict also occurs when opinions and ideas differ within the group. When this source of conflict arises, several opportunities for discussion and negotiation are available. In actuality, conflict management generally necessitates discussion, compromise, and negotiation. It is often difficult to deal with conflict based on personal interests and needs, since the actual motives may be disguised behind one of the other two sources and emerge as "hidden agendas." Although it is hard to get hidden agendas out on the table where they can be handled, this step is necessary for effective communication, conflict resolution, and change management.

Reactions to Conflict How people deal with conflict depends on their experiences, personal coping capacity, and environmental supports or constraints. Each person has a choice between dealing directly with conflict or passively reacting to it, but the choice must be made consciously after considering all possible alternatives and ramifications. Part of the decision about how to handle conflict necessitates honestly asking the question "What is the cost to me (to the group; to the organization) if I . . .?" Some situations are extremely resistant to change and cause considerable conflict for participants. When change seems impossible and personal levels of conflict are detrimental, the only solution may be to leave. The question of utmost importance is "How much conflict is tolerable for me?"

Positive Reasons for Conflict   Conflict in and of itself is not a negative force within the change process. Rather, the motives of the participants determine the organizational usefulness or destructiveness of conflict. Wood (1977) lists three reasons for encouraging conflict. First, conflict calls attention to the need for more communication and dialogue. By discussing divergent and often opposing points of view, participants can gain a "broadened understanding of the nature of the problem and its implications" (Wood, 1977, p. 116). During this phase of a conflict it may become clear that various people or subgroups hold different notions as to the issue under consideration. Conflict may be automatically decreased once problem consensus is attained.

By encouraging the presentation and discussion of different ideas, a group has more alternatives from which to choose a problem-resolution strategy. This reason for encouraging the active discussion of conflicting views may ultimately spare the decision-making group (person) the risk of prematurely arriving at a solution without considering all possible options. Choosing from carefully thought-out alternatives is the key to successful decision making. Disagreement encourages decision making to occur.

The final reason that Wood (1977) cites for encouraging the open discussion of conflict is that it serves to stimulate the interest of the participants. "Healthy noncombative disagree-

ment" promotes open conflict; individuals can comfortably offer opinions and ideas without a fear of threat from negative repercussions.

Managing Conflict   Whether conflict enriches group action, leads to a stalemate, or causes major hostilities within the group depends on how it is handled. Disruptive or restrictive conflict occurs when those who are involved do not understand the value of conflict and when they either do not know how to or choose not to direct differences into constructive channels. Environments that promote competition at the expense of participants or that communicate that all conflict must be resolved by a win/lose strategy do not encourage positive gain from the expression of differences. When a win/lose approach is taken to conflict management, the result may include personnel resignations, global dissatisfaction, the formation of subgroups or cliques, or a termination of communication. In contrast, constructive conflict resolution develops when participants do not feel threatened by the expression of differing points of view and when there is a commitment to using open dialogue to reach the desired goals.

Conflict management strategies can be categorized in a variety of ways ranging from the passive approach of avoidance to the active approach of confrontation. Each method of conflict management has positive and negative characteristics that should be considered in choosing an approach. In *avoidance,* the conflict is simply not addressed and generally the problem remains unsolved. This approach may be used in highly cohesive groups where the cost of disrupting the group's positive relationships outweighs any expected benefit gained from addressing the conflict.

Accommodation is also a passive approach to conflict management where individuals neglect their own concerns or needs to support the group. This approach is used when the issue is more important to one person than to the others or when the one opposing the idea or plan is either right or more powerful.

Compromise is midway between avoidance and confrontation. In compromise, both (or all) parties give something and move toward a "middle ground." Essentially, no one person or group gets his or her way but all participants give some and gain some. This approach is used when speed is important and when both sides in the conflict have equal power.

Collaboration as a conflict management strategy is a win-win approach in that both sides offer their perspectives so as to identify problems, examine alternatives, and search for the most effective solution. The focus is on solving the problem rather than "winning at all costs" or defeating the other side.

Confrontation is a problem-solving approach to conflict resolution that uses preplanning, considerable action or involvement in the process, and evaluation. Confrontation is essentially a three-stage process: assessment, direct confrontation, and resettlement. The first step in confrontation is to assess the situation. What is the problem? Who seems to be causing the problem? How is it personally affecting you? How does it seem to be affecting others—the total work group? What power structure is involved? What kind of changes can you expect as a result of the confrontation? What might be the cost to you of personally raising the issue? The cost to you of either confronting or ignoring the issue must be weighed. The next series of questions to ask yourself during the assessment stage of confrontation concerns "Whom do I need to confront?" Is the actual conflict between two people who are members of the same group, or is the total group involved? If the conflict is between you and one other person, the resolution should take place in private rather than in front of the group. Assessment includes "who" is involved, "where"

the discussion should take place, "when" the best time is, and exactly "how" the discussion should be handled.

Confrontation is a direct approach that deals only with the problem. Side issues are not brought in nor are the participants' personal attributes. Such an approach implies that "you say what you see, hear or experience, directly, forthrightly and clearly" (Smoyak, 1974, p. 1633). No value judgments are included in confrontation; participants must agree to stick with the issues and to present each side of the conflict in a straightforward and rational way.

Finally, during the assessment stage the other participants are apprised of the need for an open exchange about the conflict. A time and place must be decided on, and each participant must know the purpose of the meeting so that preplanning can be done.

The plan is now ready for implementation. In implementing the confrontation, basic skills for good communication prevail. First, stick to the facts, handle only one subject at a time, and avoid interrupting other speakers. No matter how much you want to interrupt to clarify, defend, or refute, it is essential to listen carefully to what the other person is saying. It is a common human tendency to want to always look good in public. Thus when a colleague is discussing how your actions have affected the group or another person, it is difficult to "hear" what is said. The tendency may be to begin defending your behavior before you have heard the speaker's complete message.

Once each participant has presented the issues, it is helpful to have each one restate what he or she heard the other person say. This form of feedback provides instant clues as to misperceptions or lack of understanding. Perception and accurate hearing may be impaired because of the anxiety level of the participants. Feedback is essential to clear, straightforward confrontation. During the feedback process, state in your words what you heard the other person say. Simply repeating what they said may not indicate understanding and the ability to find meaning in the other person's message.

The last stage in confrontation—resettlement—includes agreeing that a problem exists and jointly devising a strategy for resolution. Up until this point only one participant may have perceived a problem. The other person(s) may have agreed to talk about only "your" perception of the conflict. Now that both sides have been heard, it is time to agree that a problem exists; what the major aspects of the problem are; and that certain steps need to be taken to resolve the conflict. Once these agreements have been reached, participants need to establish goals and priorities for problem resolution and then outline a procedure to be followed. For example, after a confrontation about inconsistency in evaluation of either students or staff members, two participants may agree that inconsistency does exist, that one participant is not adhering to established evaluative guidelines, and that such behavior is not fair to either the students or the other evaluator. The next step would be to agree on a way to change this behavior and then plan checkpoints. For example, the participants may agree to complete the next set of evaluations individually and then go over them together to assess consistency before informing others of the evaluation. Follow-up should be built in to monitor continuation of new behaviors as well as to provide ongoing support and encouragement.

Nurses have two principal ways of dealing with conflict: reacting to or resolving the disagreement. Nurses react to conflict when they withdraw or defuse the situation. Withdrawing rarely solves a conflict; it only postpones the actual impact of the differences. Pent-up feelings remain and often surface in nonconstructive ways; for example, at a later

date an angry outburst may be quite out of proportion to the situation, or the nurse may react to the conflict with physical symptoms.

Managing conflict is a significant part of the role of someone leading change. Inevitably, when more than one person is involved, there will be differences about what should be done; how it should be done; who should be involved; and what the responsibility will be of each one involved. Nurses managing change may be part of the conflict, or they may be in a position to resolve the conflict.

■ KEY POINTS

- Communication takes place constantly in all organizations and serves both to coordinate and to control the functioning of the work group.
- Inherent in any communication are both verbal and nonverbal messages.
- Effective communication is blocked when one or more participants have a hearing or speaking deficit, when speakers have differing frames of reference and do not hear the same message, when the message is not clearly presented, or when the environment interferes with clear message exchange.
- Listening carefully and effectively is key to good communication and essential in the process of managing change. In any organization, people communicate in four directions: horizontally, upward, downward, and diagonally.
- Managing both collaboration and conflict is essential to organizational effectiveness and the change process.

■ CRITICAL THINKING QUESTIONS

1. Recall the typical way in which members of your family communicated with one another.
   A. How would you describe your family's amount and style of communication?
   B. When was communication about happy topics most likely to occur?

C. When did the family discuss unpleasant subjects?

2. Describe a situation in which the message you intended to send was not the one heard by the listener. What factors might have led to this incongruence?

3. Evaluate your typical communication style.
   A. Is it more masculine or feminine?
   B. Is it direct or indirect?
   C. Do you prefer to speak or write?

4. Recall a person whom you consider an effective communicator, and describe the characteristics that cause you to see this person as effective.

5. Evaluate at least three people on a television talk show in terms of their effectiveness as a communicator. What works for them? What could be improved? If you had been speaking on the topic, how would you have approached it?

■ REFERENCES

Coeling, H.V., & Wilcox, J.R. (1994). Steps to collaboration . . . essential communication elements (behaviors) necessary for collaboration. *Nursing Administration Quarterly, 18*(4), 44-55.

Cornell, Dixie. (1993). Say the words: Communication techniques. *Nursing Management, 24*(March), 42-44.

Davis, J. (1994). Body language, voice tone send nonverbal messages. *Case Management Advisor, 5*(11), 155.

Davis, K. (1972). *Human relations at work.* New York: McGraw-Hill.

Davis, K. (1975). Cut those rumors down to size. *Supervisory Management, 20*(June), 2-6.

Davis, K. (1977). *Organizational behavior: A book of readings* (5th ed.). New York: McGraw-Hill.

Gibson, J.L., Ivancevish, J.M., & Donnelly, J.H. (1976). *Organizations: Behavior, structure, processes* (rev. ed.). Dallas: Business Publications.

Hanlon, J.M. (1996). Teaching effective communication skills. *Nursing Management, 27*(4), 48B-48D.

Heim, P. (1995). Getting beyond "she said, he said." *Nursing Administration Quarterly, 19*(2), 6-18.

Liedtka, J., & Whitten, E. (1996). Building better patient care services: A collaborative approach. *Health Care Management Review, 22*(3), 16-24.

Marriner-Tomey, A. (1996). *Guide to nursing management and leadership* (5th ed.). St. Louis: Mosby.

Smoyak, S. (1974). The confrontation process. *American Journal of Nursing, 74*(Sept.), 1632-1635.

Sullivan, E.J., & Decker, P.J. (1997). *Communication and conflict, effective leadership and management in nursing* (4th ed.). Menlo Park, Calif.: Addison-Wesley.

Wood, J.R. (1977). Constructive conflict in discussion: Learning to manage disagreements effectively. In J.W. Jones & J.E. Pfeiffer (Eds.). *The 1977 annual handbook for group facilitators*, LaJolla, Calif.: University Associates.

Zak-Dance, C. (1996). The ties that bind leadership, communication, and gender. *Surgical Services Management, 2*(6), 18-20.

Leading in Times of Change

Jeanette Lancaster

INTRODUCTION

This chapter briefly addresses several of the time-honored theories about leadership as prelude to a more extensive discussion of current thinking about the skills, competencies, values, and behaviors of leaders. Leaders of today are seeking to make changes in their organizations at a time of great turbulence, unrest, and in some instances, confusion. Those who lead, participate in, and evaluate change must recognize that leaders are found at all levels of the organization and in a wide range of roles.

Although there are similarities between leading and managing, they are not the same. Zaleznik (1992, p. 126) in a *Harvard Business Review* "classic" says that "leadership inevitably requires using power to influence the thoughts and actions of other people." The leader exerts influence through a wide range of interpersonal skills to accomplish goals. In contrast, managers are problem solvers who work in a rational framework for achieving results. Managers coordinate and manage resources; they use the processes of planning, organizing, directing, and controlling to meet specific organizational goals and objectives. Although good interpersonal skills are certainly useful in effective management, the manager also has the authority, re-

sponsibility, accountability, and power given by the organization to make certain the stated goals are met. Management requires planning, priority setting, motivating, selecting the strategy for achieving the goals, and evaluating the outcome as well as providing timely feedback to those involved. Managers must be persistent, tough-minded, intelligent, and analytic to plan, coordinate, and evaluate. Management theory and the skills for effective management are discussed in detail in Chapter 17.

The most effective leadership is needed at times of transition and turbulence, which are often characterized by rapid and unsettling change. Nurses who lead today are not simply dealing with a lot of change, but rather they are managing a complex of multiple changes in their personal and professional lives, much of which is not of their making and is not necessarily considered desirable. Effective leaders create a climate that minimizes the chaos and disorder typically inherent in change. According to Kerfoot (1997, p. 384) nursing leaders face three challenges: (1) to be a change leader, (2) to settle for no less than world class excellence, and (3) to accept leadership and service to humanity as a moral imperative. These three challenges are discussed in depth in the sections that follow.

Current thinking also holds that men and women lead differently and that the talents each gender typically brings is useful for all leaders to understand; change leaders may need to learn skills that may be missing in their own current skill set. Feminine leadership styles are more likely to nurture and cultivate their teams, establish more egalitarian relationships, and put in place more of a "weblike" corporate structure than a traditional "command and control reporting hierarchy" (Entine & Nichols, 1997, p.50).

Leaders must understand the skills that will serve them best: how to communicate effectively as well as understand the importance of trust and the appropriate use of power in their roles.

Because many excellent texts in the fields of both business and nursing discuss the traditional views and theories of leadership, much of the information presented here is drawn from the works of business leaders who provide guidance for nursing leaders based on their successful business practices.

OBJECTIVES

After reading this chapter, you will be able to:

1. Utilize selected theories of leadership in leading and managing change
2. Evaluate how the qualities, attributes, and skills of successful business leaders can be used in nursing
3. Predict which use of power will be most helpful when leading during changing times

4. Describe the importance of both trust and effective communication in influencing change
5. Evaluate the ways in which effective leaders influence people and organizations
6. Describe the leader of the future, and identify those traits that you see in yourself compared with those that would need to be developed so that you could lead effectively

■ WHAT IS LEADERSHIP?

The definitions and descriptions of leadership are nearly limitless. A sampling of those that have shaped current thinking are discussed briefly here to set the stage for a later discussion of contemporary views of leadership. Over the years, questions such as these have been raised: What is leadership? Can it be learned, or is it an innate characteristic that some of us are born with and others simply do not have? Or if lead-

ership can be learned, how do you go about doing that? Fiedler (1967, p. 11) defined leadership as "an interpersonal relationship in which power and influence are unevenly distributed so that one person is able to direct and control the actions and behavior of others to a greater extent than they direct and control his."

Drucker (1996) unequivocally says there is no one best "leadership personality" or "leadership style." He has seen effective leaders who are "nice guys," disciplinarians, quick and impulsive rather than studied and purposive; some are warm whereas others are aloof. What he has found to be true of effective leaders are four simple things (p. xii):

1. Leaders have followers.
2. His or her followers do the right things.
3. These leaders set examples and are highly visible.
4. They assume responsibility.

Drucker goes on to say that the effective leaders he has known all behave the same way. That is, they begin by asking "What needs to be done?" and then move to "What can and should I do to make a difference?" Throughout their tenure as leaders, they ask "What are our mission and goals?" and "What comprises productive performance and results in this organization at this time?" (1996, p. xiii).

Bennis (1990) in his book, *Why Leaders Can't Lead,* described 5 years of study in which he spent time with 90 of the most successful leaders in the United States. He was looking for the common traits in successful leaders. Initially, he thought these common traits would not be found, since the leaders he studied seemed so different from one another. However, he actually found some common traits and concluded several things that can influence our thinking about leading in nursing. First, he found that "Leaders are people who do the right thing; managers are people who do things right" (1990, p. 18). Although that is an often-heard phrase, the immense truth in it is apparent. It is the leader who has the vision, who can see the "big picture," and who knows what is the right thing to do (and at the right time, using the right people and other resources). The leader also recruits, guides, and serves as a role model for co-workers who do things right that are consistent with the mission, goals, and values of the organization.

After much study and reflection, Bennis (1990, pp. 20-23) concluded that the leaders he studied had four competencies that differentiated them from others who hoped to lead:

- They manage attention—they draw others to them not only because they have a vision, but also because they communicate an extraordinary focus of commitment. These leaders conveyed a sense of knowing the outcome or goal they were aiming for and the direction they needed to take to achieve that goal.
- They manage meaning—they translate the vision into a language by using words, visual images, and metaphors that others can understand. Successful leaders are stimulating, not boring. You can almost see their vision, when they describe it, as clearly as they can see it.
- They manage trust—that is, they are constant in what they do and what they say; their meaning is reflected in their own actions. Think how shallow it is to talk about valuing one's team and then to shout at team members in front of others. As the saying goes, "They walk the talk." They can be counted on.
- They manage self—they know themselves, including their own strengths and weaknesses. They build a team with people whose strengths complement the leader's weaknesses. They see a mistake not as a failure but as feedback, so that they can determine what the next action should be.

Leaders, then, influence people to change, to move toward new goals through their own example and by their vision of where they and the organization are going; through their valuing and respect for their colleagues; and through their clear, straightforward communication. Kerfoot (1997) says that a useful way to describe a leader is someone who unleashes the human potential in others. Such leaders always believe their people are capable of more than the people themselves believe of themselves.

Key terms	
Term	**Definition**
Leader	Person who influences others to accomplish specific goals using effective interpersonal skills
Manager	Person responsible for efficiently planning, organizing, and evaluating the effective attainment of goals and the thoughtful use of resources
Power	Ability to produce or prevent change
Formal leadership	That which is exercised by a person with legitimate authority vested in the position
Informal leadership	That which is exercised by someone who does not have a specific management role but whom others choose to follow

■ THEORIES OF LEADERSHIP

Some people have found theories of leadership to be helpful; others have not, saying that no one theory meets everyone's needs at all times and in the many and varied organizations. However, brief sketches of several of the classic theories are summarized here to enable you to see what fits and describes you.

Trait Theories

Much of the early work in leadership research looked at those characteristics that distinguished leaders from followers. The earliest form of trait theories, referred to as the "Great Man Theory," stated that some people are born with the innate ability to be a leader. This position held that some people were simply endowed with qualities that distinguished them from others. Note in the later section on gender-related communication differences that the trait theory would likely hold that an essential characteristic is maleness.

Trait theorists thought that successful leaders would have a striking physical appearance, good speaking ability, insight, and intelligence. Further, they would be pleasant, honest, and highly energetic and have a sense of purpose. They would also demonstrate integrity, courage,

and self-discipline. Although many of these traits are seen as valuable skills in good leaders, it is currently thought that they can be learned and are not necessarily inborn.

Behavioral Theories

Dissatisfaction with the narrow scope of the trait theories led to the development of the behavioral theories of leadership. The emphasis shifted from a focus on inherent traits to that of personal qualities. This research in the early 1930s focused on the abilities and behaviors of leaders or what leaders do; and the behavioral theories posited that leaders could be developed through education, training, and life experiences.

Style of leadership One behavioral approach to looking at leadership was to consider the style of the leader. Theories that focused on style tended to describe four predominant styles: autocratic, democratic, laissez-faire, and bureaucratic. These four behaviors or styles for leading were associated with the amount of freedom that the leader provided to subordinates in making decisions. The continuum went from highly leader-centered decision making in the autocratic style to member control of decision making in laissez-faire. In general, people

Key terms	
Term	**Definition**
Leadership	An interpersonal relationship in which the leader employs style, approaches, and strategies to influence people to achieve mutually established goals
Trait theory	All leaders have certain recognized characteristics
Behavioral theories	Leaders can be developed through education, training, and life experiences, i.e., their leadership is learned rather than inborn
Styles of leadership	A behavioral approach that says each leader leans toward one of four styles: autocratic, democratic, laissez-faire, or bureaucratic

use a variety of these styles over time, depending on the situation and other participants. For example, in an ICU during a code, a directive and more autocratic style is effective. In contrast, the same nurse might shift to a democratic style during a team meeting held to look at indicators of quality outcomes for the unit.

The *autocratic leader* exerts maximal control over followers. The leader has ultimate responsibility for decision making and establishes goals for the group. In nursing, this type of leader discourages group participation and is task oriented in an attempt to ensure that goals are accomplished efficiently. This leader believes that followers are motivated by external forces, such as power, authority, and the need for approval. The leader makes all the decisions and uses coercion, punishment, and specific directions to get followers to do as told. As might be imagined, these leaders create fear among followers, and this often leads to hostility, resentment, and poor morale and performance. The autocratic leader can be ruthless in getting the job done and is unlikely to consider the feelings and needs of others. Such a leader in nursing would be seen as overbearing and demanding. In a version of this style, that of the *benevolent autocrat*, the leader maintains ultimate responsibility, is accessible to members and listens to their opinions, ideas, and suggestions, yet retains full control. The benevolent autocrat maintains power and a position as "chief" while being concerned about the needs of others as well as their attitudes. This style can be useful in busy nursing situations or when change is rapid and actions must be taken in a timely manner.

In the *democratic form of leadership,* the leader ultimately makes all the decisions but allows members to participate throughout the process. This leader assumes that people are motivated by internal drives and impulses and that they want to be part of the decision. The democratic leader requests ideas from the group and makes comments and suggestions but typically does not give orders to the group. The main function of the democratic leader is to stimulate and motivate the group. Group members are respected, and their opinions and ideas are valued. When democratic leaders praise members, it is for the work that they have done—not for their personal characteristics. Similarly, criticism is about the work—not the person. This style is often seen in nursing in work groups who function harmoniously together.

Key terms	
Term	**Definition**
Autocratic leaders	Task-focused and expect obedience from members of the group so goals can be accomplished
Democratic leaders	Ultimately make the decision but rely heavily on group involvement in establishing goals and designing plans
Laissez-faire leaders	"Laid back" and exert no direct influence over participants; allow the group to select their goals and plan of action
Bureaucratic leaders	Go "by the book," and rely on policy manuals and procedure memos to guide the group's work
Benevolent autocratic leaders	Clearly retain ultimate responsibility but are accessible to members and listen to them

To function effectively in a democratic work group, all members must understand their roles and responsibilities. The teams of today are much like the democratic theory of leadership. That is, teams comprise members who share responsibility. All are seen as valuable members with something to contribute, and each has a part in making the group cohesive and effective. This type of leadership can frustrate some members in that decision making, which is based on consensus and group interaction, is time consuming. Members may struggle with what they see as a lack of structure and a tendency to take a long time to reach a decision or develop a plan. Some people feel more comfortable being given clear and explicit instructions rather than being part of the team deciding on the plan.

In the *laissez-faire form of leadership,* it is assumed that individuals are motivated by internal drives and impulses and that if left alone, they will do good work. This style is often referred to as "hands-off" leadership, since the leader exerts no direct influence over the members. The leader provides neither direction nor efforts to facilitate the group; members are left to direct themselves. Whereas the autocratic style focuses on the leader and the democratic style focuses on the group, the laissez-faire leadership style focuses on the individual. The laissez-faire leader is not often seen as a true leader but rather a distributor of information who makes no attempt to evaluate the work of others; instead, he or she passes information from one group to another.

Jenkins and Henderson (1984) added a fourth style, the *bureaucratic style of leadership.* The bureaucratic leader assumes that employees are motivated by external forces. Neither the leader nor the followers are trusted as being reliable in making decisions, so this leader relies on policies and procedures for all decisions. This style requires limited personal interaction, and there is almost no need to reach consensus or have any discussion for that matter. These leaders simply "go by the book." The absolute source of information and authority is whatever the policy or procedure manual or minutes of committees say. Although it is often seen in nursing, this style is usually not the most effective when leading change, since it may not produce sufficient commitment to the project or plan.

The Managerial Grid Another behavioral approach to describing leadership uses a continuum called a *managerial grid.* When Blake and Mouton (1978) developed the managerial grid in the early 1960s, they defined five leadership types based on concern for production (task) and concern for people (relationships). They thought that the assumptions and concerns made about people and production were complementary—not mutually exclusive—and that the two styles on the continuum needed to be integrated for the most effective performance.

Their five leadership styles are best described as follows:

- *Impoverished*—Minimal effort and concern are devoted to both people and production, which means that the person does only what is required to sustain the viability of the organization.
- *Country club*—Minimal attention is given to production and maximal attention is paid to people, leading to a comfortable, friendly working atmosphere.
- *Task*—High concern for production and efficiency with little interest in human factors.
- *Middle of the road*—Moderate concern for both people and getting the job done.
- *Team*—Viewed as the ideal approach because it integrates high concern for both people and production; leads to mutual trust and respect in the workplace. See Figure 9-1.

The team approach is particularly suited to the change process in nursing. Employees are typically more productive when they feel valued and recognized and also when the specifics of what is expected are clear to all.

Contingency Theories

Contingency theories suggest that leaders modify their approach depending on the situation. Leadership behaviors range from authoritarian to permissive, depending on the circumstances, needs, and expected outcomes.

Fiedler's Contingency Theory During the 1960s, Fred Fiedler introduced the contingency model of leadership, which blends the behavioral approach or style with attention to the present situation. Fiedler (1967) was concerned with how a person could become an effective leader. He began by differentiating two leadership styles: the human relations or group-oriented and the task-oriented. In the former, the leader is motivated largely by a desire to maintain good interpersonal relations and to use democratic decision-making processes. In contrast, the task-oriented leader is authoritarian and concerned primarily with goal attainment; this person assumes responsibility for making decisions and directing the activities of the group.

The foundation for this theory is built on three situational factors in leadership that influence leader effectiveness: leader-member relations, task structure, and position power. *Leader-member relations* refers to the amount of confidence members have in the leader and includes support for and loyalty to the leader. *Task structure* describes the amount of routineness involved in the task, that is, how clearly defined and generally understood the task is versus how ambiguous it is. *Position power* refers to the formal authority associated with the leader's position and includes the rewards and punishments associated with the position as well as the support that leaders receive from those to whom they report. See Figure 9-2.

The key factor in determining which style fits the situation is the favorability of the situation. *Favorability* is affected by the quality of (1) leader-member relations in a group, (2) the degree to which a group's task is structured, and (3) the formal power that the leader derives from occupying the position. In general, as leader-member relations improve, a situation becomes more favorable, the task becomes more structured, and the leader's position power increases. Fiedler suggests that the leadership style needed for situations in which all three dimensions are strong or high (good leader-

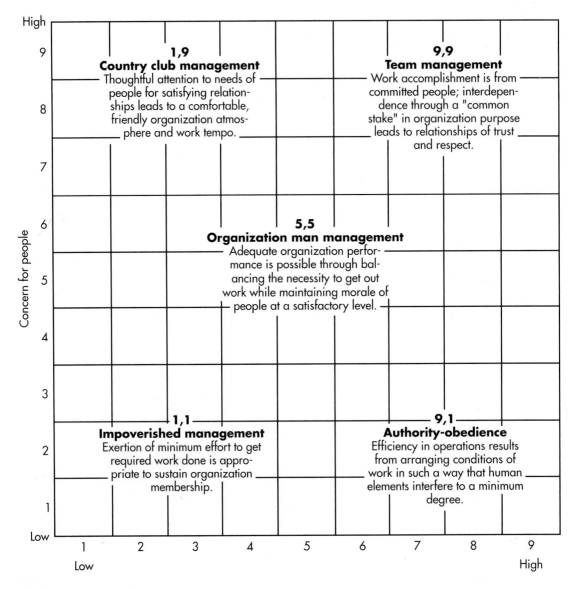

Figure 9-1 ■ The managerial grid. (The Leadership Grid® figure from Blake, R.R., & McCanse, A.A. [1991]. *Leadership dilemmas: Grid solutions.* Austin, Tex.: Scientific Methods.)

member relations, structured task, and strong position power), are much different from situations in which all dimensions are weak or low (poor leader-member relations, unstructured task, and weak position power).

According to contingency theory, task-oriented leaders perform best in extreme situations (either very favorable or very unfavorable). For example, a task-oriented leader would be recommended for handling a disaster such as a

Key terms	
Term	**Definition**
Managerial grid	A way of viewing leadership that defines five types based on concern for production (task) versus concern for people (relationships)
Contingency theory	The effectiveness of a given leader is determined by the demands of the situation
Contingency model of leadership	Includes three basic components: leader-member relations, task structure, and position power, which determine the effectiveness of the leader
Situational theory of leadership	The effectiveness of any leader is a function of the situation or context in which leadership takes place
Path-goal theory of leadership	Based on expectancy theory and says that leaders are effective when they motivate followers, coordinate their work so that they can achieve the goal, and subsequently have job satisfaction
Transformational leadership	Present when leaders are committed to the organization and people; have a vision; and enlist others to believe in the vision and work to accomplish the goals set forth by the vision

fire on a hospital unit. In this example, the leader-member relations are generally weak. The tasks are unstructured even in a hospital with regular fire drills because the same group of staff and patients is rarely present for the practice and the actual situation; often the position power is weak until someone acknowledges a leadership role in this particular fire drill.

The same leadership style would be reflected in the actions of a designated team who consistently responds to cardiac arrests. In this example, the leader-member relations are usually good because each one has a specified agreed-on role and the tasks are highly structured. Also, there is a designated team leader who holds recognized position power. In both the fire and a cardiac arrest, there is little time for consideration because each second is precious. The *consideration style* is more effective when the environment or situation is moderately certain. For example, a task force charged with developing personnel policies would generally reflect good leader-member relations, an unstructured task, and weak position power.

Situation Leadership Theory Leader effectiveness from this perspective highly depends on the situation at the time. In situation theory, leaders are generally more concerned with the needs of the group than with their own needs, since the best leaders are able to adjust their approach to a particular group at a specific point in time to deal effectively with the situation. According to Marriner-Tomey (1996, p. 270), the following variables determine the leader's effectiveness: leader personality; performance requirements of both leader and followers; attitudes, needs and expectations of leaders and followers; amount of possible interpersonal contact; time demands; physical environment; structure of the organization and the state of its development; and the extent to which the leader has influence outside the group.

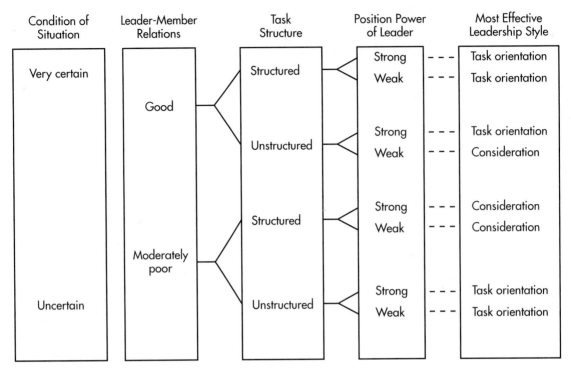

Figure 9-2 ■ Fiedler's contingency theory of leadership. (Modified from Fiedler, F. [1967]. *A theory of leadership effectiveness.* New York: McGraw-Hill.)

Hersey and Blanchard (1988) developed a theory of situational leadership whereby they identified four styles of leadership that are described according to the readiness and ability of the followers:

(1) Leaders use a telling style (S1: high task, low relationship) with followers who are unable and unwilling or insecure about performing the task (R1). (2) Leaders use a selling style (S2: high task, high relationship) with followers who are unable but are willing or confident in performing the task (R2). (3) Leaders use a participating style (S3: low task, high relationship) with followers who are able but unwilling or lacking in confidence in performing the task (R3). Finally, (4) leaders use a delegating style (S4: low task, low relationship) with followers who are both able and willing and have confidence in performing the task (R4).

Path-Goal Theory The path-goal theory of leadership attempts to match the leader's style with certain interpersonal and situational factors. Robert J. House derived the path-goal theory from expectancy theory, which says that people act as they do because they expect their behavior to produce satisfactory results. The leader facilitates task completion by minimizing obstructions to goal attainment and by rewarding followers when they achieve the goal. This is a "hands on" form of leadership in that the leader clarifies activities so people can be successful; it reduces barriers; and it provides guidance, encouragement, and positive rewards.

Expectancy theory comprises the foundation of the path-goal view. According to expectancy theory, people are motivated to produce if they believe that their efforts will be successful and will subsequently be rewarded. The concept of *path clarification,* a key aspect of leader behavior, is to clarify the types of activities that are most likely to result in goal attainment. In general, the path-goal approach to leadership has two key propositions (House, 1971):

1. Leader behavior is acceptable and satisfying to the extent that the subordinates perceive such behavior as an immediate source of satisfaction or as instrumental to future satisfaction.

2. Leader behavior will be motivational to the extent that it makes satisfaction of subordinates' needs contingent on effective performance and it complements the environment of subordinates by providing the guidance, clarity of direction, and rewards necessary for effective performance.

Key concepts in path-goal theory include motivation of subordinates to perform efficiently; the leader's responsibility to clarify activities so that subordinates can be successful; and the value of rewards as a motivating force in performance. Also, it is the leader's responsibility to clarify expectancies and reduce the barriers to goal attainment. Thus a leader can effectively combine task orientation and consideration.

Path-goal theory has considerable potential for nurses. It is basically a human-relations set of activities that recognizes the need to respect others and to provide guidance, encouragement, and clarity of directions. Such behaviors in the long run tend to motivate positive actions from followers. The application of path-goal theory can be seen in the relationship between two nurses, such as a charge and staff nurse, and in faculty-student communications.

Transformational Leadership

The current popular style of leadership, transformational leadership, fits the rapidly changing and often disquieting health care environment. James MacGregor Burns, in his book *Leadership* (1978), described transformational leaders as being committed, having a vision of what could be accomplished, and empowering others with this vision so that all would accomplish more with less.

Characteristics associated with transformational leaders include the following: being able to help one's group make changes to move the organization forward, focus on planned actions, encouraging people to take risks; listening especially to suggestions and providing feedback; coaching and role modeling; and being trustworthy. The transformational leader must recognize "that the whole culture of the workplace must reflect change as a constant, value it, and incorporate that understanding into the very culture of work" (Porter-O'Grady, 1992, p. 19). This leader also appreciates that the employee of today is a "knowledge worker" who brings knowledge and skills to the enterprise.

Transformational leadership is coordinating, integrating, and facilitating rather than directing and controlling. Because work is currently done by groups or teams rather than by individuals working alone, the effective leader must be able to work with, and bring together into teams, people from a variety of disciplines. In these multidisciplinary and collaborative units, skills in consensus building, conflict resolution, and issue mediation, as well as problem solving, solution seeking, and opportunity seeking, are essential (Porter-O'Grady, 1992). Effective leaders use community-building skills to create an environment in which many leaders can emerge. They realize that when people work as knowledge workers rather than in skilled labor or technical roles, they are more likely to work in teams, and the leadership passes from person to person depending on the timing and task to be done.

An interesting point about leadership is the view that "before people can lead others, they must lead themselves" (Gunder & Crissman, 1992, p. 7). Specifically, leaders must believe that they have power and influence and are respected and valued before they can "bring out the best in their colleagues." The successful leader in a change environment must be adaptable and flexible. This may entail the unlearning of some old skills and learning to use new skills in managing and leading through change.

■ CHARACTERISTICS OF EFFECTIVE LEADERS

Several characteristics found in successful leaders have been described already. Others will be briefly described here, and three—trust, communication, and the effective use of power—are discussed in detail because of their tremendous impact on both organizations and the people in them. Because health care, especially nursing, is "people-intensive," nurses who lead or participate in change can benefit from examining the characteristics attributed to successful leaders in other types of organizations.

Max DePree in his book *Leadership is an Art* (1989) offers some practical thoughts on what makes a good leader. First is an essential truth about leadership—leaders have ideas. The true leader is one who removes obstacles so followers can reach their full potential (see p. 237). Leaders also listen carefully, and they encourage people to share differing opinions. Leaders are responsible for effectiveness. They will ultimately be held accountable for the outcomes of the organization. The characteristics of trust, good communication, and effectively using power will enable nurses who lead change to become more like the leader DePree describes.

Trust

Trust is a basic element in the culture of effective health care organizations. Trust appears in the attitudes, beliefs, and behaviors of members of the organization and when present,

glues or bonds the people together. Traditionally, many organizations have had a hierarchic, top-down structure with a distinct pecking order in terms of rank, status, and power. This is changing. Organizations are becoming flatter and now emphasize delegating power and authority to employees.

Nurses, like other types of employees, tend to enact the expectations of the managers and leaders with whom they work; that is, if they are viewed as creative, imaginative, productive people who truly want to contribute to the organization's success, they are much more likely to behave accordingly, as opposed to their responses if they are viewed as lazy, unreliable, and unimaginative (Johns, 1996).

Health care organizations desire nurses who are committed to meeting the goals of the organization. Trust is related to commitment; that is, nurses are more likely to commit fully to their organization when they trust both their co-workers and managers. In high-trust organizations, the mission is clearly identified; there is congruence between what people say and do; people are valued and respected for what they know and contribute; and emphasis is on leading rather than managing.

The following are four traits identified in leaders who generate and sustain trust:

- *Constancy*—they do not create surprises; they "stay the course" and are reasonably predictable.
- *Congruity*—the actions of these leaders match their words.
- *Reliability*—they can be counted on when their people need them.
- *Integrity*—they honor their commitments and promises.

Leaders are constantly "on stage" and must hold trust over time. "Months of goodwill can vanish when a leader stumbles into situation that is perceived as lacking integrity" (Kerfoot, 1997, p. 152).

Communication

Communication is central to leadership. If a leader is one who has followers (one who leads, guides, and provides direction to others), it seems clear that effective leaders in nursing must be good communicators. Although an entire chapter in this text is devoted to communication, some key points need to be made here in regard to communication and leadership.

Although face-to-face, one-on-one communication is typically the most effective strategy, it may not always be possible. Other channels of communication are frequent, brief, and efficiently run meetings; newsletters; electronic mail messages; and the use of banners or posters to announce and celebrate good news, honors, or awards.

Gender Differences in Communication

Communication is affected by the culture, ages, sexual orientations, and backgrounds of the participants as well as by gender. Effective nursing leaders, during times of change, restructuring, realigning, and turbulence in the health care system, should recognize possible gender differences in styles of leading. Some writers generalize forms of behavior and communication as being characteristic of either men or women. Zak-Dance (1996) offers caution in making broad generalizations that would say boys speak and behave a certain way simply because they are male and girls speak and behave differently because of their female nature. She points out that gender is a social construction and not entirely associated with one's biologic sex; that is, people are born either male or female. They learn to be feminine or masculine. In actuality, the majority of females behave in ways associated with feminine behaviors and most males are seen as masculine. Few communication behaviors are solely associated with one's biologic sex, but many differences are learned because of one's socialization and enculturation (Ronk,

1993). Many health care organizations seem to support masculine styles of communication, yet the majority of employees are female.

To understand how enculturation leads to masculine and feminine forms of behavior and communication, especially in regard to nursing, it is useful to look back to the Victorian era and consider how women and nurses were viewed. As Moss (1995, p. 41) says: "The impact of Nursing's Victorian roots is common knowledge. However, to dismantle the glass ceiling, nurses must understand the depth of Victorian perceptions about women, as well as ways which these perceptions continue to hold the structure in place." Perhaps the most enduring is that in the Victorian era, women were viewed as serfs and considered suited for child bearing and home management and certainly they were not considered equal to the demands of running an organization. Rudiments of these ancient views are present in some current organizations and must be understood and addressed.

Tornabeni (1995, p. 30) talks about the glass ceiling metaphor by describing glass as coming in two varieties: ordinary glass that can be broken with determination; and shatterproof glass that resists all efforts to break it. Women must know the difference between these types of glass and be able to differentiate their presence in the work situation. Women must know if the glass can be broken before they rush headlong into it.

Communication is not always direct and straightforward. In fact, many messages are subtle or disguised. People, rather than explicitly stating their viewpoint or asking their questions, may communicate through what are called "hidden agendas." These hidden agendas are the real messages yet are not the message expressed. To recognize hidden agendas and other indirect forms of communication, women must understand the power structure, learn the rules of the game, and learn the language—both corporate and gender influenced.

Learn the Rules of the Game Much has been written to explain how children learn different ways to play games depending on their gender. In sports such as baseball, basketball, football, and soccer, boys learn to compete, be aggressive, play to win, and focus on the goal line. Female play is often with dolls and is more likely to teach about relationships, being fair, and getting along (Heim, 1995). In health care, style conflicts can occur when members of the team "play by different rules." For example, a manager might expect team members to "just do as I say," whereas the members expect to participate in designing the plan. Clearly, boys and girls both engage in games typically associated with the other gender. The key for nursing leaders is to appreciate the differences in masculine and feminine characteristics, especially as they affect communication and power relationships. One way to become sensitive to these different characteristics is to listen to the metaphors used at work. How often do you hear people say: "The ball is in your court"; "They are playing hardball"; or "They are really out of bounds." These metaphors are clues about the operating rules in the organization.

Understand the Existing Power Structure Many organizations have clearly defined ranks or levels of authority. People outside the vertical rank hierarchy tend not to have specifically defined powers, and people with titles like assistant have no rank in the organization. Historically, women enter organizations in the staff rather than management structure. Clearly, this is not an absolute but rather a trend. A key to success is knowing when the obstacles are within the system rather than within the person. Rather than whining about "the good old boys" having all the power, the nurse who becomes an effective leader designs strategies for getting "to the table" where decisions are made.

B O X   9 - 1

How I Learned to Let My Workers Lead

In nursing, we can learn from the successes and failures of businesses. Specifically, Ralph Strayer (1990, p. 66) decided that his family business needed to be changed when he looked around and saw a huge gap between the potential and actual performance of his employees. As he said, "I wanted employees who would fly like geese. What I had was a company that wallowed like a herd of buffalo." What he saw in his employees were people who did not seem to care; people who took no responsibility for their work. He began looking for a book to tell him how to change his company. What was the recipe for success? Of course, no such book or recipe was found that would provide a simple blueprint for the things he needed to change to effectively lead his company to become a leader in its field.

What he did learn is that he had to raise and find answers to the following questions:

- What are the company's goals?
- In the best of all possible worlds, what do I want to see happen?
- How do I learn to share responsibility when I often just tell people what to do?
- Who should make which decisions?
- Where and when should change begin?

Modified from Strayer R. (1990). How I learned to let my workers lead. *Harvard Business Review, 68*(6), 66-83.

Learn the Language Masculine communicators tend to stick more to facts, whereas feminine communicators are more likely to explain, provide more detail than may be either essential or desired on the part of the listener, and analyze more. These differences can lead to discomfort in both types of communicators when the masculine one expects a short answer and the feminine type wants to explain

BOX 9 - 2

Tips for Making the Change Journey

Observation	Action to Take
1. People want to be great. If they aren't, it is because managers won't let them.	1. Invite others to help identify and solve the problem rather than informing them of what the problem is and how it could be solved. Make people feel significant.
2. Performance begins with each individual's expectations.	2. Those who implement a decision and live with its consequences are the best people to make it.
3. Expectations are driven partly by goals, vision, symbols, semantics, and partly by the context in which people work.	3. Compensation systems, as well as decision-making structures, influence employee satisfaction.
4. The actions of managers shape expectations.	4. People watch everything you do. Be consistent in word and deed.
5. Learning is a process, not a goal.	5. You learn from both failures and successes.
6. The organization's results reflect me and my performance.	6. The leader is never a "finished product" in an evolving, changing organization.

Modified from Strayer, R. (1990). How I learned to let my workers lead. *Harvard Business Review 68*(6), 66-83.

fully so no facts will be missing. Other feminine qualities are good listening skills, compassion, empathy, pragmatism, a sense that people matter most, and an ability to focus on both the what and how of what happened (Tornabeni, 1995). Masculine qualities are usually more direct, forceful, decisive, and assertive. A synthesis of masculine and feminine communication skills will be useful in leading change; that is, an effective change leader should value team members and listen carefully while providing clear and decisive leadership. (See Box 9-1.)

The boxed material describes how one leader, who owned his own business, learned to let his workers lead. To do so, he learned to believe in his people and to both set an example by his own behavior and also set up structures to clearly support his employees. In nursing, we can learn from the experiences of successful business leaders.

As he worked to reshape his company and answer these questions, he concluded that the "change journey" could be effectively charted if he kept six observations in mind. These observations are about people and are not specific to any particular company or industry. Consider how they transfer to a health care unit or organization and what nurses leading change can learn from Strayer. The lessons Strayer learned are shown in Box 9-2.

■ POWER AS A TOOL FOR LEADERSHIP

Power is an increasingly important form of influence for nursing leaders. As has been noted, leaders are found throughout the organization and may have formal leadership responsibility as well as informal leadership within teams. Informal leadership is often derived from respect and regard for the knowledge and good judgment of the person. Power and change are ever-present in health care organizations. This discussion focuses on the nature of power; the types and sources of power; the use of power in health care organizations; and the usefulness of power in leadership.

The Nature of Power

Power is the "ability of a person or a group to require others to act as the power holder desires" (McFarland, 1982, p. 96). Power can also be defined as the "capacity to produce or prevent change" (Sullivan & Decker, 1997, p. 53). Power is the strongest possible form of influence in that the person who wields it is often in a position to exert consequences that affect others. Power is a two-way street. It cannot come into play unless those to whom it is directed acknowledge its legitimacy and are willing to behave accordingly. Power is seen in its many forms and sources in health care. Nurses who lead change must fully understand the effective use of power as well as its ineffective, manipulative, or abusive use.

Power comes from many sources. Five predominant types of power are seen in organizations: legitimate, reward, coercive, expert, and referent. *Legitimate power* is the authority vested in a role, position, or office that is accepted and recognized by others. For example, the chair of a committee has the legitimate power to lead the meetings of the committee; set the agenda; call on people to speak and participate; and so forth. Some might call legitimate power, *position power;* that is, power is determined by the person's job description with its attendant responsibilities and decision-making ability and authority.

Reward power is based on the holder's ability to offer positive endorsements or sanctions to others. This can range from compliments, letters of recognition, praise and acknowledgment of a job well done, to pay increases, bonuses, or promotions. It is important for the one with reward power to use it fairly, that is, not to give a favorite employee more rewards that other people get for the same behavior or to give rewards that far exceed the effort being acknowledged.

Coercive power is the opposite of reward power in that it uses negative sanctions such as a private or more public acknowledgment that the job was not well done; letters in the person's file; or a demotion or the withholding of a raise or promotion. This type of power is based on fear of punishment or withholding of rewards and is usually associated with a manager's or leader's perceived authority to determine the other person's employment status.

Expert power comes from the person's knowledge, skills, or expertise. For example, in most organizations some people have considerable power because they are expert in the use of a certain essential skill, e.g., the person most knowledgeable about the expectations of the Joint Commission on the Accreditation of Healthcare Organizations. (JCAHO) This type of power is related to information power. The former is more likely to be based on expert knowledge, whereas the latter is more associated with knowing what is going on, or being on the inside track for obtaining information. The person with information power will know who was at what meeting and what was said by whom, even though the person might not actually have been there.

Referent power, which is the most subtle form, is often associated with charisma or the personal charm and appeal of the person. This intangible type of power is based on respect and admiration for the holder. Followers comply with the person because they trust and believe the person knows what to do and will do what is right.

Derivative forms of power may also be valuable in health care organizations. For example, connection or associative power is based on a person's formal and informal connections or

Key terms	
Term	**Definition**
Power	The ability to produce or prevent change
Reward power	Power based on inducements such as positive sanctions or monetary benefits
Coercive power	Power based on negative sanctions or penalties if the person or group does not comply with the authority
Expert power	Power based on the knowledge, skills, and competence of the person in authority
Reference power	Power based on respect and admiration for the one with the authority
Information power	Power based on the person's access to valued and desired information
Legitimate power	The right to make requests based on one's role or designated authority in the organization

personal relationships with a powerful individual or group. Followers comply because they want to be indirectly connected to influential people. For example, a leader with position power may also have real or perceived close associations with power brokers such as members of the institution's board. Followers may comply with the nurse in the authority role with the hope of being connected to the member of the board.

Lower-participant power or the power of subordinates should not be underestimated. This has been seen in recent years in the banding together of employees to protest changes or the lack of changes in a number of industries, including airlines, automotive industries, professional sports, and nursing, via collective bargaining. The power of subordinates is collective. In a one-to-one relationship the person with position power may win, though perhaps only in the short run. The key is to avoid direct confrontations over power but rather to communicate, negotiate, and mediate conflict before the "lines get drawn in the sand" and the groups begin to take sides.

The Use of Power

The holder of power may use it constructively or destructively—for personal gain or for the good of the organization. Although power is present throughout every organization, it is typically feared and a source of concern. Power should be understood, respected, and used wisely and in accordance with the goals at hand. Improper use of power can destroy the effectiveness of the one wielding the power, and it can disrupt the group. It also may cause untold damage to the performance and career of the person who is the recipient of power used inappropriately or out of proportion to the situation. The person using power with others should focus on the behavior, not the person, and should maintain respect for the person.

Successful leaders in nursing respect the use and effects of power and use it wisely. These nursing leaders treat others with respect and as people who have inherent worth, rather than as a means to the leader's end or as objects to be manipulated. They also recognize their own potential as well as that of their colleagues and strive to find the "Olympic performance within themselves" and others (Kerfoot, 1997, p. 152).

■ LEADING IN THE FUTURE

Because change is constant, rapid, and unpredictable in health care, nursing leaders must be nimble and able to predict what is coming next. They must also openly demonstrate integrity (Brandt, 1994). Leaders lead a much more public life than do followers, and observers will readily differentiate between gestures and commitment (DePree, 1992). Leaders have to be vulnerable. It is not possible to lead effectively while taking the "easy way out"; leaders become vulnerable by acknowledging their accountability. Remember, as Depree (1992, p. 16) says, "Leadership may be good work, but it's a tough job. There is always more to do than time seems to allow."

Max DePree (1992), the former CEO of Herman Miller, a highly successful furniture manufacturer, concludes his book *Leadership Jazz* with a list of the attributes of effective leaders. He begins his list by saying that "above all, leadership is a position of servanthood" (p. 220) and nurses, like all other leaders, must be seen as people of integrity. Behavior is what counts, and actions speak louder than words. As mentioned, DePree views vulnerability as integral to effective leadership. This refers to the ability to let followers be all they can be; to let followers do their best. Leaders must be keen discerners who recognize the characteristics, needs, and qualities of their people. In nursing roles, as in others, it is important to recognize pain, beauty, anxiety, fear, loneliness, insecurity, lack of confidence, and heartbreak as well as skill, talent, potential, and intuition in others. Good leaders must also be courageous; they cannot pass off the tough decisions, actions, and risks to someone else. Followers expect a leader to face up to making the tough decisions.

In addition, nursing leaders are well-served during times of change and ambiguity by having a sense of humor. The ability to laugh at oneself and at the situation often defuses a tense event. Leaders are fortunate if they have intellectual energy and curiosity and are intrigued by the possibilities that exist; effective nursing leaders have the skill, patience, and wisdom to engage others in exploring those possibilities. Leaders in nursing should also have vision, be present and known to their co-workers, and be predictable. The last attribute that DePree lists is for leaders to respect the future, regard the present, and understand the past (1992), and this is especially true for nurses who lead change. That is, learn from those who have gone before. Box 9-3 lists seven key qualities that leaders of the future need. These qualities clearly apply to nurses who lead change.

B O X   9 - 3

Leaders of the Future Must Be:

1. People with an eye for change and a steadying hand to provide both the vision for the change and assurance that a positive outcome can be achieved.
2. Visionaries who can craft visions, inspire action, and encourage a diverse group of workers to find a common cause.
3. Integrators who can respect, understand, and bring together people from different cultures.
4. Cosmopolitans who can comfortably operate across boundaries.
5. Diplomats who can resolve conflicts among participants and influence people to work together for a common cause.
6. Cross-fertilizers who can bring the best from one place to another.
7. Deep thinkers who are smart enough to see new possibilities and who are likewise mentally agile and know when they need to change the course.

Data from Kanter, R.M. (1996). World-class leaders: The power of partnering. In F. Hessenbein, M. Goldsmith, & R. Beckhard (Eds.). *The leader of the future.* San Francisco: Jossey-Bass.

Kouzes and Posner (1996) in describing lessons for "leading the voyage to the future" say that effective leadership is needed to help overcome the cynicism and alienation of the present and move people toward hope and encouragement for their future. They describe seven lessons that effective leaders of the future must learn and use consistently (pp. 99-110):

Lesson 1:	Leaders don't wait; they are pro-active and make things happen. They think critically about what needs to be done and how to do it.
Lesson 2:	Character counts; leaders are honest and have "source credibility."
Lesson 3:	Leaders have their heads in the clouds and their feet on the ground. They have a sense of direction and a vision for the future.
Lesson 4:	Shared values make a difference; they are able to gain consensus on a common cause and common set of principles and values.
Lesson 5:	You can't do it alone; leadership is not a solo act. Leaders foster collaboration rather than create competition.
Lesson 6:	The legacy you leave is the life you lead. Leaders set an example by doing what they say they will do.
Lesson 7:	Leadership is everyone's business. Leadership is a process; a set of observations, learnable skills, and abilities.

Beckhard (1996) summarizes what future leaders must be like. They must have high ego strength, the ability to think strategically, a future orientation, and strong convictions, and they must be politically astute and know how to use power effectively. He goes on to say that (p. 129):

truly effective leaders in the years ahead will have personas determined by strong values and belief in the capacity of individuals to grow . . . they will be visionary, they will believe strongly that they can and should be shaping the future, and they will act on those beliefs through their personal behavior.

What can we in nursing learn from this? Surely the lessons learned by those who have been successful in business transfer to our business of patient care. The health care industry has as its goal to provide the best possible services in a caring, cost-effective, and accessible way. Employees are the key to success in health care, and leaders realize that and cherish, cultivate, and develop their "raw materials," which are their employees. As Kerfoot (1997, p. 152) says, "The greatest assets of any organization are the talent and energy of its people." Change leaders, then, must stimulate and awaken the inherent capacity of people in the organization to share in the tasks of leadership.

■ KEY POINTS

- Nurses who lead change will need to understand theories of leadership as well as effective tools of communication.
- Good leaders have, over time, demonstrated a consistent core of characteristics that include trustworthiness, integrity, honesty, consistency between what they say and what they do, and an inherent belief that others truly want to do a good job.
- Nursing leaders are encouraged to make evident to others their commitment to the mission, goals, and values of the organization and to lead by their example.
- Leading during times of change involves taking risks.
- Effective nursing leaders know how to use power to make it a positive force for change for the development of the people in the organization.

■ CRITICAL THINKING QUESTIONS

1. Identify a leader whom you have admired. What were the characteristics of that person that most appealed to you? Do you have some/most of these characteristics? If not, would you like to develop them? How would you go about doing this?

2. Consider a person with whom you have worked who demonstrated ineffective skills for leading change. What were the liabilities in those skills? How might those liabilities be changed?

3. Volunteer with an organization in your community. Identify who the leader(s) are. Are they leaders because of their role in the organization or because of their personal skills in leadership?

4. Design a nursing situation in which the designated manager used transformational leadership skills. What would those skills be? How would you personally respond to them?

■ REFERENCES

Beckhard, R. (1996). On future leaders. In F. Hesselbein, M. Goldsmith, & R. Beckhard (Eds.). *The leader of the future.* San Francisco: Jossey-Bass.

Bennis, W. (1990). *Why leaders can't lead.* San Francisco: Jossey-Bass.

Blake, R.R., & Mouton, J.S. (1978). *The new managerial grid.* Houston: Gulf.

Brandt, M.A. (1994). Caring leadership: Secret and path to success. *Nurse Management, 25*(8), 68-72.

Burns, J.M. (1978). *Leadership.* New York: Harper & Row.

DePree, M. (1989). *Leadership is an art.* New York: Dell.

DePree, M. (1992). *Leadership jazz.* New York: Dell.

Drucker, P. (1996). Foreward. In F. Hessenbein, M. Goldsmith, & R. Beckhard (Eds.). *The leader of the future* (pp. xi-xv). San Francisco: Jossey-Bass.

Entine, J., & Nichols, M (1997). Good leadership: What's its gender? *Female Executive,* Jan/Feb, 50-52.

Fiedler, F. (1967). *A theory of leadership effectiveness.* New York: McGraw-Hill.

Gunder, E, & Crissman, S. (1992). Leadership skills for empowerment. *Nursing Administration Quarterly, 17*(1), 17-24.

Heim, P. (1995). Getting beyond "she said, he said". *Nursing Administration Quarterly, 19*(2), 6-18.

Hersey, P., & Blanchard, K. (1988). *Management of organizational behavior* (5th ed.). Englewood Cliffs, N. J.: Prentice Hall.

House, R.J. (1971). A path-goal theory of leadership effectivemess. *Administrative Science Quarterly, 16*(Sept), 321-329.

Jenkins, R.L., & Henderson, R.L. (1984). Motivating the staff: What nurses expect from their supervisors. *Nursing Management, 15*(2), 13-14.

Johns, J. (1996). Trust: Key to acculturation in corporatized health care environments. *Nursing Administration Quarterly, 20*(2), 13-24.

Kanter, R. M. (1996). World-class leaders: The power of partnering. In F. Hessenbein, M. Goldsmith, & R. Beckhard (Eds.). *The leader of the future* (pp. 89-98). San Francisco: Jossey-Bass.

Kerfoot, K. (1997). Leadership: Believing in followers. *Nursing Economics, 15*(3), 151-152.

Kouzes, J.M., & Posner, B.Z. (1996). Seven lessons leading the voyage to the future. In F. Hessenbein, M. Goldsmith, & R. Beckhard (Eds.). *The leader of the future.* San Francisco: Jossey-Bass.

Marriner-Tomey, A. (1996). *Guide to nursing management and leadership.* St. Louis: Mosby.

McFarland, D.E. (1982). Power as a change strategy. In J. Lancaster & W. Lancaster. *Concepts for advanced nursing practice: The nurse as a change agent* (pp. 95-108). St. Louis: Mosby.

Moss, M.T. (1995). Developing glass-breaking skills. *Nursing Administration Quarterly, 19*(2), 41-47.

Porter-O'Grady, T. (1992). Transformational leadership in an age of chaos. *Nursing Administration Quarterly, 18*(3), 1-6.

Ronk, L.L. (1993). Gender gap within management. *Nursing Management, 24*(5), 65-67.

Strayer, R. (1990). How I learned to let my workers lead. *Harvard Business Review, 68*(6), 66-83.

Sullivan, E.J., & Decker, P.J. (1997). *Effective leadership and management in nursing.* Menlo Park, Calif: Addison-Wesley.

Tornabeni, J. (1995). Shake the kaleidoscope: One woman's response to gender-related barriers in health care management. *Nursing Administration Quarterly, 19*(2), 30-34.

Zak-Dance, C.C. (1996). The ties that bind leadership, communcation, and gender. *Surgical Services Management, 2*(6), 18-20.

Zaleznik, A. (1992). Managers and leaders: Are they different? *Harvard Business Review, 70*(2), 126-135.

Decision Processes and Critical Thinking

Wade Lancaster and Jeanette Lancaster

INTRODUCTION

In Lewis Carroll's story of *Alice in Wonderland,* Alice was confronted with a problem, so she pleaded with the Cheshire Puss: "'Would you tell me, please, which way I ought to walk from here?' 'That depends a good deal on where you want to get to,' the cat wisely responded" (Carroll, 1950, p. 53).

Just like Alice, throughout their lives people are continually confronted with the necessity of making decisions. When people awake each morning, they face a number of choices, such as what to wear and what to eat. In addition to the many small choices that people face throughout life, they are confronted with many decisions that must be made through critical thinking and problem solving.

Decision making, critical thinking, and problem solving are integral parts of nursing practice, not only in the design, management, and evaluation of care, but also in the process of planned change. In fact, the success or failure of nurse change managers depends on their decision-making ability; the quality of the decisions reached is a yardstick of their effectiveness. Decision-making skills are particularly needed when the environment in which nurses practice is changing rapidly.

In particular, effective nursing decision making is called for when unlicensed assistive personnel are used; the supervision and delegation of duties to nonprofessionals by registered nurses is critically important and requires keen decision-making skills.

Managed care has intensified "the focus on efficiency, effectiveness and the attainment of desired patient outcomes" (Buerhaus & Staiger, 1997, p. 316) as well as an increased use of case or care management and gate-keeping roles for nurses. For these reasons it is necessary to look at decision making as a systematic process and to find an approach that can sharpen nurses' ability to make effective decisions.

This chapter examines the various elements of decision making: the problem, the individual or group making the decision, the decision process, the decision itself, and the environment in which the decision is being made. Decision making with its components of critical thinking and problem solving is one of the principal processes engaged in by individuals, groups, and organizations. Although groups of individuals frequently engage in decision making, some individual or a small core group generally is responsible for the course of action ultimately taken.

OBJECTIVES

After reading this chapter, you will be able to:

1. Differentiate among critical thinking, problem solving, and decision making
2. Use the decision-making process in a clinical situation
3. Recall a situation in which faulty information gathering led to an ineffective decision, and evaluate an alternative that may have had a greater probability of success
4. Evaluate the values that you hold in a decision-making situation related to a specific patient care situation
5. Evaluate the usefulness of three decision-making aids for their effectiveness in evaluating a clinical problem

■ CRITICAL THINKING

The rapidly changing health care environment requires that nurses collect pertinent and appropriate data, differentiate among varying and often multiple points of view, and evaluate multiple lines of reasoning. Well-developed critical-thinking skills provide the tools for these activities (Beeken et al., 1997). Critical thinking is a process that requires both knowledge and skill in determining a course of action; it is "reasonable reflective thinking that is focused on deciding what to believe or do" (Ennis, 1991, p. 7). This brief and simple-appearing definition includes the creative art of problem solving with its formulation of hypotheses, examination of alternative ways of viewing a problem, asking varied questions, and identifying several possible solutions and plans. This definition does, however, "emphasize reflection, reasonableness (interpreted roughly as rationality), and decision-making (about belief and action)" (Ennis, 1991, p. 7). Critical thinking is a part of the problem-solving process.

Critical thinking includes the ability to challenge previous ideas and assumptions and to analyze their validity and utility at a given time. It is the "looking back" as one reconsiders the original objectives, what was actually done, and the outcome achieved. The reflective nurse "thinks while acting and responds [competently] to uncertainty and conflict situations;

this is 'thinking on one's feet' " (Sedlak, 1997, p. 12). Facione and Facione (1996) describe critical thinking as purposeful, self-regulatory judgment that gives reasoned consideration to evidence, content, conceptualizations, methods, and criteria.

■ PROBLEM SOLVING

Although problem solving and decision making have some of the same characteristics, they are not interchangeable processes. Often, decision making is a subset of problem solving, since not all decisions deal with problems, but the solving of any problem requires that one or more decisions must be made. Thus problem solving involves diagnosing a problem and solving it, whereas decision making involves selecting one of two or more alternatives to guide one's actions.

People use problem solving when they perceive that there is a gap or discrepancy between the current state or set of circumstances and a desired state. The scientific problem-solving process has a specific set of steps for gathering information to clarify the existence, extent, and nature of the problem and to set forth a variety of possible courses of action to correct the dilemma.

Before setting out to solve a problem, a nurse should ask a series of questions (Welch, 1995):

1. Is this important? If so, how important?
2. What, if anything, do I want to do?

3. Do I have the knowledge and skill to get involved?
4. Do I have the authority (or responsibility) to do something? If not, who does?
5. If I should do something and I wish to do something, do I really have the knowledge? What will it cost in time and resources to do something?
6. Can or should I delegate this to someone else?
7. What benefits, or consequences might be derived from solving this problem?

Problem-Solving Methods

A variety of methods exist for solving problems, including trial and error, experimentation, self-solving, avoidance, or using the systematic process of problem solving. *Trial and error* is the simplest method, although because of its lack of precision it may be the most time consuming if repeated failures occur. Basically, this approach means that the nurse first tries one way of doing something and then another, without carefully evaluating the situation, the options available, and the potential consequences of each option. Trial and error can have negative effects if it deals with essential patient care activities.

Experimentation is more systematic and rigorous than trial and error. For example, if nurses were designing a program to teach diabetic patients the value of regular exercise, they might do a pilot test with a few patients to see if the method being considered would really work. Specifically, 30 recently diagnosed diabetic patients could be divided into 3 groups: each group of 10 could either use printed information about diabetes, watch video tapes, or attend a series of classes. The 30 patients would keep an exercise log for 90 days to see what, if any, differences existed in their daily/weekly activity levels. Data would be carefully and consistently collected to determine which approach works the best. Experimentation can be effective if the project is carefully designed, controlled, and evaluated.

All problem-solving methods rely on the experience and intuition of the person who is solving the problem. Some problems are self-solving and may be time limited. That is, if you just wait a while, the problem will resolve itself. This approach has value when there is a high level of emotion involved. The "do nothing" or "wait and see" approach allows people to cool off and more rationally reconsider if action is required. Thus one can delay solving a problem or making a decision by "sleeping on it" or can entirely avoid dealing with the incident or problem. In this instance, making no decision actually does make a decision.

Problem-Solving Process

The *systematic problem-solving process* is a dynamic, interactive process with seven steps that may not always be linear or sequential (Box 10-1). These steps are described as follows:

1. Define the problem, issue, or situation. The most critical step is the first one. Great objectives, solutions, and evaluation for the wrong problem are a waste of time and resources. When nurses identify a problem, they are responsible for accurately determining exactly what the problem is and then dealing with it in an orderly and thoughtful manner. It is important to avoid reaching premature closure on problem identification or jumping to conclusions. Gather information to determine the problem by talking to colleagues indi-

B O X   1 0 - 1

Problem-Solving Steps

1. Define the problem, issue, or situation.
2. Gather information.
3. Analyze the available information.
4. Develop possible solutions.
5. Choose a solution.
6. Implement the decision.
7. Evaluate the solution.

vidually or in a small group and reading reports or minutes, as well as through library research or using the Internet.

2. Gather information. Once the problem is identified, more extensive information is gathered to develop a solution. The information gathered includes facts as well as opinions, perceptions, and feelings. In gathering information, one's experience and intuition are also useful sources of data. For example, Nurse Smith may complain that she does not have as desirable a schedule as three other nurses on the unit. It is known among staff that Nurse Smith tends to be self-centered and also has a pattern of finding fault with unit operations. The unit manager would be prudent to keep this information about Nurse Smith in mind while doing a 3- to 6-month retrospective analysis of her schedule to see if the claim can be verified.

3. Analyze the information. In analyzing the information, at least two key tasks exist. First, verify that the problem being solved is truly the problem and not just a symptom. For example, in receiving continuous quality improvement (CQI) records, the nurse manager finds a marked lack of documentation that the staff is making plans for discharge follow-up. The hospital has a systematic process such that when factors such as certain criteria about the patient's condition upon discharge, the level and quality of family support, and the distance from the hospital are present, the discharge-planning nurse liaison is called in. Once the data were gathered, the manager learned that the staff were, with only a few exceptions, using the appropriate criteria and resources for discharge planning. However, the liaison nurse was keeping the information in a file separate from that which held the cumulative patient record. Thus the solution dealt with record keeping. Sullivan and Decker (1997, p. 151) list six actions to use to sort data during this stage into an or-

derly arrangement that allows for useful analysis:
- Group the information in order of reliability.
- Organize the list from most to least important.
- Put information in a time sequence, i.e., past to most recent or vice versa. What happened first? What came next?
- Look at cause and effect. Did A lead to B?
- Classify information into categories such as: (1) human factors—personality, education, age, relationships, experience; (2) technical factors—type of unit, level and quality of staffing, skill of staff; (3) temporal factors—length of service, types of shift; and (4) policy factors—policies, guidelines, legal or ethical issues that pertain to the problems.
- Determine how long the situation has been going on.

Because it is never possible to gather all the information, the nurse must rely on experience, intuition, and critical thinking skills.

4. Develop solutions. Because there is rarely one right way to solve a problem, develop several options. Some people tend to see things as black or white or right or wrong when in reality they may be gray, or acceptable, but neither entirely right nor wrong. Be flexible, open-minded, and creative. Use brain-storming to identify several possible solutions. Avoid reaching closure when you are really angry or overly enthusiastic. Consider experiences with similar situations but do not allow yourself to be overly restricted, since this situation may have some slight but significant differences, such as a different mix of people or a different manager, or the dynamics of the unit have changed.

5. Select a solution. This is the time to weigh each option objectively so as to consider the potential risks and benefits. Consider costs, including time, resources, and the number of

people who need to be involved, as well as the people, traditions, or practices that will be affected, and the legal or ethical considerations, if any. Which decision is most likely to yield a solution that produces the best outcome for the predetermined objective? Then select the decision that is most feasible at this time given the people involved and those who will be affected. Because it is human nature for people to resist change, involve those people who will be affected by any change that accompanies the decision.

6. Implement the decision. The decision should be implemented with as much care and thoughtfulness as the previous steps. Some people may still resist by setting up barriers. Use the process of planned change during the implementation. Know who the supporters, resisters, and followers are.

7. Evaluate the solution. This step is the one most likely to be overlooked or short changed. Often, those involved with solving the problem are so relieved when they get to the implementation stage that they stop the process. The first step in implementation is to ask if the solution (i.e., the outcome) is still being implemented. Often a group gets excited about a solution, tries the new way for a while, and then without intending to do so, simply slips back into the old way of doing things. Ask for feedback. What worked? How closely was the desired outcome met? What could have been improved? Who needs to be informed or involved in the future?

Critical thinking and decision making are crucial parts of each stage in the problem-solving process. The remainder of this chapter deals with decision making and the process and tools that guide it.

■ **ELEMENTS OF DECISION MAKING**

Decision making frequently is defined as the selection of one alternative course of action from various alternatives that could be pursued. This definition has the advantage of being brief and easy to remember, and it focuses attention on the essential element of decision making, that is, making a choice. This definition, however, is deceptively simple; it is incomplete in that it does not emphasize the making of a decision as only one of several steps that occur in sequence as part of an intellectual process. Nor does it consider the basis for making a decision. The appropriate alternative depends heavily on the context within which decision making occurs. Moreover, this definition does not indicate that decisions, if they are to be effective, must be executed or translated into a course of action.

Regardless of whether a problem situation is a crisis or long run in nature or whether it concerns people or things, decision making consists of several elements, including the problem, the decision-maker, the decision process, and the decision itself. These elements, as well as the factors that make up the environment for decision making, are shown in Figure 10-1.

■ **DECISION-MAKING MODELS**

Decision theory consists of a group of related concepts and propositions that attempt to either prescribe or describe how individuals, as well as groups, select a course of action when confronted with a problem. Generally, people who study decision making view it from two distinctive perspectives. The first, a *normative* or *prescriptive* view, focuses on the way people should make decisions. The second, a *descriptive* or *behavioral* view, emphasizes the way people actually solve problems and make decisions. These two ways do not necessarily compete or conflict.

Normative Model of Decision Making

Early approaches to individual decision making focus on a normative model proposed by Adam Smith over 200 years ago (Kotler, 1965). This view of the decision-making process is rooted in

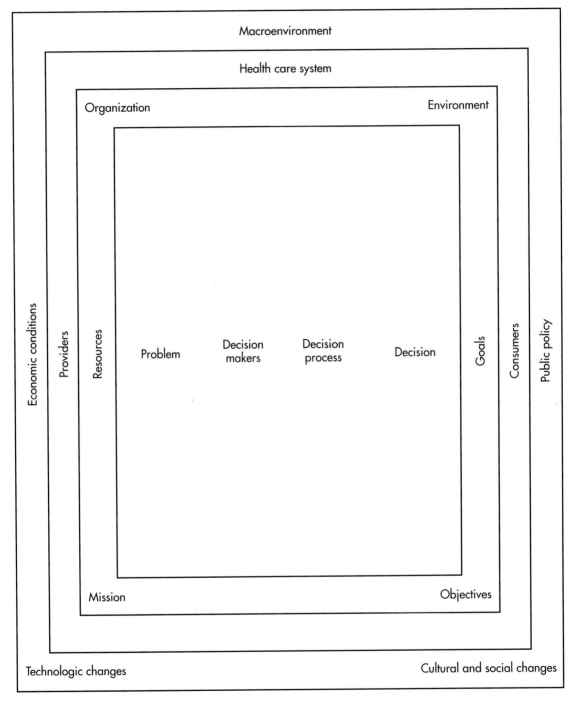

Figure 10-1 ■ Elements of decision making.

Key terms	
Term	**Definition**
Decision making	A problem-solving process that relies on critical thinking to identify and evaluate alternatives and choose the best option under the circumstances
Decision theory	Consists of a group of related concepts and propositions that either prescribe or describe how individuals or groups select a course of action when confronted with a problem
Descriptive model	Says that the decision maker will choose a satisfactory option based on the available information
Normative model	Says that the decision maker will choose the best alternative from all possible choices
Critical thinking	A process that requires reflective thinking to decide on a course of action

classical microeconomic theory and is based on two fundamental assumptions.

First, all decisions seek to maximize some predetermined goal or desired value. Whereas the original intent of classical microeconomic theory was to prescribe an analytic procedure for achieving optimal profits, a logical extension of this assumption proposed that a major goal of human behavior was to seek pleasure and avoid pain. Hence, economic man seeks to maximize pleasure. A prerequisite of the maximization assumption is perfect knowledge. This second assumption endows decision makers with the ability to know every available alternative solution and all of the possible consequences of each (Duncan, 1989).

Based on these two assumptions, the normative model of decision making characterizes the decision maker as a completely rational, all-knowing, hedonistic calculator who approaches any given problem in the following manner:
1. The problem is defined and analyzed.
2. Available alternatives are identified; evaluated according to benefits and disadvantages; ranked in the order in which they are likely to meet the desired value or objective; and the alternative that maximizes the possibility of success is selected.
3. The decision is implemented and then followed up.
Figure 10-2 depicts the normative model.

Although the normative model is analytically precise, the assumptions of maximization and perfect knowledge are unrealistic. The criticisms are valid; however, this model does prescribe a specified objective and guidelines to facilitate the application of analytic problem-solving steps.

Descriptive Model of Decision Making

The main quarrel with the normative model is with its notion of perfect knowledge. People, especially during times of great change, cannot have perfect knowledge or complete information.

Responding to what he viewed as unrealistic assumptions of the economic man model, Herbert A. Simon (1976) developed the descriptive model, which proposes that real-life decision makers cannot possibly be aware of all the alternatives, nor do they always attempt to maximize something. Instead, decision makers: (1) are sub-

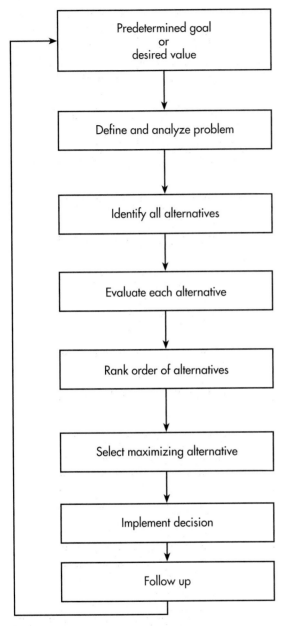

Figure 10-2 ■ Normative model of decision making.

jectively rational; (2) make decisions on the basis of incomplete information; and (3) are "satisficers," i.e., make choices that are just "good enough."

This view contends that problems are not always defined correctly, nor do people always solve problems well; instead, they solve them just well enough. Further, the descriptive model recognizes that complete information is not always available, nor is it always sought. It also recognizes the inherent costs involved in the acquisition of information. Consequently, people may consider the cost of obtaining additional information too high in proportion to the need for the information; decisions are made then on the basis of available information.

There are at least three obstacles to obtaining complete information. First, people rarely have sufficient time to acquire all available information. Second, the quantity of information available often exceeds the individual's processing capacity. Third, people frequently lack the technical knowledge required to evaluate all of the available information critically.

Faced with these three obstacles, the decision maker gathers information that subjectively appears most relevant to the problem and that will provide a satisfactory solution. Moreover, decision makers are viewed as "satisficers" rather than "optimizers."

Simon (1976) noted that if people always sought an optimal decision, the number of possible decisions they could make would be reduced to an unacceptable level. Thus instead of seeking optimal solutions, people tend to set some minimum objectives to be accomplished and they consider as acceptable any alternative that appears capable of satisfying these objectives. Etzioni (1989) refers to "humble decision making" when he says that "the flow of information has swollen to such a flood that managers are in danger of drowning" (p. 122). In earlier times, decision makers could explore every

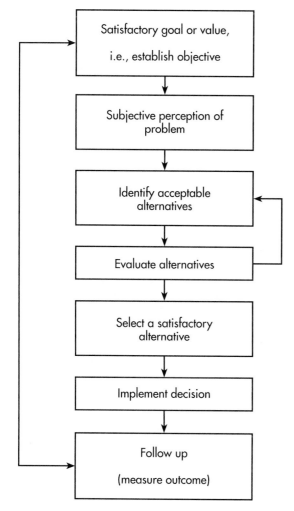

Figure 10-3 ■ Descriptive model of decision making.

1. Defines the problem in terms of subjective perceptions.
2. Identifies acceptable alternatives and evaluates each one in terms of its ability to solve the problem satisfactorily, and then selects a satisfactory alternative (this may be the first one encountered, or if several have been evaluated, the one that produces the most favorable outcomes).
3. Implements the decision and follows up.

In this section of the chapter, two general models of decision making—normative and descriptive—have been reviewed. The normative model specifies the manner in which a person should make decisions, whereas the descriptive model shows how a person actually does make decisions. In the next section, the descriptive model is explored in more detail through the decision-making process.

■ **THE DECISION-MAKING PROCESS**

When thinking about solving a problem, people often focus attention on finding the right answer. Few situations, however, have only one possible solution. Instead, several feasible alternatives exist for most problems. When multiple solutions are available, the decision maker is confronted with the problem of selecting an alternative.

In the years since Dewey (1910) first itemized the steps in problem solving, many conceptualizations of the process have been advanced. These steps, in modified form, have become accepted as the standard paradigm for the decision-making process:

1. Problem recognition
2. Information search and information-processing activity
3. Evaluation of alternatives
4. Decision selection or choice
5. Postdecision activities

The decision-making process is a sequential and reiterative series of psychologic and physi-

route that might lead to their goal; now, however, people must often proceed with only partial information for which they have insufficient time to fully analyze.

Figure 10-3 depicts the descriptive model. An examination of this diagram reveals a number of similarities as well as differences when compared with the normative model. Specifically, the decision maker does the following:

cal activities. Once decision makers recognize a problem, they collect and process information about alternative solutions, evaluate this information, and establish a preference order among the various alternatives. The establishment of an initial preference order does not, however, necessarily lead to a decision. Indeed, people often continue to search for additional information and to re-evaluate old information until they acquire sufficient confidence that their preference order will not be altered by subsequent information.

It is this reiterative process of seeking and evaluating information to achieve the required level of confidence that consumes time and differentiates various types of problem-solving behavior. Obviously, the level of confidence desired before making a decision is affected by numerous factors. When the required level of confidence is reached, the person generally makes a decision. Table 10-1 compares the nursing process, critical thinking, problem solving, and decision making. As can be seen, many similarities exist among these methods.

The stages of the decision-making process are not necessarily unidirectional. In fact, the reiterative nature of the process means that a person may move either backward or forward, or skip stages. For example, search and information-processing activities do not automatically follow problem recognition, nor do these activities lead directly to a decision and postdecision evaluation. In contrast, problem recognition always precedes the decision, which is then fol-

---

T A B L E   1 0 - 1

Comparison of Nursing Process, Critical Thinking, Problem Solving, and Decision Making

Nursing Process	Critical-Thinking Skills	Problem Solving	Decision Making
Assessment	Collect pertinent information by observing and differentiating among multiple points of view. Reflect back, and validate and organize information.	Define the problem, and gather information.	Problem recognition. Information search and processing.
Diagnosis	Identify patterns and reasonableness. State the problem. Suspend judgment.	Analyze information. Develop solutions.	Evaluate alternatives.
Planning	Transfer knowledge from one situation to another. Develop hypothesis.	Make decisions.	Select alternatives.
Implementation	Apply knowledge. Test hypothesis.	Implement the choice.	Implement the decision.
Evaluation	Decide which hypothesis worked best.	Evaluate the action.	Evaluate the decision/ follow-up.

lowed by the postdecision evaluation. In the following sections, each of the stages in the decision-making process is explored in detail. For organizational reasons, the stages are discussed in the order of their normal sequence.

Problem Recognition

The existence of a problem is a necessary prerequisite for decision making. Problem recognition is perhaps the most complex stage of the decision-making process because it is a perceptual phenomenon involving the interaction of social, psychologic, and environmental variables. Essentially the decision-making process begins when an individual believes a problem exists; that is, the person believes there is a significant difference between what is and what should be.

The ideal state of affairs, or what should be, is based on a predetermined goal or desired value. For individual decision makers, these values or goals are reflected in their perception of the ideal life, which may include preferred physical, psychologic, social, and economic conditions. In organizations, the ideal state is represented by established goals and objectives and these may include overall long-term objectives, as well as specific goals for the organization and its various subunits. For example, a hospital may view its long-term objectives as providing care for the sick and injured and serving the community through education, research, and public health activities. To meet these long-term objectives, several specific operating objectives are identified. One such objective may be to maintain excellent physical facilities so that optimum inpatient care is possible. This objective provides direction for various subunits within the hospital, such as the housekeeping department, which may have as its ultimate objective maintaining clean and sanitary facilities.

In contrast to the ideal state of affairs, the actual state is what is really taking place. For individuals, this represents a perceptual assessment of life as it is currently being lived; it is a performance evaluation of the physical, psychologic, social, and economic facets of life. For organizations, the actual state is a manifestation of its activities.

The ideal and actual states are seldom entirely congruent because both the ideal and the actual states constantly change over time, leaving both people and organizations in a continual state of incongruence.

Having recognized a problem or the presence of incongruence, the decision maker evaluates the situation to determine whether the problem is significant enough to try to solve and whether there is a feasible or possible solution to the problem. Because people have limited resources, such as time and talent, they must set priorities regarding the importance of problems. A problem such as inadequate office space or even the lack of an office may be aggravating to a nurse manager, but at the same time this problem may be of minimal importance to the success of the hospital. Hence, the manager may elect to just live with the problem while attempting to solve other ones. On the other hand, after weighing all the factors, the manager may decide that the employee who lacks an office would be more productive if this space were provided; at this point the manager's priority changes, and the lack of office space becomes the problem.

Not only do decision makers evaluate problems in terms of their relative importance, they also distinguish between those that are solvable and those that are not. Occasionally problems are encountered that are important but currently not solvable. An example of this situation is a nurse manager who is faced with a high turnover of staff nurses. The problem itself stems from a pay scale that is lower than that of competing hospitals. The hospital administration, on the advice of the chief financial officer, refuses to raise nursing salaries. The nurse manager believes that the cost of turnover (i.e., recruitment and orientation) is higher in the long run than the cost of retention (i.e., raising salaries). This problem, although important to the manager, is currently unsolvable and must be postponed or ignored. Or the manager must devise a new strategy for convincing others that a problem exists in the pay scale.

Because all identified problems cannot usually be solved simultaneously, they must be prioritized. This can be done in the order in which they occur; in terms of their complexity, i.e., handle simple problems first; in terms of the anticipated impact on the organization if the problem is either ignored or solved; or in terms of the degree to which the problem creates a crisis or emergency.

Information Search and Information Processing

Seeking and processing information are two separate yet interrelated activities. Information seeking, which takes place during the second stage of the decision-making process, involves both mental processes and physical activities

consciously used to gather information about the problem, possible alternatives, the relative merits of the various alternatives, and the consequences of selecting these alternatives. In contrast, information processing takes place in both the second and third stages of the decision-making process. In the second stage, the function of information-processing activities is to appraise the information being gathered. This appraisal function of information processing assists the individual in determining whether to continue or discontinue information seeking. In the third stage of the process, information processing focuses on discriminating and ranking the various alternative solutions identified. In short, the search process, which takes place in the second stage, gathers information about the problem, solutions, and alternatives and develops criteria for evaluating these alternatives.

No amount of effort in the subsequent steps will resolve the problem unless it is properly defined. Hasty problem analysis often leads to poor decisions when symptoms are confused with the problem itself. For example, if a physician diagnoses chest pain as a duodenal ulcer and the problem is angina pectoris, the treat-

Key terms	
Term	**Definition**
Certainty	A decision-making environment in which the available information leads to a high level of predictability
Risk	The chance of failure that exists in a decision-making situation
Satisficing	Choosing an alternative that is "good enough" but does not reflect maximal decision effectiveness
Information seeking	Mental and physical processes used to gather information about the problem, possible alternatives including the relative merits of each, and the consequences of selecting each alternative
Information processing	An appraisal of the information gathered and a determination of whether to continue the information search or to make the decision based on the alternatives identified

ment will inevitably fail. So it is in organizational settings. If a nurse manager fails to correctly and completely identify the real problem, solutions will either fail or only temporarily mask the problem.

It is not always easy to differentiate between symptoms and problems, especially those that may be the result of a variety of factors. For example, high nursing staff turnover may be the result of factors such as working conditions, wages, hospital location, or poor staff development. A good way of getting beyond the symptoms and to the root of the problem itself is to first state specifically what is wrong and what needs improvement. Then the decision maker gathers facts, investigates possible causes, and finally identifies the real problem or problems. Once this has been accomplished, the decision maker sets forth the requirements of a satisfactory solution and specifies any constraints on a solution.

Once the problem is identified, the decision maker can develop alternative courses of action and assess the potential consequences of each, that is, the search process. At first glance, it may seem that search implies the gathering of information not presently available, an assumption that is generally but not always correct. Instead, the extent of search activities varies depending on the individual as well as the nature of the situation. Consequently, the search process may be instantaneous or it may involve intensive exploration over a prolonged period. Regardless of the extent, the search process normally moves through certain steps.

Internal Search First, people must search their memories for relevant information. This process of internal search entails recalling stored information, such as the existence of an organizational policy or standard, prior experience and training, and the experiences of others. Organizational policies or standards often provide decision makers with predetermined

courses of action for a multitude of problem situations. Similarly, past experience frequently provides the necessary factual information and conceptualizations with which to make a decision (Hamer et al., 1994). Because there are limits to internally stored information, additional information gathered from the external environment is necessary.

External Search The external search, involving both mental and physical activity, is a deliberate effort to gather new information. A first step, the preliminary search, identifies alternatives and compares the attributes of these alternatives with a desired set of attributes. This preliminary sampling ordinarily results in a reconciliation of what is desired with what is perceived as being available. Full-scale external search seeks to match the desired set of attributes with those actually available by seeking information from a variety of sources including the institution's information management system. Getting the information is insufficient; the judgment of the decision maker is still key to the process.

Determinants of Search The extent of search activities depends on the individual problem solver as well as the nature of the problem situation. Numerous factors affect search behavior, and they can be grouped into four categories: the perceived value of search, the perceived cost of search, individual propensities to search, and situational variables.

Whenever people engage in external search activities, they must somehow balance the costs and benefits of search. Essentially, the amount of information sought is a function of comparing the perceived value with the perceived cost of search. Generally, when high value is accompanied by low cost, the individual will engage in extensive information-acquisition behavior. However, when the cost is high and the value of search is low, little search activity will occur. The perceived value of search is determined by the utility of information, which is influenced by variables such as the amount of information stored in memory, the quality of stored information, and ability to recall stored information.

The amount of information stored in memory is a function of knowledge and experience, and its utility is related to how closely it fits a specific problem situation (Hamer et al., 1994). The amount of stored information and the resultant perceived value of search is often influenced by the quality of stored information, which in turn is affected by satisfaction with previous experience as well as the amount of time that has elapsed between situations. When past experience has been less than satisfactory, there tends to be a greater propensity to search for new information when the same or similar problem is encountered. Similarly, the more frequently a given situation occurs, the greater the probability that a person will search for new information.

Another factor that affects the perceived value of search is a person's ability to recall relevant information. The cognitive process of assimilating new information with old varies among people; some tend to minimize differences in new information to assimilate it with stored information, whereas others tend to maximize differences, thereby enabling them to sustain recoverable stored information in an unaltered form over long periods.

Recall is also affected both by elapsed time and by the degree to which current problems resemble those that have arisen in the past; that is, the greater the amount of time between similar problems, the higher the propensity to search for new information.

Not only is the perceived value of the search affected by the quantity and quality of stored information and recall ability, it is affected by the confidence people have in their decision-making ability as well (Duncan, 1989). As a gen-eralization, search for outside information becomes more important when confidence is low, regardless of the quantity and quality of stored information, and when the perceived risk is high. Perceived risk can be financial, psychologic, social, or physical in nature, or a combination of two or more of these forms. In general, the greater the perceived risk, the more information the person gathers.

All searches cost something, and a cost-benefit analysis should be done. Searches have time, effort, and financial costs as well as the psychologic costs of frustration, tension, annoyance, and fear. These psychologic costs may outweigh the benefits of search. Another type of cost associated with search is information overload. Because there are finite limits on the quantity of information that a person can absorb and use, any information gathered that exceeds this limit becomes dysfunctional, causing frustration to mount and deterring decision-making ability. According to Etizoni (1989), people can focus on eight facts at a time.

Finally, the extent of search is also influenced by situational factors such as the availability of information, the urgency of the problem, and the type of problem itself. For example, when information is readily available, that is, an organization's information system, the extent of search is much shorter than when information has to be compiled. Similarly, an urgent situation in which a decision is needed quickly shortens the search process. Last, the type of problem often dictates the extent of search. For example, a long-range strategic problem often requires a more extensive search than an administrative problem that occurs routinely.

In summary, the search for and processing of information is usually regarded as the central phase of the decision-making process, for it is during this stage that the problem is defined, the need for additional information is determined, and the development of alternative solutions are created. Having performed these tasks, the decision maker can now evaluate alternatives.

Evaluation of Alternatives

In every problem situation the objective in making a decision is to select the alternative that provides either an optimal or a satisfactory solution. To do this, the alternatives that have been developed must be evaluated.

When the objective is to obtain an optimal solution, the decision maker should ideally know all available alternatives, the consequences of each, and their probability of occurrence. In this situation the decision maker arrays the alternatives, evaluates each in terms of its advantages and disadvantages, and ranks them in the order in which they are likely to meet the objective. Unfortunately, complete knowledge and certainty regarding the consequences and probabilities of outcomes for each alternative are not generally possible. Instead, situations exist where the decision maker is aware of only a limited number of alternatives and has only some probabilistic estimate of the outcomes of these alternatives. In evaluating alternatives under these conditions the decision maker usually relies on the tools of statisticians and operations researchers. These decision aids are used in the analysis and ranking of alternatives, and several of these techniques are discussed later in this chapter.

Even though "satisficing" appears to be a simpler approach to problem solving than "optimizing," the process of evaluating alternatives should certainly be no less rigorous. Unfortunately, our ability both to learn from experiences and to calculate probabilities is low (Etzioni, 1989). When possible, the nurse decision maker should identify the expected positive and negative outcomes for each alternative and then consider the value of each outcome and how nearly it will meet the objective. Identifying the disadvantage tends to be difficult. The benefit of delineating disadvantages is not that it forces the decision maker to reject the alternative, but rather that it provides for these disadvantages before the implementation stage, should the alternative be selected as the appropriate course of action.

Having recognized and defined a problem; having searched for alternative solutions and evaluated them; what then? At this juncture, the decision maker is ready to move to the next stage of the decision-making process and make a choice.

Selection of an Alternative

Selecting an alternative involves choosing between two or more alternatives to solve a problem and achieve a predetermined goal. Choosing an alternative should not be viewed as an isolated act; instead, it is a means to an end because it rapidly merges into a series of actions designed to implement, control, and evaluate the decision (Reitz, 1987).

Rarely are the solutions to problems either black or white, with only one right decision; more likely, they are various shades of gray. Consequently, selecting an alternative course of action is not always easy. Difficulty in making a decision is affected by several factors, such as the number and quality of alternatives, the risk involved, the interaction effect, as well as the constantly changing environment, which injects uncertainty into the probable success or failure of the projected solution.

Finally, choosing an alternative solution is complicated by the interaction of one activity on another. Rarely does a situation exist in which one activity singularly achieves the desired goal or objective without having some positive or negative influence on one or more other goals. This is especially true in organizational setting where many objectives exist. Many typically short-run objectives affect long-run objectives, for example, a hospital director who attempts to contain maintenance costs at the expense of the hospital's long-run objective of high-quality patient care in a state-of-the-art facility.

Once the decision maker has selected an alternative and established measurable objectives, it must be converted into action. Obviously, any decision is worthless if it is never implemented. Thus the final phase of the decision-making process, postdecision activities, involves not only implementing the decision, but also communicating and evaluating it.

Postdecision Activities

Effective decision making includes selecting good problem solutions and then transforming the solution into behavior. This is done by effective individual and group communicating, implementing, and evaluating. Unfortunately, not all decision makers are careful and unbiased in following up their decisions. There is no difference between no decision at all and an ineffective decision, and good decisions may become poor decisions if improperly implemented. The following questions aid in designing the implementation:

1. What must be done?
2. In what sequence must it be done?
3. Who should do what?
4. How can these activities be most effectively accomplished?

Once a plan of action is developed, the decision must be communicated to all who are involved in implementing it, as well as to those who are directly or indirectly affected by it. Several chapters in this text deal with concepts and behaviors that influence decision implementation, that is, communication, change, and leadership.

When communicating the decision, use clear, concise language, pointing out the logic of the decision and stating the reasons for making it. This communication is a measure of the probable success of the decision, since it deter-

mines the degree of commitment on the part of those who must participate in the implementation. Clearly, even the most technically sound decision can easily be undermined by those who are dissatisfied and not committed to carrying it out successfully. Once a decision has been implemented, the decision maker cannot assume that the outcome will meet the original objective but must instead have in place a monitoring system that measures the actual results or outcomes and compares them with the planned results. If deviations between the actual and planned results exist, modifications in the solution, its implementation, or the objective are necessary. Obviously, the existence of measurable objectives is an important component of the evaluation and control process, for without them, judging the performance is difficult. This control and evaluation process is illustrated by the following example:

> During the past 2 years, "Woodbrook," a hospital located in a major metropolitan area, has had difficulty hiring nurses. The chief nursing officer and nurse recruiter have reviewed their current recruiting program, evaluated several new approaches, and decided to hire professional recruiters to recruit new graduates from selected schools across the nation. To bring the nursing staff up to an acceptable level, they agree that a 15% increase in staff per year for the next 3 years is needed. Assume that at the end of the first year employment had increased only 5%: either the original objective was overstated, the use of professional recruiters (the selected alternative) to achieve the objective was not appropriate, the wrong recruiters were selected (implementation), or the wrong or an insufficient number of schools were chosen. Or perhaps they should have recruited experienced nurses—not new graduates. If the original objective must be revised, the entire decision-making process is reactivated.

There are advantages and disadvantages to choosing either an optimal or a "satisficing" alternative, which need to be determined and evaluated to select the most appropriate alternative under the prevailing conditions. The decision, when made, is converted into action, which involves the postdecision activities of implementing the decision as well as communicating and evaluating the choice. Now that the decision process has been described, the next step is to discuss the types of problems that typically require decision-making activities and the criteria used to evaluate the decision.

■ THE PROBLEM

All decisions begin with a problem, which can be either extremely simple or complex, involving many people and variables. A problem can easily be defined as an obstacle to a goal. The types of problems that decision makers face vary according to the time frame necessary to make and implement them, the degree of structure or routineness that characterizes them, whether they deal with evaluation or allocation, and whether they are organizational or individual problems.

One way to categorize decisions is under the subheadings of administrative or strategic. *Administrative* decisions deal with day-to-day activities in the organization and are concerned with short-range efficiency, such as who goes to lunch when or who has which holidays off. In contrast, *strategic* decisions refer to long-range problems that affect the organization's survival and often have some uncontrollable aspects (Reitz, 1987). Examples include economic conditions, supply of nursing manpower, or patients needing or desiring services at a specific agency.

Decisions can be categorized also as either *programmed* (structured) or *nonprogrammed* (unstructured). If a situation occurs fairly often, a routine procedure will usually be identified for solving it. "Thus decisions are programmed to the extent that they are repetitive and routine and a definite procedure has been developed for handling them" (Gibson et al., 1976, p. 342). Examples of programmed decisions are a hospital's admitting procedure and a university's standard for the grade point average that signifies academic good standing.

Other situations arise that are less structured and necessitate a novel or *nonprogrammed* decision. A nonprogrammed decision requires a creative response to a problem that has not previously occurred or that is of greater complexity than it previously was, for example, the purchase of new equipment or the construction and staffing of new facilities.

Reitz (1987) differentiates decisions as either evaluation or allocation. Basically, all decisions require some degree of *evaluation* to sort out and weigh the alternatives. Certain decisions, such as performance appraisal of employees and grading of students, as well as program appraisal, are almost entirely evaluative. In both performance and program appraisal, either people or activities are measured against a set of objective standards. Just as all decisions have an evaluative component, so also do they generally deal with the *allocation* of resources (e.g., time, people, money, physical facilities).

In health care, decisions are made at both the organizational and the individual levels. Although many of the decisions described are made at the organizational level, their effectiveness often depends on individual decisions regarding participation and production. The most noteworthy organizational goals can become dismal failures if employees fail to implement them. Whether people choose to participate in the implementation of a decision depends largely on individual perceptions—of the value, risks, and so forth of their participation. Not only are there several ways of categorizing decisions, several criteria can be noted that help to classify decisions.

■ THE DECISION ITSELF

Decisions can be classified according to *efficiency* and *effectiveness* criteria. Efficiency is a measure of what an organization gets out of a decision compared with what it puts into it (Reitz, 1987). That is, if hospital A takes 3 days and four committee meetings of 2 hours each and hospital B takes a 2-hour meeting to make the same decision, B is more efficient. Cost and time are major efficiency criteria. Cost includes hours spent in gathering information, discussing options, and reaching a decision, as well as information processing (e.g., secretarial assistance, photocopying, computer time) and the use of consultants. Time is critical, since long delays in arriving at decisions may have hidden costs such as patients seeking care elsewhere or staff turnover.

In contrast, *effectiveness* in decision making is the extent to which a decision actually solves a problem (Reitz, 1987). The effectiveness of any decision can usually be measured according to either *accuracy* or *feasibility*. Accuracy refers to how well the decision correctly evaluates the information, assesses costs and benefits of alternatives, and determines the best alternative under the prevailing circumstances. Effectiveness can also be measured according to feasibility for actually carrying out the plan. The most accurate decision will fall short of its goal if manpower or other resources are unavailable for its implementation (Reitz, 1987). Some of the conditions affecting decision making are seen in Box 10-2.

Decision making is a type of problem solving that moves through a sequence of steps. The degree to which all steps in the problem-solving

approach are used depends on the amount of predictability associated with the decision. Routine decisions made under conditions of certainty require less focusing on evaluation of alternatives than do novel, or nonroutine, decisions, especially those made under certain conditions.

■ THE INDIVIDUAL AS DECISION MAKER

The characteristics of the decision maker affect the outcome. People differ in how they perceive problems, the extent of their search for alternative solutions, the quality of the data analyzed to arrive at a decision, and ultimately the choice made. People's perceptions are affected by their experiences, goals, personal value system, ability to process information, knowledge, personality factors such as confidence, self-esteem, dogmatism, such as willingness to take risks, ability to tolerate dissonance, as well as several personal and physical factors. Personal characteristics include age, sex, and intelligence, whereas physical factors might include fatigue, alcohol, drugs, personal conflict, or stress. In clinical practice nurses continuously make decisions that are influenced by their perception of the problem. For example, if two nurses were to enter a patient's room independently and see her crying, unless they inquired about what her concern was, they might arrive at different conclusions. One nurse might assume the patient was afraid because she was scheduled for surgery the next day, whereas the other nurse might assume she was in pain. The search for the actual problem would be crucial in this example.

Intuition also plays a role in decision making. Experience can enhance intuition in that instances in the past "intuitively" provide a cue to the decision maker about what might be expected. In addition, some people are naturally intuitive. They can sense what might be going on ("they hear the unspoken word"). Benner

---

B O X   1 0 - 2

Conditions Affecting Decision Making

Certainty	Probability that a given outcome will occur
Risk	Chance of failure

and Tanner (1987) define intuition as understanding without a rationale. This is seen when a nurse walks into a patient's room and with no obvious cues that the patient's condition is worsening, just "knows" that something is not right. Rew (1988) explored intuition in nurses in critical care and home care settings and found that intuition was clearly a component of clinical decision making. Once the nurses had an intuitive feeling, they gathered additional information to support their hunch. They gathered the information from the patient, the family, the record, and reference books. They next validated their intuitions by discussing them with another nurse. Their next step was to report their findings and feelings to physicians or via the chart. Last, they performed specific interventions on behalf of the patient, such as preparing emergency medications or equipment.

Similarly, King and Appleton (1997 p. 200), after reviewing the literature on the use of intuition in nursing, concluded that "intuitive feelings appear to act as a trigger within the linear problem-solving approach of the nursing process."

The effect of differences in the ability to process and store information is most evident in the search for and analysis of data and the development of alternative solutions. Decision makers can be viewed on a continuum from open minded to close minded. The open-minded decision maker is more flexible and willing to consider both more information about the problem and more alternatives. In contrast, close-minded decision makers tend to focus on solutions that support their personal choice or are the most comfortable or expedient to make.

Thus decision making is influenced by a variety of personal factors. No two people are equally skilled in decision making. Likewise, given the same sets of information, a group of people would arrive at different solutions. The entire group might select the same solution, but there would be a unique rationale, procedures, and expectations.

■ GROUP DECISION MAKING

Although group decision making seems to be increasing, its level of effectiveness is debated. Generally it takes groups longer to make a decision than it would take an individual.

On the other hand, because a group can provide more information, sounder decisions may be made by groups versus individuals because more variables can be considered and greater "buy in" may be achieved. This, however, depends on the dynamics of the group. All too of-

Key terms	
Term	**Definition**
Dogmatism	The tendency people have to hold firmly to previously conceived beliefs, even in the presence of contrary evidence
Cognitive dissonance	The lack of harmony among a person's beliefs, thoughts, and attitudes after a decision is made
Perception	A psychologic process that helps people interpret what they see, hear, feel, taste, or smell
Values	A person's set of beliefs, attitudes, and opinions about a thought, object, or behavior

ten, open and honest group discussion is hampered by a feeling of pressure to conform, fear of reprisal, and the influence of a dominant personality or a member who is perceived as having greater status than the other members.

Certain decisions seem to be more amenable to group efforts. In particular, nonprogrammed or novel decisions usually call for pooled talent, whereas routine or more programmed decisions lend themselves to more effective individual decisions. In nonprogrammed decisions, groups are effective in the following:

1. Establishing objectives, since greater knowledge is available
2. Identifying alternatives because a broad range of potential choices can be presented
3. Evaluating alternatives because of the collective information and viewpoints of a group
4. Choosing an alternative—people are more likely to accept a risk when working as a group rather than when responsibility lies with one person

In contrast, when decisions need to be implemented, whether they are made by individuals or groups, it is the responsibility of individuals to actually carry out the actions. Few organizations function without groups, yet group participation in decision making has both advantages and disadvantages.

One of the major *advantages* of group decision making is that a potentially wider range of knowledge is available in a group than with any single member. Members bring different backgrounds, experiences, and knowledge to the decision process, which provides an increased number of choices. Also, members are more likely to accept the decision if they have been a participant; further, the chances of having commitment to the enactment of the decision are greater if all members were involved. For example, the use of unlicensed assistive personnel (UAP) is more likely to be effectively implemented if staff nurses are involved in the deci-

sion to try this form of nursing practice versus being informed by the nurse manager that professional nurse staffing will be reduced and more UAPs will be hired to assist the remaining nurses.

The *disadvantages* of group decision making include the amount of time involved and the potential for some members to pressure others into conforming with the majority view. In addition, hospitals, like other organizations, have a superior-subordinate hierarchy. Subordinates may agree to group decisions that conflict with their personal views if they fear the consequences of disagreeing or if they are seeking to obtain the favor of a superior. The desire for acceptance by other members may motivate acquiescence also. In any group there is the potential for domination by one or two members, which diminishes participation and quality of decisions. Further, some people feel less commitment to a group versus an individual decision.

Vroom and Yetton's decision theory (1973) represents an effort to integrate group and individual decision making by specifying the parameters that influence the decision about whom should be included in the decision process. They said that managers when involved in making decisions have five possible alternatives, ranging from the manager making the decision using available information at the time to the choice of sharing the problem with subordinates and requesting a group problem-solving effort. They attempted to identify the properties of the decision that would specify the best approach for effective problem solving. Basically, Vroom and Yetton conceptualized the manager's task as determining how the problem is to be solved, rather than determining the actual solution to the problem. This implies that there is no one best way to handle problems, but the strategy selected should depend on the properties of the situation.

■ DECISION AIDS

Because most decisions involve varying degrees of certainty, a variety of tools or aids have been developed to minimize uncertainty. First, computer-based data management has expanded decision makers' ability to record, store, and manipulate information. Second, a wide range of decision models aid the handling of information to make rational choices. Also, as has been implied throughout this chapter, effective decision making is enriched by creativity, an open mind, a review of past experience, and an acknowledgment of intuition or one's "gut feelings."

In thinking about creativity it is useful to recall that the human brain has two sides. The left side is considered analytic and sequential, and the right side is viewed as intuitive and conceptual and more suited to creative or "out of the box" thinking. Effective decision making requires the use of both sides of the brain. This may be accomplished most effectively by involving more than one person, since people tend to lean toward either left-brain or right-brain thinking.

Some creative thinking activities are simple things like making lists, meditating, visualizing other options, brainstorming, and using the Delphi technique.

Brainstorming is well suited to group decision making when there are simple and specific problems to be solved. If the problem is complex, it can be divided into parts with each part initially considered separately. In brainstorming, participants are asked to identify all possible choices without critiquing, screening, or censoring ideas. Some of the ideas may seem "wild" or unrealistic; however, the goal is to generate them at this point; evaluation of the ideas comes later.

The *Delphi technique* is especially useful when information is sought from people who are not in the same geographic area. Once a problem is identified, participants are asked to complete a questionnaire. The responses to the questionnaire are anonymous, and the results are tallied. Each participant is sent a copy of the results and asked to respond once more. The process continues until consensus is reached. Usually the first two rounds are the most productive. This technique is time consuming, and members do not benefit from the immediate stimulation and synergy of a face-to-face discussion.

The major categories of aids to be discussed in this chapter include PERT (program evaluation and review technique), CPM (critical path method), OR (operations research), and mind mapping.

The first two techniques, PERT and CPM, describe the components of the task, their sequencing, and the expected completion time. An example of these models is seen in Figure 10-4, where each node at the end of the arrow illustrates the beginning and end of an activity. Each sequential activity depends on the successful completion of an earlier one. For example, it would not be appropriate to work on activity four before one through three were mastered.

Specifically, *PERT* involves identifying key activities, sequencing them in a flow diagram, and

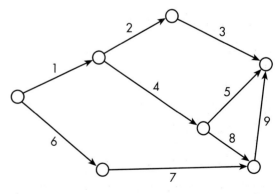

Figure 10-4 ■ Decision aid model for path analysis (PERT and CPM).

assigning the expected duration time for each phase of the project. In regard to the time component, PERT deals with uncertainty in three ways: (1) the optimistic time (t o), which refers to anticipated completion time assuming that no complications arise; (2) the most likely time (t m), which estimates completion time by taking into account the typical range of problems that can be expected; and (3) the pessimistic time (t p), which estimates completion time with the assumption that the maximum number of problems possible will occur (Marriner-Tomey, 1996, p. 8). To plan in terms of the expected time, the following formula can be employed:

$$t e = \frac{t o + 4(t m) + t p}{6}$$

If you hope to complete the project in 2 weeks, the optimistic time is (2); you may know from experience that delays such as those needed for materials to arrive from subgroups to complete their assignments must be considered, so the most likely time is (6) weeks, while your greatest fear—of encountering major resource or personnel obstacles—could cause the pessimistic time to extend to (12) weeks. Based on these projections, the estimated time is calculated as follows:

$$t e = \frac{2 \text{ weeks} + 4 \text{ (6 weeks)} + \text{(12 weeks)}}{6}$$

$$\frac{2 + 24 + 12}{6} = \frac{38}{6} = 6.33 \text{ weeks}$$

Based on this calculation, priorities can be reevaluated and extra personnel can be employed to move the project forward, or those who will be expecting or waiting for the outcome of the project can be informed of its most likely completion date. Similarly, *CPM* deals with time calculations but handles only one estimate rather than the three in PERT. CPM calculates the longest possible time estimate.

In contrast to the aids discussed earlier, *operations research* (OR) is defined as "(1) an application of the scientific method to (2) problems arising in the operations of a system which may be represented by means of a mathematical model and (3) the solving of these problems by resolving the equations representing the system" (Churchman et al., 1957, p. 18). The very term *OR*, which refers to the analysis of an entire system, calls attention to the greater scope of this tool in comparison with either PERT or CPM. The specific techniques of OR require that mathematical models be used to solve the designated problem. Specific OR techniques include linear programming, queuing theory, game theory, and probability theory.

Linear programming is most effective in situations that require that limited resources be allocated to the best possible advantage. As the name implies, linear programming deals primarily with mathematically determining the linear relationship that exists between parts and the limits that must be calculated. Three conditions must exist before linear programming is employed: (1) either a minimum or maximal value is desired in order to optimize goal attainment; (2) the variables affecting the goal must have a linear relationship; and (3) some constraints or obstacles can be determined—if no obstacles are present or anticipated then the process is unnecessary (Marriner-Tomey, 1996). Linear programming ranges from simple observations to complex computer-handled problems. Examples of nursing activities that may apply linear programming include the determination of a new health clinic within an existing network or the determination of class size based on number of students who need or desire the course, number of faculty, and the hours available to teach the course.

Queuing theory, sometimes called "waiting line theory," is especially useful in determining the correct balance of factors necessary to

Key terms	
Term	**Definition**
Brainstorming	A decision-making technique in which participants generate ideas without critique or censorship until idea generation is exhausted
Delphi technique	A decision-making technique whereby opinions on a topic are systematically gathered via a series of questionnaires from participants who are in different places
Program evaluation and review technique (PERT)	A decision-making tool that identifies and sequences key activities in a flow diagram and assigns the expected time for each phase
Critical path method (CPM)	A decision-making tool that calculates time estimates for each activity
Operations research	The use of mathematical models to solve a problem within a system
Linear programming	The use of matrix algebra or linear mathematical equations to determine the best way to get the best results given finite resources
Queuing theory	A mathematical technique used to determine the efficiency of intermittent services, i.e., "waiting line theory"
Game theory	The use of simulations, i.e., a board game, to model reality and practice solving operational problems
Probability theory	Calculating the likelihood that an event will occur
Mind-mapping	A method for organizing one's thoughts to solve a problem or write a report

handle intermittent service. It is particularly useful when the units arriving for service arrive on a random schedule but essentially require the same length of time for service. This can be seen in customers arriving at a restaurant and clients coming to a health care clinic. Queuing techniques can be used to balance the cost of waiting versus the cost to overcome the need to wait (such as employing more personnel).

In many instances, actual observations of the number of units requesting service can be made and a total can be tallied. For example, the number of people seeking services at Planned Parenthood can be recorded and staffing determinations can be made accordingly. In many instances, such observations cannot be carried out for a sufficient length of time to produce a clear picture; therefore, the Monte Carlo technique may be applied. This technique is employed to produce a sample of random occurrence of the situation. "Essentially, the Monte Carlo technique provides a large sample of random numbers that may be generated by a computer. From the large Monte Carlo sample, rather precise determinations may be made in regard to the expected servicing load for each hour of the day" (Sisk, 1973, p. 242).

Game theory is a simulation technique where a model of reality is used to simplify problems by identifying their basic parts and using trial-and-error practices to arrive at a potential solution. A well-known application of game theory is the "war game" approach that has been widely used in the military. Games allow decision makers to evaluate a variety of alternatives with minimal cost and consequences. Essentially the game provides a model for simplifying system operations where participants can try to develop strategies that will maximize their gains and minimize losses or consequences. Management games are most frequently used to train personnel rather than to solve real problems. A variety of games have been developed to help nurses make decisions in hypothetical situations, e.g., the admission, transfer, and discharge process in a complex hospital with its multiple points of entry, i.e., emergency department, ambulatory clinics, and physician offices.

Probability theory is particularly useful for determining the degree of risk involved in each potential solution. The basic assumption underlying probability theory is that factors occur in a predictable pattern. In terms of a coin toss, if a penny were tossed 10 times, it is probable that heads would occur five times and tails five times.

Limitations of operations research refers to the inability to actually make the final choice. Operations research is valuable because it contributes to the analysis and development of alternatives and potential outcomes. Its effectiveness is limited to the "analyses and comparison of relationships that may be expressed quantitatively and transformed into a mathematical model" (Sisk, 1973, p. 244).

Mind-mapping is a technique used to organize one's thoughts in order to solve a problem or to write an important report or presentation. This technique is effective since it allows you to keep your central idea clear when indicating relationships among ideas. Mind-mapping enables you to add, subtract, or reorganize ideas and provides a mental picture of an outline. This technique is especially useful for preparing oral presentations. To create a mind-map, do the following:

1. Draw a circle, and write the topic (of the paper, problem, project) or title (of the talk) in the center.
2. Write key ideas in smaller circles connected to the large circle.
3. Write supporting ideas in circles connected to the key idea circles. Use this technique to organize thoughts and prepare for important reports or presentations (Donovan, 1990).

■ **KEY POINTS**

- Decision making is a problem-solving activity that uses critical thinking skills and is at the core of planned change.
- The success of an individual, group, or organization depends on the quality of the decisions made.
- Effective decision making in nursing is a step-by-step process involving: (1) identifying the problem, (2) developing goals, objectives, and outcome criteria, (3) developing, evaluating and choosing alternatives, (4) implementing the decision and (5) evaluating the outcome of the decision.
- Although there are two general models for decision making, the normative and the descriptive, the latter is most useful in nursing since it allows full exploration of the options available under the given conditions.
- Behavioral characteristics such as perception, values, the ability to process information, and tolerance for risk and dissonance affect decision making, as do intelligence and selected physiologic factors.
- Several decision aids including, PERT, CPM, and specific types of Operations Research, i.e., linear programming, queuing theory, game theory, and probability theory, as well as the technique of mind-mapping, are useful in complex decision making situations.
- Critical-thinking skills and problem solving are integral aspects of the decision-making process.

■ CRITICAL THINKING QUESTIONS

1. Consider a decision that you made last week which had an effect on your work either in a course or in a clinical situation. (A) List the alternatives you considered. (B) Identify at least five factors that influenced your decision. (C) Describe your satisfaction or lack of satisfaction with the decision that you made. (D) As you reflect back, would another alternative have been better? (E) If yes, describe that alternative.

2. Review a decision-making situation in a clinical area in which you used a "satisficing" behavior without full reliance on the decision-making process and the outcome was less satisfactory than desired.

3. Develop a model to effectively staff a unit using one of the decision aids described in the chapter. Assume you will use no float or per-diem nurses. Be equally fair to all participants.

4. Recall a person in a clinical situation with whom you disagreed on a course of action. Ask three people to sit down with you; describe the incident as objectively as possible; use brainstorming to generate options; plan a course of action based on the group's analysis of the possible choices. How does this plan differ from what you actually did? How exactly would you evaluate the effectiveness of the plan chosen by your group?

■ REFERENCES

Beeken, J.E., Dale, M.L., Enos, M.F., & Yarbrough, S. (1997). Teaching critical thinking skills to undergraduate nursing students. *Nurse Educator, 22*(3), 37-39.

Benner, P., & Tanner, C. (1987). Clinical judgment: How expert nurses use intuition. *American Journal of Nursing, 87*(1), 23-31.

Buerhaus, P.I., & Staiger, D.O. (1997). Future of the nurse labor market according to health executives in high managed-care areas of the United States. *IMAGE: Journal of Nursing Scholarship, 29*(4), 313-318.

Carroll, L., pseudonym for Dodgson C.L. (1950). *Alice in Wonderland.* New York: Arcadia House.

Churchman, C.A., Ackoff, R.L., & Arnoff, E.L. (1957). *Introduction to operations research.* New York: John Wiley & Sons.

Dewey, J. (1910). *How we think.* New York: D.C. Heath.

Donovan, C. (1990). *Mind-Mapping.* Managers Edge Cassette Program, Managers Edge Corporation, Denver, Colo.

Duncan, W.J. (1989). *Great ideas in management.* San Francisco: Jossey Bass.

Ennis, R. (1991, March). Critical thinking: A streamlined perspective. *Teaching Philosophy, 14*(1), 5-24.

Etzioni, A. (1989). Humble decision making. *Harvard Business Review, 89*(4), 122-126.

Facione, N., & Facione, P. (1996). Externalizing the critical thinking in knowledge development and clinical judgment. *Nursing Outlook, 44*(3), 129-36.

Festinger, L. (1957). *A theory of cognitive dissonance.* New York: Harper & Row.

Gibson, J.L., Ivancevich, J.M., & Donnelly, J.H. (1976). *Organizations: Structure, processes, behavior* (rev. ed.). Dallas: Business Publications.

Hamer, J.P.H., Huijer Abu-Saad, H., & Halfens, R.J.G. (1994). Diagnostic process and decision making in nursing: A literature review. *Journal of Professional Nursing, 10*(3), 154-163.

King, L., & Appleton, J.V. (1997). Intuition: A critical review of the research and rhetoric. *Journal of Advanced Nursing, 26,* 194-202.

Kotler, P. (1965). Behavioral models for analyzing buyers. *Journal of Marketing, 29*(Oct.), 37-15.

Marriner-Tomey, A. (1996). *Guide to nursing management and leadership* (5th ed.). St. Louis: Mosby.

Reitz, H.J. (1987). *Behavior in organizations* (3rd ed.). Homewood, ILL.: Richard D. Irwin.

Rew, L. (1998). Intuition in decision making. *IMAGE: Journal of Nursing Scholarship, 20*(3), 150-154.

Sedlak, C.A. (1997). Critical thinking of beginning baccalaureate nursing students during the first clinical nursing course. *Journal of Nurse Education, 36*(1), 11-18.

Simon, H.A. (1976). *Administrative behavior (3rd ed.).* New York: The Free Press.

Sisk, H.L. (1973). *Management and organization* (2nd ed.). Cincinnati, Ohio: SouthWestern Publishing.

Sullivan, E.J., & Decker, P.J. (1997). *Effective leadership and management in nursing* (4th ed.). Menlo Park, Calif.: Addison Wesley.

Vroom, V.H., & Yetton, P.W. (1973). *Leadership and decision making.* Pittsburgh: University of Pennsylvania Press.

Welch, R.A. (1995). Problem solving and decision making. In P. Yoder Wise. (1995). *Leading and managing in nursing.* St. Louis: Mosby, pp. 108-126.

THE ENVIRONMENT IN WHICH CHANGE OCCURS

Social and Cultural Factors Affecting Health Care and Nursing Practice

Angeline Bushy

INTRODUCTION

America has been called a melting pot, but it seems better to call it a mosaic, for in it each nation, people, or race that has come to its shores has been privileged to keep its individuality, contributing at the same time its share to the unified pattern of a new nation (King Baudouin I of Belgium, 1930-1933) (*Daytona News Journal,* 1997).

OBJECTIVES

After reading this chapter, you will be able to:

1. Analyze personal cultural and ethnic preferences
2. Compare and contrast terms associated with diversity (race, ethnicity, culture)
3. Complete a cultural assessment with a patient
4. Analyze population trends and the impact of these on society and health care delivery in the United States
5. Implement interventions that are culturally acceptable and appropriate
6. Integrate a patient's cultural self-care practices with contemporary healing interventions
7. Evaluate cultural competence in nursing care rendered to patients of another background

■ RESPECTING DIVERSITY

The face of American society is changing! As we approach the new millennium, political correctness, cultural diversity, affirmative action, and equal opportunity have emerged on the forefront of political agendas, university curricula, and human resource departments of corporations, as well as the health care system. In recent years discrimination cases relating to gender, race, age, ethnicity, religious beliefs, disabilities, and nationality have escalated. From an organizational and legal perspective, discrimination of any nature is unacceptable and unlawful and can result in legal or punitive actions. In the health care system, concerns about cultural diversity juxtapose the curtailment of escalating costs while assuring quality and appropriate services to consumers. The overall focus of health care delivery has shifted from the *offering more is better* model to that of *providing appropriate and acceptable services by culturally competent providers to consumers with diverse belief systems* (Ahmann, 1994; Leininger, 1997; Morganthau, 1997; USDHHS, 1991a; 1991b; 1996). Nurses in leadership roles will work with and care for peoples from many cultural backgrounds, which makes understanding cultural diversity essential. Although this chapter explicitly focuses on nurse-patient interactions, the same principles apply in co-worker interactions.

The predominant minorities in the United States (Americans of African, Hispanic, Asian, Pacific Island, Native Indian, and Eskimo descent) differ greatly in social, political, and economic history. Moreover, there are significant differences in their cultural beliefs, behavior norms, and the extent of their acculturation into mainstream American culture (white, middle class, Anglo-European descent). This is true for other under-represented (sub)groups who live, work, and seek health care from nurses in communities across the 50 states and territories. One may even find that some mainstream

American consumers have beliefs and life-styles that appear quite unusual to health professionals who are of similar origin stemming from another ethnocultural orientation Table 11-1.

Traditional approaches to promoting diversity and a culturally aware work force have achieved varying degrees of success. Diversity in the health care delivery system is particularly challenging because efforts must focus not only on consumers, but also on providers. Development of cultural competence must begin with a self-appraisal of personal values, belief systems, and cultural stereotypes. Only then can a person become sensitive to the preferences of others who are perceived to be different, be it in color of skin, cultural beliefs, ethnicity, gender, sexual preferences, or religious beliefs.

The guiding document for public health policy, *Healthy People: 2000* (1991a) outlines goals for several vulnerable populations, specifically citing low-income groups, minorities, and persons with disabilities. Another federal publication, *Health of the Disadvantaged*, (1991b) states that some persons, because of race, ethnic background, sex, or economic status historically have been excluded from quality care and entry to the health professions. Diversity has

TABLE 11-1

Comparison of Projected Population Shifts by Race

Race	Year	
	1995	2050
White	74%	53%
Asian	3%	8%
Native American	1%	1%
Hispanic	10%	24%
Black	12%	14%

Data from USDHHS. (1996). *Health United States;* Morganthau, T. (1997). *Newsweek,* Jan. 27, pp. 58-61.

been and will continue to be integral to the national cultural fabric of the United States. Nurses in varied practice roles who provide direct and indirect care to diverse consumers must develop skills that reflect cultural and linguistic competence. This chapter examines the importance of providing culturally appropriate care in a changing society. Aspects of diversity are discussed, as well as characteristics of cultural and linguistic competence of nurses in leadership roles in a variety of settings (Barbee, 1993; Bushy, 1996; Ganey & DeBocanegra, 1996; Krieger, 1996).

■ AMERICAN CULTURE: THE MELTING POT OR A POT OF STEW

Historically, the United States has been called the melting pot of the world. Now, some metaphorically describe the national culture as being more like a "pot of stew". That is to say, each of the multitude of varied ethnic, racial, and cultural groups want to be seen as unique and distinct. (USDHHS, 1996; Ganey & DeBocanegra, 1996; DeSantis, 1990).

Predicting the shape of the future is always hazardous, but clearly the United States is in for a growth spurt (Table 11-1). By the year 2050 the population is expected to double that of 1990, increasing to about 500 million. Regional concentrations are expected to be even more pronounced. For instance, it is likely that 70% of the growth will occur in the South and West—a continuation of the trend since the 1970s. Gradual population declines are predicted for the Northeast states and parts of the Midwest. As for racial mix, the percentage of Hispanics, blacks, and Asians will jump significantly, changing the dominant majority to people of color much like what presently prevails in the state of New Mexico. The largest population growth will be in the Hispanic and elderly population, each representing nearly 20% of the country's total makeup. In brief, 25 years hence, the United States will change dramati-

cally. Figures 11-1, 11-2, and 11-3 and Table 11-2 demonstrate projected population changes over the next 25 years.

Newcomers also are entering the United States in record numbers from all over the world and this is affecting the nature of society. Of all immigrants coming to the United States, there is a slightly higher number of females than males. Immigrant women are younger than the U.S. population as a whole; more than two-thirds are of childbearing age. In many cases, these newcomers are refugees who have endured traumatic experiences associated with war, famine,

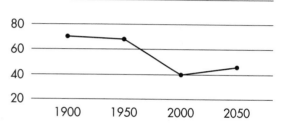

Figure 11-1 ■ Projected number of dependents age 18 and younger (per 100 persons). (Data from USDHHS. [1996]. *Health United States: 1995.* Hyattsville, Md.: Author. (DHHS Pub. No. [PHS] 96-1242); Morganthau, T. [1997]. *Newsweek.* Jan. 27, pp. 58-61.)

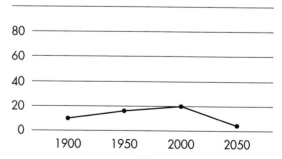

Figure 11-2 ■ Projected number of dependents age 65 and older (per 100 persons). (Data from USDHHS. [1996]. *Health United States: 1995.* Hyattsville, Md.: Author. (DHHS Pub. No. [PHS] 96-1242); Morganthau, T. [1997]. *Newsweek.* Jan. 27, pp. 58-61.)

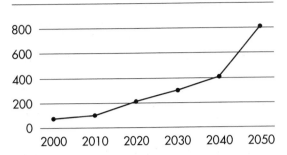

Figure 11-3 ■ Centurions: Projected number of persons older than 100 years. (Data from USDHHS. [1996]. *Health United States: 1995.* Hyattsville, Md.: Author. (DHHS Pub. No. [PHS] 96-1242); Morganthau, T. [1997]. *Newsweek,* Jan. 27, pp. 58-61.)

T A B L E   1 1 - 2

Projected Life Expectancy at Birth by Age

Race	Age	
	Born in 1995 Life Expectancy (Years)	Born in 2050 Life Expectancy (Years)
White	77	84
Hispanic	79	87
Black	69	74
Asian	82	86
Native American	76	82

Data from USDHHS. (1996). *Health United States: 1995.* Hyattsville, Md.: Author. (DHHS Pub. No. [PHS] 96-1242); Morganthau, T. (1997). *Newsweek,* Jan. 27, pp. 58-61.

loss of family and home, torture, and rape. Some have lived for long periods in refugee camps under precarious hygienic conditions. Most enter the United States in fairly good health, but their life-style and health status deteriorate after their arrival. This may be a long-term consequence of the hardships they endured before coming here, coupled with the social and eco-

nomic challenges experienced after they arrive. In addition to speaking a language other than English, newcomers from various nations possess a unique epidemiologic profile, health beliefs, and expectations about health and health care. Ethnic and cultural diversity also have major implications for the health care system with its declining resources and the concern for providing equitable access to care. Upon arriving on U.S. shores, many find the new culture a complete contrast to their home nation. For many U.S. citizens, the newcomers' belief systems and world views often are as foreign as their language (DeSantis, 1990; Ganey & DeBocanegra, 1996; Leininger, 1997; USDHHS, 1996).

Pessimists speculate that these projected demographic shifts will strain the social fabric of the nation because of ethnic tensions and the cost of supporting 33 million elderly persons on Social Security Insurance and Medicare. The gap between old and young and rich and poor will become a chasm. Some foresee decaying cities surrounded by enormous suburbs, segregated by race, ethnicity, and class. Although there seem to be ample data to support this pessimistic vision, predictions do not always become reality. Insidious driving and restraining social forces are occurring that also will affect society in unanticipated ways.

For instance, there are signs that Americans are adapting to changing cultural and ethnic diversity. Moreover, political, social, and economic forces could obscure the effects of diversity as it becomes more the norm. The current dominant racial and ethnic group of white mainstream Americans is expected to become the minority. However, no one can accurately predict when this shift will occur. Partly, it depends both on the entrance of newcomers and on the rate of interracial marriage. Currently the number of interracial marriages is not great, but each year the rate is rising significantly, as are the number of children who are of mixed racial background. Likewise, the number of Hispanics marrying across ethnic lines is increasing, thereby dissolving Hispanic ethnic identities. The federal government currently is pilot testing a questionnaire that allows millions of Americans to check some version of "other" box when asked to specify "Race." In the projected cafe-au-lait society, race-counters will have an increasingly difficult time keeping track of people's ethnic and racial origins. Politically, the nation also is adapting to the diversity. For example, the following phrases are used in the media on a daily basis, reflecting a legislated response to increasing diversity and changing societal views (Krieger, 1996; Leininger, 1978; 1991; 1997; Misener, et al., 1997; Zabara, 1996).

Ageism. Gender. Race. Ethnicity. Sexual orientation. Diversity. Multiculturalism. Discrimination. Ethnic/racial differences. Women's health. Men's health. Racial variations. Inequality. Racism. Minority health. Sexism. Nationalism. Homophobia. Poverty. Underclass. Socioeconomic status. Underprivileged. Working poor. Underrepresented. Underserved. Social class. Disadvantaged. Challenged. Marginalized. Aculturalism. Ethnoculturalism. Special populations. Vulnerable populations. At-risk groups. Discrimination. Social inequities. Cultural sensitivity. Linguistic competence. Barriers to health care.

■ WHAT DO THE WORDS MEAN?

Nurses will often find these phrases interchanged in the literature both in the popular media and in professional publications, and there is no precise definition for most of them. Several of the terms have been "federalized" in policies and programs that address specific groups, such as medically underserved communities, migrant health clinics, Indian Health Service, and the Office of Minority and Women's Health.

Reflecting on all of the terms and the essence of what they mean raises a number of questions. For instance: What do the words mean, and do they all refer to the same thing? Can *race* and *ethnicity* be used synonymously? Does *race/ethnicity* refer to skin color or a person's culture, or do the two concepts overlap? What are the characteristics that define *special population?* What makes an at-risk group different from those not categorized as such? Who are the *disadvantaged* and the *challenged?* What traits are implied in *diversity?* In health care, ethical debates center on the question of "What accounts for the social inequities?" Further, how can these inequities be addressed and by whom so as to ensure an equitable health status for the disadvantaged?

Arriving at answers to such questions no longer is restricted to the realm of academicians and ethicists. The terms now are in the public domain—used for the advantage or disadvantage of persons or communities labeled as such. In other cases, the labels are used to reveal or obscure responsibility. For instance, with concern about political correctness in our language, we may be minimizing concerns for individuals who are of minority or disadvantaged backgrounds. Or, in other instances, one or more of the terms may be used to focus on and divert attention from an issue or population. No attempt is made in this chapter to define or discuss each of the previously mentioned phrases. Background information on race, culture, and ethnicity is provided to help nurses in leadership roles better understand the meaning and implications of diversity when providing care to patients and their family, regardless of how *family* is defined. The information also is important when completing patient assessments so that the care that is rendered by nurses is culturally acceptable and appropriate for the situation. For the sake of simplicity, essentially all of the terms either explicitly or implicitly refer to disparities stemming from physical conditions, emotional status, age, race, ethnicity, gender, and a variety of social and economic factors.

Why be concerned about disparity and inequality? Epidemiologic data support the fact that cultural, racial, ethnic, and social factors interact in complex ways to affect health behaviors and the health status of individuals, families, and communities. The interaction effects often are quantified as life expectancy, mortality, morbidity, or disease etiology. As for quality-of-life measures, these data usually are described as socioeconomic status, standard of living, job satisfaction, life-style, or quality of housing. As separate descriptors, neither of the two types of data reveals much about the health and caring practices of a particular group. When both measurements are used, (epidemiologic data and quality-of-life measures), a more comprehensive view of a group's health risks can be anticipated. For instance, demographic variables such as poverty level, education, gender, race, and place of residence may provide some insights into the health of a community as a whole and perhaps individual members within the group. Measures that address quality of life also can offer insights about a group's cultural belief systems related to health, illness, and health care–seeking behaviors, whether it be a minority or the majority in a given community. At-risk, vulnerable groups are a major concern, as described in the objectives put forth in *Healthy People: 2000* (USDHHS, 1991a).

Characteristically, compared with the dominant culture, the category of *at-risk* or *vulnerable* populations often includes racial or ethnic minorities who do not have opportunities for education, employment, and economic success equal to the majority populations. Minorities are disproportionately represented in the lower socioeconomic levels; likewise they have a poorer overall health status. Cultural and social factors are highly interrelated, but they are not the same. Furthermore, health conditions and treatment outcomes sometimes are attributed to cultural preferences when these are related to social factors.

For example, consider the broad demographic category of *Hispanic;* often subcategorized according to racial background, specifically, *white* or *nonwhite.* Essentially, the general category of *Hispanic* refers to a language that continues to be used in most nations that were colonized by Spain several hundred years ago. Spanish-speaking nations are located throughout the world, including various regions in North, South, and Central America and the Caribbean and Philippine Islands. Each of these nations has distinct ethnic, cultural, and racial features. All of the nations, however, share one commonality: the people who live in those nations all speak Spanish, although with dialects associated with a specific nation's ethnicity. Hispanic cultural and ethnic diversity is particularly evident in the United States, where people who speak Spanish as their primary language immigrate from all parts of the globe—each with its own cultural, ethnic, and linguistic nuances (USDHHS, 1996).

All members of a particular group do not express the same degree of ethnicity. Individual adherence to ethnic behaviors is influenced by education and exposure to other ethnic and cultural groups. Availability and access to public transportation and communication systems have led to a highly interdependent, global society, which increases exposure to people of other ethnic backgrounds. Simultaneously, many intraethnic variations are rapidly emerging. Nurses, therefore, need to be prepared to provide competent care to individuals, families, and communities with ethnic backgrounds that are different from theirs and also to work with or lead ethnically diverse teams.

Key terms	
Term	**Definition**
Culture	Shared values, beliefs, and practices of a particular group that are transmitted from one generation to the next and are identified as patterns that guide thinking and actions
Cultural beliefs	Shared statements that individuals in a group hold to be true; all beliefs are culturally bound
Cultural values	Prevailing or persistent guides influencing the thoughts and actions of members of a group
Ethnicity	The affiliation of a group as a result of shared linguistic, racial, and/or cultural background
Race	A social classification that relies on skin color as a physical marker to define group membership

Race

Race is a social classification that relies on skin color as a physical marker to define group membership, specifically, white, Asian-Pacific Islanders, Native American, and black. Ethnicity is closely related and refers to the shared affiliation of a group based on linguistic, racial, and cultural characteristics. However, individuals who are of the same race may differ in their ethnic affiliation.

For example, persons with the race classification "black" may have been born in Africa, North America, or the Caribbean. Native Americans usually are categorized as the same race even though very few are truly full-blooded Native Americans. There are, however, more than 300 identified groups, each having its own values and belief systems. Some groups may be similar in many ways. Most are quite different from other groups, stemming from historical events, the geographic region in which they lived, the natural resources available in that region, and their exposure to other groups. It is important to stress that ethnic and cultural differences may be obscured by skin color. Consequently, misper-ceptions can emerge among the uninformed that a particular racial group is homogenous. Hence, stereotyping occurs when individual differences or preferences of individuals within a particular racial or ethnic group are not considered.

Culture

Culture is described as a set of values, ideals, and belief systems that are widely shared among a group of people. A culture emerges over time. Often, but not always, group members have a common ethnicity or race. Members in the group, in turn, incorporate cultural traditions as guides to dealing with life situations and defining their roles within that society. Cultural values and behaviors are transferred from one generation to the next. These are learned by an individual through continuous contact with the group in day-to-day interactions, as well as during special events associated with major life transitions, such as birth, childbearing, menarche, illness, and death. For a child the intergenerational transfer begins early in life and is learned from caregivers through implicit and explicit behaviors (Leininger, 1978; 1991; 1994; 1997).

Explicit cultural behaviors include verbal communication and the organization of a group's social structures. A culture, in turn, defines the manner in which family and community is organized, how they interrelate and function, and the roles for each member. Family structures vary from one culture to another. The family, however defined by the group, provides an explicit framework within which a child learns to differentiate self from others within and outside of the community.

Implicit behaviors are subtle. These behaviors include the manner in which a group views others who are not part of their community as well as members who deviate from the local norm. Nonverbal implicit behaviors often are difficult to articulate by group members and serve as a form of social control. Implicit cultural behaviors are integral to the manner in which a group defines health, illness, and how and when health care is sought and by whom. Social factors also can modify cultural practices, thereby making it difficult, if not impossible, to differentiate the two.

For example, Native American tribes and Mexican-American farm workers have a cultural preference for a highly regarded elderly woman in their extended family to care for a member who becomes ill. In cases where the person is gravely ill, the group is not opposed and even prefers to seek care from a professional provider using Western medicine models outside of their community. However, if the family does not have adequate transportation to get to the nurse or physician or cannot afford to pay for that service, they are forced to rely on the volunteered services provided by extended family members. Health care providers who do not realize the family's social and living condition, in turn, may be judgmental and critical of these culture-related practices regarding the care, or lack of it, for a seriously ill person.

Essentially, all cultures have the same basic organizational components but all cultures are not necessarily the same. Likewise, even the predominant cultural group is not homogeneous. There are wide variations within the group itself. Generally, a major proportion of

Key terms	
Term	**Definition**
Acculturation	Process of adapting or learning to take on the behavior of another group
Cultural blindness	When differences between cultures are ignored and the person behaves as if differences do not exist
Cultural relativity	Understanding the beliefs, values, and practices within the context of culture
Cultural shock	Feelings of helplessness and discomfort experienced by an outsider attempting to comprehend or effectively adapt to a different cultural group
Cultural change	Change that occurs as a result of contact between groups and forces within the culture
Stereotypes	Exaggerated beliefs and images, popularly depicted by the mass media or folklore
World view	Perspective shared by a group of general views of relationships within the universe; these broad views influence health and health beliefs

the group's members tend to conform to most of the established standards. However, there always will be a few members who will exhibit nonconforming behaviors and preferences. Consequently, stereotyping a cultural group can lead to inaccurate assessments and treatment interventions for individual members (Box 11-1).

Space constraints in this text preclude extensive discussion of the particular preferences and belief systems of various ethnic and cultural groups. A number of comprehensive guides present in more detail the ethnocultural practices and preferences of many different groups, and the reader is encouraged to refer to those publications for more information (Andrews & Boyle, 1997; Bell, 1994; Degazone, 1996; Geissler, 1994; Leininger, 1978; 1991; 1994; 1997; Rosella et al., 1994; Stanhope & Knollmuller, 1997). (See Box 11-2.)

B O X   1 1 - 1

Components of Patient's Cultural Assessment

- Name of patient
- How (by what name) does the patient prefer to be addressed
- Birthplace of patient, parents, grandparents (paternal and maternal)
- Number of siblings of the patient, parents, grandparents
- Setting where patient, parents, grandparents were raised (rural, urban, suburban, other)
- Nation/country where patient, parents, grandparents were raised
- Age upon coming to the United States (patient, parents, grandparents as applicable)
- Native language of patient, parents, grandparents; to what degree is this spoken
- Can the patient speak, understand and/or read English
- When growing up, who lived with the patient (nuclear, extended family, others)
- Who does the patient identify as his/her family (individual members of the patient-system)
- Significant other's culture, ethnic, and racial background (if applicable)
- Has patient maintained contact with other relatives (aunts, uncles, cousins; siblings; parents; own children)
- Proximity of nuclear and extended family members' residence to patient's home

- Frequency of contact with relatives (nuclear and extended family) (e.g., daily, weekly, monthly, once a year or less, never)
- Was patient's original family name changed upon arriving in this country
- Patient's and spouse's/partner's religious preferences; do they belong to a religious institution/faith; are they active members
- Frequency of attending religious services
- Religious practices engaged in within the home (specify type and frequency)
- Type of school attended (public, private, parochial); level of education
- Does patient reside in a community where neighbors have similar education, racial, ethnic, cultural, and religious backgrounds
- Are friends of similar backgrounds
- Does patient prepare foods related to ethnic background (describe)
- Does patient participate in ethnic/cultural activities (e.g., dancing, dress, holiday celebrations, rites of passage, music)
- Specific cultural/ethnic practices engaged in that relate to life-style, health maintenance, illness, and health care–seeking behaviors

Data from Geissler, E. (1994). *Pocket guide: Cultural assessment*. St. Louis: Mosby; Stanhope, M., & Knollmueller, R. (1997). *Public health and community health nurse's consultant: A health promotion guide* (pp. 211-242). St. Louis: Mosby.

Ethnocultural Barriers to Health Care

- Traditions of handing personal problems that do not fit this particular problem (e.g., self-care practices such as using over-the-counter medications, exercising, ingestion of alcohol, resting, prayer)
- Beliefs about the cause of a disorder and the appropriate healer for it (e.g., doctor, nurse practitioner, a neighborhood nurse acquaintance, chiropractor, herbologist, community lay healer, medicine man/woman, voodoo priestess, homeopathy, therapeutic touch, imagery, acupuncture/acupressure, curandero, shaman, etc.)
- Lack of knowledge about a physical or emotional disorder and the place of formal services in preventing and treating the condition (e.g., being stoic and suffering in silence rather than seeking supportive care; paying for emergency care rather than spending money on health promotion or primary prevention; expectations that one receives a prescription when paying to seek care from a doctor or nurse [e.g., antibiotic, analgesic])

- Language barriers, e.g., English as the second language; functional illiteracy (reading below the 5th grade level; note that most health care literature is written at the 10th grade level or higher); nonverbal (cultural) nuances associated with terminology that is used in health education
- Translation-related issues
- Difficulty in maintaining confidentiality and anonymity in a setting where many residents are acquainted
- Cultural insensitivity of providers or of the health care delivery system
- Confusion about publicly-funded services or third-party payer mandates
- Conflicting views regarding time perceptions
- Misinterpretations of behaviors associated with space orientation
- Previous experiences (negative in particular) with the health care system and providers

■ WHAT MAKES UP A CULTURAL GROUP?

Key components of a cultural group center on their social organizations, communication patterns, space perception, time orientation, biologic variations, and environmental-control factors. These six cultural components are important for nurses to include in a cultural assessment of patients as well as colleagues. Subsequently, these preferences also must be integrated into the treatment plan for the patient to ensure that the rendered care is culturally appropriate and acceptable. Cultural preferences and barriers to care also must be considered in evaluation models to assess the quality of care and patient's outcomes of an intervention for a health-related problem. (See Box 11-3.)

Social Organizations

The family is the basic unit of society, and cultural values influence its organization and the roles of each member within it. The term *family* is difficult to define, and there are a great many structural variations. Traditionally, mainstream American policy makers, for instance, work from the notion of a nuclear family (mother, father, children/siblings). Some cultures include large kinship networks composed of blood relatives as well as those acquired by marriage. When describing family, other cultures refer to all maternal aunts as *mother* and all maternal uncles as *father.* Some Native American tribes refer to all nonextended family members within their clan as *cousins.* Other tribes have a ritual for adopting someone with whom they have an emotional bond into the family. Adoptees, in turn, are referred to as *brother, sister, son,* or *daughter* by other family members.

In addition to nuclear and extended families, other family structures often encountered in the health care setting include same-gender couples with and without children; grandparents who are the primary care givers for grandchildren; blended-family arrangements of all types and numbers; communal arrangements with and without children; and cohabiting unmarried working or elderly persons. Consequently, it may be a challenge for nurses to complete commonly used assessment tools such as family genograms or echo-maps that diagram communication patterns among members in one household. Likewise, many well-accepted research instruments may not be culturally sensitive to family systems of various ethnic groups.

Behaviors for the various roles in the organization are culturally prescribed and vary among groups. For instance, the value placed on and the roles allocated to children and elderly persons within a group is culturally based, as are their social controls and approach to discipline. Likewise, gender role behaviors are culturally defined and affect nurse-patient relationships. As for family spokesperson and decision maker(s) regarding health care matters, in some cases a woman heads the household and decides what need to be done; in other families, such decisions are made by a man. Sometimes a family member who has had more education than the others, especially in a health-related field, becomes the designated spokesperson. In other instances, an elder extended family member may be deferred to as the final authority. Sometimes the only person who can speak or translate English in the family speaks for the rest, even if he or she may know only a few words. In some cases, the only person who can speak English is a child who has learned it in school. There may be some cultural taboos as to the topics that children can discuss, especially in regard to sensitive health and sexual problems. (Issues related to translators are examined in more detail in the section on Communication Patterns.) For this reason it is important for the nurse to ask a patient early in the assessment process who he or she includes as family and who the spokesperson is. Subsequently, those individuals also should be included in the planning, implementing, and evaluating of care for the patient (Geissler, 1994; Leininger, 1997; Rosella et al., 1994; Stanhope & Knollmuller, 1997). (See Box 11-2.)

Cultural values also influence the extent of a family's involvement in the treatment plan for a sick member. For example, in some cultures only immediate female family members are directly involved, specifically the mother or wife. In others the entire extended family (clan) may expect to be active participants when a member is hospitalized or dying. For health care providers, this cultural preference may involve extended visiting privileges for the family members, who may be many. Or it may include allowing the family to bring in foods prepared at home that they believe will help in the healing process. In some cases it is helpful to include an indigenous healer who is able to augment contemporary medicine with traditional healing rituals. All of these cultural preferences can be in direct conflict with a Western model of health care and a source of contention between nurses and their patients.

Another cultural variation related to family and community organizations is the manner in which people are addressed. For instance, in some Mexican-American families several surnames are used, such as the mother's, grandmother's, and father's. In some Asian groups, the family surname comes before a birth name. Native Americans are given a birth name; but in some instances another is taken by the person as part of the rite of passage for a life event. Immigrants with birth names that are difficult to pronounce or spell in this country sometimes select another commonly used English name to facilitate their entry into American society. In each case, confusion can result from information that is provided on official records versus word-of-mouth reports from the patient or family. If possible, individual preferences relating to name and title should be determined early on and respected by the nurse. Spelling and pronunciation should be carefully cross-referenced from verbal reports with official documents to ensure that all of the patient's health records have accurate demographic information.

Communication Patterns

One of the most obvious differences among cultural and ethnic groups is the manner in which members communicate with each other. Communication includes the use of language, vocabulary, grammar, voice qualities, intonation, rhythm, speed, pronunciation, physical gestures, and silence. In the United States the dominant language is English but this recently has been challenged in several states with large Hispanic populations. As with Spanish-speaking

groups, the English language also has terms that have different pronunciations, meanings, and nuances in the various English-speaking countries. Consequently, two individuals of different ethnicity who speak to each other in English may not completely understand, or may even misunderstand, each other.

Foreign language courses generally instruct the learner in the classic form of grammar and diction. This form often is not used in the day-to-day communication within a group, as is the case with some Spanish- and English-speaking nations. Ethnocultural nuances or regional dialects tend not to be included, and sometimes even discouraged, in formal language courses. Consequently, being able to read the written word and being comfortable with the spoken word still may not assure that a nurse can communicate effectively with all people who speak a dialect form of the language.

Communication barriers obviously are intensified in interactions between people who speak different languages. This situation can be extremely frustrating for all parties, particularly when someone is seriously injured or acutely ill and requires urgent attention. With the newcomers to a country also come their diverse and sometimes unusual languages. Ideally, all care givers need knowledge about all of the languages spoken by their patients. However, that probably is not a realistic expectation. Therefore augmenting the spoken word with gestures and pictures can be a helpful communication strategy for nurses who work with people who speak another language.

Culture rules based on age, gender, and position in the family often dictate who can or cannot discuss topics regarding personal health matters. For instance, in some cultures, children and males should not talk about health problems related to reproduction. In other cultures, male health professionals should not speak to a woman unless she is appropriately attired.

Sometimes, the rules for appropriate attire mean the woman's face being covered. Often translators' knowledge about anatomy, physiology, and the illness process is limited. Consequently, they may be unable to understand what the nurse is saying, especially if medical terms are used. The nurse may need a professional health care translator to communicate with the patient. Translators should be objective and able to provided an accurate interpretation of what is being said by both parties; however, nurses must try to use language that both the patient and the translator can understand.

Finding translators may be a challenge in some cases, especially in smaller communities or regions having a more homogeneous population. Listings of available resources and translators often are compiled by social service and public health agencies. When a significant number of foreign-speaking people reside in a catchment area, it is prudent for health care providers in that area to keep English-foreign language translation dictionaries accessible. Pocket-size, computer-operated foreign language dictionaries are inexpensive and can provide quick access to unfamiliar words. They can be used by the client-system as well as the nurse. Remember that communicating via a translator increases the time needed for the interaction.

Initiating a conversation with a stranger also is influenced by cultural preferences. For example, on the one hand a nurse may plan to complete an intake assessment shortly after meeting the patient. In a highly structured health care setting this information usually is obtained in a hasty and efficient manner using direct questioning. A patient, on the other hand, may be offended with this direct approach by a complete stranger. In the case of an elderly person, personal questions may be perceived as a sign of disrespect, especially if the nurse is younger and the other gender. Many cultures adhere to prescribed social courtesies preceding the discussion of more personal topics. Other cultural groups respond to a direct question by talking around the question or replying indirectly with a life story that metaphorically describes the health problem as it affects the person's life. Still other people talk extensively about a variety of topics, expecting the care giver to elicit the essence of a conversation. Obviously, there is no best way to initiate a conversation with persons who are of another culture. Nurses, therefore, must develop sensitivity to each patient's preferences, allocate adequate time to fulfill those expectations, and establish a mutual rapport; however, that is defined by the patient.

Nonverbal as well as verbal communication patterns are culturally based. For example, speaking softly with the head slightly bowed and eyes cast down may indicate respect and deference in some groups. For others, these nonverbal behaviors may portray shyness; for still others it communicates slyness and dishonesty. Conversely, direct and prolonged eye contact may indicate a strong sense of self for many mainstream Americans or Germans. This same behavior could be a way to communicate aggressiveness, disrespect, or contempt in another cultural group. Or, in other instances, this same behavior could be construed as an overt sexual gesture. Another example of an often misinterpreted nonverbal message is the patient who is smiling and nodding while the nurse is speaking to or explaining something to the person. Such a response does not necessarily mean that the patient understands what is being said. Rather, it may indicate a sign of attentive acknowledgment of the speaker although the person, who continues to nod and smile, does not understand a word. Another communication pattern that nurses often encounter, even in mainstream American families, is when another spokesperson provides answers to questions even when these clearly are directed to the patient.

These are but a few examples of the many culturally based verbal and nonverbal patterns that communicate a range of sometimes conflicting messages to people of diverse background. There are many others, and nurses must be sensitive to the nuances and variations in communication patterns of all patients. Although there is no best way to handle any of these communication preferences some useful tips follow:

- Speak slowly, respectfully, and in a calm, normal volume.
- Avoid speaking loudly; raising one's voice can be threatening or offensive to a patient or family of another culture.
- Ask patients to repeat in their own words what they were told; this is another way to assess the level of understanding.
- Write out what was said so that the family has a reference should questions arise about the treatment plan.

Most people, regardless of their culture or ethnicity, can sense when a person is reassuring with a well-meaning intent. This can go a long way to establishing rapport between the nurse and the patient for subsequent communication efforts.

Space Perception

Space perception is another culturally based aspect of communication and organizational structures. This concept can be described as the comfort zone, associated with the distance between persons who are interacting. Each culture has spatial preferences deemed appropriate for interpersonal interactions, and these preferences differ. For instance, compared with mainstream Americans, some Hispanic groups feel more comfortable with less space when they are speaking to another. Many Hispanics prefer to touch the person with whom they are speaking. In some cultures, it is usual practice to shake hands when meeting another person. Likewise, it is not unusual for women or men in some cultures to lightly embrace another person of the same gender as part of an initial greeting, even if the person is a new acquaintance. This gesture can be uncomfortable to mainstream Americans, who prefer more space and are unaccustomed to being touched by someone they do not know well. Inappropriate touch, in fact, may be interpreted as sexual harassment in some societies. It is important to be sensitive to each person's boundaries and avoid the inappropriate invasion of another person's comfort zone. Space preferences can be a source of conflict in health care, especially when physical examinations and nursing interventions that involve touching are performed.

Time Orientation

The manner in which time is perceived also varies from culture to culture. More specifically, cultural groups differ in having a past, present, or future orientation. Again, it is with the greatest of caution that one can make general statements regarding time perception, since there is great variation within and among ethnic groups. Several examples are offered to help explain the notion of time orientation, with the admonition not to stereotype all members in that given group.

Many people are future oriented and are willing to work hard and delay gratification for some anticipated future goal. Future orientation can affect life-style behavior in that future-oriented persons are willing to participate in activities intended to help them stay healthy, appear more physically fit, and increase their life expectancy. On the other hand, not achieving the hoped-for outcome can lead to high levels of stress and depression. Other people or groups tend to be more present oriented, and this, too, influences their choice of health behaviors. For instance, even though a person may have a chronic health condition such as hypertension or diabetes, at a family gathering he or she may decide to eat particular ethnic foods associated with the event even though these are known to be high in salt, cholesterol, or carbohydrates. Cultures that are past oriented include some Native Americans, Alaskans, Asians, and Pacific Islanders. In these cultures, the life process is viewed as a circular event and deceased relatives are viewed as part of the extended family and given great deference by the living. Deceased family members are believed to provide guidance and support to living relatives. It is not unusual for a patient with a past-oriented time perspective to incorporate healing practices that a deceased loved one suggested to them regarding a health problem. This cultural orientation can be somewhat disconcerting for nurses who are future or present oriented, especially if the patient is being treated for a mental or emotional disturbance.

Time orientation has many other ramifications that can lead to misunderstandings. Consider a patient's versus a nurse's expectations as to when an intervention is to be carried out (time-wise). On one hand, a hospitalized person may expect to have a prescribed medication at the exact moment that it is scheduled or their call-light answered shortly after it is turned on. On the other hand, a nurse may not deem that same situation to be a priority given the other urgent patient needs that exist on the hospital unit. Likewise, the nurse knows that the policy for giving medications is that they can be administered within a "window" of one-half hour of when they are actually scheduled. Or, when a person is waiting for something to happen, time is perceived to pass very slowly, especially when alone, in pain, or anticipating a major event. Conversely, an over-extended modern woman with family and work responsibilities often is heard to say, "the more work I have to do,

the faster my day passes." For this woman, the time allowed for relaxing is viewed as a luxury that, for her, occurs too rarely and passes too quickly.

In essence, mainstream Americans tend to be on tight schedules stemming from an industrialized culture. Other cultures, however, may have a time range within which they carry out life and role functions. Hence, they may not adhere as strictly to appointment schedules or preventive health protocols. Therefore it is important to learn about a patient's time orientation. Then creative consideration must be given to those cultural frames of reference when planning and implementing services. Useful strategies include anticipating late appointment arrivals, not making scheduled appointments but seeing patients upon arrival at the clinic, having clinic hours at nontraditional times, or providing outreach service at more accessible community-based sites.

Biologic Variations

Culture and biologic variations are closely interrelated and in part can be attributed to racial physiologic markers. Race, however, is becoming more difficult to differentiate because of the increasing numbers of persons with interracial origin. For example, one race may be distinguished from another by biologic markers such as color and thickness of the skin and physical and developmental patterns, emotional makeup, and susceptibility to diseases. Sometimes, though, it is difficult to determine accurately if the variation is the result of the individual's genetic makeup or of social and environmental factors such as economic systems, dietary patterns, life-style, climactic or geographic factors, or endemic health conditions.

Nurses should become aware of the more common biologic variations in their catchment area. For example, if there is a large segment of blacks, Native Americans, or other ethnic groups within the community, nurses should take the initiative to become familiar with physical and genetic variations and disease processes that occur with greater frequency in a particular group, such as sickle cell anemia, osteoporosis, diabetes, hypertension and breast cancer. State and local health status reports can provide some insights regarding epidemiologic, mortality, and morbidity data that may be associated with race, culture, and ethnicity in a catchment area (population in a given area).

Environmental Control

Environmental control refers to the relationship between humans and nature. Some groups perceive humans as having mastery over nature, whereas others perceive humans to be dominated by nature. Still other groups see harmonious relationships between humans and nature. Individuals who perceive mastery over nature believe they can overcome the natural forces of nature. Such individuals would expect a cure for an incurable malignancy with a medical or surgical intervention (Brink, 1993; Leininger, 1978; 1991; 1994; Degazone, 1996; Geissler, 1994).

Conversely, the subjugation to nature perspective, held by some blacks and Hispanics, allows the belief that people have little control over what happens to them. Those holding this view may not adhere to the treatment protocol because they believe that nothing will change the outcome of their destiny. In the case of a malignancy, these individuals are less likely than those of other world views to engage in imagery or meditation activities.

Persons who hold the harmony-with-nature world view, such as Asians and Native Americans, may perceive an illness to be a result of disharmony with nature. This perspective leads one to believe that medical interventions will only relieve symptoms rather than cure the disease. Those holding this view may, instead, use naturally occurring substances such as herbs or hot/cold treatment modalities to restore the physical and spiritual imbalance causing symptoms in the person who is ill.

■ HOW DO SOCIAL AND ETHNOCULTURAL FACTORS INTERRELATE?

Racial, cultural, and ethnic factors are highly interrelated, and it can be difficult to isolate one from the other. Moreover, socioeconomic and environmental factors also influence these three dimensions in ways that can lead to less than optimal health outcomes. More specifically, disadvantaged groups share some common characteristics, including poverty, being of a racial or ethnic minority, lower socioeconomic status, less education, a higher incidence of chronic health problems, lower life expectancies, and poorer pregnancy outcomes. Disadvantaged persons experience multiple economic, legal, linguistic, and cultural barriers when trying to access health care services. Each at-risk group has its own epidemiologically unique characteristics (USDHHS, 1991a; 1991b; 1996).

For instance, individuals of racial and ethnic minorities are more likely to work in low-paying jobs, which do not offer fringe benefits such as health care insurance. Or an employer may provide coverage for the employee but not for the family. Even if health care is available at no cost, an employed person may not be able to take the necessary time off from work to see a physician or nurse practitioner. Going to a clinic often involves taking time not only to see the provider, but also for the round-trip travel, which in many cases involves traveling a long distance. Once there, waiting in the clinic to see the provider, perhaps waiting again for diagnostic tests to be done, and then waiting for the prescription to be filled can take even more time. Consequently, it is not unusual for a seemingly short 15-minute visit with the health care provider to actually require that a person take one full day off work without pay. This example illustrates how socioeconomic and environmental factors contribute to problems in accessing health care. Ultimately, these situations also affect the health status of disadvantaged and minority groups.

Public policy also can influence the health status of disadvantaged groups in both positive and negative ways. Most nurses can cite examples of positive outcomes related to public policy, such as funding for immunization and the WIC program. Two examples of a seemingly less optimistic public policy are the Federal Welfare Reform Act and California's Proposition 187 Action. Both of these initiatives impose limitations on who can and cannot receive publicly funded benefits. Assessing the outcomes of enacted legislation is time sensitive. Moreover, since the enactment of the two initiatives is recent, the long-range impact on the health care environment and the health status of disadvantaged, at-risk, vulnerable populations is yet to be assessed (Krieger, 1996; Misener et al., 1997; Zabrana, 1996). Nurses in leadership roles need to be aware of political agendas that focus on diversity issues and be advocates to support patients who are of another cultural and ethnic origin.

■ WHAT DO WE MEAN BY CULTURALLY COMPETENT CARE?

Obviously nurses must be aware of cultural, ethnic, and racial variations in their patients and then provide appropriate and acceptable care. Cultural competence can be viewed as a continuum ranging from ethnocentrism on the one extreme to full cultural competence at the opposite extreme. Learning and achieving the highest level of competence is a process, and each individual progresses at his or her own rate. Between the two extremes, each person progresses through various levels of awareness, sensitivity, knowledge, and ability for cultural competence in caring for patients of other cultures (Bushy, 1996; Degazon, 1996; USDHHS, 1991a; 199b).(See Figure 11-4.)

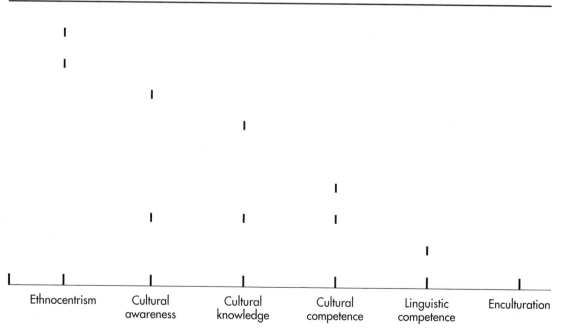

Figure 11-4 ■ Continuum of cultural competency.

Key terms	
Term	**Definition**
Ethnocentrism	Believing that one's own culture determines the standards of behavior by which all other groups are to be judged
Cultural awareness	Appreciating and being sensitive to another's values, beliefs, practice, life-style, and problem-solving preferences
Cultural knowledge	Developing insights about the organizational elements and expectations of another culture
Cultural competence	Having awareness, sensitivity, and knowledge about another culture as well as a repertoire of skills to provide care acceptable to that group
Linguistic competence	Being comfortable with the language and the cultural nuances of verbal and nonverbal patterns of communication
Enculturation	The process of acquiring knowledge and internalizing values of another culture

The Competency Continuum

Ethnocentrism refers to the belief that one's own group determines the standards for behavior by which all other cultural groups are to be judged. At this level, behaviors and beliefs of other cultural groups are devalued, treated with suspicion or hostility, or ignored. The next level on the continuum is *cultural awareness,* which is an appreciation of and sensitivity to another's values, beliefs, practices, life-style, and problem-solving preferences. Next on the continuum is *cultural knowledge,* where one gleans insights about the organizational elements and seeks information on strategies to provide care that is acceptable and appropriate for another culture.

Enculturation refers to the process of completely acquiring and internalizing the values and beliefs of another culture. All along the continuum markers, a nurse may experience cultural change or cultural relativity. *Cultural change* occurs as a result of contact between groups and forces within a culture. *Cultural relativity* refers to understanding the beliefs, values, and practices within the context of a particular culture.

Cultural competence is often described as the most sophisticated level on the continuum. At this level the person not only is aware, sensitive, and knowledgeable about another culture, but has developed a repertoire of skills to provide care that is appropriate and acceptable to the group even if it is not congruent with the care giver's own. More recently, the notion of *linguistic competence* has come into use. This level consists of even more complex skills. At this point a care giver not only is comfortable using another language, but also is sensitive and aware of all of the cultural nuances associated with the verbal and nonverbal patterns of another group.

Strategies to Provide Appropriate and Acceptable Care

A culturally competent nurse provides care that is acceptable and appropriate to patients. Several strategies to achieve this practice outcome are discussed here. *Cultural competence* has several dimensions that can be useful in planning and implementing care for diverse patients.

Key terms	
Term	**Definition**
Cultural preservation	Supporting and using aspects of another's culture to promote healthy behaviors
Cultural repatterning	Helping another person change or modify culturally based behaviors that may be detrimental to his or her health
Cultural accommodation	Ability to integrate a particular cultural practice, even if it does not have scientific support, into the patient's treatment plan
Cultural imposition	Imposing personal beliefs on another
Cultural shock	Extreme reaction to major discrepancies between cultural values

Cultural preservation is evident when a nurse can support and use selected aspects of another's culture to promote healthy behaviors. For example, when working with an extended family, the nurse would allow key members the necessary time to arrive at a decision they believe to be best in a given situation.

Cultural accommodation refers to the ability to integrate a particular cultural practice, even if it does not have scientific support, into the person's treatment plan. For example, in the patient's treatment plan, integrating family members or indigenous healers or drinking a tea or herb from the "old country" into the established Western medicine protocols for a particular diagnosis such as hypertension or arthritis is seen as cultural accommodation.

Cultural repatterning, another strategy to provide culturally competent care, refers to helping people change or modify culturally based behaviors that may be detrimental to their well-being. For example, changing eating patterns and food preferences for a particular health problem such as diabetes, allergies, or a malignancy is considered to be a form of cultural repatterning.

Several other behaviors are associated with cultural competency or its lack. More specifi-cally, *cultural imposition* is the process of imposing one's personal beliefs on another. This has particular relevance for health care providers who impose Western beliefs and traditions on patients, thereby negating the value of a patient's cultural healing beliefs, such as folk remedies or their use of an indigenous healer.

Cultural conflict refers to situations when a perceived threat arises from misunderstandings or cultural blindness between a care giver and the person of another culture because neither is aware of their differences. In some cases these kinds of conflicts may be unavoidable. However, nurses with conflict resolution skills are better able to resolve these situations and render care in a manner that fits with a patient's ethnocultural preferences.

Cultural shock occurs when interacting with patients of a particular culture to which the nurse has had limited knowledge or exposure. This type of extreme response can be a normal reaction to beliefs or behaviors that are disallowed within the nurse's culture. For example, shock sometimes occurs when a nurse cares for a patient from another culture who adheres to unfamiliar or conflicting beliefs about diet or observes practices that mutilate or disfigure the body.

Self-care and Alternative Healing Practices

An important strategy in demonstrating cultural competence is acknowledging the use of ethnoculturally based self-care practices by consumers and clients in general. In addition to seeking care from professional practitioners, when people develop a problem, they can obtain relief in a number of alternative ways, including using self-care with its folk remedies and seeking advice from alternative healers. The resources and the rationale for those behaviors may differ, depending on cultural, socioeconomic, environmental, geographic, and religious/spiritual factors. Self-care is as old as human history. Therefore self-care is a critical element of holistic and culturally competent care. Alternative healing practices have a long history and remain popular among humans for many reasons, such as the following:

- The lack of available, accessible, affordable, and acceptable health care
- Limited knowledge about body functioning and the disease process
- Reports by highly regarded family members about the effectiveness of a specific treatment or indigenous healer

For many, the major distinction between care provided by professional providers and self-care is the remuneration factor. Nurses must assume that most people, including health professionals, use self-care and folk medicine at some time. Self-treatment probably is used with greater frequency when a person feels unhealthy, is coming down with something, or is outright sick. Even though self-care practices may seem inconsistent with scientific knowledge, without these practices the already overburdened health care system would be even more taxed. Many of these products may not be harmful when used as directed, but problems often arise when they are used incorrectly or taken with other medications. Near the end of the 1980s, it was estimated that Americans spent $27 million dollars on health-related products (Miller, 1994). Now, nearly a decade later, this figure probably has doubled, with more than 40 million people using one or more over-the-counter-products within the past year. The FDA speculates that one in ten persons suffers side effects from self-treatments, yet the products are highly touted by the popular media.

Self-care, folk healing, and alternative providers must be considered by nurses as integral to the patient's treatment plan—even if these interventions are not formally acknowledged. Self-care should be viewed from two levels, that is, personal health behavior skills and social political skills. Both levels contribute to individual and family well-being. Personal self-care skills are those used to maintain or restore an individual's health. Social political skills are inherent in the self-care used by a community or a family to treat unusual conditions that occur in its members, particularly physical and emotional consequences related to social, ethnocultural, and developmental transitions.

Folk remedies can be categorized into three major groups (Bushy, 1996). The first consists of interventions to prevent or treat undesired physical symptoms and short-term or self-limiting conditions. Included in this list of conditions are warts, cold sores, minor menstrual problems, muscle aches, constipation, diarrhea, indigestion, hay fever, sore throats, ingrown toenails, colds, influenza, nosebleeds, insect bites, impetigo, hiccough, bumps, bruises, pimples, rashes, colic, dandruff, enuresis, ringworm, male itch, and athlete's foot.

The second category of self-care remedies is used to prevent and treat chronic and/or incurable conditions such as arthritis, hypertension, allergies, weight gain, weight loss, baldness, asthma, ulcers, gallbladder problems, impotence, infertility, sinusitis, and chronic pain, especially of the back and head. These conditions vary in severity depending on weather, stress, diet, and physical activity. However, the user often attributes improvement of the problem to a certain product being used during an intermittent remission of the condition.

The third category of self-treatment is to prevent or treat complex conditions that are sometimes associated with emotional, psychosomatic, or neurologic factors. Conditions in this category include persistent skin conditions (psoriasis, eczema, hives), stomach ulcers, severe persistent menstrual cramps, endometriosis, migraine headaches, seizures, insomnia, and depression. These conditions usually are long term and traditionally have been more difficult to treat. The stigma associated with mental illness is an ongoing consequence of those interventions.

Self-care continues to be popular in this country, partly because of the high cost of health care and partly because of a person's lack of faith in the effectiveness of the system. The consumer movement, too, has created a receptive audience for the distribution of a wide range of self-care literature and at-home diagnostic devices, as have escalating numbers of formerly prescribed drugs now available as over-the-counter products. Nurses also must accept that in many instances self-care may be at least as effective as Western medicine.

Because of ethnic diversity, Americans use a wide range of therapeutic systems that are alternatives to orthodox medicine. Some of the more popular are psychic healing, rolfing, chiropractic, faith healing, therapeutic massage, osteopathy, meditation, and visualization. Some of these practices, however, may interfere with or actually be detrimental to the patient. To elicit information about a patient's use of self-care and folk remedies, nurses should learn to ask tactful but pertinent questions during the cultural assessment. This information is summarized in the patient's data base and integrated into the care plan. Questioning should be nonjudgmental and should address the following areas:

- Does the patient use self-care or traditional folk practices? If so, what are these?
- Which remedies are used for health promotion? Disease prevention? Illness intervention?
- Is the patient currently being treated by a folk healer? If so, is the patient willing to share information about those interventions?
- Does the patient prefer having a folk healer as a part of the care that is planned by the nurse ? If so, who and how can this individual be contacted?
- Are there certain individuals, or relatives, a patient wishes to have present during treatment? What role are they to take during the healing process? How can these individuals be contacted?

If a patient's belief system includes folk remedies, such as drinking herb tea, eating certain foods, or using natural products or over-the-counter drugs, these beliefs should be recognized by the care giver. Recognition, however, does not require negating the use of scientifically based treatments. Rather, it implies assessing the benefits and risks of a remedy. Then, if appropriate, incorporate the self-care as an adjunct to the prescribed scientific intervention(s) or develop an educational intervention that suits the particular situation.

Nurses must be sensitive to the fact that when scientific knowledge is presented so that it appears incompatible with a patient's ethnocultural beliefs, the traditional way will probably be accepted and even the best information probably rejected. Taking time to have the patients explain, in their own words, the *negotiated* treatment plan and how to take any prescribed medicine(s) can help clarify communication and understanding. Linguistic competency on the part of a nurse is evidenced by asking another's point of view and then collaborating with the person, rather than imposing a treatment plan based on a highly structured clinical pathway protocol. Although it takes more time in the beginning, a patient-nurse collaborative model can prevent many follow-up phone calls or office visits caused by misunderstood treatment protocols.

Nurses can learn a great deal about effective teaching from consumer-oriented self-care publications. That is, instead of negating ethnoculturally based folk remedies and implementing a totally unfamiliar regimen, allow the patient something that is culturally familiar, such as folk remedies and self-care behaviors. In this way, patients are apt to adhere more closely to the scientifically based therapeutic regimen, as well, and perceive the care that they receive as appropriate and acceptable.

In essence, becoming culturally and linguistically competent is a nonlinear developmental process for a nurse. Individuals proceed at their own rate based on life experiences; exposure to other cultural, racial, and ethnic groups; and receptivity to learning about differences. As with other skills in the repertoire of nurses, ethnoculturally based interventions must be refined and modified with changing life experiences and exposure to others' belief systems (Ahmann, 1994; Andrews & Boyle, 1997; Degazone, 1996; Grossman & Taylor, 1995; Leininger, 1997).

The Self-Appraisal

Before being able to become sensitive to and accommodate another's cultural beliefs and values, the nurse must first understand something about his or her own culture and ethnicity. Self-appraisal implies reflecting on the manner in which ethnocultural origins affect personal beliefs, behaviors, and ways of interacting with diverse people on a professional and personal level. Self-appraisals tend to be composed of similar kinds of questions (Box 11-4).

Reflecting and responding to these kinds of ethnoculturally-based questions, first for one's self and then as they apply to another, is a critical element in developing awareness and sensitivity to diversity in everyday situations. A cultural self-appraisal also can offer insights as to personal expectations of people's responses when they are ill. In turn, those insights can be compared with a patient's expectations, and potential cultural conflicts possibly can be deflected.

Exposure to Other Cultures and Ethnic Groups

After developing cultural self-awareness, the nurse can expand interest to persons who are of another background. Information on diverse groups can be obtained from recreational and professional literature. An open and nonjudgmental attitude is a critical step in learning about another's cultural belief system. Talking with people who have greater knowledge and experience about another cultural group is another useful strategy to learn about the group's beliefs and preferences. Ask questions! Most people enjoy telling another person about their culture if the inquiry is made with an intent to learn. If possible, seek explanations as to how and why specific rituals are used in everyday life situations.

Community Participation

Probably the most effective strategy is to actually interact with people of a particular background—*on their turf* (natural environment)—at social events as well as in their home. If an outsider becomes highly involved and subsumed in a community's social and political activities, it is not likely that he or she will learn all of the important cultural facts about a different cultural group without making at least a few blunders. Rather, one learns gradually by work-

Cultural Self-Appraisal: Personal Reflection Inventory

- How do you identify yourself in term of race, ethnicity, religious or political beliefs, and socio-economic class?
- Identify and describe the members and roles of members of your family.
- Describe what it has meant to be part of that group and the expectations placed on you.
- Describe the customs or traditions in your family of origin that expressed your heritage. What special foods, gifts, songs, and ceremonies were related to events such as birth, puberty, starting school, graduation, marriage, divorce, illness, hospitalization, and death?
- How were feelings such as love, affection, anger, and sadness expressed in your family?
- What were the most valued and respected personal traits a person in your family could aspire to have?
- What were the roles of women and men in your family and culture?
- How were decisions made? Who had the final say in that decision? Who was the final decision maker when it came to seeking health care? Why do you believe this to be the case?

- What role did fate play in a person's life?
- How was time, work, leisure, health, and illness defined and valued in your family system?
- Reflect on your culture's perception of space and your comfort zone in interpersonal exchanges. Describe your feelings when someone gets in close proximity to you.
- How comfortable are you when someone touches you unexpectedly? Or when you touch another person with whom you are interacting? Does it make a difference who the person is?
- What is your time orientation? Are you always on time? Early? Late? Is time your friend or your enemy? How do you spend your free time? Is this congruent with what you understand about the use of time as a child in your home of origin?
- What was your first experience with feeling different?
- For what and how was discipline used? Who was the disciplinarian? What roles did other family members have in regard to discipline?

Data from Geissler, E. (1994). *Pocket guide: Cultural assessment.* St. Louis: Mosby; Stanhope, M., & Knollmueller, R. (1997). *Public health and community health nurse's consultant: A health promotion guide* (pp. 211-242). St. Louis: Mosby.

ing within a community over a period of time. Eventually, with a desire to learn, less obvious values and expectations become more obvious to the nurse. For example, through formal and informal interactions, a person becomes aware of and sensitive to a patient's manner of interacting with a health professional when the patient seeks care. The nurse also learns about the patient's self-care practices, folk remedies, and use of alternative healers.

To overcome cultural barriers to health care, nurses must acquire ethnocultural knowledge

that can explain why patients engage in certain practices to promote health or treat an illness and also why they do or do not seek professional care and follow treatment plans. It can be difficult to learn about persons who are not part of a community's mainstream unless the nurse actively seeks out those (sub)groups. Therefore when establishing a practice, it is important to assess the catchment area to define the various cultural groups within the larger community. Some under-represented groups are easy to identify because they are isolated by a geographic boundary, biologic or racial features, life-style, attire, religion, political views, language, leisure activity, or occupation.

For example, generally it is not too difficult to identify an Amish or Mennonite group in the Midwest or the Hispanic or Asian community within a large city. There are other groups that are not as obviously bound in a given region nor do they appear to have such a distinct life-style, such as Laotians, Vietnamese, Italians, Poles, Irish, Jehovah's Witnesses, Orthodox Jews, Latter Day Saints, Seventh Day Adventist, or a smaller Native American group. Nonetheless, the cultural perspectives of less noticeable groups also are critical to ensuring that services that are rendered by the nurse are appropriate and acceptable in those particular communities.

In summary, the process of becoming culturally competent involves progressing from personal awareness and cultural sensitivity to a more sophisticated understanding of the belief systems of individuals who are of a different ethnocultural origin. Becoming culturally competent requires a dedicated effort to learn about others' beliefs and life-style preferences by interacting with them in their own settings. These efforts should be augmented with outside resources that can provide accurate information about their world view, life ways, and belief systems.

Recruiting Minorities to the Health Professions

A serious problem with cultural insensitivity in the health care system can be attributed to the low percentage of individuals of minority origins entering the health professions, specifically advanced practice nurses (Barbee, 1993; Brink, 1993; Kreiger, 1996; Leininger, 1997; Rosella et al., 1994). Historically, many schools of nursing reflected a homogeneous student body, with a predominance of Anglo-Euro-American students. A number of schools have made a dedi-

cated effort to recruit and retain minority students with varying degrees of success. The latest National Sample Survey of Registered Nurses (Division of Nursing 1997) estimated that only 10% of the current 2.5 million nurses in the workforce represent an ethnic or racial minority. Current and projected demographic and social changes have challenged nurse educators to produce culturally competent clinicians as society becomes more culturally diverse. Who can better present the ethnocultural perspective of a minority group in health care than persons who are of that background? Minorities must, therefore, be encouraged to enter the health professions. Nurses in leadership roles, in turn, are in an ideal position to serve as role models to under-represented groups. Likewise, nursing programs with their own tradition-based culture must make a dedicated commitment to encourage cultural diversity among faculty and within the student body, while encouraging nursing students to practice with cultural sensitivity.

Measuring Consumer Satisfaction

In addition to planning and delivering care, a cultural perspective must be considered when measuring satisfaction and the appropriateness of services rendered to targeted consumers. Acceptability means that a particular service is offered in a manner that is congruent with the ethnocultural values of a target population and perceived as desirable and familiar to persons receiving it. As for cultural factors that evoke consumer satisfaction, these go beyond appropriateness of dietary services, access to one's preferred pastoral care provider, or the frequency with which one requests an analgesic. Ethnocultural factors are factors such as deciding the appropriate time for seeking health care services and the manner in which one interacts with a professional provider. Culturally based values also influence a person's definition of health versus illness, choice of self-care behaviors, and perception of effective and ineffective caring behaviors (DeSantis, 1990; Milburn et al., 1992).

These examples demonstrate that even if a service is available and accessible in a community, it may not be deemed as appropriate or acceptable by subpopulations or even the target population in that catchment area. Consumers' evaluations of care-related services usually are rated as "satisfactory," "unsatisfactory," "acceptable," or "unacceptable," with little attention paid to why a group perceives it as such—or even if they understand what these ratings mean. Traditional program evaluation methods may not be culturally sensitive. Hence the data that is collected is not valid or reliable. Both qualitative and quantitative methods must be used, with ongoing input from the members of the ethnocultural group to ensure that the proper questions are asked in the right way, with the right words, to assess the intervention outcomes as these are defined by the community.

■ KEY POINTS

The United States is becoming an ethnic melting pot—a mosaic of many cultures. This trend is projected to intensify in the next millennium. The effect of increasing ethnic, cultural, and racial diversity is a concern at all levels including the federal, state, and private sector, especially in the educational and health care delivery systems. For nurses the diversity phenomenon means the following:

- Reflecting on personal cultural and ethnic preferences related to health and healing.
- Becoming aware of diversity in the community and workplace and with patients.
- Routinely assessing patients' ethnic and cultural preferences related to health beliefs.
- Implementing strategies to address patients' cultural barriers to care.

- Delivering nursing care that is ethnoculturally appropriate and acceptable to patients who are of another culture.
- Integrating traditional healing practices with Western medicine as opportunities arise.
- Evaluating care to assess the level of cultural and linguistic competency in nursing services rendered to patients
- Advocating for patients who are culturally vulnerable.

■ CRITICAL THINKING QUESTIONS

1. Of what importance is cultural and ethnic diversity in the health care delivery system?
2. Differentiate among and describe the interrelatedness of race, ethnicity, and culture with socioeconomic factors.
3. Reflect on projected demographic and population shifts in the United States. How could this affect nursing in the next 20 years? What changes are projected for your geographic catchment area, and how could this affect your practice?
4. Identify a minority or under-represented group in your practice setting. What are some of the ethnocultural practices related to their health beliefs and health care seeking behaviors?
5. How can cultural assessment questions be incorporated into your existing protocols for a patient assessment?
6. What self-care practices do you and your family use? Are these for health promotion or illness prevention or to treat symptoms? Do these impede or enhance professional treatment interventions?
7. Identify a plan of action to increase your level of cultural competence when providing care. At what level of the continuum do you currently fall? What changes does this entail for you in your practice to achieve the highest competence skill level?

8. If applicable, identify specific health conditions in your catchment area that have a racial or ethnic genetic predisposition using epidemiologic health status reports. Describe how treatment protocols address ethnocultural belief systems.

■ REFERENCES

Ahmann, E. (1994). "Chunky stew". Appreciating cultural diversity while providing health care to children. *Pediatric Nursing, 20*(3), 320-324.

Andrews, M., & Boyle, J. (1997). Competence in transcultural nursing care. *American Journal of Nursing, 97*(8), 16AAA-16DDD.

Barbee, E. (1993). Racism in U.S. nursing. *Medical Anthropology Quarterly, 7*(4), 346-362.

Bell, R. (1994). Prominence of women in Navajo healing beliefs and values. *Nursing and Health Care, 15*(5), 232-240.

Brink, P. (1993). Cultural diversity in nursing: How much can we tolerate. In J. McClosky & H. Grace (Eds.). *Current issues in nursing* (pp. 521-528). St. Louis: Mosby.

Bushy, A. (1996). Cultural and ethnic diversity: Cultural competence (pp. 91-106). In J. Hickey, R. Ouimette, & C. Venegoni (Eds.). *Advanced practice nursing: Changing roles and clinical application.* Philadelphia: Lippincott.

Daytona News Journal. (1997). *Quote of the day.* Oct 19, p. 2-A.

Degazon, C. (1996). Cultural diversity in community health nursing practice. In M. Stanhope & J. Lancaster (Eds.). *Community health nursing: Promoting health of aggregates, families, and individuals* (pp. 117-134). St. Louis: Mosby.

DeSantis, L. (1990). Fieldwork with undocumented aliens and other populations at risk. *Western Journal of Nursing Research, 12*(3), 359-372.

Ganey, F., & DeBocanegra, H. (1996). Overcoming barriers to improving the health of immigrant women. *Journal of American Medical Women's Association, 51*(4), 155-160.

Geissler, E. (1994). *Pocket guide: Cultural assessment.* St. Louis: Mosby.

Grossman, D., & Taylor, R. (1995). Cultural diversity on the unit. *American Journal of Nursing, 95*(2), 64-67.

Krieger, N. (1996). Inequality, diversity and health: Thoughts on "race/ethnicity," and "gender." *Journal of American Medical Women's Association, 51*(4), 133-136.

Leininger, M. (1978). *Transcultural nursing: Concepts, theories and practice.* New York: Wiley Medical Publishers.

Leininger, M. (1991). *Cultural diversity and universality: A theory of nursing.* New York: National League for Nursing Press.

Leininger, M. (1994). Transcultural nursing education: A worldwide imperative. *Nursing & Health Care, 15*(5), 254-261.

Leininger, M. (1997). Transcultural nursing research to transform nursing education and practice: 40 years. *Image: Journal of Nursing Scholarship, 29*(4), 341-347.

Milburn, N., Gary, L., Booth, J., & Brown, D. (1992). Conducting epidemiologic research in a minority community: Methodological considerations. *Journal of Community Psychology, 19*(1), 3-12.

Miller, L. (1994). Non-traditional medical options: U.S. spends $13 million on studies. *USA Today,* Aug. 1, D1.

Misener, T., Sowell, R., Phillips, K., & Harris, C. (1997). Sexual orientation: A cultural diversity issue for nursing. *Nursing Outlook, 45,* 178-181.

Morganthau, T. (1997). America 2000: The face of the future. *Newsweek,* Jan. 27, 58-61.

Rosella, J., Regan-Kubinski, M., & Albrecht, S. (1994). The need for multicultural diversity among health professionals. *Nursing & Health Care, 15*(5), 242-246.

Stanhope, M., & Knollmueller, R. (1997). *Public health and community health nurse's consultant: A health promotion guide* (pp. 211-242). St. Louis: Mosby.

U.S. Department of Health and Human Services. (USDHHS). (1991a). *Healthy People 2000: National Health Promotion and Disease Prevention.* Washington, D.C.: U.S. Government Printing Office.

U.S. Department of Health and Human Services. (USDHHS). (1991b). *Health status of the disadvantaged: Chartbook 1990.* Washington, D.C.: U.S. Government Printing Office. (#HRSA-HRS-P-DV-90-1)

U.S. Department of Health and Human Services. (USDHHS). (1996). *Health United States: 1995.* Hyattsville, Md.: Author. (DHHS Pub. No. [PHS]96-1242)

Zabrana, R. (1996). The under-representation of Hispanic women in the health professions. *Journal of American Medical Women's Association, 51*(4), 147-153.

Labor Relations in a Turbulent Health Care Environment

Charles Braun

INTRODUCTION

There is little doubt that labor unions have been a major change agent in American society. Over the past 60 years, millions of dues-paying union members have seen their work lives enriched on both an economic as well as a psychologic level via the efforts of their bargaining agents. Nonunion workers have also benefited from the presence of labor unions in that legislation involving the use of child labor, minimum wages, overtime premiums, workplace safety, and the creation and protection of retirement programs for the average employee would have been greatly delayed—if ever enacted—without the efforts of organized labor. In short, very few workers have not benefited directly or indirectly from the American labor movement.

There are, however, individuals who insist that unions have little or no place in a professional nursing environment. In addition to potential ethical concerns regarding strikes, opponents of collective bargaining have maintained that by allowing a union contract to come between professionals and patients, nurses have regressed from the status of a "professional" to that of a "common worker." To them, this transition results in the loss of something unique to nurses that neither money nor seniority can ever replace.

In contrast to those who would argue that "professional collectivism" is a oxymoron, there are others who contend that many of the existing nursing unions have been too placid in the face of the drastic changes currently being experienced in the health care sector of the American economy. From their perspective, health care is clearly a big business undergoing many of the same financial pressures as the manufacturers of automobiles or washing machines (e.g., lowering costs). Unless the bargaining agents find ways to slow the effects of the managed care juggernaut, those who support a more active role by collective bargaining agents argue, nurses may lose whatever professionalism they still possess and become nothing more than cogs in an industrial health care machine.

This chapter describes the collective bargaining environment for nurses through discussions of the legal history of collective bargaining, the process used to select bargaining agents, and the actual negotiation process. The chapter also describes how the labor relations process has the potential to help promote positive changes in addition to minimizing undesired trends in the work lives of nurses.

OBJECTIVES _____

After reading this chapter, you will be able to:

1. Develop arguments about why some nurses support labor unions, whereas others find them undesirable
2. Integrate the effects of federal and state labor laws into the day-to-day management of hospitals and other health care facilities
3. Analyze the certification process used by union supporters to select the exclusive bargaining agent for a group of employees
4. Demonstrate how the collective bargaining process can help nurses attain personal and professional goals
5. Integrate the function and the process used in handling employee grievances in a unionized setting
6. Evaluate the American Nurses Association's role in health care labor relations
7. Theorize how nursing unions can be change agents in a turbulent, market-driven work environment

■ WHY DO NURSES JOIN UNIONS?

The literature surrounding an employee's decision to support a union is extensive, with well over 100 empirical studies having been performed over the past two decades. Although there is no one single answer to the question posed above, several trends have been discovered by researchers investigating the issue. In an attempt to summarize the driving forces behind the decision to support unionization, Wheeler and McClendon (1991) have developed a framework that categorizes employee motivation into three models.

Model A

Under Model A, employees support unionization efforts because (1) they are dissatisfied with their current work environment and (2) they believe a union would relieve some of that dissatisfaction. Within this scenario, nurses who think that they are underpaid, unfairly treated by supervisors, or have no voice in the running of their organization may see a bargaining agent as an instrument of access and/or protection. As such, the union is viewed as a means to rectify, or at least improve, an unsatisfactory employment situation.

Model B

Model B is similar to Model A in that the employee who supports unionization is trying to improve his or her work situation. However, Model B employees do not necessarily have to be experiencing job dissatisfaction to "vote

Key terms	
Terms	**Definitions**
Union	An organization that represents groups of workers with similar skills, training, interests, and concerns
Unionization	The process used to select a bargaining representative for a group of employees

union." Instead, these employees make that decision based on the utility or overall value of having a union represent them in negotiations.

Utility levels are determined by the employee's evaluation of all the possible positive aspects of unionization (e.g., higher wages, better benefits) as well as all of the potential negative attributes (e.g., sizable union dues, promotions based on seniority). If the positives outweigh the negatives, a nurse will likely vote for unionization. Conversely, nurses who believe the union alternative does not provide a net improvement to their current status would likely reject it as a low utility option. In short, the union is considered to be one of several options that could be used to advance a nurse's work life and will be supported if it offers the greatest potential benefit.

Model C

Wheeler and McClendon (1991) characterize Model C decisions as being politically or ideologically based decisions. Some workers who use this decision-making framework may consider labor unions to be an essential defender of the working class against big business in general and/or management in particular. Other individuals may oppose collective bargaining as being inconsistent with their standing as professionals while acknowledging the potential advantages of being unionized. Whereas Models A and B tend to be rational, benefit-driven processes, Model C appears to be a more philosophic belief that originates in the heart and soul of the worker.

Although most of the research regarding Model C has been based in countries where organized labor is a much greater participant in social and governmental affairs than in the United States (e.g, France, Italy), it would not be unrealistic to assume that many American workers are also affected by philosophic as well as economic criteria when voting for or against union representation. This attitude may be particularly important in areas where employees have had a long and successful history of collective bargaining and where joining a union is considered to be a natural event (e.g., cities like New York and Philadelphia; the coal fields of West Virginia).

Of these three models, it appears that Model A is the predominant decision-making scheme used by a sizable cross-section of American workers (Fiorito et al., 1987; Wheeler & McClendon, 1991). Although little current research deals specifically with nurses' decisions to support or reject union representation, the high burnout and turnover rates among these professionals actively support the argument that many nurses are not satisfied with their existing work lives (Roach, 1994).

For many of these nurses, a bargaining agent may be a viable means to achieve fairness and a voice in the way they provide care within a work environment that is increasingly concerned about cost containment and profitability. For other nurses, the potential gains of collective bargaining may be outweighed by fear of the unknown or by concerns that union representation and professionalism are conflicting concepts. In either case, the participants in the labor relations process need to be cognizant of these needs, drives, fears, and concerns when dealing with union organizing efforts, contract negotiations, and the administration of any agreement resulting from these efforts. A failure to do so raises the likelihood of undesirable consequences such as strikes and expensive litigation (Box 12-1).

■ LEGISLATIVE AND LEGAL FRAMEWORK

Labor unions, not unlike corporations, are creatures of law. They exist because the law says they can. They prosper when laws are changed to promote their existence. They also shrink when laws are enacted to curtail their powers.

Key terms	
Term	**Definition**
Collective bargaining	The process where employer and worker representatives negotiate conditions of employment
Bargaining agent	Formal organization that represents workers in the collective bargaining process
Professional	An employee whose job requires substantial amounts of advanced training and independent judgment

B O X   1 2 - 1

Why Do Workers Join Unions?

- They are unhappy with their current work environment and believe the union will help solve their problems.
- They believe the "benefits" of having union representation outweigh the "costs" associated with being a union member.
- They believe it is the right thing for workers to do.

Data from Wheeler, H.N., & McClendon, J.A. (1991). In G. Straus, D.G. Gallagher, & J. Fiorito (Eds.). *The state of the unions* (Vol 1, pp. 47-83). Madison, Wis.: Industrial Relations Research Association.

In short, labor unions depend largely on supportive laws, rules, and regulations to remain a viable part of the United States economy and society. The following sections show how the legal framework for the health care collective bargaining industry has changed over the past 70 years.

Pre–National Labor Relations Act

Before 1935, individuals seeking to bargain collectively with their employers had relatively little protection under the law. When faced with union activity, employers would contend that unions were unfair monopolies of labor and should be found in violation of federal antitrust law. Judges regularly agreed with the employers and issued injunctions prohibiting union activities. Workers thought to be union agitators or sympathizers would be routinely fired and have their names circulated among other employers so as to blackball them from working in other organizations. Workers who tried to convince their employers to accept new terms of employment through the use of strikes often found themselves doing battle with police officers and/or armed guards hired by their bosses. Unfortunately, these conflicts frequently resulted in injuries and deaths on both sides of the picket line. Ironically, these bloody battles ultimately created a positive environment for the union movement through the enactment of the National Labor Relations Act.

The National Labor Relations Act (NLRA)

In 1935, Congress enacted the National Labor Relations Act (29 U.S.C. § 169) (commonly known as the Wagner Act) in an attempt to prevent labor-management strife from affecting interstate commerce. Although other federal laws had been enacted before the NLRA (e.g., the Norris-LaGuardia and Railway Labor Acts), this piece of legislation is widely considered to be the foundation of modern labor relations law.

Among the law's chief accomplishments were the following:

- Guaranteeing a wide range of employees the right to elect a representative to bargain on their behalf.
- The prohibition of unfair labor practices on the part of employers. Examples of these practices include coercing employees not to exercise their right to vote for a union, interfering with a labor organization, and refusing to bargain in good faith with a duly elected labor representative.
- The creation of a presidentially appointed National Labor Relations Board (NLRB). The NLRB was charged with the responsibility to oversee union elections and to police the negotiation process to ensure legal compliance.

Armed with these new protections, the labor movement wasted little time in organizing workers in many industries throughout the nation. The health care sector of the economy, however, received relatively little attention during the first few years after the passage of the Wagner Act. It seems that organizing hospital or other health care workers was difficult because the NLRA applied only to organizations engaged in interstate commerce. If a labor organization could not prove that a health care facility was of sufficient size and breadth to affect several states, the National Labor Relations Board would refuse to order an election. Given the size of even the largest health care facilities operating at the time, this was a substantial legal hurdle for most unions to overcome. As a result, the number of nurses and other health care employees organized during this time was quite small.

The States Get Involved: The Creation of "Little Wagner Acts"

There is no doubt that the Wagner Act was instrumental in providing many workers with the opportunity to elect bargaining representatives. However, it did not cover all employees. Although some workers were specifically excluded from coverage (e.g., public sector employees), others ran afoul of the interstate commerce requirement (e.g., most private sector health care workers).

Several state legislatures noticed this situation and decided to plug some of the qualifying holes in the federal law with broader state laws. These state laws, commonly know as "little Wagner Acts," provided previously excluded employees an opportunity to form unions. For example, in response to the omissions found in the federal law, the Minnesota State Legislature passed the Minnesota Labor Relations Act (MLRA) in 1939.* Contained within this law were provisions that allowed—with major restrictions—health care employees the right to form unions. As a result, Local 113 of the Public Building Service Employees' Union organized 125 maintenance and service workers in the Northwestern Hospital of Minneapolis in early 1940. Even though it would be nearly 7 years before the first nurses were organized in that state, the Minnesota Labor Relations Act—like other "little Wagner Acts"—would provide nurses with protection and organizing opportunities when public sentiment began to turn against the labor movement after World War II.

The Labor Management Relations Act of 1947 (Taft-Hartley Act)

The Labor Management Relations Act (i.e., the Taft-Hartley Act) (29 U.S.C. §§ 141-197) was enacted in response to undesired behavior on the part of union organizers and officials. Although the Wagner Act greatly restricted management's freedom, it did not place many limitations on labor organizations. When some union officials

---

* The reader will notice that "Minnesota examples" are used frequently throughout this chapter. The decision to use Minnesota as an example is based largely upon that state's long and generally successful tradition of collective bargaining for nurses.

BOX 12-2

Minnesota Nurses: Early Adopters of Collective Bargaining

Shortly after the American Nurses Association adopted its first Economic Security Program in 1946, its state affiliate in Minnesota—the Minnesota Nurses Association (MNA)—began to organize registered nurses in the Minneapolis-St. Paul metropolitan area. Shortly thereafter, the MNA developed minimum standards of employment and submitted them to area hospitals for implementation. At first the hospital administrators refused to acknowledge the MNA as the bargaining agent for their nursing staffs. However, when the administrators realized the high degree of nurse support for their professional association, they agreed to enter into negotiations with the MNA. In the end, both sides agreed to a settlement that consisted of "a $10 monthly salary inrease (to $180.00 per month), the establishment of a 44-hour workweek, six paid holidays a year, three $5 length-of-service increases, and provisions for sick leave, vacations, shift differentials, and grievance machinery" (Loevinger, 1951, pp. 229-230). By the time the Minnesota Nurses Association had celebrated its tenth anniversary as a labor representative, it had become "the nation's most comprehensive program, with almost half of its more than 7000 registered nurses covered by contracts in 22% of the state's hospitals."

From Loevinger, R.H. (1951). The Minnesota story of economic security. *American Journal of Nursing, 51*(4), 228-231; French, W.L., & Robinson, R. (1960). Collective bargaining by nurses and other professionals: Anomaly or trend? *Labor Law Journal, 11,* 902-910.

used this power to abuse the rights of individual workers and companies targeted for organizing, Congress stepped in to level the playing field. The resulting legislation encumbered unions with many of the same restrictions placed on management under the Wagner Act.

The Taft-Hartley legislation also excluded several types of organizations from coverage under federal labor law. Of special importance to health care employees was the "non-profit hospital exemption" granted within the statute. Because of this clause, most health care facilities would not be considered "employers" under the law. As such, their employees would not be entitled to union representation.

For many nurses and other health care employees, this exemption was a major setback for organizing and collective bargaining efforts. However, for residents of the states that had enacted "little Wagner Acts," the effects were much less traumatic because state statutes continued to provide an alternative means for maintaining labor-management relations. As a result of Taft-Hartley, nurses in a dozen or so states could opt for labor representation, whereas most of their peers in other states were precluded from the collective bargaining process. This disparity would continue until the passage of the Health Care Amendments of 1974 to the National Labor Relations Act (Box 12-2).

Health Care Amendments of 1974 (88 Stat. 396-97)

Recognizing that (1) the health care industry was becoming an increasingly larger segment of the American economy and (2) a formal collective bargaining process could help alleviate many worker-employer disputes, Congress removed the nonprofit hospital exemption from federal labor law in 1974 (LeRoy et al., 1992). This action made it possible for employees working in hospitals, nursing homes, health maintenance organizations, and many other private sector health care facilities and organizations to seek union representation. Along with greatly expanding opportunities for unionizing health care workers, this legislation also established the following new rules for the collective bargaining process:

- Because work stoppages in the health care industry could have devastating effects on the welfare of the general public, both labor and management are required to give 90 days notice of their intention to alter contractual terms. This notice is typically given during the last year of an existing contract. Other industries have a 60-day notification requirement.

- If the sides cannot agree on contractual changes within 30 days of the notice, the Federal Mediation and Conciliation Service (FMCS) must be notified. The FMCS was created within the Taft-Hartley Act as an unbiased third-party entity whose responsibility is to help labor and management work out their differences before they escalate into full-blown labor disputes.

- Within 30 days of receiving this notice, the FMCS may create a Board of Inquiry (BOI) to investigate facts surrounding the negotiations. Within 15 days of its creation, the BOI must issue its findings to both sides. These "findings" are often considered realistic settlement goals offered by objective expert observers. The findings are not binding on either party to the negotiations.

- If the parties still cannot come to an agreement within another 15-day period, the union can approach its membership for permission to strike. If the workers vote in favor of a strike, the union must give the health care facility and the FMCS 10 days written notice of where and when the strike will take place. The function of the 10-day notice is to give both sides adequate time to finalize plans that will minimize the harm to the general public if the strike does occur.

- In addition to the negotiation-related regulations just described, the 1974 Amendments also changed the union organizing process in two ways. First, the law generally restricted union organizing efforts to public places within the health care facility (e.g., cafeterias) in an effort to keep the patients out of the process. Second, Congress ordered the National Labor Relations Board (NLRB) to avoid creating an "undue proliferation" of bargaining units (separate union groups) that may increase the likelihood of strikes. Nearly 25 years after the passage of the Amendments, the determination of "appropriate bargaining units" within health care facilities remains a major issue in the organizing process and will be discussed in greater depth in a later section.

Public Sector Labor Law

Like their peers in most private sector facilities, nurses and other health care workers employed by federal and state governments were excluded from coverage under the Wagner and Taft-Hartley Acts. Federal health care workers had to wait until Presidents Kennedy (Executive Order No. 10988, 1962) and Nixon (Executive Order No. 11491, 1969) gave them the right to form unions and to engage in collective bargaining via executive orders. Those rights were eventually codified into law by the Federal Service Labor-Management Relations Act of 1978 (Cihon & Castagnera, 1993).

State and local nurses are subject to a wide variety of state laws governing public sector labor-management relations. From an overall perspective, it is quite likely that public sector nurses working in states considered to be pro-union (e.g., Massachusetts, Minnesota, Michigan) are experiencing greater organizing rights and bargaining freedoms than those working in less labor-friendly environments. However, even employees from pro-union states may not enjoy

Key terms	
Term	Definition
The Wagner Act (NLRA) (1935)	First federal law granting employees widespread rights to form unions
"Little Wagner Acts" (various years)	State laws typically enacted to expand unionization rights to workers excluded under the NLRA
The Taft-Hartley Act (LMRA) (1947)	Pro-management federal law that restricted union activities
1974 Health Care Amendments	Federal law that expanded unionization rights to most private sector health care employees
Executive orders	Presidential edicts that generally have the force of law
National Labor Relations Board (NLRB)	Federal agency responsible for overseeing labor union elections and collective bargaining processes
Federal Mediation & Conciliation Service (FMCS)	Federal agency responsible for helping labor negotiators reach a settlement

the same opportunities as their colleagues in the private sector.

Given the dissimilar bargaining environments, differences between private and public sector health care collective bargaining systems can be significant. For example, while private sector nurses tend to select "craft" type unions containing only nurses, public sector employees can often be found grouped together in more heterogenous units that could be considered "industrial" in nature. This increased diversity of unit membership can have a substantial impact on organizing efforts in that very sophisticated bargaining agents such as the American Federation of State, County, and Municipal Employees (AFSCME) may compete with more nurse-oriented unions for representation election votes. Differences in bargaining priorities among the different employee groups may also make contract ratification more difficult. Finally, many—if not most—public sector employees are prohibited from striking and must agree to submit their bargaining impasses to a neutral

third party for resolution (Cihon & Castagnera, 1993).

Interpreting the Law: The Role of the Courts and Government Agencies

Once a law has been enacted, it is up to the courts and regulatory agencies to interpret what the policy makers have created. Because many pieces of legislation contain vague language such as "appropriate" or "reasonable," it is incumbent upon the courts and agencies to more firmly define the definitions, processes, and procedures contained within an act. Presently, many "interpretive" issues influence health care collective bargaining. Two of the more important issues are discussed below.

The Determination of Appropriate Bargaining Units A *bargaining unit* is a group of employees with common interests and objectives who have chosen to exercise their right to form a union and to bargain collectively with their employer. As noted in an earlier section, Congress instructed the National Labor Relations Board (NLRB) to refrain from creating an "undue proliferation" of bargaining units because it was feared that increasing the number of bargaining units within a health care facility would likely yield a corresponding increase of strikes and other undesired activities. Unfortunately, Congress neglected to define "undue proliferation" and left the matter in the hands of the NLRB. The result has been an ongoing redefinition as to how bargaining units should be organized.

For nearly two decades, the NLRB decided the appropriateness of health care bargaining units on a case-by-case basis using criteria that it had been developing since the 1930s. If an employer or labor organization did not approve of a particular unit determination, it could appeal the Board's ruling to the federal courts. Ultimately, a judge or (depending on the level of appeal) group of judges would rule on the issue using courtroom and/or NLRB precedent. Although this process was typically cumbersome, time-consuming, and expensive, creating the "right" voting unit was extremely important to the election process and was often pursued with great vigor by both sides.

In 1989 the Board decided to break with its existing protocols and issued rules that would define how private sector health care bargaining groups would be determined in the future (NLRB Ruling, Federal Register, 1989). Although this rule making may have affected employees within the other seven established units (physicians, clerical, technical, skilled maintenance, security guards, nonprofessional workers, all other professionals) to varying degrees, the NLRB decided to continue the practice of granting registered nurses exclusive, homogeneous bargaining units. This decision was based on the Board's belief that the position of registered nurse is truly distinguishable from the remaining job groups by virtue of its responsibilities, education, and labor markets (NLRB Notice, Federal

Register, 1988). As such, it deserved its own bargaining unit.

Even though the Board's bargaining unit decision did not adversely affect the nursing unions, it serves as an excellent example of how the rules of the labor relations process can change dramatically in a short period of time. Given the pace of the institutional changes that are occurring within this industry (e.g., redesigning nurses' job responsibilities), it remains to be seen whether registered nurses will be able to maintain their exclusive bargaining unit status (Box 12-3).

The Definition of Supervisors There are obvious reasons why supervisors are excluded from union membership under current labor law. As first-line managers, a supervisor's allegiance to the organization should be clear. Sometimes, however, the distinction between labor and management blurs when an employee has both supervisory and line duties. In other words, is this employee a worker with some supervisory duties who should be considered eligible for union status or is this employee a supervisor with some work duties who should be excluded from participation in any union activities? Box 12-4 provides the formal labor law definition.

The delineation between "workers who supervise" and "supervisors who work" is especially troublesome in the health care field, where many facilities have created positions such as "charge nurse," "lead nurse," and/or "team leader." Within these positions, nurses often have some quasimanagerial duties (e.g., leading, planning, organizing) in addition to their direct patient responsibilities. Given this status, both labor and management can easily argue that these nurses belong on their side of the bargaining table.

During the 20 years following the passage of the 1974 Amendments, the NLRB had held hospitals and other health care employers to a high

B O X   1 2 - 3

Health Care Bargaining Units

Bargaining Unit	Common Job Categories
Registered nurse	Staff nurses, telephone triage nurses
Physicians	Physicians
All other professionals	Psychotherapists, social workers, physical therapists
Technical employees	X-ray technicians, laboratory technicians, LPNs/LVNs
Nonprofessional employees	Nurses' aides, orderlies, custodians
Skilled maintenance workers	Electricians, plumbers, painters
Business office and clerical employees	Secretaries, ward clerks, transcriptionists
Security guards	Security guards

Data from the *Federal Register.*

B O X   1 2 - 4

"Supervisors" Under the Labor Management Relations Act

Section 2(11) of the Act (29 U.S.C. §152[11]) defines a "supervisor" as: "any individual having authority, in the interest of the employer, to hire, transfer, suspend, lay off, recall, promote, discharge, assign, reward, or discipline other employees, or responsibly to direct them, or to adjust their grievances, or effectively recommend such action if in connection with the foregoing the exercise of such authority is not of a merely routine or clerical nature, but requires the use of independent judgment."

Data from National Labor Relations Act. (1935). 29 U.S.C. §169.

standard when claiming employees who provided patient care were supervisors (Mahoney, 1995). This standard was shattered in mid-1994 when lawyers for a small Ohio nursing home succeeded in persuading the United States Supreme Court that the Board's definition of "su-

pervisor" was inconsistent with applicable law (*NLRB v. Health Care & Retirement Corporation of America,* 1124 S.Ct. 1778 (1994).

In early 1989, three former employees of a nursing home filed an unfair labor practice charge with the NLRB claiming that they had been fired for their involvement in protected labor activities. At the subsequent hearing, management claimed the three LPNs were supervisors and had no protection under the law. Management appealed to the federal courts after the Board decided in favor of the nurses (306 NLRB 63). In March of 1993, the 6th Circuit Court of Appeals in Cincinnati overturned the NLRB's decision (987 F. 2nd 1256). Shortly thereafter, the Board appealed to the U.S. Supreme Court to reject the appellate court's decision and reinstate its own. In a five to four decision, the Court ruled in favor of the nursing home.

A majority of the Court argued that the nurses had indeed performed many of the functions outlined in Section 2(11) and therefore met the legal definition of "supervisor." The minority claimed that it was the nurses' professional—not managerial—status (i.e., the ". . .

authority that derives from superior skill or experience" versus the "authority that flows from management") that allowed them to direct nurses' aides and other employees at the facility. Understandably, the Court's decision has caused some leaders of health care unions to be greatly concerned about future organizing and negotiating efforts (Sherer, 1994).

The *NLRB v. Health Care & Retirement* decision had an almost immediate effect on the overall labor relations environment, as at least two health care organizations (Providence Alaska Medical Center and Bozeman Deaconess Hospital) have reportedly refused to bargain with labor representatives elected, in part, by "supervisory" employees (Burda, 1994; Moore, 1996). Even though the NLRB has found both organizations to be in violation of the Labor Management Relations Act for reasons beyond those cited by the Supreme Court (321 NLRB 100 and 322 NLRB 196, respectively), the facilities will likely appeal to the federal court system for relief from the Board's ruling. Given the stakes at hand, these cases may take several years to resolve.

This case provides an excellent example of the interrelationships that exist among labor, management, the NLRB, and the United States federal court system. It also shows how the vote of one judge can affect an entire industry. It is important to remember that because of judicial and agency turnover, interest-group lobbying efforts, and the results of general elections, the law should be considered a fluid process that can change rapidly. As such, the rules of labor relations are also subject to change with little notice.

■ THE ORGANIZING PROCESS
Certification Elections

Before any collective bargaining can occur, the employees must select an organization to represent their interests. Unlike some other countries, American labor law insists on having a single labor organization represent a group of workers. The following represents a potential course by which nurses and other employees choose their "exclusive bargaining agent":

1. The first steps toward unionization are often made by management. With its many policies, practices, and decisions, most organizations have ample opportunities to anger their employees *en masse* or individually via real or perceived mistreatment. As described in an earlier section, these seeds of discontent give many employees much of the motivation they need to seek union representation.

2. Eventually, an employee or group of employees may contact a bargaining agent for information about becoming unionized. This avenue of contact may be reversed if the union has already decided to engage in a campaign to organize the facility. In that case, union organizers may hold informational meetings or distribute leaflets to generate interest for their cause. In either scenario, it is unlikely that the labor representatives will commit their resources before trying to estimate the level of potential support within a facility.

3. If it can be shown that a substantial number of employees in a facility desire union representation, a petition for an election is filed (by employees or by the union) with the NLRB. Support is usually shown through the presentation of *Authorization Cards* that have been signed and dated by employees of the facility. An *Authorization Card* may state that the individual wants a particular bargaining agent, such as the Wisconsin Nurses Association or the Teamsters, to represent her or him, or it may just state that the employee desires an election. Legally, 30% of the employee group must sign cards before the NLRB will proceed. More realistically, most unions will want to see at least a majority (50%) sign up before petitioning the Board.

B O X   1 2 - 5

Sample Authorization Card

I, (name of employee,) desire to have the (name of bargaining agent) represent me in contract negotiations with (name of employer).

(signature of employee)
(date card was signed)

Box 12-5 shows a sample *Authorization Card*.

4. If the union has been successful in securing support, it may approach the employer directly and demand to be considered the exclusive bargaining agent. In the face of overwhelming support (e.g., 80% or more), management may decide that it is useless to wage an election campaign and may opt to recognize the union without a fight. As might be expected, this capitulation happens rather infrequently.

5. When the Board receives the election petition, it will ensure that it is accurate and valid. If the petition is accepted, the Board will determine the appropriate bargaining unit and schedule an election. Once the bargaining unit is set, only those employees contained within the unit may vote in the election. Delaney and Sockell (1988) investigated how the characteristics of health care bargaining units affect election outcomes and found that small homogeneous groups are more likely to vote for unionization than larger, more heterogeneous units. Put another way, a small group of registered nurses are more likely to support unionization efforts than a large unit composed of a varied group of workers (e.g., laboratory technicians, nurses, clerks). Because the makeup of the bargaining unit can easily affect the outcome of the election, both labor and management strive to have the unit structured so as to improve their chances of winning. As stated previously, many legal battles have been fought over the determination of the "appropriate" bargaining unit.

6. Before the election date, both labor and management typically campaign hard for their respective viewpoints. Both sides have restrictions regarding what can be said, when it can be said, and where it can be said. A failure to follow the election rules can result in significant penalties to the transgressor.

7. On the assigned day, members of the bargaining unit engage in a secret ballot election that determines what labor organization, if any, will represent them in negotiations with their employer. If a bargaining agent is to win an election, it must receive a majority of the votes cast (assuming it is the only union on the ballot). In other words, if 800 nurses are eligible to vote in the election but only 400 actually cast ballots, the labor representative needs only 201 (50% plus 1) votes to become the exclusive bargaining agent for the entire group of 800 nurses. If management wins, it is generally protected from other union elections for 1 year. If the union wins, the collective bargaining process should begin soon after the election.

Voting Behavior of Nurses

Certification Elections According to Scott and Lowery (1994), 52.3% of all health care certification elections held between 1980 and 1991 resulted in victories for the labor representative. Of those elections involving only nurses, ANA affiliates were successful nearly 58% of the time. Evidently many nurses agree with the ANA's belief that "its state affiliates have more direct knowledge about actual and desired working conditions" and thus should be the preferred representative for professional nurses (Holley & Jennings, 1991, p. 510).

Key terms	
Term	**Definition**
Appropriate bargaining units	Groups of employees determined (by the NLRB) to have similar bargaining interests
"Undue Proliferation"	Congressional mandate against allowing too many unions within a single health care facility
Certification election	The process whereby employees select their bargaining agent
Decertification election	The process whereby dissatisfied employees attempt to "fire" their bargaining agent
Authorization card	Form that indicates whether an employee desires an election

Decertification Elections Whenever employees think that their labor representative is not serving them properly, they have a recall option known as *decertification.* The decertification machinery is set in motion much in the same fashion as the certification process: a petition must be sent to the NLRB requesting a decertification vote. The petition must be supported by at least 30% of the bargaining unit for the Board to go forward with the election. If a *majority of the total bargaining unit* (i.e., at least 401 nurses in an 800-nurse unit) votes against the incumbent labor organization, it loses its status as exclusive representative.

Although decertification elections are fairly rare in the health care field (a total of 608 industry-wide between 1980 and 1991) (Scott & Lowery, 1994), they can be a major disruption to the collective bargaining process. Fortunately for nurses, ANA affiliates had the highest win rate (64.3%) of all the health care unions facing decertification elections during that same time frame (Scott & Lowery 1994). When these data are compared with the average win rate for all industries (26%), it appears that many nurses are satisfied with having their professional associations serve as their collective bargaining representative.

■ THE COLLECTIVE BARGAINING PROCESS

Once the bargaining agent has been certified by the NLRB, the actual negotiation process begins. A representative example of the collective bargaining process follows.

Pre-Bargaining Stage

During this stage, both sides engage in gathering data to be used in the negotiations. Management analyzes trends and creates projections of what it can offer to the union. Union professionals survey the nurses in the bargaining unit to see what issues are high priority, moderate priority, and low priority. Both sides will also examine recently negotiated local and regional contracts in other organizations for use as benchmarks in the current negotiations.

Negotiation teams are also established at this point. Both teams will have a lead negotiator, who generally will be the chief spokesperson for her or his side. Each team will also have members possessing "on-the-floor" expertise (e.g., staff nurses for labor, first- and second-level supervisors for management). These team members are there to give input that will improve the likelihood that the contract will be workable after it is signed. It is quite likely that each bargaining team will also have experts (attorneys and other consultants) who will help deal with highly technical issues in the contract (e.g., pensions).

Most negotiations are carried out between one organization and one union. However, both sides may agree to allow "multi-employer" bargaining. Under this format, the management side may represent 10 to 20 separate organizations that desire a common contract. Management benefits because all or most of the competing facilities in the area will operate under the same set of wages, benefits, and work rules. The union side can benefit because all employees in separate facilities will share the same contract regardless of differences in bargaining power. This practice is most common in areas with an extensive health care collective bargaining background (e.g., Minneapolis, New York).

Notification of Intent to Change Contract Language

As required by federal law, any private sector health care employer or union that desires to alter an existing contract must notify the Federal Mediation and Conciliation Service (FMCS) at least 90 days before the end of a contract. (It is reasonable to expect that newly elected labor representatives will notify the FMCS as soon as they are certified as the exclusive bargaining agents for a group of employees.)

Initial Bargaining Sessions

At the first few bargaining sessions, both sides identify subject areas they wish to explore. The courts have broken the subject areas into three categories: mandatory, prohibited, and permissive. *Mandatory bargaining subjects* are major issues that affect a nurse's work life. Examples are wages, hours, and layoff procedures. *Prohibited bargaining subjects* involve language that would violate other laws. Examples of prohibited bargaining issues are pay differentials based on race or requiring employers to only hire workers who already are members of the union.

Permissive bargaining subjects are any topic that is neither excluded nor prohibited, such as color options for uniforms or hospital sponsorship of a nurses' softball team. Ultimately, the contract will likely contain many mandatory subjects along with a smaller number of clauses dealing with permissive bargaining subjects.

"True" Bargaining

After the exchange of (often unrealistic) demands made at the initial bargaining meetings, both sides get down to real negotiations. Typically, offers and counteroffers are made within package deals (e.g., management will increase its pay schedule if the union agrees to fewer vacation days and a smaller increase in shift differentials). Occasionally, both sides can come to an agreement in a fairly short time. More likely, however, the negotiations will continue to a point where both sides begin to resist further concessions. This may occur before or after the existing contract has expired. Formal mediation efforts often become necessary at this point, with the mediator serving as a neutral third-party counselor working to bring the two sides closer to an agreement. The mediator's job is complicated by the fact that the law requires the two sides only to "bargain in good faith"—not to reach a settlement.

Bargaining Outcomes

Collective bargaining outcomes typically follow one of two avenues. The first (and much more desired) route is a settlement. Under this outcome, both sides agree to a contract that gives each side some—but not all—of the language it desired. The agreement between the negotiation teams is generally a cause for celebration; however, the process does not end until the union members vote to ratify the contract. Occasionally the membership will reject the agreement and the parties will have to return to the bargaining table to try to work out a more acceptable contract.

The alternative to settlement is an *impasse.* An impasse means that both sides have bargained to a point where each side refuses to offer any more concessions to the other side. At this juncture, the union can call for a strike vote in an attempt to place more pressure on the management side. As discussed earlier, federal law requires that the union give management (and the FMCS) a 10-day written notice of its intent to strike. If the impasse cannot be resolved during those 10 days, the union is free to "go out." In nearly all cases, mediation and negotiation will continue after the strike has begun.

Strike Activity Among Registered Nurses

When the NLRB was formulating its new bargaining unit rules in the late 1980s, it asked for public comment on the proposed changes. Given Congress' concerns about the effects of having an undue proliferation of bargaining units, this should have been a tremendous opportunity for the health care industry to use the fear of increased strike activity to convince the Board of the need to limit the number of possible units. Surprisingly, representatives for hospitals and other facilities were unable to produce any significant data that suggested that strikes were a threat to either the general public or to the health care industry (NLRB Notice, p. 33908, *Federal Register,* 1988).

The reason for the health care industry's inability to generate concern is simple: strikes have been relatively uncommon events in this country's history of health care collective bargaining. According to FMCS data, "only 3.3% of all health care contract negotiations, including nurse bargaining, result in strikes" (NLRB Notice, p. 33915, *Federal Register,* 1988). More current data (1995-1990 and 1992-1994) suggest that, on average, approximately 35 strikes occur per year throughout the entire American health care industry (Burda, 1995). Given these data, it appears that the vast majority of all bargaining outcomes are settlements, not walkouts.

Unfortunately, comprehensive data dealing specifically with the incidence of nurses' strikes is rather sparse. However, some evidence does suggest that the strike proclivity of these professionals may be increasing (Burda, 1995). It is uncertain that this is indeed a trend, but nurses are currently facing increasing economic and job security pressures at the same time they are enjoying fewer legal and American Nurses Association policy restrictions against the use of strikes. If nurses and management cannot find the means to relieve these pressures, it would not be surprising to see an increase in strike votes and actual walkouts in the future.

Alternatives to Strikes

Although the strike is generally considered to be labor's most significant weapon, other job actions or alternative avenues of dispute resolution can be utilized when striking is either unlawful or undesirable. Although most of these actions have been made obsolete by the extension of bargaining rights to most private sector health care workers, some public sector employees may still engage in the following gambits.

Interest Arbitration When labor and management reach an impasse, they may decide to submit their case to an arbitrator for resolution. An arbitrator is a neutral third party jointly selected by both sides to resolve the dispute. After the arbitrator is hired, both sides present their contract demands to the arbitrator and he or she decides which side's demands will be included in the contract. This format does prevent strikes, but its existence may also improve the chance of settlement because the arbitrator's decision is rarely appealable. Interest arbitration was fairly common during the early years of private sector health care collective bargaining (1935-1974) and is commonly used in public sector labor relations whenever unions are not allowed to strike by law.

Key terms	
Term	Definition
Multi-employer bargaining	Situation where a group of employers (e.g., hospitals) bargain as one entity
Mandatory bargaining subjects	Issues that are central to the work environment (e.g., pay, benefits, seniority)
Prohibited bargaining subjects	Issues that violate labor and/or other laws (e.g., lower pay scales for women)
Permissive bargaining subjects	All other issues that are neither "mandatory" nor prohibited"
Impasse	Situation where both sides have bargained in good faith but cannot reach an agreement
Mediation	Process whereby a neutral party attempts to help bargainers work through difficult negotiations and/or impasses

B O X   1 2 - 6

Common Labor Contract Clauses

Wage rates	Holidays and vacation	Seniority
Grievance and arbitration	Hours of work	Sick leave
Funeral/bereavement	Jury duty	Part-time employees
Leaves of absence	Nondiscrimination	Retirement
Educational reimbursement	Work apparel	Joint committees
Subcontracting	Term of agreement	Union security

Sickouts A sickout is a temporary (1- or 2-day) "strike" sometimes used to show management how important the nurses are to the successful functioning of a facility. Sickouts were commonly used in cases where the nurses did not have the legal right to organize or to strike.

Mass Resignations Similar to sickouts, this is a tactic used to pressure management into concessions of some sort when other job actions are not possible or desirable. Obviously, its success is predicated upon rehiring the "resigned" nurses as a condition of settlement.

Donated Time This alternative is a ploy to bring public sentiment to bear on a health care facility. Under this scheme, nurses would con-

tinue to work their normal shifts but would refuse to accept payment for their services. Often the nurses would also inform patients that they were due some sort of discount because of the hospital's voluntarily lowered payroll.

■ CONTRACT ADMINISTRATION

Once the contract has been ratified by the union membership, the collective bargaining process now turns toward administering the document on a day-to-day basis. The complexity of the administrative process is contingent upon many variables, including the sheer number of clauses, the location and characteristics of the covered employees, and the administrative history of prior contracts. Box 12-6 lists a number

Key terms	
Term	Definition
Grievance	A formal complaint that states either labor or management has failed to follow the terms of the contract
Grievance procedure	A multistep process designed to resolve contract disputes
Union stewards	Employees who also have contract management responsibilities; usually elected by their fellow co-workers
Rights arbitration	The process by which a neutral third party (the arbitrator) decides whether an employee's (or sometimes management's) contractual rights have been violated

of clauses that can be found in many nurses' labor contracts.

The Grievance Process

The single most important section of the entire contract in terms of maintaining labor-management peace is likely to be the grievance procedure. Within this clause lies the machinery that settles disagreements of interpretation and implementation during the lifetime of the contract. Without an effective grievance procedure, unresolved conflicts would likely make the entire contract unworkable. Fortunately for both management and employees, most grievance procedures receive significant attention during the negotiation process. Box 12-7, p. 310, shows an example of how grievance machinery can operate within an organization.

As can be seen from the case in Box 12-7, the grievance procedure is a progressive system that promotes the solution of simple disputes at low levels of both labor and management organizations, while saving more complicated cases for upper-level decision makers. If this had been a real case, it is highly likely that it would have been resolved long before arbitration. Conversely, cases involving suspensions and terminations have a much stronger chance of making their way in front of an arbitrator (Box 12-8, p. 311).

■ COLLECTIVE BARGAINING ISSUES FOR THE TWENTY-FIRST CENTURY

Given the extensive turbulence present within the health care industry, nurses and the bargaining agents that represent them face pressures from many sides. Recently, union nurses have been forced to deal with several major issues that will undoubtedly affect the labor relations process for an extended period of time. A discussion of three of the more complex issues follows.

The Role of Nurses' Associations as Bargaining Agents

For over 50 years, the American Nurses Association (ANA) has, through its state affiliates, been the chief bargaining agent for registered nurses throughout the United States. Although the ANA's tradition of seeking economic security for nurses is well documented (cf. Loevinger, 1950; Flannigan, 1976; Flannigan, 1983), its role as a labor representative is being challenged from several perspectives. For example, some nurses think that unions and the practice of professional nursing simply do not mix. They prefer that the ANA get out of the collective bargaining business altogether. Another group argues that collective bargaining is a fundamental requirement for obtaining the rewards and recognition nurses deserve. This group also argues that the ANA is un-

B O X   1 2 - 7

Rita Smith's Grievance

When Rita Smith arrives at work, her supervisor informs her that because of recent changes in staffing schemes, she is to be reassigned to the third shift (11 PM to 7 AM) for the foreseeable future. Rita becomes even more upset when she finds out that nurses with less seniority are able to keep working the the highly desired 7 AM to 3 PM shift. After checking her union contract to make sure that reassignments should be seniority-driven (they are), she makes plans to challenge this obvious mistake.

Step 1. In Rita's contract, the first step is for employees to informally discuss the problem with their supervisor. When Rita is not satisfied with her supervisor's answer, she elects to move to step 2.

Step 2. Rita seeks out her Union Steward for advice. The Union Steward is another nurse who has been voted into that position by fellow nurses. As the first line of union support, the Steward accompanies Rita for a second discussion with her supervisor. When the Union Steward cannot convince the supervisor to change the decision, Rita moves to step 3.

Step 3. Rita files a formal written grievance with her Steward. The Steward will forward the grievance to the Chief Steward (another nurse voted into that position by fellow nurses). The Chief Steward will try to take care of the problem when meeting with the Director of Nursing to discuss that week's grievances. When the Chief Steward cannot prove to the Director of Nursing that the reassignment order is inconsistent with the labor contract, Rita moves to Step 4 of the grievance procedure.

Step 4. Step 4 involves the discussion of grievances by the hospital's Chief Executive Officer and a labor relations specialist employed by Rita's bargaining agent. A failure to reach an agreement moves the problem on to step 5.

Step 5. Step 5 is the final step in the grievance process and involves submitting the issue to arbitration. Whereas interest arbitration involved setting negotiation issues, rights arbitration deals with problems of contract interpretation and implementation.

The arbitration process begins by selecting the arbitrator. In this case, a list of seven qualified arbitrators was generated by a neutral third party (e.g., the FMCS). Labor and management representatives flip a coin to see who gets to strike the first name from the list. The representatives will alternate striking names until only one remains. The last name remaining on the list will be hired as the arbitrator for this case.

After contacting the arbitrator, a hearing date is set. At the hearing, both sides may offer evidence that supports their contentions. During these arguments, the arbitrator will ask questions to clarify any concerns she or he may have regarding the facts of the case. After the hearing is complete, the arbitrator compares the facts of the case with the applicable language of the labor contract. Ultimately, the arbitrator makes a decision as to which side is right and submits the decision to both parties along with the arbitration bill. (Both sides typically share the costs of the arbitration.) As with interest arbitration, the decision of a rights arbitrator rarely can be appealed through the courts.

willing and/or unable to achieve these goals and advocates the selection of a more aggressive union such as the Teamsters or AFSCME to represent them in contract negotiations. Finally, there is a group who believe that the ANA's current practice of supporting both the economic and professional interests of nurses is "just right." They argue that nurses have a unique working environment and those colleagues desiring union representation need bargaining agents staffed with personnel possessing an extensive understanding of the profession.

BOX 12-8

Advantages and Disadvantages of Using the Grievance Process

Advantages
- Provides a safety valve for workplace pressures.
- Points out problem areas in existing contracts.
- Structure helps limit arbitrary and capricious decision making on the part of managers.

Disadvantages:
- Arbitration can be expensive, especially to smaller employers or unions.
- There are inherent risks in allowing a case to go to arbitration in that neither side can be sure of the outcome, even in what appears to be "slam dunk" cases.
- Frivolous grievances based on opinions and/or individual desires instead of contract language waste time and scarce resources for both bargaining agents and employers.

BOX 12-9

The California Nurses Association Becomes an Independent Labor Organization

On October 1, 1995, the California Nurses Association (CNA) voted to withdraw from the American Nurses Association. Citing differences along patient-care and collective bargaining lines, the 25,000-member group became the first state association to leave the ANA in 99 years (Moore, 1995a; 1995b). Consistent with its campaign promises, the CNA has become an aggressive advocate for nurses and consumers.

(Please refer to the CNA website at: www.califnurses.org/cna/kaiser/index.htm.)

If the ANA were purely a labor union or a professional association, it would be relatively easy to deal with the concerns just described. However, while the ANA may not be trying to "be all things to all nurses," few, if any, labor organizations have as many nonbargaining interests and responsibilities. This semiprivate conflict recently became public knowledge when the California Nurses Association (CNA) seceded from the ANA and embarked on its own plan for representing nurses in that state (Box 12-9).

It is unclear whether the CNA defection is a one-time aberration or a harbinger of things to come. That depends largely on the organization's ability to consistently secure acceptable labor contracts for its membership. If the CNA is successful, the leadership of the ANA may need to reevaluate the group's focus and priorities. At minimum, the CNA-ANA feud will likely serve to energize future nurse-management negotiations

across the country as state nurses' associations may feel additional pressure to satisfy their memberships' needs and expectations.

Redesigning Nurses' Work

There is a massive effort within many health care organizations across the country to redesign the way nurses perform their jobs (Aiken et al., 1996). Influenced by managed-care systems, these facilities have embarked upon plans to cut costs while attempting to maintain high quality care. Because nurse wages and benefits are substantial cost items in most budgets, management may consider this area a prime opportunity in which to slash costs. As a result, many organizations have attempted to redesign nursing jobs so that "high-cost" nurses perform only those duties that cannot be delegated to less expensive personnel such as unlicensed nurses' aides (Anders, 1995). Under this work scheme, the health care facility saves money by having less-qualified (and lower-paid) employees perform as much work as possible.

This system may make financial sense to management, but it is a threat to union nurses because their work is being, in a sense, outsourced to a less expensive provider. Unless the union is careful, it may find itself with a dwindling number of working members as management continually "fine-tunes" nursing positions until they are at an optimal (for the employer, that is) level. Ultimately, this process will likely mean fewer hours and/or job opportunities for registered nurses.

Another potential pitfall within the job redesign process is the additional "managementization" of nurses. When a task has been delegated to a lower-level employee, does the nurse still have the responsibility to see that it is performed correctly? Is the nurse expected to organize, direct, and plan the work of the delegatee? An affirmative answer to either of these questions means that the nurse is probably moving much closer to the legislative definition of a "supervisor" discussed in an earlier section. If the nurse aspires to be a true supervisor, this may be a desired outcome. However, if the nurse has no intention of becoming a supervisor, he or she may be in danger of compromising many of the protections afforded under the existing labor law.

Nurses as Patient Advocates

When representatives for the Ohio Nurses Association insisted that the ANA Code of Ethics be included in collective bargaining contracts, their intention was to ensure that the labor relations process would help patients receive the care they deserved (Holloway, 1976). With the advent of managed care and other cost-containment efforts, many nurses fear that patient care has become secondary to revenue and cost projections in many American health care facilities. Some of these nurses are looking to the collective bargaining process as a lever to force their employers to manage their organization in a way that promotes high quality care (cf.

Moore, 1995a). As a result, patient-care issues are consistently being raised in labor negotiations and disputes.

Although these patient-care initiatives appear to be noble endeavors, a cynic might argue that the unions are simply trying to protect their members' jobs and salaries by feeding on the general public's growing concerns about managed health care. By portraying themselves as potential victims (along with their patients) of "de-professionalized" health care, these nurses are building a strong base of grass-roots support for their cause. However, the cynic would argue, these nurses' "cause" has more to do with maintaining staffing ratios and limiting workload transfers to nonprofessionals than with ensuring quality patient care.

Patient-care issues can obviously be a sizable "stick" when used in health care labor negotiations. However, possession of the stick is not permanent. In the unlikely scenario that a bargaining agent uses this issue solely for the benefit of its membership, it will expose itself to substantial negative publicity whenever future contracts are negotiated. To maintain the "high ground" in this area, the union must be careful to follow up on its concerns after the contract is ratified. If it fails to do so, it will likely discover the other end of the "stick."

▪ NURSING UNIONS AS AGENTS OF CHANGE: BALANCING PERSONAL NEEDS AND PROFESSIONAL RESPONSIBILITIES

When nurses first achieved the right to bargain collectively, the labor contract could be viewed as a "sword" of sorts. By using the tip of the sword to prod management into improving the work lives of nurses, unions substantially changed the dynamics within health care facilities. Among the tangible benefits of unionized nursing were professional wages and benefits, the establishment of machinery to improve workplace justice, and a greater voice in the day-to-day operation of the facilities where nurses care for patients.

Recently, however, the labor contract has also been used as a shield against what some consider to be an insidious invasion of "dollar-driven profit mongers" into the American health care system. By insisting that patient-care issues be included in negotiations, nurses have tried to minimize some of the potentially detrimental side effects of the managed-care juggernaut by raising (or perhaps by threatening to raise) consumer awareness of issues such as the prevalence of nonlicensed care givers. Under most circumstances, it would be difficult to seriously contend that nursing unions are change agents by virtue of their ability to limit change. However, it is argued here that any group that has the fortitude and ability to challenge the single largest trend in the single largest segment of the American economy is indeed a true agent of change.

The future of these unions will likely hinge on the ability of bargaining agents to offer their memberships contracts that provide adequate benefits and protections without bluntly compromising the professional facets of nursing. If these unions focus too firmly on economic matters, some nurses will reject them as being no different from the profit-maximizing managers they bargain against. If these bargaining agents see themselves as only a protector of the public and of the profession, many nurses with mortgage payments and other bills to pay will likely seek out other representatives who know much about raising wages and benefits but little about what it means to be a nurse. In the end, both labor organization and nurse will be successful if they can find the means to balance personal needs and professional re-

sponsibilities in this fast-changing, turbulent sector of the economy.

■ KEY POINTS

- Registered nurses are more likely to be "pushed" by management than "drawn" by unions into the arena of collective bargaining. In other words, satisfied nurses have less need for union contracts than their discontented counterparts.

- Changes in the health care workplace (e.g., restructuring nurses' duties) and marketplace (e.g., managed care) are creating substantial personal and professional pressures for many nurses. Collective bargaining may be viewed by some nurses as a shield against these pressures.

- Even though the history of health care labor legislation is sizable and relatively long-standing, ongoing judicial and administrative interpretations of those laws create a fragile environment for nurses seeking union representation.

- A union contract has the potential to be an effective tool in the search for a fair, professional work environment that also promotes high-quality patient care.

- The American Nurses Association is under increasing pressure from its membership and its competitors to become more aggressive in labor negotiations. It remains to be seen whether the ANA can maintain its status as the flagship organization representing nurses at the bargaining table.

- The integration of professional standards and expectancies with the realities of collective bargaining in the real world is neither easy nor neat for many nurses. With the inherent pressures associated with the "free marketization" of American health care, this struggle will likely continue for the foreseeable future.

■ CRITICAL THINKING QUESTIONS

1. Given the significant responsibilities nurses have in regard to the provision of quality care to the American public, should they be allowed to bargain collectively for their own benefit?

2. Nurses, like firefighters, enjoy a positive image in this country. Does unionization impair or diminish that reputation? Why?

3. Given what you know about its leadership and multiple missions, should the ANA be allowed to represent nurses at the bargaining table? Would nurses be better off having a more customary bargaining agent such as the Teamsters or the Service Employees' International Union represent them in negotiations?

4. The term *professional collectivism* is sometimes used when describing unions composed of employees such as nurses, professional engineers, and airline pilots. Is this term appropriate, or is it an oxymoron? Why or why not?

5. As a member of the nurses' bargaining team, you are concerned that the final contract will help to ensure the provision of high-quality patient care. Describe three realistic contract clauses that should be placed in the labor agreement to accomplish that goal. What contract language should be *avoided* to achieve the same objective?

6. Why do nurses join unions? Describe some things that nursing administrators/ managers can do to minimize the likelihood of unionization.

7. Describe the functions of a grievance procedure within a labor contract. Is it worth the costs involved with its management (e.g., arbitration costs)? Why?

■ REFERENCES

Aiken, L.H., Sochalski, J., & Anderson, G.F. (1996). Downsizing the hospital workforce. *Health Affairs, 15*(4), 88-92.

Anders, G. (1995). Medicine: Hospitals' Rx for high costs: Fewer nurses, more aides. *Wall Street Journal*, Feb 10, B1.

Burda, D. (1995). Hospital strikes fewer but nastier. *Modern Healthcare, 25*(14), 44-46.

Burda, D. (1994). Montana hospital uses court ruling to oust nurses' union. *Modern Healthcare, 24*(34), 3, 11.

California Nurses Association. (1997). *Kaiser Watch.* Internet:www.califnurses.org/cna/kaiser/index.htm.

Cihon, P.J., & Castagnera, J.O. (1993). *Labor and employment law* (2nd ed.). Boston: PWS-KENT Publishing.

Delany, J.T., & Sockell, D. (1988). Hospital unit determination and the preservation of employee free choice. *Labor Law Journal, 39*, 259-273.

Executive Order No. 11491, 3 C.F.R. 521 (1969).

Executive Order No. 10988, 5 C. F. R. 888 (1962).

Fiorito, J., Gallagher, D.G., & Greer, C.R. (1987). Determinants of unionism: A review of the literature. In K.R. Rowland & G.R. Ferris (Eds.). *Research in personnel and human resource management* (Vol. 4, pp. 269-306). Greenwich, Conn.: JAI Press.

Flannigan, L. (1976). *One strong voice: The story of the ANA.* Kansas City: American Nurses Association.

Flannigan, L. (1983). *Collective bargaining and the nursing profession.* Kansas City: American Nurses Association.

French, W.L., & Robinson, R. (1960). Collective bargaining by nurses and other professionals: Anomaly or trend? *Labor Law Journal 11*, 902-910.

Health Care Amendments of 1974. (1974). Pub. L. No. 93-360.

Holley, W.H., & Jennings, K.M. (1991). *The labor relations process* (4th ed.). Hinsdale, Ill.: Dryden.

Holloway, S.T. (1976). Health professionals and collective action. *Employee Relations Law Journal 1*(3), 410-417.

Labor Management Relations Act. (1947). 29 U. S. C. §§ 141-197.

Leroy, M.H., Schwarz, J.L., & Koziara, K.S. (1992). The law and economics of collective bargaining for hospitals: An empirical public policy analysis of bargaining unit determinations. *Yale Journal on Regulation, 9*, 1-69.

Loevinger, R.H. (1951). The Minnesota story of economic security. *American Journal of Nursing, 51*(4), 228-231.

Mahoney, M.E. (1995). Supreme Court rejects longstanding labor rule for nurses. *Health Care Supervisor, 13*(4), 13-17.

Moore, J.D. (1996). Alaska hospital disputing nurse labor law. *Modern Healthcare, 26*(34), 6, 10.

Moore, J.D. (1995a). Frustrated Calif. nurses leave ANA. *Modern Healthcare, 25*(41), 42.

Moore, J.D. (1995b). ANA fires back at California secessionists. *Modern Healthcare, 25*(39), 33.

National Labor Relations Act. (1935). 29 U. S. C. § 169.

National Labor Relations Board Notice. (1988). Second notice of proposed rulemaking—Collective bargaining units in the health care industry. *Federal Register, 53*(170), 33900-33935.

National Labor Relations Board Ruling. (1989). Collective bargaining units in the health care industry. *Federal Register, 54*(76), 16336-16347.

National Labor Relations Board v. Bozeman Deaconess Hospital. (1997). 322 NLRB 196.

National Labor Relations Board v. Health Care & Retirement Corporation of America. (1992). 306 NLRB.

National Labor Relations Board v. Health Care & Retirement Corporation of America. (1993). 987 F. 2nd 1256.

National Labor Relations Board v. Health Care & Retirement Corporation of America. (1994). 1124 S. Ct. 1778.

National Labor Relations Board v. Providence Alaska Medical Center. (1996). 320 NLRB 49.

Roach, B.L. (1994). Burnout and the nursing profession. *Health Care Supervisor, 12,* 41-47.

Scott, C., & Lowery, C.M. (1994). Union activity in the hospital industry. *Health Care Management Review, 14*(4), 21-28.

Sherer, J.L. (1994). Who's the boss? High court ruling a setback for union nurses. *Hospitals & Health Networks, 68*(14), 56.

Wheeler, H.N., & McClendon, J.A. (1991). The individual decision to unionize. In G. Straus, D.G. Gallagher, & J. Fiorito (Eds.). *The State of the unions* (Vol 1, pp. 47-83). Madison, Wis.: Industrial Relations Research Association.

Health Policy: Strategies for Analysis and Influence

Marcia Stanhope

INTRODUCTION

Workplace redesign, downsizing, resizing, cross training, the use of unlicensed assistive personnel, an emphasis on community-based practice, and an increasing demand that regulations governing practice be evaluated for appropriateness, need, and flexibility highlight the need for another look at policies that have governed the practice of nursing. New emphasis on developing practice guidelines, outcomes, or effectiveness research; information technologies; and changes in health care delivery from both national and state perspectives are aiding consumers, providers, educators, insurers, and policymakers in critically evaluating and making decisions about health care issues.

With managed care and case management as the keys to budget debates and increasing health care costs, there is a shift in the thoughts of policymakers and analysts toward a focus on disease prevention, health promotion, and preventive and primary health care. There is also a shift away from recognizing the provider as the core of the health care system to recognizing the patient as the dominant focus in all decision making about the direction the system will take.

In the 1990s the United States experienced the greatest emphasis on health care insurance reform since the advent of Medicare in the mid-1960s. Although President Clinton's plan for national health care and total system reform was unsuccessful, it served as a stimulus for changes within states themselves, with partial changes at the national level. National health care policy, burdened by fragmentation, indecision, and pretense, is not an unusual type of policy for the United States. Neither does the United States have organized, decisive national policy in other arenas in which the country spends enormous amounts of dollars, such as defense, transportation, and education.

The twenty-first century will begin with a continuing emphasis on change. All (i.e., consumers, providers, professional organizations, industry, governments) agree that change is essential. However, change in health care delivery or any other system will be unsuccessful unless it is built on a common vision, values, and virtues of the society with a guiding purpose. The past purpose of the health care system emphasized illness care. The World Health Organization (WHO) in its charter at Alma-Ata promotes a health care emphasis as the purpose for the system (WHO, 1978). To have a common purpose, the key actors in the system must consider the public interest rather than individual and political interests.

Nurses continue to be the largest provider group in the United States and can be integral to changes in policies that govern nursing practice and health care delivery. Nurses, with their emphasis on caring, their expertise in nursing and care delivery, and their recognized position in the system as consumer advocates, can readily establish credibility with consumers, volunteer organizations, professional organizations, community leaders, and government officials to effect change. Nurses can be policymakers, policy analysts, resource mobilizers, and coalition builders and can assist consumers to empower themselves to create change that will result in a healthier society. This chapter provides the framework and key steps that nurses can take to influence policy decisions and play a key role in shifting the purpose of health care from a focus on illness to a focus on health.

OBJECTIVES

After reading this chapter, you will be able to:

1. Define policy
2. Contrast health policy and healthy policy
3. Apply frameworks for policy analysis
4. Analyze research influences on policy development
5. Apply strategies to influence policy decisions

■ DEFINITIONS

Policies are simply guides to decision making that in turn governs a planned course of action to solve a problem (Rastogi, 1992). Policies exist in any environment in which individuals are involved. Policy can be aimed at preventing a problem from occurring or reacting to a situation that exists and requires change (Kessler, 1995).

Policies are essential to providing direction for problem solving and for meeting goals. Policies direct human behavior in the family, home, church, school, workplace, community, organizations, and government. There are several categories of policy: private policy, public policy, health policy, and healthy policy (Flynn, 1995; Mason et al., 1993; Stanhope, 1995). Box 13-1 describes these four types of policies.

All types of policies are important to the functioning of society. Policies are viewed as a means of raising an issue on a public or private agenda. The policy process is a mechanism for passing laws or making rules that commit resources to situations that affect peoples' lives. A policy may be developed to impose regulations or rules that interpret laws or that withdraw previous policies. A policy guides the process of implementation and evaluation of the usefulness of a program (Patton & Sawicki, 1993). The remaining discussion focuses on expanding the constructs of health policy and healthy policy.

■ PURPOSE OF HEALTH POLICY

The purpose of health policy is to clearly define measurable and obtainable objectives that can guide changes in health care delivery that will effectively and efficiently produce a healthy society by improving the health of individuals (Sultz, 1991).

BOX 13-1

Four Types of Policy

Private policy   A purposive course of action to deal with concerns in the family and in private sector voluntary organizations and businesses. Such policies provide guidelines for spending money, for lines of communication, and in organizations providing service and employee conduct (Hanley, 1993).

Public policy   A purposive course of action to deal with concerns at all levels of government, educational systems, and publicly owned corporations. Public policy comprises legislation, statutes, regulations, court actions, and institutional guidelines, including provider licensure, Medicare agency conditions of participation, annual academic sessions, and profit sharing in corporations (Hanley, 1993).

Health policy   Actions developed by the public sector or private sector and related to the how, when, where, why, and to whom health care is delivered, how much money is spent, and who is considered a health care provider, including scope of practice (Mason et al., 1993; Stanley, 1994).

Health policy   Public or private sector actions developed by consumers in collaboration with others through a collective approach to improve the health of the patient (individual, group, or community). This approach to developing policy assists consumers to take interest in their own health and in the health of others (Mason et al., 1993).

One of the most identifiable examples of the development of health policy for the United States is the evolution of national health objectives. In 1979 the surgeon general of the United States, Julius B. Richmond, published a report on health promotion and disease prevention entitled *Healthy People.* In the first *Healthy People,* the target date for reaching the goals was 1990. The goals and subgoals were developed by governmental personnel; they were organized around five major age-groups (infants, children, adolescents, young adults, and older adults) and were directed toward reducing mortality within the first four age-groups while focusing on improving health and life quality of the older adult (Branch, 1994; U.S. Department of Health and Human Services, 1979).

Based on lessons learned from the development of these first objectives, *Healthy People 2000* was developed and published in 1991. In contrast to the development of the first document, *Healthy People 2000* was the product of 22 expert working groups, a consortium of 300 national organizations, all states' health departments, the Institute of Medicine of the National Academy of Sciences, and additional testimony from 750 individuals and organizations. Ten thousand persons participated in public review and comment before finalizing the 300 objectives and 284 subobjectives to increase healthy life spans, to reduce health disparities, and to achieve access to preventive services for all Americans (U.S. Department of Health and Human Services, 1990). The process was changed from 1979 to 1990 as a result of a philosophy that the more people who were involved, the more likely the "buy in" to implementing the objectives. Such participative methods of change are used to overcome resistance and to use the two most important sources of wealth for creating change: the knowledge individuals and groups bring to the situation; and their ability to communicate the change (Swansburg, 1996).

■ PURPOSE OF HEALTHY POLICY

In contrast to health policy, healthy policy places health as a priority by developing shared responsibility among persons to identify the strengths and resources of people as a collective and of their environment. This approach emphasizes the physical environment; community connectedness; access to services and resources; social, educational, occupational, and economic viability; and health status rather than emphasizing individual problems and pathologic conditions for directing actions (Chapin, 1995; Flynn, 1995).

A prime example of a healthy policy approach to problem solving is the healthy communities/healthy cities concept that developed from a conference in Toronto in the 1980s. This concept was based on the *WHO Health for All Framework by the Year 2000* (Flynn, 1995; Takarangi & North, 1990) (Box 13-2).

The European Healthy Cities Project was launched by WHO in 1984 to bring cities together to collaborate in the development of urban health promotion initiatives. In the begin-

ning, six cities were involved, addressing concerns such as substance use, nutrition, health, and environment. By 1988 it had grown to an international movement, and by 1995 more than 1000 cities worldwide were participating (Flynn, 1995; Takarangi & North, 1990).

Healthy Cities began in the United States in Indiana and California in 1988. In Indiana a project was developed by faculty and staff of the Institute of Action Research for Community Health at Indiana University School of Nursing. Funded by the W.K. Kellogg Foundation, the staff of the project collaborated with six Indiana cities. This project, now called CITYNET, is based on a nine-step initiative and has continuing success locally and nationally. The CITYNET program has five objectives (Flynn, 1995):

- Health first
- Shared responsibility for community-wide health
- Involvement of local people
- A focus on hard-to-reach populations
- Promotion of healthy public policy

Involvement of local people and promoting shared responsibility among community members for increasing the health of the community create a feeling of ownership in the change. This is referred to as *participative evaluation* (Swansburg, (1996).

As a result of this project and based on community needs assessments, healthy policy developments in Indiana include reductions in crime rates for some cities, annual family health awareness projects, recycling programs for solid waste, and a teen pregnancy initiative (Flynn, 1995).

Such efforts focus the attention of lawmakers on problems within a community or state. Other examples of healthy policy developments include seat belt laws, helmet laws, immunization programs for children, and nonsmoking policies in public areas (Flynn, 1995). Although this example has focused on the development of

---

B O X   1 3 - 2

Nine-Step Initiative to Develop Healthy City

- Orient community to process.
- Build partnership and community commitment.
- Develop community structure for change.
- Develop community leadership.
- Assess community strengths and needs.
- Institute community-wide planning.
- Implement community action.
- Provide data-based information to policymakers.
- Monitor and evaluate progress.

Data from Flynn, B. (1995). *Nursing Policy Forums,* 2(6), 6.

healthy policy in the public arena, healthy policy may also be developed within private arenas, such as within organizations. In the development of policy for healthy living, nurses and other health providers often play a supportive, advocacy role and/or a consulting role as persons in a community come together to identify what their priorities are and write policy to make those priorities become reality.

■ FRAMEWORKS FOR POLICY DEVELOPMENT

The development of policies involves choices: decisions to do or not to do something to resolve a problem. The development of policy follows an organized and deliberate process. This process involves specific steps through which an issue progresses from problem identification to resolution. In the process of the development of a policy there are no absolute truths. Seldom are "new" policies developed. Most policies are replacements for past policy. A policy grows from an identified need or problem that someone or some source wants to do something about: an individual, a public interest group, a researcher, a professional or voluntary organization, or a governmental entity. An analysis of the policy issue defined as a problem or need is essential to the development of an acceptable policy to resolve the issue.

Policy Analysis

There are a number of models proposed in the literature to analyze an issue for the purpose of developing a policy. This analysis process has been described as requiring compromise, argument, persuasion, judgment, and the art of influence: politics (Patton & Sawicki, 1993; Stanley, 1994).

Anderson (1975), McRae and Wilder (1979), Quade (1982), and Stokey and Zeckhauser (1978) all describe a policy process framework that mirrors the rational decision-making pro-

cess found in many fields, including nursing (Patton & Sawicki, 1993). This framework includes the following:

- Defining a problem
- Identifying alternatives to addressing the problem
- Quantifying the alternatives
- Analyzing aids for evaluating alternatives that will assist in making decisions
- Choosing an alternative
- Implementing and evaluating a decision

The above authors describe the process as an iterative one with policy analysts working back and forth between steps until objectives are classified, the problem is redefined, alternatives are redesigned and evaluated, and better approaches are found to solving the problem (Patton & Sawicki, 1993). This is a very comprehensive approach to policy analysis.

Weimer and Vining (1989) describe a framework that focuses on problem analysis and solution analysis because they feel both are equally important, and once a problem is defined it is thought that the road to the solution has already been paved (Backer, 1991).

The incremental approach to policy analysis (Lindblom & Woodhouse, 1993) is an alternative framework to the rational decision-making framework. The incremental approach focuses on a process whereby changes can be made using smaller steps in a relatively short time span versus seeking immediate radical changes at once. Lindblom and Woodhouse suggest focusing on analyzing a few policy alternatives to the most pressing problem rather than trying to be comprehensive as in the rational models. Their model advocates strategies of trial and error and revised trials based on what is a manageable solution and politically feasible.

Etizioni (1967) suggested another framework that is a compromise between the incremental and the rational approaches and that focuses on looking comprehensively at the problem while

Key terms	
Term	**Definition**
Coalition building	When groups join together in a temporary relationship to build consensus around a common issue
Collaboration	Joining forces with others to pursue an agreed-on goal
Empowerment	Giving oneself permission to participate in decision making and change that affects the individual self
Key actors	May be referred to as stakeholders; individuals affected by policy decisions: nurses, patients, other providers, administrators, insurance companies, governments
Health policy	A way to change one's institution, community, state, and nation
Policy process	A complex, organized, and deliberate approach to decision making that results in selecting a course of action to address an issue; requires knowledge, skill, and input from many sources (Stanley, 1994)
Policy analysis	A means of pulling together information, including research, to produce a set of alternatives for decision making
Policymaker	One who can make a decision to implement change: a patient, a parent, an agency, an administrator, a public official, or a health care professional
Politics	The art of influence

focusing only on the alternatives that seem most promising as a solution.

Kingdom (1984) proposed a framework for policy analysis that involves three concepts: (1) problem stream, (2) policy stream, and (3) political stream. In the *problem stream* the nurse looks at the problem complexities and gets policymakers to focus on the problem. In the *policy stream* goals and objectives are set based on ideas from others: researchers, staff, agencies, public interest groups, professional organizations. In the *political stream,* political factions are considered that can influence the political agenda: media attention, inflation, special interest groups (Mason et al., 1993; Parsons, 1995). Each of these concepts interacts with the others, and as opinions or environmental circumstances change, issues change.

Although there are numerous other frameworks in the literature, this discussion will fo-

cus on (1) the rational decision-making model, called a stagist approach, using steps from agenda setting to policy evaluation and termination; and (2) a communities or network approach, called a subsystem approach, which focuses on relationships, connectedness, dependencies, and informal networks for policymaking. This approach purportedly allows a more fluid and realistic analysis of how people interact at different levels (Parsons, 1995).

Rational Model   The rational model described by Patton and Sawicki (1993) involves a six-step process to analyze a policy issue (Figure 13-1). The model depicts an interactive, iterative process between the steps, all of which may or may not be followed in the development of a policy, depending on time available for the analysis. This process is used to develop health policy by nurses and other professionals and organizations. It is a top-down approach for devel-

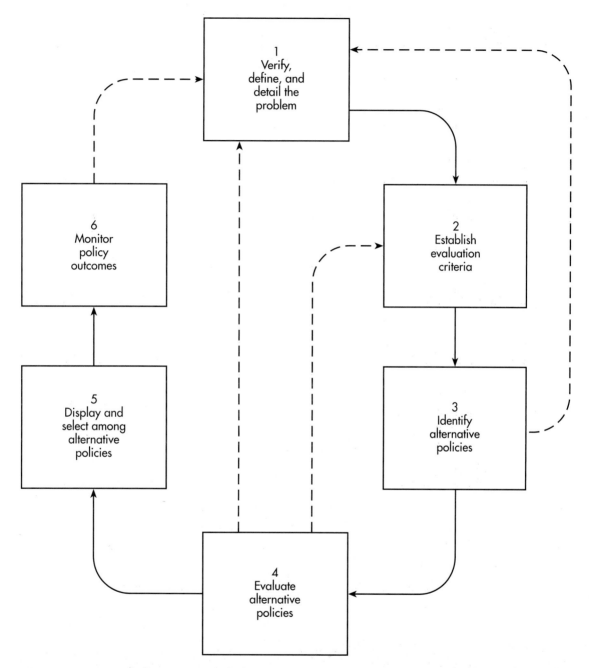

Figure 13-1 ■ **Six-step process to analyze a policy issue.** (From Patton, C., & Sawicki, D. [1993]. *Basic methods of policy analysis and planning* [2nd ed.]. Englewood Cliffs, NJ: Prentice-Hall.)

oping health policy. This is a method of thinking about problems, organizing data, and presenting findings.

For all steps in the process, needed data must be identified and gathered. Library searches, reviews of past policies aimed at solving the problem, interviews of key persons, and quick surveys are all means to gather data. At each step, data analysis and communicating the analysis to others are essential to the process. Depending on the step, one may communicate to other team members involved in the analysis, to interested parties (e.g., consumers), to funding sources, to political figures, to managers, or to family members.

Step 1: Verifying, Defining, and Detailing the Problem At step 1 the problem's concrete terms are defined, based on the values of the person or persons affected. These persons are the key actors. Their motivations to have the problem solved and their beliefs are important. The boundaries of the problem are also defined. A fact sheet is a useful aid in discussions with others, and the use of numbers is helpful to justify the problem when possible. In addition, the problem is stated in measurable terms and goals and objectives are listed for resolving the problem. The resources available, usable, and needed are determined. It is important to find out who will make decisions about the problem. The problem statement is reviewed for accuracy. In some instances a needs assessment may be required to define the problem (Patton & Sawicki, 1993).

Step 2: Establishing Evaluation Criteria Step 2 will help to develop outcomes for each objective to be met by a policy and to compare alternatives to determine which will be acceptable to the key actors, including the decision makers. Rules will need to be established to evaluate alternatives to avoid choosing a favorite option. Criteria may include evaluation of costs, risks, legalities, effectiveness, political viability, administrative ease, equity, and timing. It is important to attempt to determine whether the alternatives will meet the objectives defined in step 1; the cost benefit of the alternative; its acceptability to power groups, legislators, administrators, citizens, neighbors, and unions; and whether it can be implemented within the political, social, administrative, or community environment (Patton & Sawicki, 1993).

Step 3: Identifying Alternatives In step 3 the process revolves around choice. Many options should be considered. One option that should be included in this step is *no action.* One can consider types of alternatives that have been used in similar situations. Taking suggestions from talking with others is a good approach. One can determine individual, group, and organizational reactions to alternatives and find out how past problems were solved. Also it is good to compare alternatives with an ideal solution in the literature. Several alternatives may be considered in solving a problem:

- Keep what is.
- Modify an existing system or method.
- Use someone else's design.
- Create a new system or method.

Above all, one will want to be creative in thinking about possible alternative solutions (Patton & Sawicki, 1993).

Step 4: Evaluate Alternative Policies Step 4 determines whether any policies will work to solve the problem. One can look at what has happened in the past when the options identified have been chosen; look at the links between the variables that may affect the desired outcomes: social, political, economic, ethical, and environmental; talk with key actors to determine what may happen; describe what outcome is desired; and find data in the literature or through a survey to predict what will happen. It is necessary to consider the time, resources, and cost to implement each alternative (Patton & Sawicki, 1993). Each alternative has uncertainties and unintended consequences. It is impossible to predict what may happen if one alternative is chosen over another. Look at which alternative has the most positive outcomes as well as those options with the greatest possible risks.

Step 5: Displaying Alternatives and Selecting Among Them Step 5 involves ranking the alternatives and comparing them with each other based on the criteria in step 2. It is necessary to determine which of the criteria established in step 2 are the most important for each of the alternatives to meet and to select the one alternative that meets the most criteria. A matrix to display all criteria and how each meets the criteria provides a picture for evaluating the alternatives. The preferred option is chosen, and the others are priority ranked in the event that the preferred option is unacceptable to the policymakers (Patton & Sawicki, 1993).

Step 6: Monitoring and Evaluating Policy Outcomes Step 6 is very important because it allows a comparison of the problem situation before and after the policy implementation. This step answers the question of whether the target goal was met. These comparisons can be made by looking at a situation where the policy remained the same and one where the policy was changed. If the policy resulted in an intervention for a health problem, a look at before and after morbidity, mortality, incidence, or prevalence data will show any change in outcome after the intervention. This step assists in learning about what works, what does not work, what was done well, and what improvements can be made to techniques for future analysis (Patton & Sawicki, 1993).

Quick Decision Analysis The quick decision analysis using a decision tree (Figure 13-2) is a process that can be used to look at the deci-

sion dilemma, to think about the problem and alternatives. There are four possible outcomes to any problem based on alternatives chosen (Patton & Sawicki, 1993):

• Do nothing, and get outcome anyway.
• Do nothing, and get nothing.
• Do something, and get outcome.
• Do something, and get nothing.

Figure 13-3 shows a decision tree looking at the need for children to be immunized.

The Strengths Approach Whereas the rational decision-making model emphasizes an iterative analysis of the problem, problem definition, and assessment of alternatives to resolve the problem, the strengths approach focuses on assessing the strengths of the people and their environment that the policy targets. This is an approach for developing *healthy policy* and is based on the subsystems approach previously described. This is a social policy model based on the beliefs that people continue to grow, develop, and change and should have equal access to resources; that truth and reality can be and have regularly been negotiated; that the understanding of problems is based on society and reasonably constructed views of reality; that policy that reflects the reality of its intended recipients is more likely to be successful if policymakers are also the people directly affected by the policy; and that inclusion of patients in policymaking is essential (Chapin, 1995). This is a grassroots approach to policy development with support and facilitation by the nurse. As stated earlier, the *Healthy Cities* projects by Flynn is a fine example of a strengths approach to policy development. The nurse is the facilitator, getting groups together; the advocate, showing individuals and groups how to make systems work for them; and consultant, providing knowledge and information that individuals can use to make decisions.

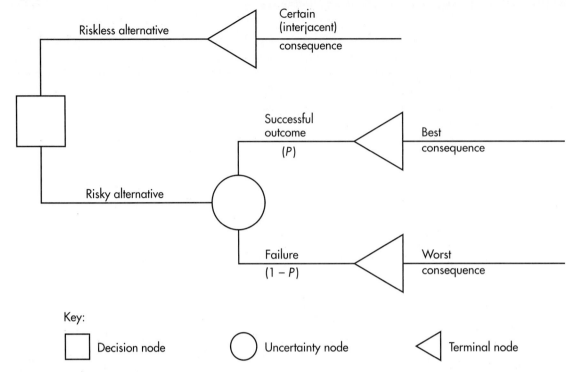

Figure 13-2 ■ The quick decision analysis using a decision tree. (From Behn, R.D., & Vaupel, J.W. [1982]. *Quick analysis for busy decision makers* [p. 41]. New York: Basic Books.)

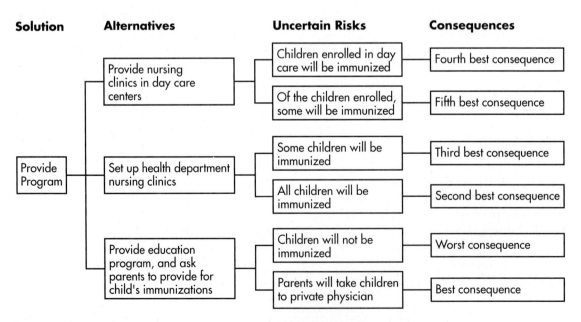

Figure 13-3 ■ Decision tree: providing a preschool immunization program to low-income children.

B O X   1 3 - 3

Comparison of Health Policy Analysis and Healthy Policy Analysis Frameworks

Rational Decision Making	Strengths Approach
Define problem	Identify common/collective strengths
	Identify basic needs and barriers
Determine evaluation criteria	Define need(s) with patients
Identify alternative policy choices	Identify program, community, or patient approaches to barrier resolution
	Identify opportunities and resources essential to meet needs
Evaluate alternative policy choices	Formulate policy
	Negotiate policy consensus
Select preferred policy	Design program policy
Implement preferred policy	Implement policy
Monitor and evaluate policy	Evaluate and assess patient outcomes

Data from Patton, C., & Sawicki, D. (1993). *Basic methods of policy analysis and planning* (2nd ed.). Englewood Cliffs, N.J.: Prentice-Hall; Chapin, R. (1995). *Social Work, 40*(4), 508.

The strengths approach process involves the following (Chapin, 1995):

- Focusing on common or collective strengths
- Identifying human needs and barriers to meeting needs
- Negotiating definitions of needs and barriers
- Valuing the input of persons
- Searching for opportunities and resources to support persons' efforts in resolving needs
- Building on personal and environmental strengths
- Giving a voice to the patient perspective
- Helping negotiate definitions and goals that include patient perspectives
- Focusing on the patient as collaborator from the beginning of policy development through the evaluation phase

The strengths approach highlights the interconnectedness of patients within groups or communities. It focuses attention on those areas that make a group or community healthy: social, economic, educational, health services, physical, as well as living, work, and play environments. This approach does not negate the need for the nurse in the policy process; rather, it changes the role from one who informs others and develops the goals to be met to one who advocates for the patients, assists in negotiating definitions, and collaborates with patients throughout the policy process. This model truly reflects the values and vision of those affected by the policy. An evaluation of the outcomes of policies developed using this model will be based on the extent to which ideas of the patients are included and on the patient outcomes that occur as a result of the policy implementation (Chapin, 1995). The CITYNET model previously described is indicative of a strengths approach. Box 13-3 contrasts the two approaches to developing policy. All strategies previously described for policy analysis and collecting data may be used in either framework.

Practical Tips for Policy Development

Health policies are typically developed for four reasons: (1) to increase public knowledge of relationships between a behavior and health; (2) to promote unified, organized approaches to an issue among all interested parties; (3) to educate the public, including lawmakers, about the best practice or practices for resolving an issue; and (4) to encourage the development of new technologies or methodologies that may result in more healthful, more accessible, more affordable living (Kessler, 1995).

The following principles (Patton & Sawicki, 1993) are useful in assisting nurses to practice policy analysis and development. Reading extensively helps to focus on problems confronting patients: the professional literature, the popular literature, and the daily news are all helpful resources.

- Learn to focus quickly on problems and criteria. Who is affected, what is the cost, who will make the decision?
- Think about possible actions to take. Vote; check the Internet for pending bills to see what is going on currently in the political arena.
- Learn to live with uncertainty. Uncertainty is present in every problem.
- Avoid a "tool box approach." Avoid using a favorite method to analyze a problem. Let the problem situation dictate the method.
- Use numbers. Try to quantify the problem: how many, how much, how often, what size. Compare to other situations.
- Use simple and clear analysis. Make certain the analysis is simple and clear so that others understand and can repeat the process.
- Be factual. Check sources, use more than one source, and understand how facts were generated.
- Be an advocate for the patient's position. Learn to provide a convincing argument.
- Present the analysis to the patients. Let the patient make the final decision.
- Push beyond the "policy envelope." Do not accept initial problem definition and alternative solutions. Be creative.

- Recognize that all analyses are incomplete. There are not enough time and resources to do a perfect analysis.

To make relevant policy decisions, one will want to monitor all events related to a policy. Be aware of the internal and external environmental issues that are ever changing and that forecast emerging problems. For example, as the health care system moves toward managed care networks, one can forecast the need for more nurses to be prepared to work in the community. Analyze the problem situation using methods previously discussed. Always critique current policies to determine what has succeeded and what has failed. Redefine the problem based on the criteria given, analyze the policymaking process, and know how one can influence the policymaking process (Abdellah, 1991). The staff nurse can apply this same process in the health care agency when a policy about nursing care is being changed, for example, use of more unlicensed assistive personnel instead of RNs.

Pitfalls to Policy Development

When attempting to analyze a policy issue, people often rely too heavily on past experiences to find solutions for a current problem. This leads to stereotyping an issue and trying to fit it into a previously used mold. Be creative and explore all possible options for problem resolution. In discussions with others or in reading materials, jot down ideas and insights about a particular issue. Be diligent and record all thoughts. They will be useful in creating a wide variety of options. Allow time to move back and forth in the steps of the policy process to avoid incorrectly defining the problem. When trying to state objectives to be met, it may become clear that the problem has not been defined correctly. In reviewing the policy alternatives, provide time to analyze each option with the stated criteria for evaluation. This will avoid bias and a preference for one alternative versus another. When talking with patients or others involved in the policy analysis, be accepting of all suggestions and avoid criticizing others' suggested options.

If suggestions of others are criticized, they may fail to offer a suggestion that could have been the best option. Include all possible alternatives, and do not rule out any based on the beliefs or bias of self or others included in the process. Reconsider alternative options previously discarded if it appears that conditions and problem definition have changed during the process of analysis (Patton & Sawicki, 1993).

Stanley (1994) has described a number of pitfalls to successful policy development:
- Inadequate knowledge about the issue
- Limited data
- Choice of inappropriate approaches
- Unclear goals and changing objectives
- Multiple approaches applied to problem resolution
- Systems resistant to change
- Problem complexity

Stanley suggests that a complex society means complex problems with no one right solution. Often decisions are delayed by policymakers for political reasons or personal choice. Also time, money, and other resources may limit how well a problem can be analyzed, resulting in less than perfect solutions. One must be prepared to use an organized approach to policy analysis, recognizing that as patients' values and interests must be considered, so must the values and interests of the policymakers.

Common Evaluation Criteria

A very simple approach to evaluating alternatives for solving an issue is that proposed by Bardach (1972). Bardach's typology includes four concepts to assist in determining whether a policy will work as intended: technical feasibility, political viability, economic/financial possibility, and administrative operability (Bardach, 1972; Patton & Sawicki, 1993). The technical feasibility of alternatives can be measured by whether one can determine that the policy outcomes will achieve their purpose. For example, will a certain program approach achieve the purpose of immunizing 80% of the children in the community? The economic/financial possibility must include an analysis of the cost of choosing an alternative in conjunction with the benefits of the alternative. Benefits may include, for example, a needed health service, reduced mortality, new knowledge, or better health. When considering political viability, one must think of the impact and reaction of power groups, such as decision makers, legislators, administrators, and citizen coalitions. Will the alternatives be acceptable or made to be acceptable? In considering administrative operability, one must consider the resources needed for each alternative: people, money, time, supplies, and space (Patton & Sawicki, 1993). As previously indicated, drawing a matrix and evaluating each alternative using four criteria are useful in prioritizing the alternatives. A point system (e.g., from 1 to 4) may be used, with 1 being lowest and 4 being highest and points ascribed to each criterion per each alternative. Summing the points will give an idea of the potential for using a particular alternative.

Policy Development and Research

Policy development is initiated via several means: the individual patient, public stimulus, substantive research, governmental entities, or organizations. The more entities involved in identifying the issue as a problem, the more likely change will occur. When many parties are interested in the issue, however, there are also diverse views, opinions, values, and competing objectives and uncertainties (Stanley, 1994).

In such instances, research can play a key role in substantiating data, evaluating documents, identifying the relevancy of a proposed solution, and analyzing past actions. Some individuals view research and policy as direct opposites. One focuses on knowledge development, whereas the other focuses on setting a course of action. Research usually takes an extensive amount of time to complete, whereas policy analysis and development are usually short term. However, research findings can play a key role in policy analysis by providing the foundation for policy development. For example, the Agency for Health Care Policy and Research has been developing clinical practice guidelines for a variety of common health problems using expert panels of providers and consumers. The primary technique used by these panels for this policy initiative is to review all research done on the common problem being considered. This research with input from power groups and other experts serves to assist these panels in developing the guidelines to be used in practice when managing a patient with the identified problem. One of the first such guidelines published was on urinary incontinence (Gaus, 1996; U.S. Department of Health and Human Services, 1992). The guidelines were based primarily on nursing research.

There are a number of stumbling blocks to using research for policy analysis. Researchers engage in a rigorous activity that involves scientific reasoning and evidence. They develop scientific and reasonable arguments to justify their research outcomes. Since researchers often disagree with one another about research outcomes and since research generally does not offer easy, quick-fix solutions to a problem, communication difficulties and differences of opinion about societal responsibilities often exist among researchers, policy developers, and policymakers. The policymaker wants a quick solution to the policy problem, whereas the patient needs ready information on staying healthy, recognizing his or her own problem, and taking an active part in treatment. Therefore it is essential for nurses to find ways to assist policymakers in valuing research findings. The researcher can do this by making information

available to policymakers through personal contact when priorities are first being set. Researchers can also influence policy decisions through consumers by presenting their research in such a way that it will be published in popular magazines and newspapers and discussed on radio and television. It is important for researchers to attend professional and political meetings to talk about their research findings (Kessler, 1989; McKeever, 1996; Orosz, 1994; Young, 1994).

The issue paper is one of the best approaches to the development of a reasoned argument for defining a problem that requires a policy resolution. Although the issue paper is often used for quick policy analysis, it may also be used by the researcher to present a solution to a problem based on prior research findings. At a minimum the issue paper includes a history of the issue, a definition, an analysis of the issue, a review of past policy to resolve the issue, and research findings to support a solution.

Issue papers should be simple because they are generally not being read by the scientific community but by consumers and policymakers. Accuracy is a must. It is important to be factual and accurate, report any inconsistencies, and refrain from going beyond the data. In documenting your analysis be certain that the analysis can be replicated by others, own any assumptions that are made, report all alternative views on the subject, cite the work of others, and pay attention to the format of the paper (Patton & Sawicki, 1993).

Although the prior discussion has focused on using patient research to support what is commonly referred to as quick policy analysis and development, there is another facet to health policy called *policy research.* Policy researchers engage in scientifically rigorous studies of policies in four areas: *content,* which are studies aimed at explaining how a policy emerged and was implemented; *process,* which are studies aimed at analyzing the influence of different factors on policy formulation and implementation; *output,* which analyzes policies in relation to social, economic, political, and other environmental factors; and *evaluation,* which analyzes the impact of a policy on a population (Orosz, 1994).

Such research assists policymakers and others in knowing the impact of policies on changing the health of a population and on solutions that have worked and do not work. Nurses are intricately involved in policy development and in recommending to others changes needed in education and practice, in accessibility of care to others, and in health care financing. Clinical research as well as research on past policies used by nursing to make practice decisions is essential to influencing the continuing practice of nurses and the importance of health policies on patients.

■ STRATEGIES FOR INFLUENCING HEALTH POLICY

Governments are significantly involved in making health care decisions. Like other systems within society today, health care is increasingly complex and officials are bombarded by issues and points of view from consumers, health providers, insurers, special interest groups, and others about the "right" policy decision. As a result these officials often turn to experts for guidance in making these decisions. At the national level officials have staff people to assist them with researching topics, writing issue papers, and analyzing policies. At the state and local levels nurses may need to be the voluntary staff to get information to officials for decision making (Box 13-4).

Health policy decisions are made in government at the federal or state level, whereas *healthy policy* is more likely to occur at the local level. Nurses' involvement in influencing such policies is critical to health care system organization, to patients' ability to afford and find

B O X   1 3 - 4

Components of Issue Paper

- History of problem
- Problem definition
- Analysis of issue
- Past policies addressing issue
- Research to support solutions
- Summary

accessible and equitable health care services, and to the nursing profession's continuing role in the delivery of preventive care and health-promoting activities.

Collaboration

Although occasionally one individual can effectively create change, it is more likely to occur when individuals with similar values collaborate with each other (Johnson, 1994). When nurses collectively join forces with one another to pursue an agreed-on goal, they empower themselves to take action. The key to success in collaborating with others is that "the sum of the whole is greater than its parts" and that a spirit of cooperation and collegiality with one another is critical in influencing policy (Mason et al., 1993).

Coalition Building

Effectiveness in influencing policy decisions increases when several groups of interested parties join together, usually temporarily, reach consensus, and are willing to support key issues. The coalition is identified as one of the most effective ways to initiate and sustain change and to garner community support. As one builds support, the chances of success increase. Coalition building requires trust building, mutual respect, a willingness to support group consensus, streamlining communication processes, building relationships with lobbyists, and making friends with public officials (Haber, 1996a).

The American Organization of Nurse Executives (1992) described the development of a unified coalition of nurse executives and managers so they could represent the best interest and concerns of nursing administrators in policy decision making. This coalition uses the following five basic strategies.

Political Advocacy Political advocacy involves lobbying legislatures on an issue, promoting agreed-on policy goals, monitoring the progress of legislation, counting congressional votes, drafting legislatures' amendments to bills to assist legislators in promoting a policy, and networking with coalition members about the happenings in government to determine the support or lack thereof by legislators debating health policy issues.

Grassroots Networking Grassroots networking is based on the philosophy that "all politics are local"; that is, politicians listen to their constituents or next-door neighbors. Thus coalition members across the United States are pulled together in a network; they are individually apprised by the coalition office of pending policy issues, and in turn the network members contact their legislators or other officials to articulate the coalition members' position on the issue.

Policy Board Membership Organizational policy boards, health care agency policy boards, governmental policy boards (e.g., state Medicaid boards), or local public health boards provide opportunities for nurses to deliberate with others and to provide nursing's perspective on an issue in order to influence the outcomes of policy decisions.

Political Action Committee Participation Many organizations or a group of organizations will come together for the purpose of supporting identified policy issues or raising awareness of the organizations' members, or the public,

about policy issues. Primarily the goal is raising awareness of public officials about problems and issues supported by the PAC. PACs raise money to support campaigns of public officials, including presidents, based on the officials' stands on issues of interest to the PAC. Nurses can influence policy by joining PACs to assist in the education of officials and the public and by contributing money to the PAC for campaign support.

Multiorganization Coalitions Joining forces with other groups in nursing, other disciplines, or consumer groups to strive to arrive at consensus on policy issues is an excellent strategy for influencing policy decisions. The greater the number of individuals represented when promoting a policy issue, the more likely a positive outcome will occur (American Organization of Nurse Executives, 1992).

• • •

Any or all of these strategies can be used for building a coalition.

Self-Empowerment

Nurses are "resource mobilizers" who can empower themselves to exert control over their own environment (Wood & Ranson, 1994). All too often, nurses, as the local constituents of public officials, underestimate their own influence in policy decisions. Nurses often think they are separated from the legislators and other public officials by distance from Washington, D.C., or their state capitol. Although nurses are the largest provider group in the United States, they do not go to the polls to vote in any greater numbers than other citizens, yet that is where influence can be duly made (Bocchino & Wakefield, 1992).

Individual nurses can use many strategies to influence policy decisions. Meetings by appointment with public officers are important contacts for expressing policy issue views. Telephone calls and correspondence that describe a problem and offer a solution can be helpful to the official in developing a proposal for change. Inviting public officials or their staff to visit a clinic for the homeless may help the officials to better understand what policy changes are needed to provide better care for that population, for example. Using local, state, and national media can make a difference in a policy outcome. Few will forget the "Harry and Louise Go to Washington" commercials on television in the mid-1990s that so effectively encouraged consumers' negative views about President Clinton's plan for health care reform (West et al., 1996). Writing a letter to the local newspaper editor praising the local congressperson who supported a bill to require insurance companies to provide comprehensive health insurance coverage for children will make the nurse a new friend in the legislature, or joining the local radio talk show host to discuss the harmful effects of secondhand smoke on children and requesting listeners to call their legislators to vote "no" to tobacco subsidies will create major influence. Legislators often count the number of phone calls and letters received to determine their vote on a particular issue.

Haber (1996b) provided guidelines that are helpful for developing relationships with public officials:

1. Make an appointment by calling or writing your legislator at home or at the capitol.
2. Clearly identify the issue you want to discuss and rehearse what you plan to say. Decide how many people should go with you and who should go to visit the official.
3. Set a definite agenda; prepare examples and facts to illustrate your position.
4. Use facts, figures, and consumer-driven vignettes to support the desired change.
5. Arrive on time, and identify yourself as a constituent and a nurse. If the legislator is busy, meet with one of his or her aides, par-

ticularly the staff person for health care issues.
6. Be prepared to discuss the issues. Familiarize yourself with your legislator's previous position on this issue.
7. Keep the atmosphere open and friendly. You are there to exchange ideas and gain your legislator's support; if that is not possible, keep the lines of communication open.
8. If you do not know the answer to a question that the legislator asks, say so. Explain that you will get the information, and then be sure to follow through. That is an opportunity for another contact.
9. Leave some literature on the subject and your business card with the legislator.
10. Follow up your visit with a thank-you note and perhaps more information on the issues discussed.

There are a number of ways to get your message to those involved in making decisions about health policy (Box 13-5). One cardinal rule is to never threaten to withhold votes or money if the official does not agree with your position.

B O X   1 3 - 5

Carrying Your Message: the Menu of Choices

Face to face	Fact sheets
Letters	Executive summaries
Mailgrams	Letters to the editor
Fax sheet	News releases
Telegrams	Speeches
E-mail	Forming coalitions
Providing testimony	Demonstrations
Issues report	Litigations
Position papers	

Developed for policy workshop presentation by Cary, A., & Stanhope, M. (1992). Workshop at Eastern Kentucky University. Richmond, Ky.

It is important to be involved individually, collectively with others, or through coalitions. Timing is critical in the delivery of messages, and diplomacy is essential. The ability to influence policy is primarily one of communication, using critical thinking and problem-solving abilities to define and analyze the issue and present a reasoned argument for change.

■ KEY POINTS

- Policies are essential during times of rapid change, and they are simply guides to decision making that govern a planned course of action designed to solve a problem.
- Health policies are needed because they set forth measurable and obtainable objectives to guide the scope of health care delivery.
- Healthy policy, in contrast, places health as a priority, and it focuses on identifying the strengths and resources of the group and its environment.
- Policies can be analyzed in a variety of ways. Methods of policy analysis in this chapter include the following: the rational model for policy analysis that is a six-step iterative problem-solving process; the quick decision analysis that uses a decision to think carefully about the problem and possible alternatives; and the strengths approach that focuses on an assessment of the strengths of the people and their environment and is largely used for developing a healthy policy.
- There are a variety of useful hints when one becomes involved in the development of health policy, including learning to focus quickly on problems and criteria and thinking about possible actions. Living with uncertainty, being factual, advocating for the patient's position, presenting the analysis to the patient, and recognizing that all analyses, no matter how good, are incomplete are just some of the useful principles for policymakers.

- Policymaking can fail when there is insufficient information, none of the possible approaches are useful, the goals are unclear or the objectives keep changing, the problem is complex or the systems are resistant to change, and multiple approaches are tried for handling the same policy.
- An issue paper is an excellent way to focus on the work that needs to be done to influence policy. Such a paper would include a history and definition of the problem, an analysis of the issue, and an understanding of past policies that pertain to the issue, as well as research that will support possible solutions and a summary.
- Some of the most useful strategies for influencing health policy include collaboration, coalition building, and self-empowerment.

■ CRITICAL THINKING QUESTIONS

1. Identify an issue that you have observed in one of your clinical areas. What are the concerns that led to this issue? If you were going to devise a purposive course of action to deal with the concerns you have observed, how would you proceed? Specifically, what is the concern? Who should be involved in the design of a policy to resolve this concern? In a stepwise fashion, develop a plan for policy development.

2. Similarly identify an issue or concern in a social group to which you belong. Who would you engage in your pursuit of a new policy? Using the strengths approach, devise a strategy for designing a policy to achieve a positive outcome for the identified issue or concern.

3. Assume you are going to be actively involved in the development of a healthy policy that affects the community in which you live. Pick a particular concern in that community, such as the high rate of hypertension or diabetes among men aged 35 to 50 years, lack of

safe playgrounds for children younger than 5 years, or the high rate of teen drinking that appears related to automobile accidents. Once you have picked an issue, describe how you would do the following:

A. Increase public knowledge about the relationship between health and one's behavior.

B. Develop a unified, organized approach to interest others in the policy you wish to develop.

C. Educate the public, including your elected officials, about ways to solve the problem.

4. Using the issue or concern selected for question 3, apply the tips for avoiding pitfalls to outline your specific plan of action. How would you know you had sufficient data? Where would you get it? Who would be available to help you? What type of resistance might you expect? Given that resistance is likely, how would you counter it to achieve a positive outcome?

5. Using the issue above or selecting another issue of keen interest to you, write an issue paper that will help you both clearly identify the problem and design a policy to solve it.

■ REFERENCES

Abdellah, F. (1991). *Health policy.* Washington, D.C.: American Academy of Nursing.

American Organization of Nurse Executives. (1992). Influencing health care policy. *Nursing Management, 23,* 18-19.

Anderson, J. (1975). *Public policy making.* New York: Holt, Praeger.

Backer, B. (1991). You can get there from here: Guide to problem definition in policy development. *Journal of Psychosocial Nursing, 27(10),* 24.

Bardach (1972). *The implementation game.* Cambridge, Mass.: MIT Press.

Bocchino, C., & Wakefield, M. (1992). Forces influencing public policy. *Nursing Economics, 10(1),* 53.

Branch, L. (1994, Spring). The development of health promotion guidelines and recommendations. *Generations,* p. 24.

Cary, A., & Stanhope, M. (1992). Workshop at Eastern Kentucky University, Richmond, Ky. Unpublished.

Chapin, R. (1995). Social policy development: The strengths perspectives. *Social Work, 40(4),* 508.

Etizioni, A. (1967). Mixed scanning: A third approach to decision making. *Public Administration Review, 27(5),* 385.

Flynn, B. (1995). Building partnerships for healthy public policy. *Nursing Policy Forums, 2(6),* 6.

Gaus, C. (1996). Future directions for the Agency for Health Care Policy and Research. *American Journal of Medical Quality, 11(1),* 526.

Haber, J. (1996a). Coalition building: An effective vehicle for achieving legislative changes. *Journal of the American Psychiatric Nurses Association, 2(4),* 127.

Haber, J. (1996b). Cultivating grassroots political savvy. *Journal of the American Psychiatric Nurses Association, 2(2),* 58.

Hanley, B. (1993). Policy development and analysis. In D. Mason, S. Talbott, & J. Leavitt (Eds.). *Policy and politics for nursing* (2nd ed.). Philadelphia: Saunders.

Johnson, K. (1994, March/April). Influencing public policy through collaboration. *Nursing Policy Forum,* p. 31.

Kessler, D. (1995). The evolution of national nutrition policy. *Annual Review of Nutrition, 15(1),* 22.

Kessler, T. (1989). Research & policy formation: Is there a fit. *Journal of Professional Nursing, 5(5),* 246.

Kingdom, J. (1984). *Agendas, alternatives and public policy.* Boston: Little, Brown.

Lindblom, C., & Woodhouse, E. (1993). *The policy making process* (3rd ed.). Englewood Cliffs, N.J.: Prentice-Hall.

Mason, D., Talbott, S., & Leavitt, J. (1993). *Policy and politics for nurses* (2nd ed.). Philadelphia: Saunders.

McKeever, P. (1996). The family: Long term care research and policy formulation. *Nursing Inquiry, 3,* 200.

McRae, D., & Wilder, J. (1979). *Policy analysis for public decisions.* North Scituate, Mass.: Duxbury Press.

Orosz, E. (1994). The impact of social service on health policy. *Social Science & Medicine, 39(9),* 1287.

Parsons, W. (1995). *Public policy: An introduction to the theory and practice of policy analysis.* Cheltenham, U.K.: Edward Elgar.

Patton, C., & Sawicki, D. (1993). *Basic methods of policy analysis and planning* (2nd ed.). Englewood Cliffs, N.J.: Prentice-Hall.

Quade, E. (1982). *Analysis for public decisions.* New York: Elsevier Scientific.

Rastogi, P. (1992). *Policy analysis and problem solving for social systems.* London: Sage.

Stanhope, M. (1995). Primary health care practice: Is nursing part of the solution or the problem? *Family & Community Health, 18*(1), 49.

Stanley, S. (1994). Crafting mental health policy. *Nursing Clinics of North America, 29*(1), 19.

Stokey, E., & Zeckhauser, R. (1978). *A primer for policy analysis.* New York: Norton.

Sultz, H. (1991). Health policy: If you don't know where you're going, any road will take you. *American Journal of Public Health, 81*(4), 418.

Swansburg, R. (1996). *Management and leadership for nurse managers* (2nd ed.). Sudbury, Mass.: Jones & Bartlett.

Takarangi, J., & North, P. (1990). Healthy cities on international movement: Are we ready to participate? *Nursing Praxis in New Zealand, 5*(2), 7.

U.S. Department of Health and Human Services. (1979). *Healthy people: The surgeon general's report on health promotion and disease prevention.* USPHS pub. no. 79-55071. Washington, D.C.: The Department.

U.S. Department of Health and Human Services. (1990). *Healthy people 2000.* USPHS pub. no. 91-50213. Washington, D.C.: The Department.

U.S. Department of Health and Human Services. (1992). *Urinary incontinence: Clinical practice guideline no. 1.* AHCPR pub. no. 92-0041. Rockville, Md.: Agency for Health Care Policy and Research.

Weimer, D., & Vining, A. (1989). *Policy analysis: Concepts & practice.* Englewood Cliffs, N.J.: Prentice-Hall.

West, D., Heith, D., & Goodwin, C. (1996). Harry & Louise go to Washington: Political advertising and health care reform. *Journal of Health Politics, Policy & Law, 21*(1), 35.

Wood, S., & Ranson, V. (1994). The 1990s: A decade for change in women's health care policy. *Journal of Obstetric, Gynecologic, and Neonatal Nursing 23*(2), 139.

World Health Organization. (1978). *Primary health care report* (3rd ed.). Geneva: WHO UNICEF.

Young, D. (1994). Using research plus community action to change national health policy. *Birth, 21*(1), 2.

Ethical Issues in Nursing Practice

Lynn Noland

INTRODUCTION

Moral questions are fundamentally questions about what to do. . . . Moral knowledge is knowledge about what to do or what attitude to take toward what has been done, is being done, or is intended (Nelson, 1967, p. 130).

We are born within covenants of life with life. By nature, choice or need we live with our fellowmen in roles or relations. Therefore we must ask, what is the meaning of the faithfulness of one human being to another . . . This is the ethical question (Ramsey, 1970, p.xiii).

Health professional education encompasses a rich blend of knowledge from multiple disciplines. The basic sciences are clearly crucial for the education of nurses and physicians; however, other areas of study, such as ethics, are equally important to be a successful practitioner in today's complex health care environment. Because ethics is an important but at times underemphasized component of nursing curricula, it is useful to review and supplement ethical subject matter for nurses and other health professionals. This chapter assists nurses to acquire a minimal working knowledge of ethics by introducing basic elements of ethical knowledge and an approach for analyzing ethical issues and by using case examples to display ethical thought and analysis.

It is clear that in the years ahead there will continue to be unprecedented ethical challenges for health care professionals. A major concern will be whether nurses and others can continue to practice ethically in the wake of health care reform and ongoing fiscal restraint that at best places tension on key covenants with patients. Questions such as "What should be done if patients cannot obtain needed referrals from their health maintenance organization (HMO)?" or "How do I respond if patients are not offered care because they cannot pay?" will probably increase in number. Solutions for these and other ethical problems in today's complex settings are elusive without a working knowledge of health care ethics.

Health care ethics is a subset of normative philosophic ethics. The subject matter of normative ethics provides guidance for and knowledge of how people ought to live, what behaviors might be considered good or bad, and how those behaviors are to be justified. When the subject matter of normative ethics is used in a health care context to resolve ethical problems, it is referred to as *health care* or

Key terms	
Term	**Definition**
Ethics	Formal study of ways of conceptualizing and understanding the moral life; the subject matter of ethics helps to determine what is meant by right, wrong, good, or bad behavior; this is accomplished in part by defining ethical terms
Normative ethics	Area of inquiry that seeks to determine which approach or action is the most ethically desirable in a given situation
Health care ethics	Use of the methods of normative ethics to resolve ethical issues in health care settings

biomedical ethics. Understanding health care ethics assists nurses to make informed ethical choices. Ethics in this context is used to determine objective standards for judging professional behaviors to be right or wrong in health care settings.

These are difficult times for health care professionals, and as such the need for the content and guidance of health care ethics is especially important. Rachels (1995, p. 3) writes ". . . moral guidance is most needed when times are hardest and temptation is the greatest." The current environment fits well with Rachel's imagery of hard times and great temptations. There are growing pressures in health care environments to make quick, cheap, and ethical decisions. Responding to these pressures may present goals that are in constant tension with one another, and some may be mutually exclusive. The reasons for ethical tensions are varied: the pace of the work has accelerated, there are competing priorities and agendas, technologic innovation has broadened the possibilities of intervention, and radical changes have occurred in health care financing and delivery because of economic necessity. The list continues indefinitely, and these and other reasons are certainly important, but by far the most significant reason is that a major paradigm shift has occurred in the way health care is conceptualized and delivered.

OBJECTIVES

After reading this chapter, you will be able to:

1. Explain relevant concepts and theories of ethics
2. Evaluate common ethical conflicts associated with the current practice environment
3. Analyze the dominant ethical principles, rules, and values of nursing
4. Use at least one method for resolving ethical conflicts
5. Explain ways to practice preventive ethics in nursing practice

■ WHAT DOES THE NEW PARADIGM LOOK LIKE?

Health care is currently viewed as a commodity to be traded like any other, with patients or their insurers being the purchasers of the product, which is health care. For-profit HMOs view patients as desirable assets—that is, as long as patients use minimal services. This means that ever-expanding patient enrollment and strict cost containment are necessary to maintain the solvency of the HMO. There is no legislated universal right to health care access in the United States, and there probably will not be in the near future. It is now clear that in the United States, health care is distributed for the most part according to ability to pay rather than need. Health care is available primarily through employment or as an entitlement for limited populations such as very poor patients, elderly patients, and patients with end-stage renal disease. Health care delivery is increasingly seen as a profitable industry operated according to business principles. If there is any doubt about this, consider the number of lucrative health care stocks currently traded on Wall Street.

These characteristics of the new health care paradigm may initiate radical changes in the way nursing care is delivered to patients. There is nothing inherently morally good or bad about many of these changes. What makes them ethically questionable is the way that they are enacted and who wins or loses in the process. If the most vulnerable people in society are the sole losers, the changes that have been made are problematic according to nursing's professional code of ethics. If all citizens share equally in the sacrifices to be made, perhaps there is no ethical problem. Although nurses may not like the way the health care delivery system is changing, these changes may not reflect an unethical system. At present there is limited objective evidence that ethical standards are being consistently compromised. At best, only isolated cases can be found. It is crucial, however, for nurses to be able to critically evaluate proposed plans and actions and to be knowledgeable enough to determine whether the suggested changes are ethically sound or reflect ethically questionable practices in the delivery of health care.

■ NURSES AS ACTIVE PARTNERS TO CHANGE

Nurses should be active partners in bringing about change that is enacted for the right reasons and in the right ways. The historical legacy of nursing, the American Nurses Association's (ANA's) *Code for Nurses,* and the public's trust in the profession require that nurses be a party to change only if it can be seen ultimately to benefit and in no way harm patients. To assist with this goal and to ensure that public trust is not violated, nurses need to be able to actively analyze the environment in which they work to determine if proposed changes will enable them to meet their ethical obligations to patients. To do this effectively, nurses need to know their obligations, be familiar with ethics in general, and understand ethical issues that specifically relate to their area of practice.

The first part of the chapter reviews general ethical knowledge by briefly discussing ethical concepts, such as theories of ethics, ethical principles and rules, professional values, and ethical decision-making frameworks. This information serves as background material for the second half of the chapter, which focuses on how to think through ethical problems associated with three common types of ethical issues. This section ends with a brief discussion of strategies for preventive ethics. The chapter is designed to assist nurses to both lead change and adapt to it and to find ways to practice ethically regardless of the type of change that occurs.

■ UNIQUE NATURE OF ETHICAL KNOWLEDGE

There is an assumption in the health professions that a technically proficient practitioner is an ethical practitioner; that if one understands the science of the field, the rest of the knowledge needed to become an expert practitioner will follow. Both of these assumptions are naive. Analysis of ethical problems requires a different database than is found in either clinical professional education or the scientific disciplines. Clinical knowledge, technical knowledge, and scientific knowledge are only part of the knowledge needed for sound professional practice. Ethical knowledge is also necessary and unique in its contribution. For health care professionals to obtain needed ethical knowledge, ethics should be studied separately or, at the very least, aggressively integrated into professional education. Simply put, practitioners require a critical mass of ethical theory to make sound ethical decisions. There is no substitute for formal ethical knowledge; practitioners who do not have the benefit of ethical knowledge are at increased risk for unethical practice. Understandably this possibility is magnified as the pace at which decisions are made is accelerated. The following section briefly describes some of the key elements of formal ethical knowledge commonly used to construct a sound professional ethic.

■ CONSTRUCTING A PERSONAL AND PROFESSIONAL ETHIC

For most people a primary personal existential goal is to lead an ethical life. Likewise, professionally, a primary goal is to practice as ethically as possible. It is reasonable then to think that nurses can develop a strategy for linking both goals; the use of a metaphor is helpful. Developing an ethical practice or leading an ethical life requires careful construction; in fact, it can be compared to building a house. A house is constructed with clear intent from a distinct plan. If the plan is well conceived, the outcome is a predictable, desirable structure. Likewise, leading an ethical life requires a carefully thought-out plan. If the plan is followed, the outcome should be logically consistent and reflect justified responses to ethical dilemmas. Building a house also requires a variety of materials chosen for strength and performance. The same is true of one's ethical life; that is, the materials must be thoughtfully chosen to meet the goal. The materials for constructing the ethical life are cognitive materials and coherent ethical standards, not bricks and boards. To extend the metaphor, both the house and one's ethical life must be built on a firm foundation, or they will not stand the test of time. The foundation of a house is engineered to support the activities that need to occur in it; not to do so conjures up images such as the clear fate of a house of cards or of a house built on shifting sand. The same is true of an individual's ethical life. The foundation must be sound; if it is not, decisions and actions that result will be inconsistent, incoherent, and unjustifiable. Clear ethical standards form the foundation and superstructure needed to lead an ethical life. Foundations adequately constructed, whether real or metaphoric, support one's actions in life and help to provide sufficient justification for ethical decisions.

The above discussion demonstrates that there is nothing magical or mystical about making ethical decisions. It is a planned cognitive process. One of the most effective ways of assisting in this process is to work for consistency between one's personal and professional ethic. The ethical concepts and ideals that serve in one part of life can and should serve well in all other aspects of life. If choices across life's varied contexts are justified by consistent and well-thought-out ethical concepts, making ethical decisions becomes a matter of relating and expanding familiar standards to new situations. For example, to believe that it is wrong to lie to patients but acceptable to lie to one's spouse is inconsistent logic and does not help to establish coherent internal standards needed to become adept at making ethical decisions. Achieving consistency between personal ethics and professional ethics does not mean that variations in interpretation of ethical standards will not exist across contexts. For example, the magnitude of ethical decisions and their consequences is likely to be different in professional practice than it is in social relationships. What constitutes beneficence or the intent to do good in one situation may be somewhat different in another. Helping a friend make decisions during an illness certainly requires different obligations than providing professional support and guidance to a patient or family making a decision to stop or start a new therapy. However, the intent and the basic generic idea of beneficence remain the same—to do good or to actively benefit the person or the patient involved. One thing is certain, a *prior* commitment to upholding a principle such as beneficence will allow for more intentionality and consistency of behavior across personal and professional relationships. Also, nursing practice will be more comprehensive the more informed and thoughtful nurses are about ethical concepts and principles. Pragmatically, once ethical knowledge is obtained, it is truly transferable across all life circumstances.

■ ETHICAL CONCEPTS: BUILDING BLOCKS OF THE ETHICAL LIFE

To expand the building metaphor: whereas the foundational elements of a house are block and mortar, the foundational elements of ethics and ethical practice are basic moral concepts, such as values, rules, and principles.

In science or any other discipline a foundational element is the most basic unit of any compound, organic structure, or organism. For example, oxygen is a foundational element of the

Key terms	
Term	**Definition**
Value	A cherished belief that one is willing to act on
Rule	A specific prescriptive action guide, usually expressed as an imperative; many ethical rules exist
Principle	An action guide that is more universal and general than a rule; only a few broad-based ethical principles exist

compound water, and amino acids are foundational elements of a protein molecule. Foundational elements are simply building blocks for more complex structures. Foundational elements in ethics are building blocks for the construction of sound moral responses. Purtillo (1993, p. 17) refers to ethical norms as elements because they are similar to chemical elements. She reasons that chemical elements, like ethical elements, have different properties both alone and in combination. For example, they may have different weights, or they may conflict or interact.

By definition, values are cherished beliefs that a person is willing to act on. If people do not act on what they say that they value, all that they really have are noble ideas. Ideas alone are insufficient support for the grounding of a person's ethical life. To embrace an ideal as a value there must be an observable compatible action. For example, if nurses say that patient confidentiality is a value but then read the records of a well-known person out of curiosity, patient confidentiality is a nice idea but not a value. This conclusion is consistent with the knowledge that ethical values not only involve thoughts and decisions about what constitutes right or wrong

B O X   1 4 - 1

Ethical Values

Values are beliefs, purposes, and attitudes that are:
- Freely chosen
- Prized
- Acted on

Data from Raths, L., Harmin, M., & Simon, S. (1978). *Values and teaching* (2nd ed.) (p. 28). Columbus, Ohio: Charles E. Merrill.

behavior, but also, by definition, have an action component that is consistent with the cognitive element of the decision (Box 14-1).

There are both moral and nonmoral values. One way to identify a moral value is that when the value is violated, the individual who does so will likely experience pangs of conscience or feelings of guilt or wrongdoing (Rokeach, 1973). This outcome can usually be anticipated in advance. By contrast, food, color, and reading preferences are examples of nonmoral values, and action in regard to these preferences does not evoke strong emotion if violated. In the examples of moral values that follow, note the requisite action component of each:

- If a nurse subscribes to the value of truthfulness, this means, among other things, that patients will not be knowingly deceived.
- If a nurse embraces the value of mercy, part of what this value means is that she or he will not allow a patient to suffer unnecessarily if the means and authority to prevent suffering are available.
- If a nurse says that she or he values mercy but takes a work break before administering requested pain medication, maybe mercy is a nice idea but not yet a confirmed value.

■ HOW DO PEOPLE ACQUIRE VALUES?

People acquire values in a number of ways. They first are learned from parents. As a sense of

reason and judgment begins to develop in young children, parents teach them that some behaviors are desirable or good and other behaviors are undesirable or bad. Good behaviors may include telling the truth, sharing with others, or demonstrating kindness. Initially, children are not always sure why they should conform to ethical teachings. Generally, they do so primarily because parents and other authority figures advocate for certain behaviors, reinforce them, and punish children for the absence of these expected behaviors. Eventually good behaviors are internalized and become habits. A person's value system is influenced by the education system, peer group, spiritual groups, religious institutions, and culture. These sources help form a value system that is firmly established by the time students enter a nursing education program. Nursing education deepens participants' moral values by conveying an understanding of what it means to practice ethically and by providing objective justification for what is believed to be morally correct. This ability to think through situations and provide justification for moral values develops mature moral agents. If early values education is thorough, professional ethics will seem like a natural extension of the student's ongoing personal ethics education. People are not born knowing how to be ethical personally or professionally; instead, behaving ethically is a learned skill that can be modeled and taught just as clinical skills are taught. This is a lifelong learning experience because the acquisition of values is dynamic—not static. This means that values change with maturation, time, and exposure to people and situations (Uustal, 1987).

■ CLARIFYING VALUES

To effectively act on values, the values must be consciously accessible. Values are tools that are used to construct ethical practice, and as such, several authors think that to properly use them it is important to actually clarify them to oneself.

"The clearer you are about what you value, the more able you are to choose and initiate a response that is consistent with what you say you believe. The quality of your decision making is a direct reflection of a clear vision of your values" (Uustal, 1987, p. 151). Uustal offers a series of values clarification exercises that are useful to further explicate and shape values. In these exercises she addresses such areas as philosophy of nursing, childhood value messages, and comparison of emerging trends in health care with personal value systems. This type of self-reflective process is highly recommended because it allows more effective preparation for the times when value conflicts occur.

■ HOW DO PROFESSIONS CONVEY VALUES TO THEIR MEMBERS?

Each profession by definition has a code of ethics. Ethical values are contained in the code, and members of the profession are expected to incorporate the values into their practice. For example, there are several obvious values in the ANA's *Code for Nurses* (1985), such as respecting human dignity, protecting privacy, maintaining competence, and being honest with patients. By reading the code a nurse knows generally how to practice ethically. The code, however, should not be viewed as the sum total of what it means to practice ethically. It is a skeleton, with sound but minimal guidance for ethical practice. Special cases may require more knowledge on the part of the nurse to ensure ethical practice.

One area that the code does not assist in is how to make an ethical decision when ethical values are in conflict. For example, the code does not help to determine what to do ethically when there is a difference of opinion between the patient and any of the involved health care professionals. This situation requires ethical conflict resolution, an acquired skill. This type of skill is developed by obtaining formal ethical knowledge as taught in ethics courses, semi-nars, and lectures and through mentoring and role-modeling situations. The fine points of ethical reasoning and justification are not self-evident in these settings and situations but are learned.

■ ETHICAL RULES AND PRINCIPLES: FLESHING OUT THE BOUNDARIES

Values are one of the primary foundational elements of the ethical life. Rules and principles are additional elements that provide further structure for ethical practice. Rules and principles establish boundaries that provide context and content for an individual's work. Rules are not foreign to nurses; in the health professions, nurses constantly practice under the guidance of rules of clinical practice. There are pharmacologic rules, such as "Do not mix certain drugs together in an intravenous solution or they will precipitate." There are physical rules, such as "Use hot packs on a patient's arm to vasodilate a vein before venipuncture." There are also ethical rules, such as "Do not violate patient confidentiality; keep your promises to patients; do not deceive patients." Behind the rules lies a professional value system that enables nurses to create generally agreed-on ethical rules to guide and justify behavior in relation to patients. Rules are basic action guides that are frequently expressed as imperatives (Nelson, 1967, p. 131) (Box 14-2).

Ethical rules are part of the body of knowledge referred to as *general moral belief* or *common morality.* Their purpose is to provide common ground to begin deliberations about what should be done in any given case. Without commonly agreed-on rules as starting points for discussion, decisions may appear subjective. Rules as starting points for ethical discussion provide a standard other than one's own opinion that allows others to argue for or against a specific ethical position. If that were the case, why should one opinion be any more convincing than another? The response is that the best opin-

BOX 14-2

Rules of Conduct

Morality or ethicality involves rules of conduct. Just as there are rules of conduct for various forms of human interaction, such as a baseball game, a board game, or a formal dinner party, there are rules of conduct for professional interaction with patients . . . moral behavior is also a rule-governed activity . . . [moral behavior is] a complex cluster of practices with procedural rules that define those practices.

From Nielson, K. (1967). Problems of ethics. In P. Edwards (Ed.). *The encyclopedia of philosophy* (Vol. 3). New York: MacMillan.

BOX 14-3

Four Ethical Principles for Health Care Decision Making

1. Respect for autonomy: an obligation to respect competent individuals' inherent right to make their own decisions
2. Nonmaleficence: an obligation to avoid inflicting harm
3. Beneficence: an obligation to positively benefit another
4. Justice: an obligation to fairly distribute benefits (goods) and burdens (risks or harms) to people who have a legitimate claim to a given benefit or good

From Beauchamp, T.L., & Childress, J.F. (1994). *Principles of biomedical ethics* (4th ed.). New York: Oxford University Press.

ion is supported by the best ethical reasoning and rules are a significant part of sound ethical reasoning. Thus both values and rules are important foundational elements of ethical decision making. There is another crucial ethical element that should be discussed as well—ethical principles.

Ethical Principles

Ethical principles are more universal action guides than ethical rules or values. Whereas rules and values are more restricted and narrow in scope, principles are general and fundamental. Jonsen (1994, p. 18) says of moral principles that ". . . they are not unlike sky marks used in celestial navigation: A position is determined and a course marked by continual reference to fixed points such as sun, stars, and planets. . . . The principles provide an indispensable general guiding direction." They do not define the course precisely like mathematical coordinates would, but they serve as ever visible guides to keep people on course.

Beauchamp and Childress (1994) refer to principles as general guides that leave consider-

able room for judgment in specific cases. As such they provide guidance for the development of more detailed rules and policies or, to use the navigation metaphor, coordinates. Principles are the framework, the skeleton of ethical decision making. Ethical values and rules flesh out the more specific meanings of the principles and by doing so provide more specific guidance for action. Principles provide boundaries that should not be exceeded without justified reasons. Rules and values define the terrain. Bound together, ethical principles, rules, and values give substance or specific meaning to the ethical life.

Beauchamp and Childress (1994) described four primary principles (Box 14-3) with corresponding norms. These are the standards that guide nurses (and physicians) in ethical decision making. Other authors use these four principles as a foundation for what counts as ethical behavior. Some add or subtract one or more principles, but most agree that principle-driven decision making is logical and functional. The principles themselves rarely guide specific actions. The more specific action guides or the ethical rules that are generated from the principles are, the more effectively can they guide action. The rules help people arrive at specific judgments. In fact, the four principles are described as being more like clusters of ethical guidelines in that each is the embodiment of a group of norms or rules that when adhered to will give moral substance to the principles (Beauchamp & Childress, 1994, p. 38). Rules then are necessary ethical standards that give content and specificity to the broader principle. An example of rules giving specificity to principles is the rule that nurses ought not to deceive patients about the expected benefit of a particular intervention. The rule gives content to the principle of respect for autonomy. With this rule in place intentional deception would then clearly violate the principle. Without these types of specific rules the principles are idyllic and somewhat vacuous. The four principles and associated ethical rules are represented in Box 14-4. The four principles are consistent values in nursing practice. The ANA's *Code for Nurses* states clearly that nurses base their decisions on consideration of these principles and rules. The code, however, takes the position that respect for persons is the most important principle for nursing, thus setting it above the other three.

Should ethical principles be thought of as absolute? Beauchamp and Childress (1994) suggest that principles should be considered binding but *not* absolutely so. Instead, principles (and rules) are considered to be prima facie binding, meaning that they should be adhered to unless a strong moral argument is offered to override them. Further, if they are overridden, they do not disappear; they leave what Nozick (1968) refers to as "moral traces" or moral repercussions. To illustrate the serious nature of setting aside moral principles, Beauchamp and Childress (1994, p. 53) say that overriding moral

---

B O X   1 4 - 4

Ethical Principles and Corresponding Rules

Nonmaleficence: refrain from inflicting harm of any type especially in the form of suffering, death, or disability

Beneficence: be kind, merciful, competent, safe, and helpful (This includes prompt treatment of pain, nonabandonment, and promotion of health and well-being.)

Respect for individual autonomy: keep promises, maintain confidentiality, be truthful, avoid coercion, preserve dignity, provide informed consent

Justice: provide indicated treatment regardless of differences; allocate resources according to a logical, fair, and objective method

---

principles or rules should be undertaken not only conscientiously but also with regret on the part of the agent doing so.

As nursing's patient populations become more diverse, it is of interest to note that because principles are more general in nature, it is likely that they may generate more consensus across cultural boundaries than values or rules. This would help to explain how nurses can speak generically of a concept such as human rights and have a broad notion of what a violation of human rights might mean (i.e., an infringement of the principle of respect for the autonomy of every person). Logically this makes ethical principles an ideal starting point when working in an international setting. However, it is important to recognize that specific rules that arise from these same principles might be quite different in different cultures. For example, in a conversation the author had with a Chinese graduate student, the student said that in her culture people often considered it a benevolent act to deceive patients about

Key terms	
Term	**Definition**
Theory	An organized explanation of particular phenomena; basic components of a theory: principles, or basic assumptions believed to be true
Consequentialism	Set of ethical theories that assume an act is ethical if it produces desired outcomes; the right act is the one that produces the best overall outcome or outcomes
Kantian deontology	Ethical theory that assumes an act is right when the agent behaves according to prescribed duties and obligations that preserve the dignity of each person
Utilitarianism	Most well-known consequentialist theory that assumes an act is right if it produces the greatest possible value over disvalue; the definition of what is to be valued might vary according to who is interpreting the issue

the gravity of their illnesses, whereas in the United States this type of deception violates the principle of autonomy and would not be considered beneficent generally.

In summary, ethical principles and rules are the raw materials, the foundational elements for constructing ethical responses to ethical conflicts. How principles, rules, and values are configured and conceptualized and how they are specified, weighted, or prioritized will determine which option is selected. The most ethically correct option in a given case can be decided in a variety of ways; several will be discussed here after a brief review of how to think about ethical theory.

Ethical Theories

A theory in any field is an organized explanation of particular phenomena. Explanation in a theory is accomplished by principles or basic premises assumed to be true based on evidence. Scientific theory with which professionals are well familiar in the health sciences is used to explain natural phenomena. For example, the germ theory of disease uses principles of microbiology to explain the etiology of infectious dis-

eases. The theory of solutions and their movement across membranes uses the physical principles of osmosis and diffusion to explain how dialysis clears metabolic waste products from the blood. Ethical theories use ethical principles and their corresponding rules to explain what constitutes ethical behavior. Several ethical theories are proposed. This chapter discusses two of the most prominent: utilitarianism, a form of consequentialism; and kantian deontology. Each emphasizes a different principle in an effort to explain what counts as ethical behavior.

Consequentialism   Consequentialism involves subtheories that state that an act is ethical if it produces desired outcomes. The outcomes may take different forms; for example, an act is ethical if it produces the greatest good for the greatest number of people or if it yields the greatest net benefit over burden. The right act is simply the one that produces the best overall outcome regardless of how the best outcome is defined. A predominant subtheory of this sort is utilitarianism. Only one principle, utility, receives consideration in the context of utilitarianism. In utilitarian theories, the interests of all parties are weighted equally. Utility asserts that "we ought always to produce the maximal balance of positive value over disvalue (or the least possible disvalue, if only undesirable results can be achieved)" (Beauchamp & Childress, 1994, p. 47). One might already begin to anticipate how this premise would influence ethical decision making. Some of the questions that are commonly asked in relation to this theory are as follows: Who determines what (or whose) good is of greatest value in a given situation? Does the theory bias decision making in the direction of the majority and knowingly sacrifice the interests of the few in favor of the many? If it does, is this morally acceptable in the context of the patient/provider relationship? Certainly nurses will face these sorts of questions more frequently as they enter more deeply into managed care reimbursement systems.

Deontology The second type of theory is deontology, specifically for purposes of this chapter, kantian deontology. In 1781 Immanuel Kant, a German philosopher, wrote the supreme counterpoint to utilitarian moral theory. He rejected utility as a primary moral principle and proposed instead that the rightness or wrongness of human actions is to be considered totally independent of the goodness or badness of consequences (Mappes & Zembaty, 1981, p. 6). At the heart of kantian deontology (deontology is derived from the Greek *deonto* meaning duty) is the notion that people are acting correctly when they act according to prescribed duties and obligations that respect the dignity of each human being. Persons are to be respected because, as humans, they stand alone in the created order. They occupy a special place in the world and consequently are owed certain generic responses. Given this, Kant proposed several maxims (Box 14-5) to help decide how to know what is ethically correct. His first maxim, referred to as the *categorical imperative,* was

---

B O X 1 4 - 5

Maxims of Kant

1. An act is morally right if and only if it is universalizable.
2. An act is morally right if and only if the agent performing it refrains from treating any person solely as a means to an end.

---

that an act is morally right if and only if it is universalizable. This means that if people say that an act is right, they would want it applied to all persons and to similar situations without reservation. His second maxim is one that he argued should be consistently followed and applied as well. "An act is morally right if and only if the agent who is performing it refrains from treating any person merely as a means." These two notions are the crux of morality for Kant. If you never see people as objects for personal gain but instead see them as "a sacredness in the social and political order" (Ramsey, 1970, p. xiii), then theoretically all persons' (and patients') autonomy should be respected. This for Kant would equate to ethical treatment. Kant's theory has a few limitations, but it is still a primary starting point for persons who reject the idea that all that is important in ethical decision making is the end result. In deontologic theories, both intent and how people achieve the end result are important, not just the end result itself, as in consequentialist theories. The principle of autonomy becomes a supreme value in deontologic theories, in contrast to the principle of utility, which is of greatest import in consequentialist theories.

A discussion of theory is useful in that it helps to demonstrate how educated people can end up so far apart on ethical matters. In fact, it is somewhat amazing that people ever find common ground. This brings up an important point, namely, that the object of ethical reflection is to find common ground while preserving as many important values and principles as possible. This is done using a process of deliberation and justification.

Deliberation and Justification When nurses acquire a foundation of basic ethical knowledge, they are in a much better position to make sound ethical decisions. Even so, there is still a missing component—a method for justifying and objectifying thinking. Every day nurses function as members of a health team, responsible for decision making and problem solving on behalf of patients. As they perform this aspect of their jobs, it is not sufficient to decide what is believed to be the best ethical solution; they need to be able to justify their decisions to the patient, the family, and all members of the team. They need to be able to say *why*.

On a day-to-day basis, justification of decisions is generally not necessary. Beauchamp and Childress (1994, p. 54) explain that "we commonly make moral judgements about everyday issues without difficulty. We know we are to be truthful, honest etc. . . . When uncertainty occurs over right and wrong, deliberation and analysis are required to determine one's ethical obligation or what should be done according to moral action guides." A deliberative process is essential for proper resolution of today's complex ethical problems, and nurses are accountable to patients to engage in as thorough analysis of their ethical issues as they do those of a clinical nature. Predictably, weak analysis yields simplistic and ultimately unsatisfactory results.

Philosopher Rachels (1995, pp. 17-18) said of the importance of a careful deliberative process:

> Aristotle, Butler and others emphasized that responsible moral judgment must be based on a full understanding of the facts; but, they added, after facts are established a separate cognitive process

is required for the agent to fully understand the import of what they know. It is necessary not merely to know the facts but to rehearse them carefully in one's mind.

Rachels, with support from time-honored philosophic giants, advocates the use of critical analysis and formal justification. Nelson (1967, p. 126) explains that "justification in ethics involves the process of stating, elucidating, and defending a sound procedure for determining the truth of conflicting moral claims and the soundness of moral arguments." It is a complex process but one that is infinitely worth nurses' time.

Justification means that acceptable grounds can and should be given for desiring one course of action over another and that the desirable course will be the one that is backed by the best reasons (Rachels, 1995, p. 11). The best reasons involve logical consistency to support why nurses believe a particular reason to be the best reason. If a nurse is willing to apply a certain option in one situation, it should also seem applicable and reasonable in similar cases. Regardless of the soundness of the overall deliberative process, it is clear that the best reasons (and responses) will be found only if the facts of the conflict are accurate, so establishing factual parameters of the case is always the starting point. All forms of bioethical dispute resolution begin with urging the parties involved to carefully assimilate the facts. In clinical ethics cases, facts should be methodically accumulated and would include items 1 to 5 in Box 14-6, which is a framework for ethical decision making.

This framework can serve as a guide for ethical decision making. It is similar to the critical pathways or algorithms used for clinical decision making. Although ethical decision-making frameworks such as the one in Box 14-6 cannot be as specific as critical paths, they can provide a realistic general guide for decision making.

BOX 14-6

Framework for Bioethical Decision Making

To use the framework for bioethical decision making, identify the following:

1. Relevant patient and family demographics, including pertinent social data
2. Medical facts, including course of illness, diagnosis, prognosis, quality-of-life information, and a statement as to patient's or family's understanding of these data
3. Name of the legally designated decision maker
4. Persons who should be present for the discussion of options
5. Available legal or ethical options
6. How the available options are justified ethically: the specifications of the ethical norms involved and the pros and cons associated with each option (i.e., principles and rules at risk in each option)
7. The most ethically sound option and justification for it

BOX 14-7

Nursing Process as a Framework for Ethical Decision Making

Assessment: composed of problem identification and information gathering
Plan: selection of a strategy for resolution
Implementation: putting the agreed-on moral plan into effect
Evaluation: analysis of the process and the efficacy of the plan

From Reigle, J. (1996). Ethical decision-making skills. In A. Hamric, J.A. Spross, & C.M. Hanson (Eds.). *Advanced nursing practice.* Philadelphia: Saunders.

They serve as useful starting points for beginning ethical analysis. When an ethical problem becomes apparent, the framework helps to assimilate and organize case information for proper analysis. Once the facts, values, preferences, possibilities, and so on are laid out, deliberation and justification can be simplified.

The framework in Box 14-6 is an outline of a deliberative process that is not unlike the nursing process used to resolve clinical problems. Reigle (1996), in fact, advocates the use of the nursing process to resolve ethical problems because it is a framework for decision making that is already familiar to nurses. She conceptualizes it as shown in Box 14-7. Although Reigle did not use the nursing process as it is currently conceptualized, current nursing process models involve a nursing diagnosis. This is a useful step

that can help to state the ethical problem in concrete terms. Listing the various nursing diagnoses can also assist to delineate all aspects of the often complex ethical dilemmas confronted by nurses in the current environment. These might include patient and family coping, grief, and body image issues.

Fry (1994) offers another form of problem resolution based on values clarification. Fry's method is especially useful when trying to resolve problems in multicultural settings. In fact, her model was developed as part of an international guidebook on nursing ethics for the International Council of Nursing. When ethical conflict arises, Fry advocates that the parties involved ask four questions (Box 14-8). Fry's model, a narrative approach, may be used alone or in conjunction with other decision-making frameworks. Obviously its strength is found in its ability to explicate, understand, and protect diverse values while still finding acceptable solutions to ethical conflicts.

Another useful method is advocated in a publication by the United Hospital Fund of New York. Dubler and Marcus (1994) in their guide entitled *Mediating Bioethical Disputes* present a model derived from a demonstration project at

Values Clarification Approach to Problem Resolution

What is the story behind the values conflict?
What is the significance of the values involved?
What is the significance of the conflict to the parties involved?
What should be done?

From Fry, S.T. (1994). *Ethics in nursing practice.* Geneva, Switzerland: International Council of Nurses.

Tasks of Mediators in Resolving Bioethical Disputes

Assessment phase: investigate and characterize the conflict, identify the parties, and reach agreement on medical fact

Development phase: distinguish and clarify the relevant legal and ethical principles and make sure that all parties understand the facts and the rights of parties in the same way

Resolution phase: help patient and family think through the options, articulate values to caregivers, and ensure that the agreed-on solution is carried out accordingly

From Dubler, N.N. & Marcus, L.J. (1994). *Mediating bioethical disputes.* New York: United Hospital Fund.

Montefiore Hospital in New York. The model is based on the premise that a truly neutral trained third party (not a stake holder) can best assist the health team to work through the complex issues generally involved in bioethical disputes. The panel that developed the framework encourages use of a three-stage process: (1) assessment, (2) development, and (3) resolution. The most important aspects of each stage for the mediator are shown in Box 14-9.

The final model and the one the author commonly uses is Beauchamp and Childress' approach (1994). They advocate a framework for analyzing ethical problems using the foundational ethical elements previously described. They specify and weigh these elements in each situation. Their framework is sound but not simple. To use Beauchamp and Childress' framework, the nurse needs a sound basic knowledge in ethics and critical thinking. This is certainly true regardless of the approach used but perhaps even more so in the Beauchamp and Childress approach. The reason, of course, is that today's ethical conflicts are often complex and cannot be easily simplified or summarized; to attempt to do so generally yields unsatisfactory results. Ethical problems take time to develop, and they are commonly entrenched in the complexities of human relationships. Hence they take

time and thought to sort out, and there are generally no reasonable shortcuts that prove adequate.

Beauchamp and Childress (1994) use a model for ethical dispute resolution called the *coherence model.* The basic idea is that the best ethical option is the most logically coherent option, or the one in which all elements of the selected decision are supported to the degree possible by fact, accuracy of terms, and the best ethical reasons. Based on their understanding of ethical problem solving, abstract ethical principles are made into more functional tools or action guides by a process of specifying and balancing the ethical principles involved. This is necessary because, as they point out, "Every general norm . . . contains regions of indeterminacy that need reduction through further development and enrichment" (Beauchamp & Childress, 1994, p. 28). Meaning is established by further defining abstract or hazy elements of any question whether the problem is one of ethics or any other topic of deliberation. For example, in prin-

Key terms	
Term	**Definition**
Specifying	Process of shaping more abstract norms (i.e., principles) so they can be developed into more useful concrete action guides by defining them both in a given situation and ultimately overall
Balancing	Deliberation and judgment about the relative weight of norms; the purpose is to locate the greatest balance of right over wrong (Ross, 1930, p. 33)

ciple no one would argue about the wisdom of avoiding flammable liquids; however, it is important to specify that there are exceptions (i.e., the use of gasoline for the automobile and lawnmower or propane for the gas grill). The abstract principle alone is certainly true but almost unusable in modern society. To put the principle to work, whether in ethics or in the natural world, it has to be shaped and further defined. This is Beauchamp and Childress' point (1994), namely, that usability is accomplished primarily through specification or the conceptual shaping of ethical norms so that they connect with more concrete action guides and thus yield practical judgments.

Specification of principles is frequently the function of rules, and often rules themselves need to be further shaped and defined. An example is when the rule honoring patient confidentiality lends definition to the principle of respect for the autonomy of the person. The rule itself has been further shaped to mean that confidentiality is to be maintained unless doing so places another person at risk. This specification

of the rule of confidentiality occurred with the Tarasoff case (*Tarasoff, V. et al. v. The regents of the University of California*, 1976), in which a psychologist maintained patient confidentiality and did not warn a third party whom he thought to be a target of attack by his patient. The psychologist notified only the police, and unfortunately his patient murdered the third party after police decided that the patient appeared rational and should be released. The courts found that in this and similar cases a duty to warn did exist and in all instances should supersede the requirement to maintain patient confidentiality. This finding by the court adds specificity to the rule of patient confidentiality (*Tarasoff, V. et al. v. The regents of the University of California*, 1976).

As demonstrated by the Tarasoff case, the process of specification adds definition to the ethical conventions of the society and can actively change commonly understood meanings of a prevailing ethical norm. It should be noted that specification of ethical norms can also eventually lead to policy formation or change, as in the case of end-stage renal disease and the public provision of universal access to dialysis. In this case the public understanding of two principles (*beneficence* and *justice*) changed to encompass a requirement to publicly provide a particular life-sustaining technology, *dialysis,* according to need and not according to ability to pay or social standing. Previously, dialysis was offered based on the social worth of the individuals in need of the technology. The public found this ethically unacceptable. Hence public pressure provided impetus for universal Medicare dialysis reimbursement provisions, which were quickly passed into law by Congress in the mid-1960s. These provisions allowed for everyone in need of the technology to have an equal chance of receiving it as long as potential benefit was shown. This ruling changed society's understanding of what it means to benefit patients and what criteria for distribution of the benefit should be used.

In summary, Beauchamp and Childress (1994) suggest that careful deliberation yields several ethical options. The identified options may then be properly analyzed, specified, and balanced to find a solution that compromises the least number of ethical norms (principles, rules) and protects (to the degree possible) the values, first of the patient but also of all involved moral agents.

These frameworks illustrate several of the many proposed methods of deliberation and justification available in the ethics literature. There are a variety of methods because any number of ways of reasoning are meaningful to individuals. Everyone should be able to find and use a method that makes sense to him or her. The important thing is not which method is used but that *a* method is used to facilitate careful and effective ethical problem resolution. Further, any reputable approach will generally advocate similar features, such as accumulation of facts, identification of options, provision of ethical justification for the options, and examination of the adequacy of ethical justification before making a decision. This is the essence of the deliberation/justification process.

■ ETHICAL ISSUES

The remainder of this chapter discusses three types of ethical issues: ethical problems associated with (1) informed consent, (2) withholding and withdrawing treatment, and (3) resource allocation. Conflict surrounding these issues is virtually always related to tension between two or more of the four ethical principles outlined above. Ethical analysis is needed to decide which principle takes priority in a given case. Discussion of each of the three types of problems begins with a brief case, proceeds to a background summary of relevant ethical concepts, and ends with a brief analysis of the case.

Informed Consent

Discussion: Informed Consent The doctrine of informed consent has a long and contentious historical and legal legacy. It is an important ethical standard in both Western clinical practice and research and a rule that is central to the principle of autonomy. It requires accurate communication with patients regarding what the health team proposes or intends to do with the patient and his or her body and psyche. The basic assumption is that no one is in a better position to make decisions about therapeutic or research procedures than the person who will be directly affected (the patient or subject). When every effort is made to provide patients with adequate information, the humanity of the person is protected and his or her status as an autonomous individual confirmed, thus preserving important ethical standards.

Why is the rule of informed consent so important? One reason informed consent is needed is found in history. Humankind's global record for ethical treatment of patients and research subjects is darkened by actions such as those of Nazi nurses and physicians during World War II or the investigators and staff in the Tuskegee syphilis experiments and human radiation experiments, both conducted in the United States in the 1940s and 1950s. The Tuskegee study lasted into 1972, and similar abuses continue today. In these cases patients or subjects were deceived, coerced, sickened, and, in the case of the Nazi nurses and physicians, even tortured and murdered in the name of science.

The Nazi experience in fact was the catalyst for the Nuremberg Code, a compendium of standards developed to protect future research subjects. The first sentence states that "the voluntary consent of human subjects is absolutely essential." Ten basic tenets follow and serve as a modern-day foundation for the rule of informed consent (Capron, 1997).

CASE STUDY

Informed Consent

Mrs. W., 72 years old, has been treated for metastatic cancer of the uterus. The prognosis for this type of advanced cancer is grim, with a less than 20% likelihood of survival at the end of 6 months. Her physician recently obtained permission to use an experimental protocol for patients with this diagnosis who had not responded to conventional therapy. She informed Mrs. W. about the drug trial in the presence of one of the oncology nurses, who was asked to witness Mrs. W.'s signature on the consent form. The nurse agreed to serve as a witness. After they were finished discussing the study, the nurse asked the physician to leave the consent form so that she might review it for her own information. On review, the nurse thought that the study was represented to the patient in terms that were too optimistic and that the patient was led to believe that there was a good possibility of cure or at least an extended life span. The form was accurate in its discussion of the scientific merit of the research and the fact that there may not be any benefit, but the nurse believed that the physician's description did not coincide with the consent form. When asked about this, the physician said, "Look, it's all she's got. Neither you nor I know if this will be helpful, but if she starts out thinking that it won't be, it will compromise the potential for the therapy to work at all. I think that I gave her a fair description of the drug and its toxicity. Besides, she can read it herself and get the full range of potential side effects of the drug. She needs for me to be hopeful. She's from the old school and really wants her physician to make decisions for her that are in her best interest; she's told me as much. We also need to know whether this has any hope of being a beneficial treatment for future patients."

What should the nurse do now? She has witnessed only that the patient actually signed the consent form, not that the consent was fully informed. Does she have any further obligation to the patient? Will further discussion with the patient do more harm than good? Should the patient receive a more candid explanation, or should she just be expected to read the consent form for further information if she desires it?

As discussed more fully in Chapter 15, standard legal elements of true informed consent evolved this century through case law. In the early 1900s patient consent was sought for pragmatic, not legal or ethical, reasons. Medicine was anything but a science, and physicians needed as much help as they could get to bring about successful healing. The patient's endorsement was considered essential for the treatment to succeed. A 1914 legal case changed the justification for obtaining patient consent from a concern with therapeutic efficacy to one of an individual's legal right to self-determination. Judge Cordoza, the presiding judiciary in the 1914 case, stated that "Every human of adult years and sound mind has a right to determine what shall be done with his own body" (*Schloendorff v. Society of New York Hospitals,* 1914). In this case the ruling was that a surgeon who performed an operation without the patient's consent committed an act of assault. After the ruling in this case the human body began to be conceptualized as personal property and as such was not to be touched or subjected to intrusion without permission.

The 1914 ruling simply required patient permission. It was not until 1957 that another case (*Salgo v. Leland Stanford Jr. University Board of Trustees,* 1957) stated that patient understanding was also required by law to fulfill the obligations of informed consent. This meant that specific types of information were to be provided to meet the informed consent mandate. This elevated the doctrine beyond simply requiring a signature on a page to actually determining that a sufficient explanation was given.

The present understanding of the doctrine has been strongly influenced by philosophers and theologians writing from the 1960s to the present. Usually their agenda was to shape and define more clearly the principle of autonomy in the health care realm and to move the physician/patient relationship away from its paternalistic tendencies (paternalism is evidenced when someone other than a competent person presumes to be able to act on that person's behalf without full discussion with the individual to be affected) to one in which the patient was seen as more of an equal partner with health care team members (including the physician). Shoring up the rule of informed consent was an expedient way to do this. It was also a way to support two important patient values: well-being and self-determination. It was during this era that informed consent became a cornerstone of health care ethics.

The current understanding of informed consent for research subjects is derived mostly from federal regulations passed in the 1970s and 1980s in which the doctrine of consent was specifically defined in relation to research subjects. In fact, these guidelines are still used to write patient consent forms for research protocols today. Modifications of the consent standards used for research subjects are used to obtain consent for purely clinical or therapeutic procedures. Informed consent is now an expected part of all human research protocols and many clinical patient encounters. There is little doubt that informed consent is valued by the public. In a national survey done in the 1980s, the majority of physicians and members of the public agreed that patients have a right to all information regarding their conditions and treatments and that the public universally desired to have that information provided. Further, the desire for information is universal—not restricted by age, gender, race, or class (President's Commission for the Study of the Ethical Problems in Medicine and Biomedical and Behavioral Research, 1983). To meet the need for standard information, fundamental elements or general requirements of informed consent have been developed (Box 14-10).

To summarize the procedure, true informed consent is obtained only if a mentally competent person is provided sufficient information to clearly understand what is to occur, the alternatives, the associated risks, and why the procedure is necessary and preferable and then voluntarily agrees to what is proposed (Beauchamp, 1997). The agreement is expected to be in writing for purposes of documentation and contract law if it involves research or clinical risk to the patient. Consent is thought to be necessary especially when invasive therapy is proposed.

An important question is where nurses stand in the process of providing informed consent? It is not always easy to determine, but perhaps the best response is that it is clear where nurses *should* stand. They should guarantee that patients have the information that they need to make informed decisions. The ANA code (American Nurses Association, 1985, p. 11) is unequivocal on this topic: "Clients have the moral right to determine what will be done with their own person; to be given accurate and complete information so that they may make informed judgments; and to be assisted with weighing the burdens and benefits of options."

B O X　　1 4 - 1 0

Fundamental Elements of Informed Consent

Disclosure
Comprehension
Voluntariness
Competence
Consent

If patients have a right to be informed, every nurse has an obligation to see that they are informed. Nurses should be clear about this, since in practice nurses often spend precious time trying to determine what patients know instead of what they need to know to make a sound decision. When nurses make a choice to contribute actively to the process of informed consent, ethical obligations to patients are much more likely to be met.

Discussion: Case Study   The case described on p. 353 illustrates a conflict between the principles of beneficence and autonomy. One way to resolve it is by better specifying the meaning of *beneficence* and *autonomy,* the two principles in question. A direct way to accomplish this is to delineate the rules associated with the principles and to determine if there is sufficient justification to set them aside. The options that exist are (1) to do nothing, (2) to talk further with the patient or the physician, or (3) to do both. The goal is to select the option that best preserves the patient's values and the integrity of the staff and protects the ethical principles and rules involved to the greatest degree possible.

When considering options it is clear that in this case all the requirements for the rule of informed consent (a foundation of the principle of respect for autonomy) have not been met and hence the principle of respect for individual autonomy is violated. The physician did not determine that the patient actually understood the risks and benefits of the procedure. The physician operated from a well-meaning but paternalistic perspective. The physician believed that the proposed treatment was in the best interest of the patient whether the patient understood all the nuances of the therapy or not. As long as a signature was obtained, informed consent had been obtained. The nurse recognized the knowledge deficit of the patient and knew that the basic informed consent element of patient understanding was lacking. Once the nurse recognized this lack of understanding, she was ethically obligated to act to correct the patient's comprehension deficit. One way to do so is to ask the patient what her understanding of the protocol was and then to correct any misunderstanding that existed. Another way to proceed is to have an additional discussion with the physician in a collegial manner about the comprehension requirement of informed consent. The patient could be encouraged to confirm that she was willing to assume the involved risks for such uncertain benefit. A discussion of this sort is possible only if there is sufficient familiarity with the requirements of the rule of informed consent.

Adequate ethical knowledge is imperative in this type of situation and can be used to justify successful further discussion with the physician about the concerns that the nurse has. In this case, identifying and specifying the rule of informed consent were instrumental in clarifying the nurse's ethical obligation.

Another rule that adds tension in this case is that of the obligation to avoid deceiving patients. Although the physician might be justifying mild deception for what she considers the patient's good, overriding the rule of avoiding deception of patients is difficult to justify in this case or any case. Modern ethical thought suggests that patient deception is rarely if ever justified and should not be resorted to in most instances. The argument is that there is reasonable certainty that more good is to be gained by deception than by telling the truth and for some reason the patient would prefer it. In this case, this point would be difficult to argue because there is no evidence that either qualifier to the rule is true.

An additional consideration is whether benefit to future patients is sufficient to justify deception. The answer, at least from a deontologic perspective, is *no.* Patients must be completely aware that a study will likely be of more benefit to others and they still choose to participate. A negative response is compatible with a specific understanding of the principle of respect for autonomy that includes the kantian rule that persons should never be used solely as a means to an end but only as ends in themselves.

The best choice in this case (and the choice that appears to preserve the greatest number of important ethical principles and rules) is to make sure that the patient fully understands the risks and benefits of the research. The most respectful way of accomplishing this is to first have a conversation with the physician regarding the current interpretation of what constitutes fully informed consent and then encourage the physician to more fully explain the study to the patient. Suggest that patient understanding be tested by using a series of questions, such as "What do you hope to gain from participation in this study? Would you mind reviewing your understanding of the risks of the study?" This approach preserves the principles and rules of autonomy and informed consent and also is a respectful approach to the physician colleague in the scenario. In using this approach, an ethically sound option can be selected that more closely preserves the patient's, nurse's, and physician's values.

Withdrawing or Withholding Life-Sustaining Treatment

Discussion: Withholding and Withdrawing Treatment In March, 1983 the President's Commission for the Study of the Ethical Problems in Medicine and Biomedical and Behavioral Research (1983, pp. 15-16) submitted a report on one of its assigned topics, foregoing life-sustaining technology. The following is an excerpt from that report:

> Physicians realize . . . that the mission of vanquishing death is finally futile, but often they and their patients are determined to do all that is possible to postpone the event. Sometimes this objec-

---

C A S E   S T U D Y

Withholding and Withdrawing Treatment

In a now well-known case, 25-year-old Elizabeth Bouvia petitioned the court to allow her to die and requested to have her physicians assist her in the process by not force-feeding her. Bouvia, almost completely paralyzed and wheelchair bound, was by her own report in constant pain from muscle spasm and arthritis. She at one point said that ". . .death is letting go of all burdens . . .being free of my physical disability and mental struggle to live" (Pence, 1990, p. 30). Because Mrs. Bouvia was physically at the mercy of her caregivers, the only way that she could proceed with her plan was to pursue her wish for noninterference in her dying process by enlisting the help of the court.

---

tive so dominates care that patients undergo therapies whose effects do not actually advance their own goals and values. Specifically the drive to sustain life can conflict with another arguably more fundamental objective of medicine—the relief of suffering. . . . The attempt to postpone death should at times yield to other, more important goals of patients.

The report sets the stage for the beginning of an era in which doing everything available at all costs to preserve life might be seen to severely violate other important existential patient goods, such as being without pain or not having to endure profound disability to maintain life or a poor quality existence. In fact, it is now common practice to withdraw life support when the health care team, the patient, and the family believe that it is appropriate. On this point most members of the public and the health care team agree. What is not agreed on is how to determine when that point has arrived and how it should be approached by the team.

At the heart of any disagreement associated with end-of-life care is determining what is beneficial for the patient. Increasingly it is recognized that the best person to decide this is the patient. This has become more the case in the last several years as emphasis has been given to individual rights of patients and the role of the principle of autonomy in health care. Today it is well accepted that competent patients have a right to accept or reject intervention. A problem occurs when a patient needs members of the health care team to assist the patient to carry out his or her wishes and those wishes will bring about the end of life. Such was the case with Bouvia.

The President's Commission for the Study of the Ethical Problems in Medicine and Biomedical and Behavioral Research (1983) identified several values that health care professionals should consider when attempting to resolve this type of conflict (Box 14-11). The commission further concluded that in spite of a predisposition to respecting individual patient choice, the preferences of patients, family members, and health care providers may legitimately be limited on grounds of public policy, professional judgment, and considerations of resource scarcity. Basically the commission advocated decision making within a communal context with priority but not absolute supremacy given to the patient's life goals and preferences. The commission attempted to answer the question of who should have the right to make these types of decisions, the patient or the health care team.

Brock (1997, p. 367) in a recent discussion of the withholding and withdrawing controversy shed further light on the issue by pointing out that until recently it was assumed that the only legitimate ends of health care were preservation of life and health. Now there is a third contender, patient well-being. This third goal of health care can in fact at times be at odds with the first two. Consider Brock's statement (1997,

---

BOX 14-11

Values Identified by President's Commission in Relation to Life-sustaining Treatment

1. Respect the choices of individuals who are competent to decide to forego life-sustaining treatment.
2. Provide mechanisms and guidelines for decision making on behalf of patients who are unable to do so on their own.
3. Maintain a presumption in favor of sustaining life.
4. Improve the medical options available to dying patients.
5. Encourage health care institutions to take responsibility for ensuring that adequate procedures for decision making are available for all patients.

From President's Commission for the Study of the Ethical Problems in Medicine and Biomedical and Behavioral Research. (1983). *Summing up.* Washington, D.C.: U.S. Government Printing Office.

---

p. 367) that health and life extension are of value in so far as they facilitate the patient's pursuit of his or her life plan or the aims, goals, and values important to that particular person.

Take, for example, the situation in which life and a baseline of health could be preserved but the cost is continuous suffering or a life of profound disability. Does preservation of life in this situation continue to support any of the patient's life plans? If faced with these options some would say no, that death is preferable to being condemned to live in such a state. This is the decision that some patients and families have made in several of the more controversial legal cases involving withdrawing treatment. Brock (1997) argues rightly that there is no single correct answer to how such conditions (e.g., disability, pain, intubation) should be valued; there are only actual answers that real

BOX 14-12

Spectrum of Treatment Options

Obligatory————Optional————Mandatory
                                    foregoing of
                                    treatment

From Beauchamp, T.L., & Childress, J.F. (1994). *Principles of biomedical ethics* (4th ed.). New York: Oxford University Press.

people give for themselves. This is why many persons have urged that health care decision making be a shared function among physician, nurse, patient, and family and not the one-sided paternalistic model of past decades.

How should withdrawing and withholding life-sustaining treatment be viewed? Beauchamp and Childress (1994) make a distinction between obligatory versus optional treatment. They endorse a spectrum of responses that include those in which provision of certain types of therapy would be wrong. In the middle of the spectrum is optional treatment, and at the opposite end is obligatory treatment. Box 14-12 shows a schematic of treatment options. The type of situation that would fall to the far right of the spectrum might be a patient in severe pain or with disability that would make life continuously burdensome to the patient, who has no hope of improvement and is requesting an end to treatment. Treatments would be considered optional when they are elective procedures, such as cosmetic surgery or when it is unlikely but remotely possible that they will change the course of events to a positive outcome. Obligatory treatments are those with unquestioned benefit, such as antibiotics for sepsis or intubation for an acute asthma attack for patients who have a reasonable chance to recover. Once medical fact and clinical judgment firmly indicate that the outcome of therapy would only further suffering and death, the obligation to treat falls off proportionate to the likelihood of patient benefit. Obviously the more likely a treatment is to yield beneficial results, the more obligatory it becomes. In light of this, how should the Bouvia case be interpreted?

Discussion: Case Study The facts of the Bouvia case are that a mentally competent adult with a great deal of emotional and physical pain made a decision not to eat or drink. The staff did not agree and so forced their value of life at all costs on Mrs. Bouvia and force-fed her. Because of her disabilities and her family situation, she could not physically resist, but she did appeal to the American Civil Liberties Union (ACLU) to protect her right to self-determination. This right of self-determination is a cherished American value derived from the principle of respect for individual autonomy. What guidance is available for this case? For example, does the ANA's *Code for Nurses* or the ethics literature offer direction?

Actually the Code gives a somewhat mixed message. In the first interpretive statement the following wording is found: "Nurses are morally obligated to respect human existence and the individuality of all persons who are the recipients of nursing actions. Nurses therefore must use all reasonable means to protect and preserve human life when there is a reasonable hope of benefit from life-prolonging treatment" (American Nurses Association, 1985, p. 1). In the Bouvia case one cannot do both things advocated by the Code, that is, respect individuality and preserve life if there is any hope of meaningful existence. So what action should take precedent? If nurses depend on the Code alone for guidance, it is difficult to make a decision. Further ethical knowledge is needed. This could take the form of ethical consultation, certainly a review of the ethics literature of related cases, and finally careful deliberation. In the actual case the courts were utilized as final arbitrators, and the decision was to force-feed Mrs. Bouvia on the grounds that there would be a profound negative effect on others (primarily the hospital staff and other disabled persons) to do otherwise.

After enduring months of force-feeding in a local hospital, Mrs. Bouvia left the hospital and went to Mexico, where she was eventually convinced to give up her plan to starve herself. She admitted herself to a private care facility for further care. She led a reclusive life after that, and follow-up information is not available. The preamble to the ANA's *Code for Nurses* (American Nurses Association, 1985, p. ii) actually stands in opposition to the court's decision:

> Since clients themselves are the primary decision makers in matters concerning their own health, treatment, and well-being, the goal of nursing action is to support and enhance the client's responsibility and self-determination to the greatest extent possible. In this context, health is not an end in itself but a means to a life that is meaningful from the client's perspective.

This statement makes a case of this type especially difficult for nurses. However, it is encouraging that since the 1980s when this case occurred, there has been more recognition of the importance of respecting patients' values and nontreatment decisions, especially when faced with intractable pain or significant disability. It is reasonably clear that, in Bouvia's case at least, she should not have been force fed.

The Principle of Justice and the Right to Health Care Access

Discussion: Access to Health Care Resources In the health care realm, access to care is generally presumed to be a benefit and obstacles to access are considered a burden. Ill health prevents the pursuit of one's life goals, so subsequently people seek to resolve illness. Access to health care involves interpretation (specification) of the ethical principle of justice. The question that is usually asked is how much

---

C A S E   S T U D Y

Access to Health Care Resources

R.H. is a 36-year-old manual laborer of African-American descent who has moderate hypertension. He discovered this at a free blood pressure screening conducted by a nurse (J.S.) who had also employed him occasionally in the past. R.H. is married with a child and has no health insurance. His salary of $19,000 is insufficient to pay the 60% fee that he would be charged at the public hospital for a clinic visit. Given these financial constraints, J.S. convinced one of the physicians at the hospital where she worked to examine him for free. The physician confirmed R.H.'s moderate hypertension and prescribed an antihypertensive medication. Although J.S. counsels R.H. about a variety of ways to influence his blood pressure, including diet changes, exercise, and effective ways to handle stress, R.H. unfortunately cannot afford $55 per month for medication. What accountability does J.S. have to help R.H. obtain his medication? Is this an ethical issue of justice, beneficence, or both?

---

health care access the principle of justice requires. At present the debate continues.

The reason for the intensity of the debate is that in the United States there is a quirk of logic. Most people agree that everyone should have the opportunity to seek and receive affordable quality health care. When asked if they would be willing to contribute more taxes toward this goal, most say no. When asked if quality or type of care should be compromised to reach the goal of universal access, most again reply no. What is left is a nice *idea* but not a *value* of universal access (i.e., a value by definition means that people are willing to act to preserve it). As Purtilo (1993, p. 199) writes, "Western societies are experiencing a tension that derives from believing that health care belongs to everyone, but for various reasons it must be rationed." Rationing, of course, means that everyone cannot have what is being rationed, that some will be excluded from participation or benefit.

Is there guidance for nursing practice in the ethics literature? First, what does the principle of justice require from the perspective of the ANA Code? Statement 11 of the Code states that "the nurse collaborates with members of the health professions and other citizens in promoting community and national efforts to meet the health needs of the public"; Statement 11 further states that "nursing care is an integral part of high quality health care, and nurses have an obligation to promote equitable access to nursing and health care for all people." It is clear that the authors of the Code believed that it is a part of a nurse's ethical obligation to ensure equitable access to health care. Given this, what should J.S. do when a patient cannot pay for what is clearly beneficial therapy?

In fact, there is little specific guidance in the literature regarding this common dilemma. Miles (1993) expressed a concern that there is the common question of what to do when a patient cannot afford to pay for conventional therapy such as medications for high blood pressure. Miles goes on to say that the ethics community has not addressed these more common issues effectively but instead has focused on some of the more exotic and also less frequently encountered dilemmas. This is an identified gap in contemporary ethical knowledge. So where can individuals find more specific guidance? In R.H.'s case the options are as follows:

1. One can assume that it is solely R.H.'s responsibility to obtain the drug and that J.S. fulfilled her ethical obligation when she assisted with affordable (free) access to an appropriate provider.
2. Based on the ANA's *Code for Nurses,* more assistance is required. A means for obtaining the drug should be secured.

3. Not only is assistance with obtaining beneficial therapy indicated for this patient, but also J.S. should begin to actively work to ensure that all persons would be able to obtain clearly beneficial therapy regardless of ability to pay.

Which of these options guarantees the preservation of the greatest number of ethical principles and rules? How should the option be implemented?

Option 1 seems to clearly violate Statement 11 of the ANA Code as described above. The fact that R.H. cannot afford medication to treat an otherwise treatable disease seems inherently unfair. Thinking about the case in relation to Aristotle's formal principle of justice (i.e., that similar cases be treated similarly) illuminates why there is a problem. R.H.'s life will be shortened through no fault of his own because he is not as skilled or fortunate as someone who earns more money and who can pay to have his or her high blood pressure treated. He is certainly no less worthy of treatment as a human being than someone who is wealthy or has insurance, but yet he will not receive treatment if the material criterion of justice (ability to pay) is used to decide allocation issues in health care. Option 1 seems to border on harming R.H. through abandonment. Thus option 1 seems undesirable because it violates the principle of justice as conceptualized by the nursing profession and standard ethical theory. It also seems to border on abandonment, which would violate the principles of nonmaleficence and beneficence.

How does option 2 compare with established professional ethical standards? If J.S. finds a way to provide R.H.'s medicines, the formal principle of justice has been preserved in this case. Resources were provided based on need and ability to benefit. Option 2 conforms with Statement 11 in the ANA Code, and it also helps to avoid the problem of abandonment as outlined above.

Is option 3 an improvement over option 2? Yes, in that it addresses overall inequity in the system and mobilizes a grassroots initiative to move toward a more just system. This is certainly a more complete solution to the problem of access to health care resources. It is difficult to justify being a party to a system that condones the type of inequity illustrated by the case, unless one is trying to become part of the solution as well.

Implementation If option 3 is selected, J.S. might convince the manufacturer to provide the drug, either free of charge or at cost. She might then write her legislators or involve professional nursing organization lobbyists in the case. She could urge them to consider a way to address obstacles to better health through the legislative process. Finally, until a more permanent solution is negotiated, she might help to organize a free clinic in the area by pooling talent and resources from community health agencies.

It is important to note that there are several sound ethical reasons why J.S. is obligated to find a way to provide this particular treatment. Primarily, pharmacologic therapy has proven efficacy, and it is not exotic but quite commonplace. It seems inherently wrong that this therapy would be rationed based on ability to pay. It is also important to note that J.S.'s obligation would be different depending on the type of resource that her patient needed. For example, if R.H. needed a liver or kidney, she would only be expected to see that he had a fair opportunity to receive an organ.

Discussion: Case Study This case illustrates an ethical dilemma involving the principles of justice and beneficence. Bioethical issues of justice generally involve fair distribution of societal benefits, burdens, goods, and services. Conflicts associated with this principle will probably involve how "fair distribution" is defined. In health care the question often involves distribution of health care services to all citizens. The problem is often referred to as one of access to care and leads to one of the most controversial ethical questions in health care today: How should society distribute health care services?

• • •

As is apparent in these three cases, finding and doing what appears to be the most ethical thing might lead to more effort and responsibility on the part of a nurse who is concerned with practicing ethically or leading an ethical life generally; however, this is simply part of the role of a professional nurse. Given the historical professional legacy of nursing and the advocacy role that is often promoted and written about in the nursing literature, who more than nurses should be willing to thoughtfully consider ethical dilemmas and work for the best ethical option? One of the most effective approaches to reaching the goal of identifying the best ethical option is to practice preventive ethics.

■ PREVENTIVE ETHICS

Five fundamental strategies assist nurses to practice ethics preventively:

1. Ethical problems often develop because of ineffective communication between patient and provider around ethical issues. The best time to determine what patients value is before a health crisis occurs. Use of a values history and an advance directive, preferably taken in the primary care nurse practitioner's or physician's office, is an excellent way to generate a dialogue around these issues. If this is done, when crises occur, patients have had an opportunity to consider what they do value in a less stressful setting.

2. Establish clear hospital or workplace policies associated with ethical issues. For example, what is the proper way to determine the appropriateness of a *Do Not Resuscitate* order? Or how does the institution recommend

withdrawing life support? A response to these questions and similar ones can be facilitated by an on-site ethics committee.

3. The establishment of relationships with patients and families based on trust that encourage dialogue is crucial to implement preventive strategies. Enter into partnership with patients and their families, and encourage them to take an active role in developing solutions and options. It is the patient's life; nurses are just part of the journey. Help the patient to chart his or her own course of action.

4. Be an active participant in developing an ethical environment. Respect others, and work to construct a work environment that *is* respectful of everyone. Encourage free flow of information and candor up and down the organizational ladder. Celebrate the right and good things that are accomplished, and foster collaboration so that everyone can succeed in doing his or her job on behalf of patients. A working knowledge of ethical behavior is imperative for all members of an organization.

5. A final strategy involves participation in the policy formation stage whenever it is appropriate and likely to be efficacious. Nursing involvement in local and state activities relevant to ethical health care practices is an important preventive health strategy and one of the better ways to practice preventive ethics. Anticipation and prevention of unjust practices are an effective way to help to ensure that the public health is protected for all persons, not just a select fortunate few. Nursing holds a unique perspective within the health care realm, and it is always desirable to have nursing's perspective represented in the legislative process.

• • •

In conclusion, while teaching a graduate nursing seminar recently, the author asked the students what percent of their professional problems had an ethical component. They estimated that 50% to 60% of the problems that they confronted in their practice were ethical problems or had ethical elements associated with them. They also concluded that they found themselves less prepared than they would prefer to confront these types of problems. During discussion of what it would require to be comfortable with ethical problems, the consensus was that a working knowledge of ethics and ethical issues in the nursing field would be the minimal requirement.

Access to a formal deliberative process is mandatory. There is no substitute for this content. Nurses who take this responsibility seriously will have a much better opportunity to meet their obligations to patients. The work of nurses is privileged work. They enter people's lives at times of great vulnerability. Patients give nurses their trust and in turn are entitled to excellent clinical and ethical judgment. Both are possible with ethical knowledge and careful skilled deliberation.

■ KEY POINTS

- Ethics and an understanding of the principles of ethics and their role in guiding behavior are an integral part of nursing practice.
- Normative ethics is an area of inquiry that seeks to determine which approach or action is the most ethically desirable in a specific situation.
- It is essential that a nurse construct both a personal and a professional ethic based on his or her values and knowledge of ethical concepts, principles, and rules.
- Four key ethical principles for health care decision making are respect for autonomy, nonmaleficence, beneficence, and justice. Each of these ethical principles has corresponding rules.
- Two prominent ethical theories that have particular relevance to nursing practice are utili-

tarianism, which is a form of consequentialism, and kantian deontology.

- People use deliberation and justification as guides to making day-to-day decisions about the actions they should take.
- Steps can be employed to make thoughtful ethical decisions, and a variety of frameworks exist to guide one's steps.
- Some of the most important ethical issues for nurses to deal with include informed consent, withdrawing or withholding life-sustaining treatment, and the question of who has the right to health care.
- Preventive ethics, much like health promotion, helps nurses participate in a way that reflects an understanding of and valuing of ethical principles and rules.

■ CRITICAL THINKING QUESTIONS

1. If you were faced with an ethical dilemma that arose from having a difference of opinion with another health care provider about the best course of action to take on behalf of a patient, what would you do? Prioritize the steps that you would take, and describe your rationale both for each step and for the order of the steps.
2. What ethical dilemmas may be posed as managed care becomes an increasingly predominate way to finance health care? How might each of the dilemmas you list be reduced or eliminated?
3. Think carefully about 10 core values that you learned from your family. How might each of these values influence your actions as a nurse? What is the relationship between each of these values and principles of ethics?
4. In the case of Mrs. W. described in this chapter, what course of action would you have taken? Given your selection of a course of action, list the steps in the order in which you would have taken them. What family values can you recall that would explain your course of action?

5. In the case of R.H. described in this chapter, in addition to assisting him to find funds to purchase the prescribed medication, what other nursing actions, including patient education, would you have employed to help R.H. get his blood pressure under control?
6. Think back to a recent clinical situation. What preventive ethics might have been used, and how might they have changed the course of events that occurred?

■ REFERENCES

American Nurses Association. (1985). *Code for nurses with interpretive statements.* Kansas City, Mo.: American Nurses Association Press.

Beauchamp, T.L. (1997). Informed consent. In R.M. Veatch (Ed.). *Medical ethics* (2nd ed.). London: Jones & Bartlett.

Beauchamp, T.L., & Childress, J.F. (1994). *Principles of biomedical ethics* (4th ed.). New York: Oxford University Press.

Brock, D.W. (1997). Death and dying. In R.M. Veatch (Ed.). *Medical ethics* (2nd ed.). London: Jones & Bartlett.

Capron, A.M. (1997). Human experimentation. In R.M. Veatch (Ed.). *Medical ethics* (2nd ed.). London: Jones & Bartlett.

Dubler, N.N., & Marcus, L.J. (1994). *Mediating bioethical disputes.* New York: United Hospital Fund.

Fry, S.T. (1994). *Ethics in nursing practice.* Geneva: International Council of Nurses.

Jonsen, A.R. (1994). Clinical ethics and the four principles approach. In R. Gillon (Ed.). *Principles of health care ethics.* New York: John Wiley & Sons.

Mappes, T.A., & Zembaty, J.S. (1981). *Biomedical ethics.* New York: McGraw-Hill.

Miles, S.H. (1993). Clinical ethics and reform of access to health care. *Journal of Clinical Ethics, 4*(3):255-257.

Nelson, K. (1967). Problems of ethics. In P. Edwards (Ed.). *The encyclopedia of philosophy* (vol. 3). New York: Macmillan.

Nozick, R. (1968). Moral complications and moral structures. *Natural Law Forum, 13,* 1-50.

Pence, G.E. (1990). *Classic cases in medical ethics: Accounts of the cases that have shaped medical ethics, with philosophical, legal, and historical backgrounds.* New York: McGraw-Hill.

President's Commission for the Study of the Ethical Problems in Medicine and Biomedical and Behavioral Research. (1983). *Summing up.* Washington, D.C.: U.S. Government Printing Office.

Purtilo, R. (1993). *Ethical dimensions of the health professions* (2nd ed.). Philadelphia: Saunders.

Rachels, J. (1995). Can ethics provide answers? In J.H. Howell & W.F. Sale (Eds.). *Life choices: A Hastings Center introduction to bioethics.* Washington, D.C.: Georgetown University Press.

Ramsey, P. (1970). *The patient as person.* New Haven, Conn.: Yale University Press.

Reigle, J. (1996). Ethical decision-making skills. In A. Hamric, J.A. Spross, & C.M. Hanson (Eds.). *Advanced nursing practice.* Philadelphia: Saunders.

Rokeach, M. (1973). *The nature of human values.* New York: The Free Press.

Ross, W.D. (1930). *The right and the good.* Oxford: Claredon Press.

Uustal, D. (1987). Values: The cornerstone of nursing's moral art. In D.M. Fowler & J. Levine-Ariff (Eds.). *Ethics at the bedside.* Philadelphia: Lippincott.

■ LEGAL CASES

Salgo v Leland Stanford Jr. University board of trustees, 317 P 2d 170 (1957).

Schloendorff v Society of New York Hospitals, 211 N.Y. 125, 105, Nebr. 92 (1914).

Tarasoff, V. et al. v The regents of the University of California, 551 P 2d 334, 17 Cal. 3d 425 (1976).

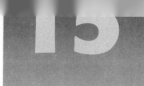

Legal Issues in Nursing Practice

Sheryl Feutz-Harter

INTRODUCTION

This chapter provides information about legal principles as they relate to the practice of nursing. Nurses are held responsible for personally complying with laws that affect their area of practice; nurse managers and administrators are held accountable for assuring that their staff understand the laws and are compliant with them.

As nurses move into advanced practice roles and nontraditional health care settings, they will be exposed to increased liability under a variety of legal theories. They may find themselves in situations where there is little or no legal guidance and must be able to make well-reasoned judgments based on their clinical and legal knowledge.

These are exciting and challenging times for nurses clinically; they are equally challenging legally. Being knowledgeable of the laws will best prepare nurses to meet their many challenges. This chapter is intended to serve as a resource to be used in conjunction with the laws in the state in which the nurse is practicing. Nurses need to identify legal resources available to them and seek them out for assistance when confronted with specific client situations.

OBJECTIVES

After reading this chapter, you will be able to:

1. Identify sources of laws, and discuss the elements necessary for nursing liability
2. Describe mechanisms for maximizing the defensibility of nursing care through patient care documentation
3. Discuss appropriate actions to take when there are staffing issues
4. Evaluate the legal significance of clinical practice guidelines
5. Analyze the process for informed decision-making

■ OVERVIEW OF LEGAL FUNDAMENTALS

The term "law" is derived from the Anglo-Saxon *lagu,* which means *that which is laid down or fixed.* Laws are established as a means to regulate how society conducts itself.

In the United States, the supreme law is the United States Constitution. The purpose of the Constitution is to define the operation of the federal government and differentiate between powers and limitations of the federal and state governments. The first ten Amendments to the Constitution are the Bill of Rights, which affect primarily individual rights such as due process of law, privacy, religion, and speech.

All other state and federal laws flow from or expand upon the Constitution. These laws include statutes, regulations, court decisions or case law, and attorney general opinions. Laws must be read and applied in conjunction with other laws, considering both state and federal laws.

Standard of care is a legal term meaning that level of conduct that a reasonably prudent nurse would undertake under the same or similar circumstances. Most states now recognize that there is a minimum standard of care required throughout the country and no longer use what was commonly referred to as the "locality rule" or "community standard." A nurse working in a given area is required to meet the minimum standards of care for that specialty practice, regardless of whether the nurse is practicing in California, Montana, or Alabama. Laws are one source of the standards of care for which a nurse will be held accountable. Other sources of standards of care include the American Nurses Association, the various specialty nursing organizations, the Joint Commission for Accreditation of Healthcare Organizations (JCAHO), the National Committee for Quality Assurance (NCQA), and professional journals.

In addition to the above external standards, internal standards of care are those standards established by a health care facility. These may include job descriptions, policies, procedures, protocols, clinical practice guidelines, and critical paths. These standards will be deemed the primary basis for accountability in the event there are allegations of nursing malpractice.

A deviation from the established standard of care is an element that must be proven for a plaintiff to prevail in a lawsuit alleging nursing malpractice. This is referred to as *negligence* or *malpractice.* The nurse must act or not act in a way that fails to meet the standard of care. An expert witness, usually another nurse, must testify how the nurse's action deviated from the standard of care. In addition to the required element of negligence, three other elements are required to find a nurse liable in a malpractice action.

One of these elements is that of *duty,* which is the legal relationship between a nurse and a patient. This duty will typically arise when a nurse is assigned to a specific patient or as a result of the nurse's employment responsibilities. Duty can also arise because a nurse voluntarily assumes a duty to an individual outside of the employment setting, such as rendering assistance in an emergency, volunteering at a health fair, or giving advice to a neighbor.

Key terms	
Term	**Definition**
Duty	Legal relationship with patient
Malpractice	Failure to meet requisite standard of care
Causation	Cause or contribute to cause injury to the patient
Damages	Physical, financial, or emotional harm suffered by patient and family

The second key element for liability to be found is the *causation* of an injury. The nurse must cause or contribute to cause the patient's injury; the injury must be as a direct result of the nurse's negligence. An expert witness must testify that it is more probable than not that the injury was attributable in whole or in part to the nurse's negligence.

The third and final element is *damages* that the patient and family members sustained as a result of the injury to the patient. These may include physical, financial, and emotional damages, both past and future. The other type of damages is punitive damages, which are awarded to punish grossly negligent or intentional conduct. These include nursing actions that are willful and wanton, flagrant, or done with malice, fraud, or oppression.

Liability may be placed on the nurse in two different capacities. The first is individual liability—nurses are accountable for their own actions. They are required to exercise independent judgments and apply their knowledge consistent with the applicable standards of care. Although historically physicians were held responsible for the actions of nurses, it is evident that nurses now may be found liable with absolutely no liability placed on a physician. In fact, a physician may offer as a defense that the physician acted reasonably based on the information provided by a nurse. The physician is entitled to rely on nurses to provide necessary and appropriate information. Failure of a nurse to meet the standard of care for notifying a physician will negate any liability of the physician (*Glassman v Saint Joseph Hospital,* 631 NE 2d 1186 [Ill. Ct. App. 1994]).

The other means by which a nurse can be held liable is if the nurse has management or administrative responsibilities for other health care providers. However, this expansion of liability does not relieve the health care provider from personal liability. The nurse has two responsibilities for health care providers whom the nurse is managing or supervising: (1) appropriate delegation of duties; and (2) providing adequate supervision.

Appropriately delegating duties means giving tasks to those health care providers who are qualified to implement them. This applies to any health care provider, including an RN, LPN, LVN, nurse's aide, unlicensed assistive personnel, or orderly. The significance of this is that the nurse has a right to rely on other health care providers to competently carry out assigned tasks. If a health care provider is not competent to complete an assignment and the nurse is or should be aware of this lack of competence, the nurse must provide adequate supervision. This could encompass having appropriate policies and procedures available for the health care provider to refer to, providing direct supervision of the health care provider, or having the provider's skills validated before making the assignment. A nurse who assigns a task to a competent health care provider who is appropriately supervised will not be held liable for the acts of the provider.

Liability may be avoided if there is a legal or factual defense. Contributory or comparative negligence is a defense if the acts of the patient caused or contributed to the injury sustained by the patient. Contributory negligence of the patient was substantiated in *Marottoli v Hospital of St. Raphael,* 1992 WL 257758 (Conn. 1992). When Mr. Marottoli was admitted to the hospital, he had problems with his knees, requiring him to use a cane. A nursing note on February 20 at approximately 2 AM indicated that the siderails on Mr. Marottoli's bed were kept up while he was in bed. Mr. Marottoli claimed that on the evening of February 20, Nurse Saunders raised only the left siderail of his bed. Mr. Marottoli claimed that he needed to defecate, pressed his call button, and after obtaining no assistance within 10 minutes, proceeded to get out of bed.

As he rose to his feet, he grasped a bedside table that slid away and he fell to the floor, fracturing his hip.

The court determined that Mr. Marottoli's testimony was not credible. Mr. Marottoli described the call button as being located on the opposite side of the bed from where other testimony had it located. If it had been where Mr. Marottoli claimed, a coiled wire would have been stretched from a console across his chest as he lay in bed. Mr. Marottoli further described the call button as being on the top of a lowered siderail, located even with the mattress. If the siderail had been down, the call button would have been well below the level of the mattress, according to other evidence. Mr. Marottoli testified that he heard nothing after he pushed the call button; there is evidence that once activated by the bedside button, the call system emits a steady beeping sound. According to Mr. Marottoli, after his fall he "blacked out" and was not alert until the next morning. Yet in his medical record, there were notations of conversations he had with nurses and no indication that he received any care typically required by an unconscious patient.

Nurse Smith, who took over for Nurse Saunders, testified that she asked Mr. Marottoli what had happened and he admitted that he had put down the siderail so that he could go to the bathroom by himself. This conversation was documented in the medical record, and there was nothing questioning the reliability of the entry. Based on all of the evidence, the court concluded that the nurses had taken adequate precautions to discourage Mr. Marottoli from getting out of bed unassisted and that he attempted to do so even though he knew that he should not.

Another potential defense in a nursing malpractice action is that the statute of limitations has expired. This is the time period established by state legislation limiting the time for an injured party to file a lawsuit. The time limit begins running on either the date of the incident causing the harm or when the patient knows or should have known that an injury may have been caused by negligence. When the statute of limitations expires, the patient is legally barred from filing a lawsuit.

■ TECHNIQUES FOR DEFENSIVE DOCUMENTATION

A comprehensive and accurate medical record can provide the most effective defense in nursing malpractice actions. Jurors believe the medical record is the most credible evidence of what happened and will take time to read it to verify the accuracy of testimony given by witnesses. Unfortunately, frequently the medical record is inconsistent with the testimony and may actually make a competent nurse appear negligent. It has been shown that the better the quality of documentation, the better the quality of care (Phaneuf, 1976).

The cardinal rule regarding documentation is that if it isn't charted, it did not occur. It is virtually impossible for a nurse to convince a jury that observations or actions or thoughts can be recalled with any reliability years after the fact. The adequacy and accuracy of nursing documentation can be a significant factor for an attorney in deciding whether to sue a health care provider for medical malpractice, as the following statements reflect (Nurse liability, 1988, p. 99):

> In a case of suspected negligence, nurses' documentation should be carefully scrutinized. . . . When evaluating medical negligence against hospitals, doctors, or nurses, the nurses' documentation (or lack of it) can help prove plaintiff's case.

Documentation must reflect pertinent information about the patient based on what a nurse sees, hears, thinks, says, and does regarding that patient. Nurses continue to strive to develop the perfect documentation system. In this author's opinion, this has not yet been achieved, although many of the current documentation systems are an improvement over previous systems. The "perfect" documentation system will achieve a balance in creating the most comprehensive and effective documentation to benefit the patient, while also being time-efficient and defensible in a legal action. All of the current documentation systems, problem-centered charting, PIE (Problem Intervention Evaluation), FOCUS®, and charting by exception, have their advantages and disadvantages (Kerr, 1992). Many difficulties arise because of the complexity of the documentation system and because nurses are not adequately trained in how to use it.

An extremely significant issue is having a documentation system that maximizes reimbursement. Some documentation systems do not incorporate care plans or protocols in the permanent medical record. Third-party payers, including Medicare and Medicaid, have indicated that the lack of these documents may result in denials of reimbursement. In a personal communication received from Medicare, the following was expressed (Aug. 4, 1991):

> As stated in HIM 15-1, Section 2304, sufficient detail for the services furnished to patients must be available for the determination of proper payment to the provider. The determination of proper payment includes claims audits as needed. Without access to . . . protocols, it is not possible to trace charges and perform a claims audit. Furthermore, a system that requires an enormous amount of checking back and forth between various records and protocols in order to conduct an audit is not reasonable. The provider is required to maintain auditable records and the medical records should be complete and able to stand alone without reference to other documents. Unauditable records will be denied.

The charting by exception documentation system was criticized by the court in *Lama v Borras,* 16 F 3d 473 (1st Cir. 1994). The United States Court of Appeals upheld the jury's con-

clusion that the hospital had been negligent in using the charting by exception method of recording notes in the patient's medical record.

The patient, Romera Lama, suffered from back pain and was referred to a neurosurgeon, Dr. Borras. On April 9, 1986, Mr. Lama had surgery, at which time Dr. Borras attempted to remove an extruded disk. Either Dr. Borras failed to remove the material or he operated at the wrong level because Mr. Lama's symptoms returned several days after the operation. On May 15th, a second operation was performed. No preoperative or postoperative antibiotics were ordered by Dr. Borras.

On May 17, a nurse's note indicates that the bandage covering Mr. Lama's surgical wound was "very bloody," obviously indicating the possibility of infection. The following day, Mr. Lama experienced pain at the site of the incision, another symptom consistent with an infection. On May 19, the bandage was "soiled again." Based on these entries, the court noted (*Lama v Borras,* pp. 475-476):

> A more complete account of Mr. Lama's evolving condition is not available because the hospital instructed nurses to engage in charting by exception, a system whereby nurses did not record qualitative observations for each of the day's three shifts, but instead made such notes only when necessary to chronicle important changes in a patient's condition.

Mr. Lama began to experience severe discomfort in his back on the night of May 20, and spent the night screaming in pain. The next morning, Dr. Piazza diagnosed discitis and initiated antibiotics. Discitis is extremely painful and very slow to cure, resulting in Mr. Lama being hospitalized for several additional months.

Mr. Lama sued Dr. Borras and the hospital. He alleged the hospital failed to prepare, use, and monitor proper medical records and failed to provide proper hygiene. At trial, one witness testified that a regulation of the Puerto Rico Department of Health required qualitative nurse's notes for each nursing shift. In the opinion of the court, the nurses attending to Mr. Lama did not supply the required notes for every shift even though they followed the hospital's policy of charting by exception. In its defense, the hospital argued that there was no evidence the nurses had observed but failed to document any material symptoms that would have caused Dr. Borras to investigate the possibility of an infection at an earlier stage. Pursuant to the charting by exception policy, the nurses regularly recorded Mr. Lama's temperature and vital signs and medications given to him.

However, the damaging evidence was that in documenting pursuant to the charting by exception policy, the nurses did not regularly record certain information that is important in diagnosing an infection, such as the changing characteristics of the surgical wound and Mr. Lama's complaints of pain. A nurse who took care of Mr. Lama testified that she would not document a patient's pain if she either did not administer any medication or simply gave the patient an aspirin-type medication as opposed to a narcotic.

According to the expert witness who testified on behalf of Mr. Lama, his medical record contained scattered possible signs of infection that deserved further investigation, including the excessively bloody bandage and local pain at the site of the wound. In the expert witness' opinion, Mr. Lama acquired the infection as early as May 17 when the very bloody bandage was first noted, or possibly May 19 when he complained of pain at the site of the wound. The infection progressed into discitis on or about May 20 when Mr. Lama experienced excruciating back pain. Although the initial infection may not have been preventable, the significant issue is whether early detection and treatment would have prevented the infection from developing into discitis. According to the

plaintiff's expert witness: "Time is an extremely important factor in handling an infection; a 24-hour delay in treatment can make a difference; and a delay of several days carries a high risk that the infection will not be properly controlled" (*Lama v Borras*, p. 481).

In upholding the jury's verdict, the court reasoned (*Lama v Borras*, p. 477):

> As to Hospital del Maestro, it was entirely possible for the jury to conclude that the particular way in which the medical and nursing records were kept constituted evidence of carelessness in monitoring the patient after the second operation. Perhaps the infection would have been reported and documented earlier. Perhaps the hospital was negligent in not dealing appropriately with wound inspection and cleaning, (and) bandage changing.

It was the hospital's "substandard record keeping procedures (that) delayed the diagnosis and treatment of Romera's wound infection at a time when controlling the wound infection was likely to prevent the development of the more serious discitis" (*Lama v Borras*, p. 481). The jury thus awarded Mr. Lama $600,000 in compensatory damages.

This case represents how a jury might perceive such a documentation system that does not clearly reflect knowledge and attentiveness of the nursing staff. The nurse will be challenged to comply with new documentation systems while also validating that standards of care have been met.

In an attempt to make documentation more efficient, there has been a trend to develop flow sheets in lieu of the traditional narrative nurse's notes. (Box 15-1 gives criteria for flow sheets.) Although flow sheets are likely to reflect a more accurate and complete record and require less time for documentation, there are also certain pitfalls.

All *blanks* must be filled in or noted as "N/A." Otherwise, it appears there was an oversight in

B O X   1 5 - 1

Criteria for Flow Sheets

No blanks
Specific times of events
Provider identification
Complement narrative entries
Patient identification

making that assessment or performing that function. A blank box on an emergency room record resulted in a verdict of $1,304,984 in favor of a 30-year-old man.

On April 6, 1993, the patient came to the hospital's emergency department and was first seen by a nurse. The nurse documented that the patient was experiencing a recent onset of "pain all over" the abdomen. However, the patient testified that he had told the nurse the pain was localized on the right side. The emergency physician did not identify any localized tenderness and documented, "no peritoneal signs." There was no laboratory workup, and the patient was given Donnatol and discharged.

At trial, the issue was what discharge instructions, if any, were given to the patient. The testimony was that the patient should have been given a set of computerized instructions that advised him to return to the emergency department or obtain other medical care "if you don't get better." They also would have directed the patient to return if the pain localized in his right lower quadrant. On the emergency department record, there was a box that the nurse was to check if the patient was given the computerized instructions. On the patient's emergency department record, the box was blank.

The hospital's position was that the patient must have received the computerized form, since it was the nurse's habit to give it to patients and she was very responsible. Yet the patient testified that he was given no information that alerted him to the possibility of a serious condition; he was told only that he had gastroenteritis, which was the diagnosis in his medical record.

When the patient did not improve, he went to a different hospital, where he was found to be extremely septic. He was taken to surgery, and a ruptured appendix was discovered, with a portion of the large bowel gangrenous. The surgeon resected the bowel, but three subsequent operations were required over a period of 7 weeks. A portion of the right scrotum had to be removed. The patient had an ileostomy for a time, and his residual disability includes a short bowel syndrome.

The issue at trial was not whether a diagnosis of appendicitis should have been made on April 6; the issue was the adequacy of discharge instructions. The patient testified the only information given him was a photocopied form that indicated that he should return "if worse." Thus, because his complaints were no better but no worse, the instruction did not prompt him to seek further medical care. The patient's treating surgeon testified that the patient was meticulous about following instructions, as reflected by him having made 26 trips from the San Francisco Bay area to the surgeon's office in Yuba City for follow up after his hospital discharge, never missing a single appointment. It was the surgeon's opinion that the patient had a literal mind and if he had been instructed to return if he was not better, he believed the patient would have done so.

The jury apportioned 60% of the fault to the patient for his failure to seek care more promptly, and apportioned 40% of the fault to the hospital defendant. The emergency physician won a defense verdict. The jury thus concluded that it was the nurse's oversight in failing to give the patient the computerized instruction sheet that resulted in its verdict.

The specific *time* of the assessment or activity must be noted rather than a general time frame encompassing hours. If that parameter is reassessed, that should also be noted, even if it is not otherwise required to have been done. It must be clear *who* performs each assessment or activity. If initials are used, the provider's full name and credentials must be documented on the page. Make certain that the patient's name and the date are written on each flow sheet or page of a multipage document, including the front and back.

Although the intent of flow sheets is to minimize narrative documentation, they do not eliminate the need for such entries. The goal is to have these documentation tools complement one another without duplicating information charted. For those entries that are in a *narrative* format, several significant criteria will make that documentation more effective and provide a better defense in malpractice actions.

Entries must be written objectively, not subjectively. Objective information is that information within the personal knowledge of the nurse who documents the information. These are the facts as seen, heard, or done by the nurse. An opinion or characterization of an event is subjective documentation. An example of subjective documentation is the entry, "patient has pain." It is the nurse's perception that the patient is experiencing pain, since "pain" is not a direct observation. The nurse may be observing the patient crying, moaning, holding a part of the body, or exhibiting a behavior that may be interpreted as pain. The patient may state: "My head is causing me extreme pain." These are the objective findings and what must be documented. Documenting specific statements made by a patient is effective and is encouraged.

If a nurse documents what someone else has seen, heard, or done, the identity of that person must be reflected in the medical record. It must be clear that the nurse documenting has no personal knowledge of the accuracy of those events or information. Otherwise, the nurse documenting the information may be held legally liable for the events, since that nurse's name is in the medical record associated with the events.

Patient medical records must contain accurate and complete information. The failure to do so may result in liability, as occurred in a California case brought against an HMO, Family Health Program (FHP) (Los Angeles County Superior Court, No. SOC76558, July, 1990). The patient, a 23-year-old pregnant woman, went to FHP's outpatient clinic for her first prenatal visit. A nurse practitioner examined the patient and obtained a history, upon which she estimated delivery on January 31, 1984. Subsequently, the patient had two ultrasound examinations, both ordered by the nurse practitioner. A due date of March 7 was given based on these examinations. However, even though the sonogram reports were sent to the nurse practitioner, she did not correct the clinic record to reflect the changed due date.

On December 25, the patient felt she had leaking amniotic fluid and went to the hospital. She was seen by an obstetrician whom she had not seen before. Because the sonograms were not in the patient's medical record, the only information available to the obstetrician was the January 31 due date and thus he assumed the patient was at 35 weeks. The obstetrician hospitalized the patient, anticipating she would soon go into labor. Twenty-four hours after hospitalization the patient still had not begun labor; because of the ruptured membranes, the obstetrician thought there was a risk of infection. He started an intravenous solution of Pitocin, and the patient delivered 12 hours later. The baby weighed 3 pounds, 4 ounces. Two days after birth, the baby exhibited apnea of prematurity and subsequently developed a small intracranial bleed. He then developed a periventricular leukomalacia with consequent spastic quadriparesis, most profoundly involving the lower extremities.

The primary negligence issue at trial was the accuracy of the estimated due date. Although there was some testimony supporting the original due date of January 31, the stronger testimony supported the due date of March 7 based on the sonograms at 16 weeks and 23 weeks. The focus then was on the fact that the nurse practitioner did not document the correct due date based on the sonograms, which resulted in the obstetrician relying on the wrong due date. The jury agreed that it was the nurse's negligence that caused the significant damages to the infant and returned a verdict of $9.8 million.

A frequent problem with documentation is that it lacks specificity as to when observations or actions occurred related to a patient. In addition, documentation is not accurately timed when the entry is made in the medical record. The entry must be timed when it is being documented in the medical record. Within the context of the entry, indicate the time of the observations or events being reported. Depending on the event, it may be important to document specific times that events occurred, such as telephone calls to physicians, a patient's sudden change in vital signs or condition, or a patient activity. More general observations can be noted over a time frame of one or several hours, such as a patient visiting with family, sleeping, or complaining of pain. The specificity required is generally associated with the patient's acuity level and whether the patient is in a long-term care facility, in the ICU, or at home.

Because the critical purpose of documentation is to record and communicate information about the patient, the documentation must be legible. An illegible entry can result in malpractice. In conjunction with legibility, only abbreviations that have been approved within the facility should be used so that entries can be interpreted by other readers. This is a require-

ment for some health care facilities by the Joint Commission on Accreditation of Healthcare Organizations and state laws (Box 15-2).

Although the medical record is considered a legal document, corrections and additions can be made provided they are accurately reflected. There is no time limit as to when a correction can be made or information can be added to a medical record. The only caution is where it is either known or suspected that the medical record may become the subject of litigation or involved in other legal action. Under those circumstances, any errors in the medical record should be brought to the attention of the attorney or risk manager for the health care provider or facility.

Entries are deleted by drawing a *single line* through the entry; avoid obliterating what is written. The deletion is noted with the *initials* of the person making the deletion, and the *date* and *time* of the deletion. This eliminates any allegation that a deletion was made subsequent to a claim or lawsuit.

If correct or new information needs to be added, *date and time the entry* when it is being made. Within the context of the entry, document the date and time of the event to which the entry refers.

An example of how the failure to appropriately correct an error in charting a medication can result in liability is demonstrated in *Georgia Osteopathic Hospital v O'Neal,* 403 SE 2d 235 (Ga. App. 1991). George O'Neal was admitted to Georgia Osteopathic Hospital on December

---

B O X   1 5 - 2

Corrections and Additions

Single line through error
Date, time, and initial error
Correctly identify when information was added

12 because of complaints of head and neck pain and numbness in his right hand. Mr. O'Neal was also exhibiting symptoms of hypertension, creating a concern that he might have a stroke. Over the next 3 days, Mr. O'Neal received numerous central nervous system depressant drugs.

At approximately 12:25 AM on December 15, the nursing staff first became concerned about Mr. O'Neal's behavior. He was exhibiting an "inappropriate laugh" and refused to take his medications because they were aggravating his pain. During the next hour and a half, it was documented that Mr. O'Neal complained of feeling short of breath and of experiencing numbness "in the back of his head." Finally at 2:10 AM, after Mr. O'Neal again refused his medication, his nurse notified the house intern. The nurses were then instructed to discontinue several of the medications for Mr. O'Neal.

Later that morning, Nurse McKenzie observed that Mr. O'Neal appeared confused and disturbed, and she spent several hours with him during the morning attempting to reassure and comfort him. Nurse McKenzie also called Dr. Boecker several times to express concerns about Mr. O'Neal and related that he threatened to leave the hospital. Dr. Boecker saw Mr. O'Neal at 12:40 PM and observed that Mr. O'Neal had an "inappropriate affect and uncharacteristic confusion regarding time and events." Dr. Boecker then requested a neurologist, Dr. Lara, to examine Mr. O'Neal, which he did at about 2 PM. Dr. Lara concluded that Mr. O'Neal was "suffering from a confusional state secondary to medication effect." However, he concluded that Mr. O'Neal was not dangerous at this time. Based on this recommendation, by 3 PM, Dr. Boecker had discontinued all of Mr. O'Neal's prior medications.

At approximately 10:15 PM, Mr. O'Neal called the nurses' station and asked for someone to come and look at his arm. When Nurse Branch responded, she found Mr. O'Neal sitting in a chair beside his bed. As she touched his arm to look at it, he jumped back in a manner in which she found alarming. She said she would have someone else look at his arm. Mr. O'Neal responded, "Well, I'm going to die anyway," and grabbed a pocket knife and charged at Nurse Branch. Although Nurse Branch escaped uninjured, Mr. O'Neal ultimately stabbed and wounded another nurse, a security guard, and himself before the police arrived and shot him to death.

Mr. O'Neal's family filed a lawsuit against the hospital, alleging the following:

1. Its pharmacy was negligent in failing to monitor the various medications being provided to Mr. O'Neal for possible adverse interactions.
2. Its nurses were negligent in failing to keep Mr. O'Neal's physicians, as well as their own superiors, adequately informed about Mr. O'Neal's deteriorating condition.
3. Its nurses were negligent in failing to apply physical restraints to Mr. O'Neal before he went berserk.
4. Nurse Branch had given Mr. O'Neal a discontinued drug, Dalmane, approximately a half hour before he went berserk.

At trial, the plaintiffs' psychiatric expert witness testified that Dalmane was a very potent central nervous system depressant drug. His opinion was that the co-administration of the numerous central nervous system depressant drugs precipitated an anticholinergic drug reaction in Mr. O'Neal that ultimately caused him to go berserk. If, in fact, Dalmane was administered on the night of December 15, it "was probably the straw that broke the camel's back."

Nurse Branch, however, testified that she had not administered Dalmane to Mr. O'Neal on the night of December 15; that she had administered it to him only on the previous night, before it was discontinued. Yet she acknowledged having previously testified in her deposition that she had given Dalmane to Mr. O'Neal on the night of December 15.

In Mr. O'Neal's medical record, it was noted that on December 15, the entry for Dalmane was written with a line drawn through it and the notation "D/C" written beside it. As the court reasoned, it was "within the jury's province to determine whether this entry contradicted or supported the witness' original deposition testimony." "There can be no question that hospital nurses are under a duty to refrain from giving patients unauthorized medications" (*Georgia Osteopathic Hospital v O'Neal*, p. 242).

The court further noted that a prior inconsistent statement of a witness is admissible as substantive evidence and thus the jury was authorized to conclude that the original deposition testimony of Nurse Branch had not been the product of confusion about the dates, but that she had fully intended to testify that she administered Dalmane to Mr. O'Neal at 9:45 PM on the night he died. Substantive deposition testimony may not be erased from the record through the mere submission of an errata sheet or subsequent attempt to change the testimony (*Georgia Osteopathic Hospital v O'Neal*, p. 242).

Had the entry been corrected appropriately by Nurse Branch, with her initials and the date and time of the correction, the hospital would have had no liability for the death of Mr. O'Neal.

The medical record is the primary source of communication among health care providers. However, frequently an urgent situation requires the information to be communicated verbally as well as in writing. These verbal communications must be clearly documented to reflect when another health care provider is notified about a significant event or change in a patient's condition. The specific time of the phone call should be documented and the entry should include to whom information was given, what information was given, and the response. Avoid

making vague references to the patient's condition; the specific concerns about the patient's condition must be documented.

Physicians and other health care providers have a right to rely on nurses to notify them when there are significant events with their patients. If a nurse attempts to reach a health care provider who does not respond in a timely way, it is the nurse's responsibility to find another individual who can provide the necessary assistance. It is the nurse who will ultimately be held accountable for obtaining the appropriate treatment for the patient.

▪ STAFFING

Nurses have been significantly affected by the changes in the delivery of health care services that have occurred over the past 30 years. Many of the changes are directly related to reimbursement as well as to the increased costs for health care services. Health care facilities and nurses are expected to comply with the applicable standards of care, regardless of what staff are available to provide patient care. Inability to have adequate staff in terms of training and numbers is not a viable defense.

There has been much speculation that current staffing levels in health care facilities are inadequate to meet patient care needs, and that patient care is suffering as a result. However, no reliable study or other data demonstrate a direct correlation between what the nurses are perceiving staffing levels to be with objective measures of quality of care (Institute of Medicine, 1996). Neither are there data that establish at what staffing level quality is achieved.

Unlicensed Assistive Personnel

Many of the concerns regarding current staffing also result from the increased use of unlicensed assistive personnel. Such health care providers have always been used in health care facilities. As the scope of nursing practice has expanded, so has the scope of practice for unlicensed assistive personnel. They now have skills and competencies to perform tasks that were traditionally assigned to nurses. As nurses have invaded the scope of medical practice, these providers are now invading the scope of traditional nursing practice.

In using unlicensed assistive personnel, the important determination is whether that provider is competent to perform the delegated task. It is the unlicensed assistive person who will be liable for the appropriate performance of the assignment (Box 15-3). As discussed above, the nurse has the right to rely on other providers to carry out their assignments competently. There is no automatic or vicarious liability placed on the nurse who is making the assignment. It is also not required that a nurse validate that every assignment was performed competently.

The nurse is responsible for providing adequate supervision over those persons to whom assignments have been made. "Adequate supervision" has been defined by the American Nurses Association (ANA) as (American Nurses Association, 1992):

> the active process of directing, guiding and influencing the outcome of an individual's performance of an activity. Supervision is generally categorized as on-site (the nurse being physically present or immediately available while the activity is being performed) or off-site (the nurse has the ability to provide direction through various means of written and verbal communication).

B O X   1 5 - 3

Unlicensed Assistive Personnel

Unlicensed assistive personnel, adequately supervised, will be held personally responsible for the appropriate performance of their assignments.

Supervision includes such activities as providing an adequate orientation to the unit, providing appropriate policies and procedures, providing inservice training and continuing education opportunities, and performing effective and timely competency evaluations. In effect, supervision is a process that is continuous but also flexible to meet the needs of each staff member.

Making Assignments

Several factors are important to consider when making assignments. The patient must be assessed to determine the knowledge and skills a provider needs to treat that patient. This includes the status of the patient physically, psychologically, and emotionally. Based on the patient's assessment, the minimum needs for that patient are identified, including teaching and discharge planning. Another issue is the extent to which other professional staff are available to provide assistance to the nurse, such as clinical nurse specialists, pharmacists, residents, intravenous therapy nursing teams, respiratory therapists, and laboratory personnel. Obviously, the availability of such personnel will decrease some of the nursing responsibilities and workload. Finally, the nurse needs to examine what health care providers are available from the perspective of numbers, their level of education, their experience, and their familiarity with the unit.

It is unnecessary to document every staffing judgment; however, the process used in making staffing decisions must be delineated in internal documents. These should not be written as mandatory staffing patterns but provide an anticipated range of staff required. The criteria to be considered in making staffing decisions must be defined. The following are suggested criteria (Feutz-Harter, 1997):

1. The number of patients
2. Patient acuity levels
3. The number of available RNs, LPNs, LVNs, and unlicensed assistive personnel

4. The experience of the available staff
5. The familiarity of the nursing staff with the unit
6. What shift it is
7. What day of the week it is
8. Other resources available to the nursing staff to provide assistance

The mechanism used frequently to maximize staffing is to require nurses to float from their regular assignments. However, nurses must be advised before they are employed if floating will be used at the facility. Courts have upheld the appropriateness of floating and determined that it is not unlawful nor does it constitute serious misconduct.

In *Francis v Memorial General Hospital,* 726 P 2d 852 (N.M. 1986), an RN sued the hospital for suspending him for failure to float from his regular assignment in the ICU to the orthopedics unit. The basis for the nurse's refusal was that he was unfamiliar with this area and felt incompetent to be the charge nurse there. The court noted that floating was an established policy at the hospital, which was made known to the nurse at the time of employment. He had been offered the option of orienting to other units so that he would feel more comfortable if requested to float to one of those units. Yet the nurse refused this offer.

As the court reasoned (*Francis v Memorial General Hospital,* p. 855):

> Requiring a nurse to "float" is not the kind of unlawful or serious misconduct for which recognition of the tort of wrongful discharge was intended. Moreover, the hospital is quite correct in responding that "floating" in fact implements another important public policy, that of maintaining an adequate staff on all patient floors in a cost-effective manner.

Thus the court upheld the nurse's discharge.

The Wisconsin Supreme Court issued a somewhat different opinion in *Winkelman v Beloit Memorial Hospital,* 483 NW 2d 211 (Wis.

1992). Betty Winkelman graduated from nursing school in 1947, obtained a bachelor's degree in nursing in 1953, and obtained a master's degree in nursing service administration in 1956. She was employed part-time at Beloit Memorial Hospital from 1971 to 1987. During this time, she worked exclusively in the nursery.

In October 1987, the hospital developed a specific policy requiring all nurses in the maternity ward to float when not needed there. The guidelines stated that "the responsibilities of floating will be to do nursing care on a prn basis, not in a team-leading capacity."

On November 24, 1987, when Nurse Winkelman arrived at the hospital, she learned that the maternity ward was overstaffed and she was requested to float to the postoperative and geriatric care unit. Nurse Winkelman met with Supervisor Nurse Linebarger and told her that she had never floated, that she was exclusively a nursery nurse, that she was unqualified to float to that area of the hospital, and that floating would put the patients at risk, her license at risk, and the hospital in jeopardy. Nurse Winkelman testified that Nurse Linebarger gave her the options of floating, finding another nurse to float in her place, or taking an unexcused absence day and going home. That testimony was contradicted by Nurse Linebarger, who said she told Nurse Winkelman to either accept the assignment or find a replacement. Instead, Nurse Winkelman went home.

Nurse Winkelman then received a letter from the hospital stating that it construed her actions as a voluntary resignation of her employment. Although Nurse Winkelman denied that she had resigned and requested reinstatement, the hospital refused. Nurse Winkelman then filed a lawsuit alleging that the hospital's actions constituted a wrongful discharge "contrary to a fundamental and well-defined public policy."

At trial, the hospital argued that its floating policy did not require Nurse Winkelman to offer or perform services for which she was unqualified. Nurse Winkelman disagreed and testified that her 40-year history of nursery-only work made her unqualified for even the simplest tasks on a postoperative and geriatric floor.

The Court took judicial notice of the Wisconsin Administrative Code, which stated the following (*Winkelman v Beloit Memorial Hospital*, p. 217):

> A nurse is not necessarily qualified or competent to practice in any area of nursing simply because the nurse has graduated from a school of nursing and has passed the licensure exam. Therefore, employers and nurses themselves are accountable for determining competence to practice in a particular area of specialty. If a particular area is not a nurse's major area of employment, the nurse has a right to refuse assignment to the questionable area. If an employer wants a nurse to rotate to an area that is not the nurse's usual area of assignment, then the employer should provide for the nurse's further education and training to prepare the nurse to work in the area

The Court's opinion was that there was sufficient evidence to show that Nurse Winkelman was not professionally trained or qualified to be assigned to the postoperative and geriatric unit or even to select a nurse to float to the unit.

The troubling aspect of this case is that there was no evidence that Nurse Winkelman was asked to perform services for which she was unqualified. This was focused on in a dissenting opinion of one of the judges, who noted that the obstetrics nurse who accepted the assignment in place of Nurse Winkelman testified that she was at the assigned unit about half of a day. When she felt uncomfortable with an assigned task, she merely refused to do it and was not disciplined in any way for such refusal. The judge further noted that all of the other obstetrics nurses were willing to render their assistance elsewhere; it was only Nurse Winkelman who refused to be floated. This seems somewhat strange in light of Nurse Winkelman's numerous

years of nursing experience, teaching experience, and her advanced education.

This judge concluded that the conflict between Nurse Winkelman and the hospital constituted a difference in professional judgment (*Winkelman v Beloit Memorial Hospital*, p. 220):

> The hospital had a legitimate purpose in attempting to control health care costs by maximizing its work force in a flexible manner while at the same time assuring a basic level of quality care to its patients. The majority opinion here allows a professional employee, such as Winkelman, to exercise a vital power over the professional judgments of an employer. Id. at 220.

What this case demonstrates is the need for a specific policy on floating that delineates the scope of activities to be performed by a nurse who is asked to float to another area. The emphasis must be on assigning tasks within the nurse's level of competency. Identify techniques to facilitate the usefulness of nurses who are floated. Requiring nurses to attend orientations on the various units to which they may be floated familiarizes the nurse with the layout of the unit, equipment routinely used there, types of patients, and staff and decreases the nurse's anxiety if requested to float to that unit.

Agency Personnel

Many health care facilities have found it necessary to use agency personnel on a regular basis. The use of agency personnel is frequently criticized, based on perceptions that care provided by them is substandard. In 1980 the Department of Health and Human Services began a study on use of agency personnel and found no evidence that agency personnel caused detrimental effects on the quality of nursing care (Department of Health and Human Services, 1993). The study demonstrated that many of the nurses working for agencies did so as a second job and that the average nurse had worked 9 years. Whereas some facilities using agency nurses increased their costs, other facilities reported their use decreased costs.

Health care facilities should have written agreements with temporary agencies delineating the responsibilities of each organization. Such an agreement increases the effectiveness of agency nurses as well as decreases the potential liability to the health care facility. The facility should provide job descriptions and special requirements for practice areas that the agency can use in selecting nurses. Other issues that should be addressed in the written agreement include the following:

1. Requiring the agency to screen and assess nurses before assigning them to the health care facility, including performing a skills assessment and health screening for communicable diseases
2. Requiring mandatory orientation to the health care facility
3. Designating supervisory staff at the health care facility to evaluate the agency nurse and make a report to the agency
4. Establishing the right of the health care facility to dismiss a nurse immediately and without recourse if the nurse is found unacceptable for the assignment
5. Requiring the agency to carry worker's compensation insurance for its nurses
6. Requiring the agency to carry professional liability insurance coverage for itself and its nurses, or requiring the nurses to personally carry professional liability insurance with minimal levels of coverage

The health care facility can be found liable for the acts of agency nurses even though they are not employees. Although an employer is automatically liable for the acts of its employees, under a theory of vicarious liability or respondeat superior, there is a different relationship between a health care facility and an agency nurse. Because the agency nurse is being held out to the public by the health care facility, it has a duty to provide a competent nurse; patients have a right to rely on the health care facility to provide it with competent nurses. An important responsibility is the appropriate selection of the nurse. The health care facility is not in a position to make that determination and therefore must rely upon the agency to appropriately screen and assess nurses before assigning them. The health care facility will then have some responsibility for assessing the nurse's performance. The basis for imposition of liability on the health care facility is whether it knew or should have known of an agency nurse's incompetency.

Liability

In medical malpractice actions, allegations of improper staffing assignments or lack of staff are increasing. A mistake by an unqualified nurse that caused severe injuries to a mother and her newborn baby resulted in a verdict of $12.7 million against a Texas hospital. *Chan Lee and Lisa Lee, Individually and as Next Friends of Alexander Lee v Chin H. Lee,* No. 93-31897 (Tex. 151st Jud. Dist. 1995). Nurse Tarriman injected Mrs. Lee with Pitocin when it was not ordered by her physician. Because Mrs. Lee had already started labor, the Pitocin caused spasms and shock to her system, resulting in severe brain damage to her son, Alexander. Mrs. Lee also required emergency removal of her uterus and other life-saving measures.

The significant evidence at trial included testimony that Nurse Tarriman had only 4 months of experience; questions were raised regarding whether she was qualified as an obstetrics nurse. Also, the hospital produced documents that reflected that it had reduced the nursing staff to save money. The jurors were angered by these documents, which caused them to award such substantial damages.

Managing Assignments

When a nurse is reassigned to an unfamiliar unit, the immediate response is to object to the assignment, claiming a lack of competency. Instead, the nurse should begin by clarifying what tasks the nurse may be asked to perform and what other staff will be available to provide any necessary care beyond the nurse's competency. If at that point the nurse truly believes that the assignment is unsafe for the patients, the nurse should know what procedure needs to be followed within the health care facility. The facility must have written guidelines identifying how these issues will be resolved so that they can be dealt with, and dealt with uniformly (Box 15-4).

In the guidelines, delineate the mechanism for resolving questionable assignments. There must be a mechanism for immediate intervention as well as an appeal or review process of assignment decisions. Identify the factors the nurse should consider when being given an assignment. Recognize the right of a nurse to reject an unreasonable assignment. Explain how a rejection is to be communicated, to whom the rejection is to be communicated, the documentation necessary to support that decision, and to whom copies of the documentation are distributed. Identify who will have the immediate authority to make decisions regarding assignments.

Specific disciplinary actions should be outlined that may be taken when a nurse refuses an assignment. What actions are available may depend in part on state laws regarding the rights of employees or the existence of any contract or collective bargaining agreement. These disciplinary actions must be complied with to avoid allegations of discrimination by treating one nurse differently from how another is treated for refusing an assignment.

It is recommended that before employment, nurses be specifically advised of the policy regarding assignments. This will avoid any potential allegation that the nurse might make of being unaware of the health care facility's policy regarding assignments in the event the nurse sues relating to an assignment. Perhaps more important, it provides an opportune time for the issue of assignments to be discussed with the nurse. Through recognition of a nurse's right to reject an inappropriate assignment, which is balanced by the facility's policy regarding prevention or resolution of problematic assignments, this promotes a cohesive and professional atmosphere among the nurses and the health care facility's administrators.

■ CLINICAL PRACTICE GUIDELINES

Two of the hot terms in health care are *clinical practice guidelines* and *critical paths.* In actuality, these are not new. The twentieth century will be known for the emphasis on identifying optimal methods of practice. Numerous professional organizations have developed guidelines to reflect this knowledge, such as the Joint Commission on Accreditation of Healthcare Organizations and the National Committee for Quality Assurance. In 1977 the federal government became involved when the National Institutes of Health established its Consensus Development Conference Program to reach consensus on a wide range of medical problems and treatments. These documents have been identified by an assortment of terms: *algorithms, clinical indica-*

B O X   1 5 - 4

Managing Assignments

When a nurse questions an assignment, consider:

Factors for evaluating an assignment
Procedure for rejecting an assignment
Who has decision-making authority
What are the disciplinary actions for rejecting an assignment
What is the appeals process

tors, guidelines, practice parameters, protocols, and *standards.* Finally in 1989 these documents became codified as *clinical practice guidelines.*

The Agency for Health Care Policy and Research (AHCPR) was created with the passage of Public Law 101-239 and the Omnibus Budget Reconciliation Act of 1989. The AHCPR was challenged with a bold mission (42 U.S.C. §299[b]):

> The purpose of the Agency is to enhance the quality, appropriateness and effectiveness of health care services, and access to such services, through the establishment of a broad base of scientific research and through the promotion of improvement in clinical practice (including the prevention of diseases and other health conditions) and in the organization, financing and delivery of health care services.

In implementing its duties, the AHCPR focuses on the following (42 U.S.C. §299a[a]):
1. Effectiveness, efficiency, and quality of health care services
2. Outcomes of health care services and procedures
3. Clinical practice, including primary care and practice-oriented research
4. Health care technologies, facilities, and equipment
5. Health care costs, productivity, and market forces
6. Health promotion and disease prevention
7. Health statistics and epidemiology
8. Medical liability

The first accomplishment of the AHCPR, in conjunction with the Institute of Medicine (IOM), was to define clinical practice guidelines: "systematically developed statements to assist practitioner and patient decisions about appropriate health care for specific clinical circumstances" (Field & Lohr, 1990). As this definition reflects, the intent is to focus on clinical conditions rather than on technical procedures. With this definition forming the structure for its

work, the AHCPR and IOM have attempted to meet their legal charge: to develop and periodically review and update (1) clinically relevant guidelines that may be used by physicians, educators, and health care providers to assist in determining how diseases, disorders, and other health conditions can most effectively and appropriately be prevented, diagnosed, treated, and managed clinically; and (2) standards of quality, performance measures, and medical review criteria through which health care providers and other appropriate entities may assess or review the provision of health care and assure the quality of such care (42 U.S.C. §299b-1[a]).

The clinical practice guidelines are to be based on the best available research and professional judgment regarding the effectiveness and appropriateness of health care services and procedures. They are to be treatment-specific or condition-specific and presented in formats appropriate for use in clinical practice, for use in educational programs, and for use in reviewing quality and appropriateness of medical care. Another aspect of the clinical practice guidelines are that they are to include information on risks and benefits of alternative strategies for prevention, diagnosis, treatment, and management of a given disease, disorder, or other health condition, along with the cost of each alternative strategy.

The legislation requires that each clinical practice guideline be formatted into four documents to meet the needs of different audiences. They are as follows:
• *Clinical Practice Guideline.* This version contains the specific guideline statements and recommendations, algorithms, summary of evidence tables, and pertinent references. It is intended for use by health care practitioners as a reference for clinical decision-making.
• *Quick Reference guide for Clinicians.* This document is an abbreviated version of the *Clinical Practice Guideline.* It includes a summary of the points of prevention, diagnosis,

and treatment. It is for day-to-day use by health care practitioners.

- *Consumer Version.* This version is for patients, care givers, and parents of young patients and describes the condition, presents treatment options with benefits and risks in easy-to-understand terms, and suggests questions to ask health care practitioners. The information is intended to help patients make decisions about treatment alternatives. This version is published in English and Spanish.

- *Guideline Technical Report.* This technical version contains all background and supporting materials for the clinical practice guideline, including algorithms, methodology, literature review, summary of scientific evidence tables, references, and a comprehensive bibliography. It is for health care practitioners, researchers, educators, and professional organizations.

The AHCPR clinical practice guidelines are developed by expert panels, consisting of approximately 15 members who represent a broad range of professional disciplines and clinical experience relevant to the clinical condition under study, as well as representing a diversity of geographic locations and ethnic origins. The panels also include health care consumers. A significant characteristic of the AHCPR clinical practice guidelines is that they address patient preferences and are specifically drafted so that patients will actively participate in the decision-making process. The procedure used in developing the guidelines includes the following steps:

1. Define the scope of the guideline.
2. Define the major questions regarding the clinical condition that the guideline will address.
3. Review and analyze the available scientific research for each question.
4. Review estimates of important patient outcomes that will be influenced by the interventions for the clinical condition.
5. Review benefits and harms of each intervention.
6. Review current and potential health care costs associated with the guideline. Where cost information is available and reliable, provide costs of alternative strategies.
7. Invite information and comments on the guideline topic from professional and consumer organizations, researchers, and others at a public open meeting.
8. Prepare the guideline draft on the basis of available empirical evidence, and professional judgment when empirical evidence is insufficient.
9. Submit the draft guideline for independent review by outside experts.
10. Revise the draft guideline on the basis of analysis of comments and information received.
11. Prepare the guideline in the required formats appropriate for use by providers, consumers, educators, and researchers.
12. Periodically review the new scientific evidence related to the clinical condition, and update the guideline when such evidence indicates a need.

The same criteria and process that is used in developing the AHCPR clinical practice guidelines should be used by health care facilities in developing their own internal guidelines. A multidisciplinary team must be involved in their development, implementation, and evaluation for them to meet the eight attributes of clinical practice guidelines as defined by the IOM. These are as follows: validity; reliability and reproducibility; clinical applicability; clinical flexibility; clarity; multidisciplinary process; scheduled review; and documentation (Field & Lohr, 1990). Especially important is the inclusion of alternative acceptable treatments to avoid perceptions of the guidelines as an attempt to establish cookbook medicine.

Nurses have used clinical practice guidelines for decades in delivering patient care; these guidelines have been in the form of care plans and protocols. These are now evolving into more scientifically grounded documents with a greater emphasis on specific patient outcomes. Another significant change is that they are developed in collaboration with other health care providers, which streamlines and increases the effectiveness of patient care. Clinical practice guidelines are not intended to be used in a vacuum but must be considered in the total context of that patient, in that environment, with those providers. Deviations from clinical practice guidelines should not be interpreted as automatically representing a breach of the standard of care. It is expected that alterations in treatment will occur because of specific patient variances, needs, or desires or because of clinical differences.

The actual legal effect of clinical practice guidelines is currently unknown. There has been much speculation that the likely impact of clinical practice guidelines will be to increase liability exposure of health care providers and facilities. The theory is that such documents will be used in medical malpractice cases to prove that the defendant provider deviated from the standard of care because there was a deviation from the clinical practice guidelines. Although it is true that courts look to statements by professional groups and health care facilities as defining standards of practice, this is precisely as it should be. The strength of these documents is that these are standards of care drawn from the consensus work of informed, competent providers with appropriate experience. Their use may actually prevent the retrospective expert witness battles that are currently prevalent in the courtroom.

A legitimate function of clinical practice guidelines is to establish a quality baseline with which professional conduct is compared. Although the clinical practice guideline may establish evidentiary presumption of what constitutes appropriate care, the defendant provider

will then be offered an opportunity to rebut or overcome the presumption by showing that the clinical practice guideline was not applicable to the facts of the particular case. At a minimum, the provider will know the conduct for which the provider will be held accountable and will understand the need to justify any deviation from that guideline rather than anticipating what standard of care may be argued by expert witnesses.

There is also a potential benefit: compliance with clinical practice guidelines may be presumptive evidence of appropriate conduct as a defense in medical malpractice actions. The clinical practice guideline will become recognized as a standard of care and preempt other standards. Thus the more reasoned analysis is that clinical practice guidelines have a greater potential to reduce rather than increase liability exposure.

■ INFORMED CONSENT

Patients today are much more personally involved in making health care treatment decisions and less likely to blindly accept a decision by a health care provider. This is reflected by the significant rise in the number of lawsuits involving allegations of failure to obtain consent or lack of informed consent. In a study conducted on informed consent issues with endoscopists, 42% reported that in lawsuits brought against them, the informed consent process was an issue (Levine et al., 1995). It is clear that the doctrine of informed consent needs renewed attention.

The following premises form the legal basis for requiring that adequate information be provided to patients so that they may make informed decisions (*Cobbs v Grant,* 502 P 2d 1, 9 [Ca. 1972]):

1. Clients are generally persons unlearned in the medical sciences and, therefore, except in rare cases, courts may safely assume the knowledge of the client and physician are not in parity

2. An adult who is competent has the right to exercise control over what medical treatments are personally rendered
3. To be effective, a client's consent to treatment must be an informed consent
4. The client has an abject dependence upon and trust in the physician for the information which is relied upon during the decision-making process

Before touching a patient, the patient must consent. All states and the District of Columbia require consent, either by statute or by case law. This includes touching related to bathing, administering medication, listening to breath sounds, or performing a diagnostic test or surgical procedure. For many of these touchings, the consent is implied; patients voluntarily acquiesce to these activities, which can be interpreted as consent. This implicit consent applies for those activities and procedures that are not invasive and present very few risks. Yet a patient may revoke that implicit consent at any time. Any touching subsequent to that revoked consent constitutes a battery which is the unauthorized touching of another.

For those treatments, procedures, or diagnostic tests that have potentially serious side effects or complications or are invasive, specific informed consent is required. Examples include the following:

• Major or minor surgery that involves entry into the body
• Procedures in which anesthesia is used
• Medications
• Chemotherapy
• Hormone therapy
• Myelograms
• Intravenous pyelograms
• Arteriograms
• Radiologic therapy
• Electroconvulsive therapy
• Experimental procedures
• Transfusions of blood or blood products

If there is any doubt as to whether a treatment or procedure needs specific informed consent, err on the side of giving information to the patient and allowing the patient to decide whether to undergo the proposed procedure or treatment. More frequently, courts are ruling in favor of patients who allege treatments or procedures have been performed without the patient's specific consent.

There are four exceptions to the requirement for informed consent. If the patient has an *emergency medical condition,* consent is implied, either by statute or as a matter of public policy. What constitutes an emergency medical condition may be defined by state law or otherwise should be very broadly interpreted to extend to situations in which immediate treatment is necessary to prevent jeopardy of the patient's life, health, or limb; disfigurement; or impairment of faculties. If withholding a medical procedure or treatment may result in greater harm to the patient, consider it to be an emergency. In the patient's medical record, the nature of the emergency and why consent cannot be obtained must be documented to proceed under the implied consent law.

Another exception is the *therapeutic privilege,* which permits a physician to withhold information from a patient when it is believed that more harm will result by disclosing that information. This exception is much more difficult to defend in light of the recognition that patients have a right to accept or refuse treatment, regardless of the consequences. Obviously, withholding information will interfere with the patient's ability to make an informed decision. Thus, to defend an assertion of therapeutic privilege, the evidence must be substantial that the truth will create a greater harm than the lie.

A patient may choose to personally *waive* the right to consent and rely upon the decision of the health care provider. The issue will be whether this is a voluntary waiver of the right to consent. The waiver must be documented, perhaps through an authorization for the health care provider to consent on behalf of the patient.

The other exception to the informed consent requirement is where a patient has *knowledge* about the proposed treatment or procedure based on previous personal experiences or because the information pertinent to the decision is within the patient's common knowledge. If relying upon this exception, document how the patient is knowledgeable about the elements required for informed consent. It is also recommended that one not assume that the patient is knowledgeable. Rather, at a minimum, verify that the patient believes that he or she has the necessary information to make an informed decision (Box 15-5).

Although different people are frequently involved with each step, the same person can give the information as well as obtain consent. This is actually the preferred method.

It is generally accepted that the duty for giving information to the patient is that of the person ordering or the person performing the treatment or procedure. In acute care facilities that is usually a physician; in other practice settings it may be a nurse. In addition, a physician may delegate that responsibility to a nurse, who then assumes that duty and that liability for the information given to the patient.

BOX 15-5

Informed Decisions

Steps in obtaining an informed decision are:
1. Providing the information to the patient so that an informed decision can be made
2. Obtaining consent

In *Hoffson v Orentreich*, 543 NY Supp.2d 242 (N.Y. Sup. 1989), the patient alleged that the nurse failed to obtain her informed consent for a procedure. The patient, Ellen Hoffson, was diagnosed as having acne. During a visit to her dermatologist, Ms. Hoffson requested advice or treatment of her acne. Nurse Burke consulted with Dr. Kalman, and he ordered Nurse Burke to incise and drain three acne cysts and remove blackheads. The testimony was that Nurse Burke was trained in dermatologic procedures and performed the procedures appropriately with the consent of Dr. Kalman. Ms. Hoffson alleged that the procedure caused the formation of three disfiguring, permanent, depressed scars. The defendants asserted that the scars could not have resulted from or been produced by the procedure performed by Nurse Burke. In their opinion, they were self-induced by Ms. Hoffson's picking at her face, resulting in necrotic excoriation, for which she failed to obtain prompt medical treatment. The incision sites became infected, and scars developed.

As the court noted, Ms. Hoffson did not cite any authority for her allegation that Nurse Burke could not act as an agent for Dr. Kalman in obtaining her informed consent. The jury agreed that Nurse Burke had appropriately obtained consent and performed the procedures and that she had not engaged in the unauthorized practice of medicine (Box 15-6).

To make an informed decision, the patient must have a general *understanding* of what the proposed treatment or procedure will involve: How will the patient's body be invaded? Where will the incision be? How long will the surgery take? How much time will need to be spent at the clinic receiving chemotherapy treatments? The amount of information given to the patient will depend upon the patient's level of education, understanding, and interest. It should be sufficient so that the patient feels comfortable in knowing what is being proposed.

B O X   1 5 - 6

Elements for Informed Consent

Nature of the proposed procedure or treatment

Expected outcome and the likelihood of success

Material risks and the likelihood of occurrence

Alternatives and supporting information regarding those alternatives

Effect of no treatment or procedure, including the prognosis and material risks associated with no treatment

The patient should understand what the *purpose* and expected *outcome* of the treatment or procedure are—what is hoped to be accomplished. The patient also needs a realistic assessment of the likelihood of success. This may be based on general statistics as well as the provider's personal clinical experience with that treatment or procedure.

The third element is advising the patient of the potential material *risks* or complications. The failure to disclose material risks is the most common basis for alleging lack of informed consent. Whether a risk is "material" has not been defined by courts in view of either the frequency or severity of that risk. One court has held there is no duty to disclose a risk of death if it is considered minuscule (*Pauscher v Iowa Methodist Medical Center,* 408 NW 2d 255 [Ia. 1987]). Deciding materiality of a 1% possibility of paralysis resulting from a laminectomy was the issue in *Canterbury v Spence,* 464 F 2d 772 (D.C. App. 1972). As the court noted: "There is no bright line separating the significant from the insignificant; the answer in any case must abide by a rule of reason" (*Canterbury v Spence,* p. 787). Material risks have been defined as including "the risks or hazards that could have influenced a reasonable person in making a decision to give or withhold consent" (*Barclay v*

Campbell, 704 SW 2d 8, 9 [Tex. 1986]). There the court concluded that the materiality of a risk is based on how the condition manifests itself, the permanency of the condition caused by the risk, the known cures for the condition, the seriousness of the condition, and the overall effect of the condition on the body. As with the expected outcome, the frequency of occurrence of the material risks must also be discussed with the patient. What the patient will engage in is a balancing of the potential benefits versus the potential risks. That is in essence the thrust of the informed consent process. This is also where patients may differ in their decisions. Whereas one patient may conclude that the potential benefits outweigh the potential risks, another patient may conclude the opposite.

Advising the patient of any reasonable *alternatives* is the next element for informed consent. This also includes the supporting information about each of those alternatives: what it will involve, the expected outcome and likelihood of success, and the material risks and their frequency of occurrence.

The final element is explaining to the patient what may happen if no treatment or procedure is undertaken. This includes the risks or *prognosis* if the patient chooses to not receive treatment or a procedure.

The failure to so advise a patient of the potential risk of refusing a diagnostic procedure was the issue in *Truman v Thomas,* 611 P 2d 902 (Ca. 1980). The patient had presented to her gynecologist for her yearly examination. Although the physician recommended a Pap smear, the patient refused. When the patient subsequently died from cancer of the cervix, a lawsuit was brought against the physician alleging that he failed to inform the patient about the material risks of not consenting to the Pap smear. The evidence was that there were no references to any discussions regarding the Pap smear in the patient's medical record. The court's opinion was the following (*Truman v Thomas,* pp. 905-906):

> Material information is that which the physician knows or should know would be regarded as significant by a reasonable person in the patient's position when deciding to accept or reject the recommended medical procedure. . . . If the physician knows or should know of a patient's unique concerns or lack of familiarity with medical procedures, this may expand the scope of required disclosure.

The court concluded that the physician had a duty to apprise the patient of the risks of deciding not to undergo the Pap smear and the physician's failure to do so constituted medical malpractice.

The health care provider who engages in giving the information to the patient so that an informed decision can be made must document exactly what information is provided. General statements in the medical record such as "the procedure, its benefits and risks, alternatives, and prognosis without treatment were discussed with the patient" are no longer sufficient to defend an allegation of lack of informed consent. A recommendation is to develop consent forms specific for procedures or treatments that include all of the required information but also allow for modifications to be made as applicable to that patient. The consent form then constitutes the required documentation to support what the patient was told. Other suggested documentation includes the following:

- Whether anyone else was present during the discussion
- That the patient was given an opportunity to ask questions
- That the patient indicated his or her understanding
- The amount of time spent discussing the proposed treatment or procedure with the patient

---

B O X   1 5 - 7

Obtaining Consent

The person who obtains consent, whether verbal or written, is attesting to:

Authenticity of the signature, if written consent is obtained

Patient has decisional capacity for that treatment decision

Patient is authorized to personally consent, or the person is authorized to consent for the patient

Consent is being given freely, voluntarily, and without coercion

A reasonable belief that the patient has been informed so that an informed decision can be made

---

- Whether any materials were used in providing the information, such as videos, anatomy drawings, or pamphlets
- Whether further discussion with the patient is warranted before a decision is made

After giving the patient the necessary information to make an informed decision, consent then must be obtained. The important concept is "obtaining consent," not "obtaining a signature on a consent form." In most states, a signed consent form is not presumptive evidence that consent is informed, although a few states have legally established that presumption (Box 15-7).

The *authenticity* of the signature means that the signature is that of the person signing and is not being forged. On any authorization or consent form, the patient's name should never be written by another person. If the patient is unable to write his or her name and uses a mark, the witness should document on the consent form that it was the patient who made the mark.

The *capacity* of the patient to make the specific treatment decision must be assessed at the time consent is being obtained. This is a critical determination and must be carefully made. The determination of capacity is to be made based upon the client's ability to do the following:

1. Comprehend the information relative to that decision
2. Deliberate regarding the available choices, considering the patient's own values and goals
3. Communicate a decision, verbally or nonverbally

There are no fixed standards for determining decision-making capacity. Licensed health care providers have the skills necessary to assess capacity in most patients. If there is a concern because of a possible underlying neurologic or psychologic condition, it may be appropriate to request an evaluation by a neurologist, psychiatrist, or psychologist. It is usually beneficial to have capacity determinations made as a collaborative effort by the most informed and experienced providers who have had contact with the patient.

The standard for evaluating capacity must be based on the importance and complexity of the clinical decision. As the risks of the decision increase, the standard should be higher. Decision-making capacity should be task-specific—the patient may have the ability to make some decisions but not others. It is imperative that a patient not be found to lack decision-making capacity because the patient prefers an action that is different from what the average person would choose. What some might perceive as an irrational decision is not inherently evidence of incapacity.

Where a question may be raised as to a patient's capacity, document how the determination was made and by whom. That may also provide important information as to how frequently capacity needs to be reevaluated or whether it is expected to change in the future.

It must be verified that the patient is *authorized* to personally consent or that the person consenting for the patient is authorized to do so. Who has authority to consent is set forth in state laws. If the patient is an adult (a person 18 years of age or older), the patient is authorized to consent to personal treatment. A parent or guardian of a minor patient (a person under the age of 18 years) may consent to treatment for the minor patient. Most states have authorized minor patients to personally consent for treatment related to specific health conditions, such as drug and alcohol abuse, sexually transmitted diseases, and pregnancy and to consent if the minor patient is married or the parent of a child. If a patient has been declared incompetent and a guardian appointed with the authority to make health care treatment decisions, state law will also identify what treatment decisions can be made by the guardian.

Some states have enacted legislation designating family members as having authority to consent for the patient, but in the majority of states, no such authority exists. However, traditionally consent from family members has been accepted. It is clear that accepting such consent creates some legal risk, although the alternative of seeking guardianship may not always be in the patient's best interest because of the time involved, stress on family members, and costs. This is an issue that needs to be very carefully examined with input from legal counsel to determine whether it may be appropriate to accept the potential legal risk and obtain consent from an unauthorized person.

When a husband consented to a surgical procedure for his wife, she subsequently sued the hospital (*Mahurin v St. Luke's Hospital of Kansas City*, 809 SW 2d 418 [Mo. Ct. of App. 1991]). Mrs. Mahurin was admitted to St. Luke's Hospital for childbirth. A cesarean section was performed. Although Mrs. Mahurin had consented to the cesarean section, she had not consented to any other surgical procedure. During the surgery, consent was obtained from

Mr. Mahurin to perform a bilateral tubal ligation on Mrs. Mahurin, rendering her sterile. There was no evidence that it was otherwise medically indicated. Mrs. Mahurin testified that she did not at any time request, authorize, or consent to a bilateral tubal ligation, nor was she advised postoperatively that a tubal ligation had been performed.

The court pointed out that an operation performed without a patient's consent is a battery; consenting to one operation does not constitute consent for any other operation where there is no evidence that a necessity arose during the authorized operation (*Mahurin v St. Luke's Hospital of Kansas City,* p. 422). The court concluded: "There is no agency between a husband and wife merely because of the marital relationship and neither is empowered to act as agent for the other simply because they are married" (*Mahurin v St. Luke's hospital of Kansas City,* p. 422). Thus Mr. Mahurin's consent was not binding upon his wife, since he had no authority to consent to the nonessential tubal ligation.

Consent must be given *freely and voluntarily* and not because a physician or family member prefers that course of treatment. With elderly patients who may be more easily subjected to and influenced by these pressures, great attention must be focused on this element.

When obtaining consent, there must be a *reasonable belief* that the patient has been given the information required for an informed decision. This does not require that the witness be present while information is discussed with the patient; however, the witness must verify there was a discussion, the patient can communicate a basic understanding of what treatment is being consented to, and the patient is asked whether any further questions need to be answered before a decision can be made.

There are some special consent requirements when conducting human research. Two sets of federal regulations exist regarding clinical re-

search: one set enacted by the Department of Health and Human Services (DHHS) (45 C.F.R. Pt. 46); and the other by the Food and Drug Administration (FDA) (21 C.F.R. Pt. 50). These regulations specify in detail what information is to be disclosed to a prospective research subject, which includes the following:

- A statement that the study constitutes research, an explanation of its purposes and the expected duration of subject involvement, and a description of the procedures involved, with experimental procedures identified as such
- A description of risks and discomforts that are reasonably foreseeable
- A description of possible benefits to the subject and others
- Disclosure of appropriate alternative treatments, if any
- A statement describing the extent of confidentiality of medical records
- An explanation of whether compensation or treatment will be available if injuries occur
- Who can be contacted with questions or reports of injury
- A statement as to the voluntary nature of participation and the subject's right of withdrawal at any time

Six optional elements of information also may be included if appropriate:

1. A statement that unforeseen risks may arise
2. A description of circumstances in which the subject's participation may be terminated without the subject's consent
3. A notice to any additional costs to the subject as a result of participation
4. A description of the consequences of premature withdrawal
5. A statement that subjects will be informed of any findings that may affect their willingness to continue
6. The number of subjects to be involved in the research

Review and approval by an institutional review board (IRB) is required for any experiment involving human subjects that is conducted by the DHHS or funded in whole or in part by it, or if non-FDA approved drugs are involved.

Although health care facilities are deemed to have no accountability for obtaining informed consent unless the physician or individual required to obtain consent is an employee of the facility or that responsibility has been delegated to an employee, two recent cases have held otherwise where medical research was involved.

Richard Kus brought an action against Sherman Hospital, Dr. Vancil, and the manufacturers of the intraocular lenses that were implanted in Mr. Kus (*Kus v Sherman Hospital,* 644 NE 2d 1214 [Ill. Ct. App. 1995]). The allegation against the hospital was failing to obtain informed consent. Dr. Vancil had recommended cataract surgery and a lens implant to Mr. Kus. Mr. Kus testified that Dr. Vancil never told him that the lens to be implanted was under investigation for its safety and effectiveness. Before surgery, in Dr. Vancil's office, Mr. Kus was presented with an informed consent document to read over and sign, which Mr. Kus did. This consent form was then placed in his medical record at Sherman Hospital. Eye surgery was performed, during which time Dr. Vancil implanted an intraocular lens into Mr. Kus' left eye. Subsequently, Mr. Kus' vision deteriorated in his right eye and Dr. Vancil again recommended the implantation of an intraocular lens. Surgery was then done on the right eye with allegedly no consent form in Mr. Kus' hospital medical record. Mr. Kus claimed that he signed a consent form 2 to 10 days after the surgery and the form then appeared in his hospital medical record.

The hospital's IRB had reviewed and approved the investigational study with the intraocular lenses and had approved a consent form. In the consent form there was a paragraph on "clinical investigation" that informed patients that the lens was under investigation as to its safety and efficacy. Dr. Vancil's receptionist testified that the consent forms he used had this section on "clinical investigation" deleted as directed by Dr. Vancil. This removal was done for all of Dr. Vancil's 43 patients who underwent intraocular lens surgery at Sherman Hospital.

The issue was whether the hospital had any liability for the defective consent. Although the court agreed that a hospital generally has no duty to obtain informed consent from the patient in that it is the duty of the physician, in this case involving experimental intraocular lenses, Sherman Hospital had become a participating institution in the study and was therefore charged with assuring that "legally-effective informed consent" was obtained before the experimental surgery (*Kus v Sherman Hospital,* p. 1221). As a participating institution, the federal regulations require Sherman Hospital to conduct "continuing review of research," which includes the duty to review the informed consent process (*Kus v Sherman Hospital,* p. 1221). The court concluded that Sherman Hospital had the minimal duty of verifying that the form its IRB had approved was being used by Dr. Vancil.

A similar decision was reached in *Friter v. Iolab Corp.,* 607 A 2d 1111 (Pa. Sup. 1992). This also involved the implantation of an intraocular lens. Mr. Friter was never informed before surgery that he was about to become a participant in a clinical investigation and to have an unapproved medical device implanted in his eye. Here the court also agreed that under Pennsylvania law there is not a duty on a nonphysician to obtain a patient's informed consent in the traditional surgical setting. Yet the facts of this case caused the court to conclude the following (*Friter v Iolab Corp.,* p. 1113):

[We] are not here addressing the duty owed by a physician to a patient, but rather a duty owed by the hospital to the client. In this instance, the hospital, as a participant in a clinical investigation for the FDA, specifically assumed a duty to ensure that informed consent was obtained by any patient participating in this study.

This hospital had an affirmative duty to "assure that the rights of human subjects were properly protected, that legally-effective informed consent is obtained, and that the methods of obtaining consent properly informs the human subject of the significant aspects of the study," as required by the federal regulations (*Friter v Iolab Corp.,* p. 1114).

■ KEY POINTS

- The scope of nurses' accountability has grown in recent years and has become more difficult to define as roles within health care shift and change. Given the shifting roles and greater need for accountability, nurses must be knowledgeable about basic legal principles. Ignorance of the law is not a defense; rather nurses must assume responsibility for being well-informed about legal issues that will affect them and their practice.
- A key legal principle relates to the "standard of care" or that level of conduct that a reasonably prudent nurse would undertake under the same or similar circumstances.
- There are four key elements of liability for nurses: duty, malpractice, causation, and damages.
- A comprehensive and accurate medical record is the most effective defense against a charge of malpractice. There is no more credible evidence than the record of what actions the nurse took; what observations the nurse made; and who else was involved in the care of the patient.
- Criteria for flow sheets or nursing record forms include such points as: leave no blanks; be specific about the time of events; identify the providers involved; identify clearly who the patient is; make corrections or additions

to the record carefully and follow recommended protocol for doing this; and provide the appropriate amount of quality of narrative to accurately document the events that occurred.

- Staffing is a key issue in nursing in terms of the use of unlicensed assistive personnel, the guidelines that must be followed with regard to adequate delegation and supervision, and the quality and thoughtfulness in making assignments, which include floating nurses to other units and the use of agency personnel.
- In recent years clinical practice guidelines or critical paths have become more popular. These guidelines are based on the best available information about the effectiveness of health care services and procedures, and they provide useful guides for nursing practice.
- Nurses are part of the team responsible for making sure that patients are adequately informed before a treatment is begun. Nurses need to know what exceptions exist to informed consent, and if none of these exceptions are present, to make certain that patients do get adequate information in a manner they can understand before treatment begins.
- Nurses should be knowledgeable about steps to getting informed consent and key elements for the consent.

■ CRITICAL THINKING QUESTIONS

1. When you think of standards of care and consider the concept of a "reasonably prudent person," who comes to mind as an example of a reasonably prudent person? What are the most obvious, positive characteristics of that person?
2. Consider the example of Mr. Lama in this chapter. If you had been his nurse, exactly what would you have done to avoid the untoward outcome? Be precise, and list your actions in the order in which you would have taken them.

3. Write a sample medical record in which you made a change. Pay attention to the guidelines for making corrections and additions.

4. Using the example of Mr. O'Neal in this chapter, describe a step-by-step set of nursing actions that would have prevented what ultimately occurred. Evaluate what went wrong in the actual case that led to the lack of sufficient nursing actions.

5. Consider the issue of staffing on the unit with which you are most familiar. Are assignments made in ways that could be supported legally? If no, how so? What would you do differently? What do you think leads to any decisions that you would change if you could?

■ REFERENCES

American Nurses Association. (1992). *Position statement on registered nurse education relating to the utilization of unlicensed assistive personnel.* Washington, D.C.: Author.

Department of Health and Human Services. (1993). *Study of the utilization and effects of temporary nursing services.* Washington, D.C.: Author.

Feutz-Harter, S. (1997). *Nursing and the law* (6th ed.). Eau Claire, Wisconsin: Professional Education Systems.

Field, M.J., & Lohr, K.N. (1990). *Clinical practice guidelines: Directions for a new program.* Washington, D.C.: Institute of Medicine.

Institute of Medicine. (1996). *Nursing staff in hospitals and nursing homes: Is it adequate?* (pp. 116-124). Washington, D.C.: National Academy Press.

Kerr, S.D. (1992). A comparison of four nursing documentation systems. *Journal of Nursing Staff Development, January/February,* 26-31.

Levine, E.G., Brandt, L.J., & Plumeri, P. (1995). Informed consent: A survey of physician outcomes and practices. *Gastrointestinal Endoscopy, 41,* 448-452.

Nurse liability. (1988). *Trial, January,* 98-101.

Phaneuf, M. (1976). *The nursing audit and self-regulation in nursing practice.* New York: Appleton-Century-Crofts.

Credentialing in a Changing Health Care Environment

Ann H. Cary

INTRODUCTION

The health of the public is enriched by professional nurses, including advanced practice nurses (APNs) who demonstrate the relationship between the processes of care, provider competencies, and subsequent health outcomes. In the rapidly shifting health care environment, consumers, employers, and health systems are struggling to meet the competing demands of cost effectiveness, quality, and access to services. Traditionally, the authority to practice nursing has been based on a social contract with the public that acknowledges professional rights, responsibilities, and processes for public accountability (ANA, 1995). Self-regulation is at the heart of the social contract and remains central to professionalism.

This chapter reviews key issues and trends in credentialing of the registered and advanced practice nursing work force. Credentialing processes for both providers and systems of delivery and education are described. Finally, the proposition of a historical shift in public protection processes is offered as the context for change in the credentialing marketplace.

OBJECTIVES

After reading this chapter, you will be able to:

1. Evaluate the factors driving the evolution of credentialing for nurses
2. Analyze the roles of federal, state, and voluntary organizations as well as the marketplace in credentialing of APNs
3. Differentiate the credentialing options available to entry level and advanced practice nurses
4. Evaluate the status of credentialing options by accessing websites for specific organizations
5. Explain the challenges facing the credentialing system in the twenty-first century

■ CREDENTIALING: TRENDS AND ISSUES

The notion of credentialing remains central to the protection of the public as the twenty-first century dawns. However, multiple state processes, discipline-specific licensure, and a lack of uniformity in language among the regulatory bodies, professions, and institutions confuse the public. The 1990s are characterized as the decade of "unfreezing." The assumptions and traditions of isolated professional regulation contrast starkly with an era of global, integrated, and interdisciplinary systems development. "Traditional" credentialing mechanisms are largely being shaped by three interrelated influences. These include the Pew Health Professions Commission report *Reforming Health Workforce Regulation: Policy Considerations for the 21st Century* (Finocchio et al., 1995); the globalization and market reform of health care services; and telehealth delivery options.

Agenda Setting for Policy: Regulating Reform of the Nursing Work Force Regulation

By early 1996, the Pew Health Professions Commission report on work force regulatory reform challenged consumers to demand more protection from regulatory bodies as well as to actively participate in the public bodies entrusted with protection of the public's health. Acknowledging that the current credentialing system, created in the twentieth century, had evolved around fifty separate state systems, the report lamented that public protection through credentialing was tied to political boundaries rather than provider competency (Safriet, 1994). Box 16-1 lists the major issues that warrant examination and reform in credentialing of the health work force as noted by Pew. In light of these concerns the Pew study (Finocchio et al., 1995) proposed five principles to guide the reform of health professions regulation. These take the acronym SAFE:

- *S*tandardized (where appropriate)
- *A*ccountable (to the public)
- *F*lexible (access, safe, competent providers)
- *E*ffective and *E*fficient

Five guiding principles were described by the Pew Health Professions Commission to serve as a platform for reform (Finocchio et al., 1995, p. vii):

1. Promoting health outcomes and protection of the public
2. Assuring accountability of regulatory bodies to the public
3. Respecting consumer choice among safe options
4. Encouraging effective working relationships among health care providers within a rational, cost-effective system
5. Promoting geographic and professional mobility among competent providers

These guiding principles promote standardization of regulatory reform and preserve flexibility for health providers, thereby supporting planned change options in line with these principles. Experimentation among the federal, state, professional, and market entities is encouraged by this approach to allow for the emergence of new regulatory systems in the twenty-first century that will address the issues identified in Box 16-1.

To date, actions reflecting these principles are apparent in the following examples:

- The vision statement by the National Council of State Boards of Nursing (NCSBN, 1997, p.1) "A state nursing license recognized nationally and enforced locally." NCSBN is exploring diverse models of licensure and credentialing and endorsed the notion of mutual recognition among states of a national licensure approach similar to the state driver's license mechanism (Woodward, 1997).
- Public members on regulatory health profes-

sion boards are rapidly becoming the rule rather than the exception (Finocchio et al., 1995, p. 16).

- States are exploring the creation of consortia of health profession boards to address interprofessional issues and to promote communication and coordination of principles (Finocchio et al., 1995).
- Alternative dispute mechanisms are being established to address complaints that may not require public protection but that require attention to maintain public confidence in providers. In addition, establishing a triage/priority system that will address "worst cases" to expedite appropriate responses is being implemented in many jurisdictions—thus assuring timely responses.
- Laws are being developed in some states that require critical review of any request to regulate new professions ("sunrise laws") and to review the benefits of continuing regulation of existing ones ("sunset laws").
- Outside the United States, the province of Ontario in Canada has identified 13 "controlled acts" potentially dangerous to consumers. Each regulated profession contains "authorized acts" among the controlled acts that are within that profession's scope of practice. Subsequently, more than one profession may perform the same acts.

These examples reinforce the implementation of innovative processes to reduce the barriers to professional credentialing and public protection. Each of the issues and examples stimulated in the landmark Pew report (Finocchio et al., 1995) is important to nurses if they are to practice within legal boundaries; to consumers for access to cost-effective providers; and to systems that provide care across continuums. These principles rest on the collaboration and competencies of many professional team members supporting a system that assures public protection.

B O X   1 6 - 1

Issues of Twentieth Century Health Work Force Credentialing (Pew, 1995)

- Lack of uniformity in language, laws, and state regulations
- State-specific, nonstandardized limits to professional practice
- Barriers to practice mobility among states
- Barriers to integrated delivery systems effectiveness
- Barriers to use of telehealth
- Near-exclusivity in scopes of practice to a few professions regardless of competency evidence by others
- Reduced access to care from providers demonstrating competencies "belonging" to exclusive scopes of practice
- Barriers to full disclosure of practitioner information for consumers to make informed choices
- Lack of full public representation on regulatory boards
- Barriers to complaint identification, processing, comprehensive investigation, and public disclosure
- Lack of mandatory, effective continuing competence assessments, performance measures, and performance improvement mechanisms
- Conflicts of professional preservation to the exclusion of public protection principles
- Escalating regulation costs to providers
- Escalating costs to consumers and systems because of regulatory barriers
- Lack of data to establish relationships between regulatory processes and quality-of-care outcomes

From Finocchio, L.J., Dower, C.M., McMahon, F., Gragnola, C.M., & Taskforce on Health Care Work Force Regulation. (1995). *Reforming health care work force regulation: Policy considerations for the twenty-first century.* San Francisco: Pew Health Professions Commission.

Globalization and Market Reform

Both globalization and market reform represent a second trend supporting reform in the credentialing process. The demand for nurses has expanded to global markets where there are inadequate numbers of providers in many countries. Global communities, governments, and businesses are seeking health system partnerships with U.S. health corporations to design, implement, and evaluate health services. Developing countries use "expatriate" nurses and other providers to staff delivery systems, and the demand for nurses with U.S. credentials exceeds supply in many developing countries. Opportunities for nurses come not only from international sources, but from private U.S. corporations that are expanding from traditional Western or Canadian markets to the emerging markets in Latin America, Asia, and the Caribbean. Multinational corporations are increasing employer-sponsored insurance benefits for their employees worldwide, thereby increasing the ability of employees in other countries to pay for health care. Much of the growth in RN jobs internationally is in the private sector. As an example, the market for private home health care services in the United Kingdom (UK) is expanding dramatically. Private home health nursing services constitute 36% of the market now versus 2% of the market 4 years ago. All home health and subsequent home health nursing position growth in the United Kingdom is now in the private sector (Financial Times, 1997).

Dramatic global shifts in epidemiologic patterns and health status indicators accelerate the demand for the skills of nurses, in particular credentialed APNs in developed, developing, and underdeveloped nations (Choski, 1997):

- Child mortality is 10 times higher in developing countries.
- Maternal mortality is 30 times higher in developing countries.
- As communicable disease rates decrease globally, emerging sources of morbidity and mortality will be linked to the chronic disease burdens experienced by a global aging population.
- Global tobacco deaths are at 3,000,000 annually and are expected to triple in the next 25 years.

International purchasers of health and nursing services are likely to require credentialing data that assure knowledge, skill, judgment, and applications reflecting competence with "controlled acts" or other regulatory mandates at the site of practice or patient locations globally. International trade agreements now challenge individual states within the United States to examine the similarities and differences in education, accreditation, regulation, and utilization of the health care work force internationally. As nurses encounter global employment opportunities and as international trade agreements provide employment opportunities for a globally credentialed work force, the shift in the globalization of nursing will identify and dismantle the barriers to international mobility and uniformity in credentialing processes (Finocchio et al., 1995, p. 42). U.S. and international credentialing will be essential to global health care delivery in the twenty-first century.

Market reform has an equally powerful impact on the globalization of health care providers and credentialing of nurses. Market competition shapes the rapid formation of integrated delivery systems in an attempt to decrease redundancy in care, improve coordination of services, and decrease gaps in continuity of care. The ultimate impact of competition is on cost of service delivery and quality outcomes based on restructuring, re-engineering, and work force redesign. Cost constraints, practitioner competency, and accountability are central tenets to the success of market reform efforts, if cost, access, and quality are prevailing principles. All dimensions of the health professions work force are being examined in the market reform paradigm: education, training, financing, credentialing, distribution, and continued competence.

Market forces influence many opportunities for the APN provider within integrated delivery. The APN adds value to systems that emphasize primary care and prevention, disease management, population-based care, and interdisciplinary teamwork. Meaningful outcomes generated by APNs are evident in clinical effectiveness research and financial performance reports. However, regulatory and credentialing processes today appear to be a mismatch with the rapidly changing delivery system needs. Specifically, credentialing currently reinforces geographic boundaries, yet markets demand a semipermeable boundary of expanding geographic delivery. Disciplinary boundaries of practice now exist, but the demand is for an interdisciplinary, competency-based provider. These concerns are amplified by a Federal Trade Commission report indicating that occupational licensure frequently escalates the price of service, which in turn increases consumer costs without necessarily increasing the quality of professional services (Cox & Foster, 1990).

Clearly the values of the market are escalating the concerns of credentialing applicable to the nursing work force. For all providers, the trends in regulatory and credentialing reform in the future will likely address the issues posed by both globalization and market reform: costs; restrictions on professional performance and flexibility as well as managerial operation; barriers to provider access and care; and the equivocal relationship of the credentialing process to quality.

Telehealth Delivery of Nursing Practice

The third major factor in the tripartite confluence of change in nursing credentialing, especially for APNs, comes from the information superhighway, the emerging health technologies,

and the rapidly developing capacity to provide telehealth services to distant sites globally. All of these technologies are an integral part of access to appropriate health services. Currently, most of the telehealth legislation at the state level allows only physicians to deliver services and receive reimbursement for electronically delivered care. However, beta testing is occurring in the home health care industry in the use of televisiting by nurses to patients in the home. Several other prototype systems are also being tested in this delivery mode. For example, one system uses ordinary telephone lines and a laptop computer with a digital camera and a software package that captures images and then transfers and stores information. Video and audio conferencing are used to connect the diagnostician to the home care patient and provider. The computer used in the home is voice-enabled, which allows information to be collected without using a keyboard. Another system adds diagnostic tools (blood pressure testing; camera ability to view wounds). Both systems report decreased acute care utilization and fewer in-home nursing visits (*Business Briefs,* 1997).

Whether identified as telemedicine, telehealth, telenursing, or telecare, the new technologies constitute a highly visible model of service delivery that has the capacity to increase access, improve quality of care, and reduce avoidable costs. A flurry of experimental, legislative, and application activity is under way. Professionals, the public, legislators, and global investors view telehealth as *the* vehicle to global market expansion.

As revised models of health delivery and credentialing emerge, the public's health must be protected. Reduced barriers to nursing practice and use of technologies that deliver quality service across state and national boundaries must be assured. Practice competencies in telehealth must be visible and measured and demonstrate their usefulness to the public and regulatory bodies. The penetration of international boundaries for routine service delivery by nurses requires credentialing elements for cultural competency and continuing technologic competency, as well as evidence-based practices.

The twenty-first century will likely commence with incremental changes in the credentialing mechanisms offered to nurses. Examples of experimental models and serious discussions in health professions communities are evident in the 10 summary recommendations applicable to regulatory reform as seen in Box 16-2. In all likelihood, the actions will approximate the Pew guiding principles to assure public protection, provider access to service options, and uniformity of competence. The impact on a nurse's credibility will be enhanced if the principles for credentialing, as envisioned, are met.

B O X   1 6 - 2

Pew Health Professions Commission Taskforce on Health Care Workforce Regulation: Summary of the 10 Recommendations

Recommendation 1 States should use standardized and understandable language for health professionals regulation and its functions to clearly describe them for consumers, provider organizations, businesses, and the professions.

Recommendation 2 States should standardize entry-to-practice requirements and limit them to competence assessments for health professionals to facilitate the physical and professional mobility of the health professions.

Recommendation 3 States should base practice acts on demonstrated initial and continuing competence. This process must allow and expect different professions to share overlapping scopes of practice. States should explore pathways to allow all professionals to provide services to the full extent of their current knowledge, training, expeience, and skills.

Recommendation 4 States should redesign health professional boards and their functions to reflect the interdisciplinary and public accountability demands of the changing health care delivery system.

Recommendation 5 Boards should educate consumers to assist them in obtaining the information necessary to make decisions about practitioners and to improve the board's public accountability.

Recommendation 6 Boards should cooperate with other public and private organizations in collecting data on regulated health professions to support effective workforce planning.

Recommendation 7 States should require each board to develop, implement, and evaluate continuing competency requirements to assure the continuing competence of regulated health care professionals.

Recommendation 8 States should maintain a fair, cost-effective, and uniform disciplinary process to exclude incompetent practitioners to protect and promote the public's health.

Recommendation 9 States should develop evaluation tools that assess the objectives, successes, and shortcomings of their regulatory systems and bodies to best protect and promote the public's health.

Recommendation 10 States should understand the links, overlaps, and conflicts between their health care workforce regulatory systems and other systems which affect the education, regulation, and practice of health care practitioners and work to develop partnerships to streamline regulatory structures and processes.

From Finocchio, L.J., Dower, C.M., McMahon, F., Gragnola, C.M., & Taskforce on Health Care Workforce Regulation. (1995). *Reforming health care workforce regulation: Policy considerations for the twenty-first century* (p. ix). San Francisco: Pew Health Professions Commission.

■ CREDENTIALING OPTIONS: THE 1990s AND BEYOND

Credentialing is defined by Seppanen (1995, p. 3) as "a process by which individuals or institutions or one or more of their programs are designated by a qualified agent as having met minimum standards at a specified time." Both providers and institutions are subject to credentialing measures as a covenant of public protection when participating in direct or proxy services. Most of the discussion in this chapter pertains to provider credentialing; however, methods of credentialing for institutions of employment as well as credentialing of the credentialers are briefly reviewed.

Constitutional authority is conveyed to states to regulate activities that affect the health, safety, and welfare of citizens. Each of the 50 states, the District of Columbia, and 5 U.S. territories define their process and procedures for granting licensure, renewal of licenses, and regulation of provider practice. In contrast, the Federal government, including the military and the Veterans' Administration, has the authority to establish national licensure standards. Examples are the Medicare and Medicaid programs, in which conditions of participation specify the credentials and standards of practice under these respective programs. Institutions or providers accepting reimbursement for services from Medicare and Medicaid must meet the "conditions of participation" to be eligible for reimbursement. In the rare cases for which it is evoked, the U.S. Constitution mandates that even "state regulation designed to protect the state's interest must give way to paramount Federal legislation." (Joint Working Group on Telemedicine, 1997, p. 4) For example, should Congress desire to regulate telemedicine by licensure, the Federal preemption could apply to the states (Joint Working Group on Telemedicine, 1997).

Uniformity of terms and definitions for the more common mechanisms of credentialing are listed in the Key Terms box. Although not exhaustive, these illustrate the issues noted in the PEW report on regulation. Standardization of terms can assist readers in the future to understand the regulatory classifications. Regardless of the definition, credentialing criteria are commonly based on an individual's current license, education, training, experience, competence, and/or professional judgment (Cericola, 1996).

To practice as a registered nurse in the United States, providers must first be licensed. Generally, in the past a nurse has been required to obtain a separate license for each state in which he or she sought to practice. However, in late 1997 the NCSBN endorsed the mutual recognition model of licensure, providing alternatives to separate, state licensure. Under this model, a nurse will possess a license in one state (state of residency) and will be able to practice in any state that has implemented the agreement known as an *interstate compact*, as long as the nurse follows the laws and regulations required by the state in which the practice occurs. Each state can choose whether to enact the interstate compact legislation. The interstate compact is a legal vehicle or piece of legislation adopted and implemented on a state-by-state basis, enabling nurses to practice across state boundaries. The contract among the states specifies shared licensure authority and disciplinary jurisdiction and shared data and information to accomplish this authority. Between 1998 and 2000, states will be developing the infrastructure essential to coordinate the licensure system and the necessary supportive services to operate the new model of mutual recognition. It is expected that no state will implement the interstate compact legislation before January 1, 2000. Therefore nurses will likely be able to use this new licensure process, if adopted by a respective state, at the turn of the century (Woodward, 1997).

Key terms

Term	Definition
Certification (types) • Issued by professional organization	Statement declaring a nurse has met predetermined qualifications to practice in a specialty area
• Issued by the state	Legal endorsement by a state board of nursing certifying that legal requirements for practicing the specialty scope of practice are met
• Issued by an institution	Statement issued by an academic or service institution recognizing a nurse has completed requirements of the program of study for specialty practice (Bulechek & Maas, 1994)
• Certificate	Statement of completion of a specific program awarded to graduates (Finocchio et al., 1995)
Certified (as in Medicare certified)	Statement from a certifying body that the organization has met standards
Clinical privileges	Authorization granted by a governing body to a practitioner to provide specific patient care in an organization based on practitioner's license, ability to perform the privileges requested, judgment, education and training, and experience (Cericola, 1996)
Competence/Competency	Capacity is equal to requirements (Cericola, 1996); a single, observable or definable skill consisting of knowledge, skills, aptitudes, attitudes, and intellectual strategies (i.e., problem-solving; ability to deal with ambiguity) (Callahan, 1988)
Credentialing	Process of validating the qualifications of a licensed independent practitioner to provide services in an organization (Cericola, 1996)
Credentials	Documents that state that a provider has a right to exercise a certain power or authority (Cericola, 1996)
Accreditation	Statement issued by an accreditation organization recognizing that the organization has met the criteria and requirements specified in the standards of the accrediting organization
Registration	Submitting required documents to a state authority without necessarily meeting standards for entry-to-practice or continued competence; provider's name appears on an information list
Licensure	Permission granted by government to engage in businesses or occupation or in an activity otherwise unlawful; the most common form authorizes a specific occupation or profession to provide services; practice acts can be exclusive and monopolistic; a carved-out section of another profession's scope of practice, or combination of various scopes of practice (Finocchio et al., 1995)

Key terms—cont'd

Term	Definition
Reciprocity	Mutuality; the term is used to denote the relation existing between two states when each of them gives the subjects of the other certain privileges, on the condition that its own subjects shall enjoy similar privileges at the hands of the latter state (*Black's Law Dictionary,* 1990); based on state-to-state contract with no review of individual credentials (NCSBN, 1996)
Endorsement	To sanction, approve, or support (Webster's Ninth New Collegiate Dictionary, 1984); applicant information evaluated by state based on individual state criteria (NCSBN, 1996)
Mutual recognition	A method of licensure in which licensing entities voluntarily enter agreements to legally recognize the licensure policies and processes of a licensee's home state so as to permit the exercise of the licensee's privileges within the host state's borders; a separate license issued by the host state's competent authority is not required (waive rights to [my] standards and accept other state's standards); not based on core requirements or need to harmonize standards (NCSBN, 1996)
Drivers license model	Each state issues license; other states allow holder to drive in their state but require adherence to laws in that state; within a specific time frame after relocation, a license is required in the state of residence (NCSBN, 1996)
Corporate credentialing: possibilities	(1) Standards for nursing license (or permission to practice) could be authorized by state (or federal government) with corporate implementation; (2) licensure of delivery system (corporation) granted by state (or federal government) with corporation determining individual practice credentials; or (3) corporation decides who practices and standards upon which practice is based with no government role (NCSBN, 1996)
Veterans Administration (VA) model	Nurse must be licensed in at least one state and may practice in any federal property/agency; state law does not apply (NCSBN, 1996)
Multistate license (MSL)	A hybrid composed of elements from other models; could be implemented by all states/jurisdictions or only by states/jurisdictions choosing to participate—would authorize practice in all participating states/jurisdictions (NCSBN, 1996)
Interstate compact	In agreement between two or more states, established for the purpose of remedying a particular problem of multistate concern (*Blacks Law Dictionary,* 1990, p. 820)

In addition to licensure, registered nurses who meet eligibility requirements of a specific certification organization may add certification credentials so that they are both licensed and certified in a specific field of practice.

APNs who engage in practice that may be beyond the identified scope of nursing practice must do so under legal authorization for the practice in accordance with state law. Any title and authority to practice, even if issued by a national certification body, carries legal status *only* if the title is recognized or authorized by state statute or regulation. State authorization to practice as an APN may require certification by a national professional body (e.g., American Nurses Credentialing Center, American Academy of Nurse Practitioners, National Association of Pediatric Nurse Associates and Practitioners). Any certification body can fulfill its obligation to protect the public by meeting the test of "Regulatory Sufficiency." *Regulatory sufficiency* is based "upon examination designs geared toward entry level competencies, exclusively job-related knowledge and skills, pass/fail scores at the point of the minimum essential level for safety and effectiveness, and use of generally accepted testing practices" (NCSBN, 1997, p. 1).

According to Pearson (1996), the regulation of APN legal authority to practice varies among states although current state rules and regulations are moving toward the support of independent APN practice with decreasing physician involvement. As of the 1996 report, APN practice in 23 states was regulated by the board of nursing with no requirements for physician collaboration or supervision. In 17 states, APN practice was regulated by state boards of nursing and with some form of physician supervision, collaboration, and/or written protocols. In 10 states, regulation of the APN was by the state board of nursing and jointly and collaboratively with boards of medicine. Summarily, APNs in some states may be regulated by multiple boards within a state such as nursing, medicine, pharmacy, and medical examiners (O'Malley et al., 1996). From 1987 to 1997, the number of APN providers doubled (Kendrick, 1997). This swell of the APN workforce can be expected to influence the political impact of APN practice issues in states, promoting continued independence in practice based on data to support effectiveness and quality of APN practice.

Since 1995, NCSBN has participated in collaborative efforts with representatives of nurse practitioner certification programs to establish legally defensible and psychometrically sound nurse practitioner examinations consistent with the concept of regulatory sufficiency. To establish this condition, all collaborative parties have agreed to a review process by the National Commission of Certifying Agencies (NCCA), an arm of the National Organization for Competency Assurance (NOCA). NCCA performs the reviews along with NCSBN supplemental criteria that apply to regulatory use for authorizing state approval. Following the full recognition reports issued by NCCA, the NCSBN responds to each individual certifying organization that fulfills the regulatory sufficiency criteria and disseminates the report of results to state boards of nursing. State boards of nursing consider these reports in specifying which certifications meet state authorizations to practice as an APN.

The stewardship issues of various credentialing bodies are reflected in this model. The NCSBN protects the public through mechanisms that meet the assurance notion of regulatory sufficiency. This is the essential uniform criteria used by the NCSBN to recognize the contribution of voluntary certification bodies to uniform principles of protecting public safety. Once a certifying body fulfills the NCSBN criteria, the board of nursing in the provider's state of licensure can issue title/regulatory coverage for the APN to practice within the extended scope of practice.

In summary, unlike physicians, the scopes of practice for nurses are not sufficiently expansive to include all components of advanced practice nursing. Therefore legal authority to function as an APN is required through nursing statutes or regulation at the state level. As of 1997, all states reported that they regulate APNs in some manner: 18 states license nurse practitioners; 32 additional states authorize practice through certificates, recognition, registration, or similar mechanisms. To date, 38 of the 50 states and 5 U.S. territories rely on national certification programs to measure APN competency (NCSBN, 1997, pp. 5-6). Because the status of APN regulation within each state changes intermittently, the reader can access current information through NCSBN, voluntary organizations, or state regulatory body Web Sites as shown in Box 16-3.

In addition to the nurse practitioner category of APNs, the NCSBN conducts other activities. It monitors the role of clinical nurse specialists (CNS); it serves as a clearinghouse of information provided by certifying bodies and reviews disciplinary actions against certified registerd nurse anesthetists (CNRAs) by boards of nursing; and it provides the same services for certified nurse midwives (CNMs) as for CRNAs, as well as assessing regulatory implications of admitting nonnurses to the CNM certification program. The NCSBN anticipates changes in regulatory models to strengthen the unified impact of state boards of nursing on protection of the public. These changes acknowledge the following:

- The increase in number of nurses who are practicing across state boundaries
- The number of nurses practicing in a variety of settings and with new technologies
- Consumer expectations to expedite access to qualified nurses
- Employer expectations to expedite authorization to practice
- The inefficiency and costs associated with demonstrating comparable authority and qualifications to practice in multiple states

B O X   1 6 - 3

Selected Web Sites for Current Credentialing Information on Rapidly Evolving Policies and Regulations.

http://www.ncsbn.org	National Council of State Boards of Nursing
http://www.aacn.nche.edu	Commission on Collegiate Nursing Education
http://www.nursingworld.org	American Nurses Association and Online Journal
http://www.jcaho.org	Joint Commission on Accreditation of Healthcare Organizations
http://www.nln.org	National League for Nursing
http://www.nlnac.org	National League for Nursing Accrediting Commission
http://www.ncqa.org	National Committee on Quality Assurance
http://www.nursing.org/ancc/ancc.htm	American Nurses Credentialing Center
http://futurehealth.ucsf.edu	The Center for the Health Professions—Pew Health Professions Commission
http://www.napnap.org	National Association of Pediatric Nurse Associates and Practitioners
http://www.aanp.org	American Academy of Nurse Practitioners

Consult state regulatory Web Sites of each state and/or U.S. territory with jurisdiction for regulation of nursing practice to access the most current information for that state.

• Emerging practice modalities and technologies pushing the boundary of state licensure laws

The notion of multistate and mutual recognition licensure mechanisms, endorsed by NCSBN in 1997, addresses these trends and issues. The federal vehicle of interstate compact encourages uniformity in regulations between states, subsequent to congressional consent. At the turn of the century this new model appears to meet the advantage of uniform public protection and state sovereignty; for providers, care standards are consistent among participating states and provider mobility is enhanced.

Credentialing for Continued Competency: The Debate

Once the nurse receives an initial license as a registered nurse and adds the required credential (typically, certification acceptable to the respective regulatory board) for APN practice, the issue of validating continued competence during a lifetime of practice becomes salient.

Several different mechanisms are used to support life-long learning needs; however, many of these methods provide no assurance of continued competence among providers. When continued competence is not assured, protecting the public's health is a challenge. The debate concerning what constitutes a psychometrically strong assurance of provider competency continues to be fueled by consumer concerns, employer concerns, and the values of mandated and voluntary criteria. The Citizen Advocacy Center (1996, p. 3) proposes six elements necessary to establish programs of continued competence:

1. Identification of key factors that lead to competence
2. Development and assessment of continuing education courses
3. Assessment of licensee needs—strengths and weaknesses
4. Assignment of required courses

5. Evaluation of licensee performance
6. Evaluation of the effectiveness of the continuing education program

Most state licensing boards have chosen mandatory continuing education requirements to address the issue of assuring continuing competence of licensees. These boards may require a certain number of contact hours of continuing education (CE) by accredited providers of CE for relicensure. The American Nurses Credentialing Center (ANCC) and Commission on Accreditation awards accreditation to programs that approve CE activities offered by others or who provide CE activities—all within standards designated by ANCC. However, the Citizen Advocacy Center (1996) cautions that continuing education programs generally do not possess the necessary components to ensure continued competence, since most licensees must only demonstrate attendance. Regulatory review does not determine the relevance of courses to the licensee, the level of knowledge obtained, or whether the licensee's skill and decision-making capacity is acceptable.

Voluntary and private certification processes have demonstrated greater consistency with the elements of continued competence. Requirements for recertification by health profession organizations often reflect multimodel processes to establish a sense of competence. These include the following:

• A recertification process
• Continuing education
• Reexamination
• Self-assessment
• Peer review
• Office record review
• Computer recertification examination
• Choice of modes among multimode options (from one to more than three methods)

These combinations approach the comprehensive nature of measurement and reduce several concerns in competency testing. However, nonstandardized approaches among professions continue to raise policy questions concerning protection mechanisms for consumers. The Citizen Advocacy Center (1996) has published 11 policy questions confronting the viability of the competency assessment system for APNs and other professionals (Box 16-4). These bear dialogue and action plans to ultimately resolve concerns about the lifelong competencies of health professionals. Incremental shifts in the regulatory process for RNs and APNs are gradually addressing demands for uniform public protection, access to APN providers, and geographic mobility. These small but essential changes in licensure and certification contribute to the shift-

ing credentialing landscape for practice in the twenty-first century. Equally dynamic are the credentialing mechanisms developing at the institutional level to assure the public's health through institutional performance measures (e.g., length of stay, readmissions, patient falls), including those related to provider credentialing and performance.

Accreditation: Institutional Credentialing Mechanisms

The accreditation process for health care delivery and work force education are proxy measures of individual and team-based provider performance. Accreditation criteria include pro-

B O X   1 6 - 4

Citizen Advocacy Center: 11 Policy Questions to Address Regarding Continued Competence

1. What techniques should be employed to evaluate continuing competence?
2. Should practitioners be given the option of demonstrating continuing competence by a variety of approved techniques, or should licensing boards specify the one or ones to be utilized?
3. How frequently should licensees be required to demonstrate competence?
4. Should *all* licensees be required periodically to demonstrate their continuing competence, or only those whose performance cause the licensing board to question their competence? If the latter, what criteria (markers) should apply?
5. What relationships should exist, if any, between licensing board continuing competence requirements, and those of specialty certification boards? On what basis might licensing boards recognize and accept the findings of specialty boards?

6. Is recertification a *de facto* limited license? If so, is it fair or good policy to grant a general license to first time licensees, but only a limited license at the time of recertification?
7. What needs to be done to assure that a recertification system meets the required legal standards of a state?
8. How should continuing education needs assessment be accomplished? Are all methods equally viable?
9. Who should pay the costs of recertification? Licensees? The State? What is affordable?
10. What rules of confidentiality, if any, should apply to recertification information? What information should be provided to the public concerning the results of needs assessment?
11. What is the legal status of licensees who cannot meet recertification standards? Should they be given a period of time to upgrade their skills. How long? What is the legal status of their license during this interim period? Is the fact that the licensee has not been recertified public information?

From Citizen Advocacy Center. (1996). *Excerpts* (pp. 1-2). Washington, D.C.: Citizen Advocacy Center.

vider performance elements, which together with the remaining system elements convey the degree of quality and public protection both consumers and employers can expect in these systems. APN credentialing is consistent with institutional accreditation outcomes. Institutional credentialing of delivery and educational systems is discussed below.

Health Care System Accreditation

Since 1951 the Joint Commission for the Accreditation of Healthcare Organizations (JCAHO) has viewed its purpose as improving public access to quality health care through the administration of health care accreditation and related services that support performance improvement and outcomes. JCAHO is an independent, not-for-profit, voluntary organization that accredits more than 16,000 health care organizations in the United States. The accreditation programs include the following:
• Ambulatory health care
• Home care
• Hospitals
• Long-term care
• Provider networks (health plans, integrated delivery networks, and provider-sponsored networks [PSOs])
• Behavioral health care
• Laboratories

Nurses participate as representatives to the Professional & Technical Advisory Committee (PTAC) of JCAHO to assist in the development and evaluation of accreditation processes; they may also serve as JCAHO site surveyors.

In 1996 the Joint Commission announced a plan for integrating data from multiple, qualified performance measurement systems into the accreditation process. Performance measurement is an integrated set of process measures, outcome measures, or both that reveal internal and external comparisons of an organization's performance and trends. The JCAHO believes that the new data sources and configurations permit health care organizations to demonstrate accountability to patients, communities, and purchasers of care. The new process also assists the Joint Commission to link standards compliance with measurements of actual performance (Loeb & Buck, 1996).

In 1997 the Joint Commission announced the new ORYX initiative to integrate outcomes and other performance measures into the accreditation process. The JCAHO has approved 60 performance measurement systems from which hospitals and long-term care organizations must choose, in addition to at least two clinical performance indicators. Data based on these measures are to be submitted to JCAHO no later than the first quarter of 1999.

Organizations meeting the provider network accreditation program designation will be required to choose 10 separate measures from one or more of the specified consensus-based measurement sets in 1997; 20 measures in 1998; and 30 measures in 1999. By 1999, health plans/provider networks will need to demonstrate improvement in outcomes and other measures.

Ambulatory care, behavioral health, home health care, and laboratories seeking JCAHO accreditation are expected to meet the same initial criteria for hospitals or long-term care organizations by December 31, 1998. The new ORYX initiative is expected to increase the revenue and value of accreditation, support systems, and process improvements in those organizations that are accredited and allow expanded, comparative performance evaluations among health care organizations (ORYX, 1997). These new initiatives answer some of the concerns of advocacy critics that JCAHO presents a conflict of interest because it is operated and funded largely by the industry it regulates, that patient safety may not be its top priority, and that the Joint Commission has been too lax in monitoring organizations (Prager, 1996).

The predominant accrediting body for managed care organizations (MCO) is the National Committee for Quality Assurance (NCQA), an independent not-for-profit organization that measures and reports quality and services for MCOs. NCQA accreditation is required by most businesses for the selection and purchase of managed care contracts and products. The standards used by NCQA assist purchasing organizations and providers to prioritize initiatives and focus on quality.

Several functions involving APNs may have a proxy linkage to NCQA standards. These include the following:
- A clearly documented process for credentialing and recredentialing in the organization
- Accession of the National Practitioner Data Bank for credentialing, education, training, and liability (NCQA, 1996).

Other drivers of performance improvement in MCOs will likely identify, incorporate, monitor, and evaluate the contributions of APNs to the quality indicators in MCO accreditation processes. The Health Plan Employer Data and Information Set (HEDIS) currently includes provider performance measures for physician board certification, types of trained specialists, availability of obstetrical and prenatal care providers, children's access to primary care providers, and availability of primary care providers. As APNs fulfill provider service positions in the MCO environments, they too will become essential components of explicit credentialing status and performance measures in HEDIS (Parisi, 1997).

Finally, employer and business mandates for performance processes and outcomes may be tied to the accreditation status of the provider organization or may specify unique data ele-

ments to use as selection criteria by mechanisms such as the request for information (RFI) and request for proposal (RFP) process (Parisi, 1997). MCOs that employ APNs will want to respond completely, accurately, and competitively to demonstrate proper credentialing and performance measures for the system, providers, and consumers. Credentialing data on APNs and their relationship to productivity and performance will likely contribute to cost-effective responses as well as active contracts between MCOs and purchasers of health care in the near future.

Numerous accreditation programs award accreditation status to health care organizations employing APNs (e.g., Community Health Accreditation Program [CHAP] for hospice and home health services; Commission on Accreditation of Rehabilitation Facilities [CARF]). In addition, accreditation is available through the American Nurses Credentialing Center for organizations providing continuing education activities to APNs either as freestanding educational delivery systems or within health service provider systems.

Academic Educational Programs: Accreditation

Academic educational programs preparing nurses are typically approved and/or licensed by each state government, often represented by the state board of nursing. Accreditation by private voluntary organizations may also be required. In 1996, thirteen state boards of nursing recognized professional accreditation in lieu of state approval (NLN, 1996). To access data for the current year, consult the NLN Web Site.

These independent voluntary organizations that accredit academic educational programs are themselves subject to recognition by the U.S. Department of Education (DOE). The DOE monitors accreditation bodies and offers initial and renewed recognition status of an accreditation organization based on DOE parameters.

Both the accreditation of academic educational programs and recognition by DOE of the accreditation bodies are nationally recognized seals of approval, since they influence eligibility for federal nursing education funds. Toward this end, two accreditation services are now emerging to be recognized as accrediting bodies for nursing education programs.

In 1996 the National League for Nursing (NLN) established a separate accreditation en-

tity in response to DOE scrutiny. The National League for Nursing Accrediting Commission (NLNAC) is the independent accreditation entity responsible for nursing education programs. These include practical nursing; associate degree, diploma, and baccalaureate degree programs to prepare candidates for RN licensure; and programs leading to the master's degree. There is not a recognized accreditation process for doctoral programs in nursing (the caveat being where the doctorate is the first nursing degree of which there are few programs to

---

C A S E   S T U D Y

Credentialing

As a new advanced practice nurse graduate you are exploring the job market in a rural Midwestern region. You anticipate that the interview will be divided into two areas:
- The organization will be seeking to understand your credentials and practice boundaries
- You will be seeking to understand the practice parameters of the organization along with the organizational credentials it possesses.
1. Explain the credentialing process used by the educational institution from which you completed the APN coursework.
2. Explain the credentialing process required for you to practice as an advanced practice nurse in your state of residence, state of employment, and state of practice delivery. (Remember, if you engage in any form of telehealth delivery—telephone case management, consultation, or televisiting—you may have legal practice concerns in many states).
3. Generate two questions to ask during the interview process to understand
   a. The credentialing processes applicable to the employer
   b. The specific aspects of the organizational credentialing process that will influence your practice

Accessing contemporary resources

Access two Web Sites listed in Box 16-3 or others you have discovered.
1. What issues and developments are noted in the organizational Web Sites?
2. What new products/processes are they reporting?
3. Bring these issues to light through discussion and debate with your colleagues.
   a. What issues and recommendations from Boxes 16-1 and 16-2 are addressed by the on-line information?
   b. What additional issues are likely to evolve from those identified in the boxes, based on the Web Site information?
   c. What new Web Site sources on credentialing did you discover, or to what other sites were you "hot linked?"

What recommendations can you make to address the concerns and issues raised by the Citizen's Advocacy Center in Box 16-4?

date). APNs graduating from master's programs through 1998 are likely to have graduated from programs accredited by the NLN/NLNAC.

Likewise, in 1995 the American Association of Colleges of Nursing (AACN) began to explore and plan for the implementation of another option for academic accreditation. By late 1998 the Commission on Collegiate Nursing Education (CCNE) plans to conduct its first accreditation process and site visit, after which it can request DOE recognition. CCNE will offer accreditation to both baccalaureate and master's nursing education programs (C. Padham, personal communication, September 9, 1997). Because of the preliminary status of the CCNE accreditation process as of this writing, readers are encouraged to contact the Internet source for current information on CCNE. (See Box 16-3.)

Academic educational programs preparing nurses are likely to have choices among accrediting bodies should both NLNAC and CCNE exist in the twenty-first century. State approval, licensure, and national accreditation are important vehicles for identifying, monitoring, and improving the performance of nurses' educational programs and subsequently the graduates from these program.

The issues embedded in the concept of credentialing for nurses are not easily resolved given their competing values. Such values include protection for the health of the public; assurance of safe provider practices; mobility; reduction in restraint of trade; entry into practice; costs; provider effectiveness; employer/purchaser mandate; uniform data reporting; performance and outcome improvements; federal and state rights; market competition; globalization of demand; escalation of telehealth delivery; and, immediate access by consumers to appropriate services of nurses. Box 16-4 lists a variety of policy questions.

The twenty-first century sets the stage for change, establishing and refining the relationship among credentialing mechanisms and health service costs, quality, and access. Nurses will create the solutions to these challenges by identifying, creating, monitoring, and evaluating both the data and the research processes that assist those involved to make informed choices for healthy futures.

■ **KEY POINTS**

- Traditional processes for credentialing health care providers appear inadequate to meet the needs of organizations and clients distributed among diverse locations for care.
- New models of licensure and certification are emerging for discussion and implementation among bodies that regulate and certify nurses.
- Continuing competency remains an unresolved issue for regulators who rely on evidence after an adverse incident occurs. Educational processes to assure continued competence before errors are evident are preferable to protect the public.
- Accreditation standards for delivery systems and academic educational institutions are evolving toward outcomes that are measurable.
- Although changes are evident, both governmental and voluntary regulatory processes are likely to remain essential to the goal of public safety and protection in health care delivery.
- Access to the most current information concerning the status of a state, voluntary, and/or federal body processes of credentialing is found through Web Site resources. (See Box 16-3.)

■ **CRITICAL THINKING QUESTIONS**

1. Read the nurse practice act in your state, and evaluate to what level it serves to assure safe practice. If you could change any part of the act, what specifically would that be?
2. Secure copies of two sets of criteria for specialty certification. Examine how this form of

credentialing differs from or is similar to the original licensure of a nurse.

3. Secure copies of what is used to credential the practice of nurses in either Canada or Mexico. Examine how these counterparts to our state-based nurse practice acts differ or are similar.

4. Describe a hypothetical plan for credentialing the use of telehealth. How can this be regulated across state lines? What is a solution for the issue of credentialing telehealth care?

5. Interview at least three people in a hospital with which you are familiar. Ask them in what ways the accreditation process by the Joint Commission for the Accreditation of Healthcare Organizations is useful. Ask them how they would change this process to improve it. Ask also if they believe the advantages of a process such as this one outweigh the cost in time and labor to prepare for it.

6. Debate the pro and con perspectives of whether there should (should not) be institutional licensure versus individual licensure.

■ REFERENCES

American Nurses Association. (1995). *Nursing's social policy statement.* Washington, D.C.: Author.

American Nurses Association. (1996). *The American Nurses Association response to the Pew report on healthcare workforce regulation.* Washington, D.C.: Author.

Black's Law Dictionary (6th ed., p. 820). (1990). St. Paul, Minn.: West Publishing.

Bulechek, G.M., & Maas, M.L. (1994). Nursing certification: A matter for the professional organization. In J. McCloskey & H.K. Grace (Eds.). *Current issues in nursing* (4th ed., pp. 327-335). St. Louis: Mosby.

Callahan, L. (1988). Competence models: From theory to practice application. *Journal of the American Association of Nurse Anesthetists, 56,* 387-389.

Cericola, S.A. (1996). What is the credentialing process? *Plastic Surgical Nurse, 16*(4), 257.

Choski, A. (1997, June). *Global economies and health opportunities.* Paper presented at the NCSBN Public Policy Conference, Washington, D.C.

Citizen Advocacy Center. (1996). *Excerpts: Continuing competence requirements of selected licensing boards and health professional voluntary credentialing bodies.* Washington, D.C.: Citizen Advocacy Center.

Commission on Collegiate Nursing Education. (1997). *Mission statement and goals.* Washington, D.C.: AACN.

Connors, H.R. (1997). Telecommunication and health care: Interest escalates as potential benefits are recognized. *Issues, 18*(2), 1-7.

Cox, C., & Foster, S. (1990). *The costs and benefits of occupational regulation.* Washington, D.C.: Bureau of Economics of the Federal Trade Commission.

Finocchio, L.J., Dower C.M., McMahon, F., Gragnola, C.M., & Taskforce on Health Care Workforce Regulation. (1995). *Reforming health care workforce regulation: Policy considerations for the 21st century.* San Francisco: Pew Health Professions Commission.

Joint Commission on Accreditation of Healthcare Oraganizations. (1997). ORYX: The next evolution in accreditation. *Nursing Management, 27*(5), 49-50, 52, 54.

Joint Working Group on Telemedicine. (1997). *Telemedicine report to Congress* (on line). Available at *http//www.ntia.doc.gov/reports/telemed.execsum.ntm.*

Kendrick, J.M. (1997). The advanced practice movement in nursing: Impact on perinatal care. *Journal of Perinatal and Neonatal Nursing, 10*(4), 20-27.

Loeb, J.M., & Buck, A.S. (1996). Framework for selection of performance measurement systems: Attributes of conformance. *Journal of the American Medical Association, 275*(7), 508.

National Committee for Quality Assurance (NCQA). (1996). *HEDIS 3.0 health plan employer data and information set: Draft for public comment.* Washington, D.C.: NCQA.

National Committee for Quality Assurance (NCQA). (1996). *National committee for quality assurance standards, 1997.* Washington, D.C.: NCQA.

National Committee for Quality Assurance (NCQA). (1995). *HEDIS 2.5 updated specifications for HEDIS 2.0.* Washington, D.C.: NCQA.

National Council of State Boards of Nursing. (1997). *Issues, 18*(2), 1-3.

National League for Nursing. (1996). NLN accreditation q&a. *NLN Update, 2*(3), 7-10.

NCSBN. (1996). *Concepts and models of regulation: Draft.* Chicago: National Council of State Boards of Nursing, pp. 1-2.

Olson, D.K., Verrall, B., & Lundrall, A.M. (1997). Credentialing. *AAOHN Journal, 45*(5), 231-238.

O'Malley, J., Cummings, S., King, C.S. (1996). The politics of advanced practice. *Nursing Administration Quarterly, 20*(3), 62-73.

Parisi, L.L. (1997). What is influencing performance improvement in managed care? *Journal of Nursing Care Quality, 11*(4), 43-51.

Pearson, L.J. (1996). Annual update of how each state stands on legislative issues affecting advanced practice nursing. *Nurse Practitioner, 21,* 10-70.

Prager, L.O. (1996). Private accreditation too lax, consumer group charges. *American Medical News, 39*(28), 15.

Private home care: United Kingdom. (1997, April 28). *Financial Times,* p. 4.

Safriet, B.J. (1994) Impediments to progress in health care workforce policy: License and practice laws. *Inquiry, 31*(3), 3107.

Seppanen, L. (1995). Accreditation: Differentiation from regulations. *Issues, 16*(2), 3-13.

Telemedicine or Telecare: What's next for home care? (1997, June/July). *Business Briefs, NAHC Report,* p. 3.

Using nurse practitioner certification for state nursing regulation: An update. (1997, March 24). *National Council News Release.* Chicago: NCSBN, p. 1-7.

Vaughan, C.E. (1997). Why accreditation failed agencies serving the blind and visually impaired. *Journal of Rehabilitation, 63*(1), 7-15.

Waters, R.J., & Shotwell, L.F. (personal communication, July 22, 1996).

Webster's ninth new collegiate dictionary. (1984). Springfield, Mass: Merriam-Webster, p. 411.

Woodward, S. (1997, Dec 16). Boards of nursing approve proposed language for an interstate compact for a mutual recognition model of nursing regulation. *NCSBN Press Release.* Chicago: National Council of State Boards of Nursing, pp. 1-2.

EFFECTING CHANGE
IN THE HEALTH
CARE SYSTEM

CHAPTER 17

Management Skills

P.J. Maddox

As is discussed in other chapters, the health care industry is undergoing great change at a rapid pace and the environment in which health care organizations must operate is complex, uncertain, and continuously changing. Amid expectations for continued change in health care, the need for competent leadership is high. Nurses need strong leadership and management skills to effectively manage and support patient care in a variety of organizational circumstances. Increasingly, nurses in direct patient care are being held accountable as individuals or leaders of teams for decision making and actions that determine health service quality, efficiency, and effectiveness. No longer do staff depend on managers for information and supervision of direct service providers. Indeed, according to Porter-O'Grady (1997), emerging health systems require only two levels of leadership: systems integration leadership and coordination of service leadership. It is the nurse, working at the point of service in providing care, who assumes the new leadership role in the coordination of service.

To prepare themselves to work effectively in such capacities, nurses need knowledge of the financial, technical, sociopolitical, cultural, and ethical dimensions of the health care envi-

ronment. In addition, they need to have knowledge about the organization and its environment and possess a variety of leadership and management skills that are discussed in detail in other chapters, such as systems thinking, negotiation, implementation of planned change, communication, conflict resolution, delegation, and group dynamics (Krejci & Malin, 1997).

This chapter presents an overview of historical and contemporary leadership and management concepts and discusses skills useful to nurses who are expected to provide quality, efficient patient care in a variety of health care settings and circumstances. The focus is on the *practice* of leadership in contemporary health care organizations without regard to a particular organizational position. Content is organized into five sections:

1. Differentiation of leadership and nursing management
2. Evolution of management thought and practice
3. Evolution of organizational architecture
4. Changing views on work, organization, and leadership
5. Leadership skills at the point of service

OBJECTIVES _____

After reading this chapter, you will be able to:

1. Differentiate and integrate leadership and management functions
2. Explain the management process and its use in leadership and management roles

3. Analyze interpersonal, informational, and decisional roles in nursing management
4. Relate trends in the evolution of management thought to current nursing leadership and management functions
5. Discuss trends in management of health care services and systems

■ DIFFERENTIATION OF LEADERSHIP AND MANAGEMENT

As discussed in Chapter 9, leadership and management skills are necessary for the success of any organization. There are a wide variety of ideas about what constitutes leadership and management and what distinguishes effective performance. Some notions draw sharp distinctions between the two concepts; others call for integration. Beginning with identification of the characteristics of managers and leaders, this section of the chapter explores selected historical and contemporary theories that have guided the practice of leadership and the development of management roles and skills.

According to Marquis and Huston (1996), the following characteristics differentiate managers from leaders:

• *Managers*
  • Are always assigned a position within an organization
  • Have a legitimate source of power based on the delegated authority that accompanies the position
  • Are expected to carry out specific functions
  • Emphasize control, decision-making, decision analysis, and results
• *Leaders*
  • Do not necessarily have delegated authority; may obtain their power through other means

  • Have a wider variety of roles than do managers
  • Are not part of the formal organization
  • Focus on group process, information gathering, feedback, and empowering others

This perspective represents a traditionally differentiated distinction between leadership and management roles in organizations. It also represents the perspective that hierarchic assignment of power by delegated authority differentiates managers from leaders and thus explains the difference in their roles and functions. Until recently, this has been the most widely held viewpoint—differentiating leadership and management practice. This notion is being challenged by a number of futurists (Russell Ackoff, Peter Drucker, and Timothy Porter-O'Grady) by proposing a different paradigm for management and leadership practice. The "new age" perspective on leadership and management thinking are discussed later in the chapter (Ackoff, 1994; Drucker, 1995; Porter O'Grady, 1997).

Many experts in nursing contend that traditional definitions of management and leadership practice do not fit health care organizations and the management of the work of nurses. Some contend that every nurse is a leader and manager at some level and effective performance of professional nursing roles requires both leadership and management skills (Blouin & Crabtree Tonges, 1996; Marquis & Huston, 1996; Spitzer-Lehmann, 1996). They see such skills as integral to a wide variety of work responsibilities performed by clinical and advanced practice nurses alike. An explanation of leadership and management terms are shown in the box below.

According to Spitzer-Lehmann, there is less agreement about what constitutes and differentiates leadership than what constitutes management (1996, p. 80):

> The core components of leadership and management are circular, dynamic, and interrelated. In management the requirements may be to manage a particular process, whereas leadership's role is to assure the process is being managed, or the right problem being solved, while focus is kept on the outcome.

She contends that knowledge-based workers, such as nurses, are often called on to fulfill managerial functions and believes that professional nurses should acquire the knowledge and skills to be capable of doing so. According to

her, a "fine line" differentiates leadership and management, and successful leaders and managers cross between leading and managing, depending on the situation and need. The definition of nursing management used in this chapter subscribes to this view.

An observable shift in leadership styles and skills is evolving in health care organizations and other industries. Rigid hierarchies, control, and organizational motivation from the top are being replaced by decentralized units, interdisciplinary teams, group decision making, and leaders who support innovation and entrepreneurship (Aroian et al., 1996, part I). This is known as the "new age" leadership paradigm (Porter-O'Grady, 1997). Before elaborating on the new paradigm as it relates to nurses in health care organizations, it is important to understand some of the thinking that has contributed to the evolution of leadership and management from the early 1900s to the present. Appreciating how we got to where we are will help us to fully appreciate this continuous process of change and improvement.

■ EVOLUTION OF MANAGEMENT THOUGHT AND PRACTICE

To appreciate current leadership and management concepts, it is useful to examine selected important developments that have shaped leadership and management thinking since the turn of the twentieth century. Several management theories form the basis for such an understanding. Among them, classical and contemporary theories illustrate how management thought has evolved and helps support the basis for predicting what will be useful in the future. The classical theories of management have focused on a variety of phenomena: management functions, bureaucracy, and scientific management. The contemporary theories of management typically include the second generation human relations, systems, and contingency theories. Selected theorists and their contributions are summarized

Key terms	
Term	**Definition**
Leadership	The ability to influence others in the determination and achievement of goals
Management	The coordination and integration of resources through planning, organizing, coordinating, directing, and controlling to accomplish specific organizational goals
Nursing management	The coordination and integration of nursing resources by applying the management process to accomplish nursing care and service goals and objectives

and briefly explained in the next section. These selected perspectives help to explain current leadership and nursing management practice.

Classical Management Theories

Beginning in the early twentieth century, classical management theorists were interested in explaining organizational phenomena, particularly responses to management interventions. Each has contributed to leadership and management practice today. Scientific management, bureaucracy, functional management, and human relations schools of thought comprise classical management theory.

Taylor (1856-1915): Taylor is considered the father of Scientific Management (also known as *traditional* or *classical organizational theory*). He was concerned primarily with improving the efficiency and productivity of employees by timing, measuring, simplifying, and defining individual tasks. He viewed the organization as a machine with the primary goal of increasing production and efficiency by decreasing wasted human effort. His insistence on assembly line production methods was one of the underpinnings of the Industrial Revolution. The techniques first introduced by Taylor are still used in industrial engineering studies and productivity improvement projects (e.g., time and motion studies of nurses' work) (Taylor, 1911).

Weber (1864-1920): At a time when organizations were in chaos, Weber proposed an organizational structure to create the "ideal" bureaucracy. Bureaucratic Theory addressed the processes that organizations applied to increase work performance. Weber suggested that clearly defined and exacting processes would eliminate confusion and uncertainty and would increase efficiency while making workers more comfortable on the job. His system of organization created authority structures that were designed to support more rational, efficient, and systematic organizational operations. He believed that five "ideals" of organizational authority could improve organizational performance: (1) a division of labor with well-defined re-

sponsibilities; (2) a hierarchy of authority with a clear chain of command; (3) employee selection based on qualifications rather than favoritism; (4) salaried managers with a career orientation; and (5) clear rules uniformly and fairly applied (Weber, 1947).

Fayol (1841-1925): Fayol identified the functional approach to management, calling it Administrative Science (a systematic practice of management functions). The original five management functions were planning, organizing, commanding, coordinating, and controlling. Today, the five functions of management are identified as organizing, planning, leading, controlling, and staffing. The management process is a rational, logical process based on repetitive performance of management functions. Because of the importance of this concept and its influence on management education and practice, further explanations of Fayol's management functions are included in the definition of terms that follows this section. Administrative Science supports the traditional differentiation of management and leadership (Fayol, 1925).

Mayo (1880-1949): Mayo is considered the founder of the human relations school of thought and industrial sociology. His research in the 1920s and 1930s demonstrated the importance of groups in affecting the behavior of individuals at work and enabled him to make deductions about what managers ought to do. His work led to a fuller understanding of the "human factor" in work situations. Central to his understanding of human behavior in organizations was the discovery of the importance and influence of the informal group (i.e., an outlet for the aspirations workers). The most renowned of Mayo's research projects involved General Electric's Hawthorne Plant (from which the term *Hawthorne Effect* was derived). These contributions have been important in helping to develop insight into what motivates employees and how to influence work force/worker motivation (an important consideration for leaders and managers alike) (Mayo, 1933).

McGregor (1906-1964): McGregor developed a human relations management theory that was built upon Mayo's understanding of worker motivation: Theory X and Theory Y. He described two types of managers: Theory X managers believed their employees to be lazy, under-motivated, and indifferent to the needs of the organization (thus assuming them to require constant direction and supervision); Theory Y managers believed their workers enjoyed work, were self-motivated, and were independently responsive in pursuing personal and organizational goals.

Quality Gurus: In the 1950s, based on the application of mathematical modeling and statistical design of processes, the early Quality Management Gurus (Deming, Juran, and Crosby) introduced several quality management constructs. It was not until the 1970s, however, that the influence of quality management thinking was felt in organizations in the United States. With the importance of outcomes management and data-driven decision making, along with increased organizational participation, quality management concepts are making a substantial and important contribution to leadership and management today. Refer to Chapter 19 for further reading on the influence of quality management theories.

Contemporary Management Theory

Contemporary theories of management comprise systems and contingency theories. They have had considerable influence on current thinking related to the management and development of organizations and the practice of management and leadership in contemporary organizations. Although many theories belong in this category (including general systems theory), the following are particularly notable for their recognized impact on current management and leadership practice.

Mintzberg (1973): Through an observational study, Mintzberg characterized the varied work of managers in 10 roles. He suggested that these ten roles cluster under three major categories: *interpersonal, informational,* and *decisional.* Within the interpersonal category are *figure head, leader, and liaison* roles; within the informational category are the *monitor, disseminator,* and *spokes-*

person roles; within the decisional category are the *resource allocator, entrepreneur, negotiator,* and *disturbance handler* roles. Many of these roles will be recognized as useful to both leaders and managers; they are summarized and explained with reference to practice by nurses in Box 17-1.

Burns (1978): In studying leaders and followers, Burns found that both have the ability to raise each other to higher levels of motivation and morality. He is recognized as developing the concept of *transformational leadership.* He described leaders as one of two types: those concerned with the day-to-day operations of the organization (transactional); and those who create a "vision" and empower others to pursue their work through the vision (transformational).

Senge (1994): Senge is recognized for popularizing the construct of *learning organization.* He focuses on decentralizing the role of leadership in an organization to enhance the capacity of all people to work productively toward common goals. He describes three elements of "Context" that create meaning and set perspective in learning organizations: vision, values and integrity; dialogue; and systems thinking. In his popular text on learning organizations, *The Fifth Discipline* (1994), he posits that organizations work the way they work because of how they think and interact. He believes that by fundamentally changing how members in an organization think, they change deeply embedded practices. By changing how organizations interact, they have the capacity to become learning organizations in that they have established shared visions, shared understandings, and new capacities for coordinated action.

Management theory has developed over time under influences from a number of disciplines (e.g., psychology, anthropology, business, engineering) The variety of backgrounds and constructs attributable to these selected management theorists illustrates the phenomenon. Management thinking continues to evolve as a function of changing circumstances and as a result of the process of discovery from research findings and practical experience.

BOX 17-1

Mintzberg's Managerial Roles

Interpersonal Roles
Figurehead

Presides over or conducts organizational ceremonies. Nurses commonly distribute certificates, pins, and acknowledgement for committee, departmental, and institutional award and recognition events.

Leader

Engages in a variety of behaviors that serve to influence and motivate. Nurses interact and supervise a variety of members on the health care team. They commonly use verbal praise to acknowledge notable work efforts and contributions/participation on challenging assignments, whether they be team projects or at the point of service for patients.

Liaison

Involves representing a work group's interests or preferences in working on organizational initiatives. Nurses often participate in establishing a policy when the concerns of their unit or work groups must be conveyed or to support patient services. In addition, they interact with peers (internal and external) for networking purposes.

Informational Roles
Monitor

Involves the collection of information from a wide variety of sources to serve a variety of purposes. Data may be related to patients or clinical processes or may be administrative in nature. Monitoring detects problems and opportunities. Nurses who oversee point-of-service care or traditional shift or unit operations are continuously collecting administrative and clinical data and assessing situations for intervention or follow-up.

Disseminator

Involves dispensing information. Nurses receive considerable amounts of information and use dis-

cretion about what amount and level of information to pass on, and to whom. As knowledge-based workers, disseminate information to support communication related to clinical, administrative, or professional needs.

Spokesperson

Involves transmitting information to individuals external to the organization. Nurses regularly transmit information from physicians or hospital management to patients' families and to other health care institutions.

Decisional Roles
Resource allocator

Involves the distribution of human or capital resources to accomplish the organization's work. In the new management paradigm resource allocation is done by point-of-service leaders and system managers with budget authority. Nurses to allocate staffing and supply resources at point-of-service units.

Entrepreneur

Involves focusing on change and innovation. Nurse regularly have opportunities to improve clinical services or develop new clinical and educational programs.

Negotiator

Involves bargaining with others. Nurses often bargain to resolve conflicts with other professionals around patient care–related work or to resolve nursing work group or organizational conflicts.

Disturbance handler

Involves taking charge when a conflict impedes necessary work. Opportunities for disturbance handling are common around interemployee/work unit arguments, morale problems associated with personnel changes, or even institutional disasters.

Key terms	
Term	**Definition**
Management functions	First identified by Fayol, as the essential components of management practice: organizing, planning, commanding, coordinating, and controlling; currently recognized as organizing, planning, leading, controlling, and staffing
Organizing	The management function that mobilizes human, material, and capital resources into an orderly system for purposes of supporting the achievement of organizational goals and objectives
Planning	The management function associated with determining the short-term and long-term future direction (goals and objectives) for an organization
Directing	The management function (also called *coordinating*) that involves motivating and leading individuals and groups to carry out desired organizational actions; contemporary management writers often replace this term with the term *leading*.
Leading	Influencing and motivating employees to willingly pursue organizational goals
Controlling	The management function that seeks to ensure that the work of the organization occurs in conformity with established rules; it compares the results of work with predetermined standards of performance and takes corrective action when needed
Staffing	The management function of establishing human resource and personnel capabilities to achieve the organization's goals and objectives
Management process	A systematic approach to management that seeks to advance the organization's goals and objectives through an iterative process employing Fayol's five management functions

The Evolution of Management Practice

The *Harvard Business Review (HBR)* asked consultant David Sibbett to synopsize the most important changes in management thinking and practice since the inception of the *HBR* in 1922. Over a 75-year timeline, he found that management science and thinking had evolved to produce changes in the focus and practice of management.

The *HBR Timeline on the Evolution of Management Practice* (1922-1997) identified three key periods of change resulting in new developments in the focus of management for each period. From approximately 1922 to 1945 the practice of management focused primarily on administration, personnel, sales, production, accounting, and finance. From 1946 to the 1980s management practice focused on business policy, human resources, sales and marketing, operations, accounting, and finance. Since the mid-1990s the focus of management has been reported to be on people, sales and marketing, adding value, measuring results, and finance (Box 17-2). This most recent development is particularly significant as it supports a broader philosophic and methodologic change in the management of organizations (one focused on purpose, process, and people). This concept is discussed later in the chapter.

Seventy-five Years of Management Practice: 1922-1997

Foci of General Managers

1922-1944	1945-1990	1991-1997
Personnel	Business policy	Leadership
Sales	Human resources	Managing people
Production	Sales and marketing	Sales and marketing
Accounting	Operations	Adding value
Finance	Accounting	Measuring results
	Finance	Finance

From Sibbet, D. (1997). Seventy-five years of management ideas and practice: 1922-1997. *Harvard Business Review, 75* (Suppl. Reprint No. 97500).

As the focus of management has changed, so have the skills needed for effective management practice. Change in management ideas and practice has followed a complex, evolutionary route; the impact/effect in organizations can be seen in everything from organizational structure, to work and role design, to communication, decision making, and relationship management. The practice of leadership and management in health care organizations has likewise changed over time and will continue to do so. This means that nurses will continue to see changes in management and leadership thinking and practice as knowledge is acquired and as health care organizations and their environments change. The uncertain environment in which health care organizations are operating and the nature of the work and work force in health care organizations explain the drivers of change in the focus of leadership and management practice in the 1990s.

Because of the unique characteristics of the work and responsibilities of highly educated, knowledge-based workers (nurses), distinctions that explain traditional staff and management functions do not fit (Lawler, 1988). The com-plexity of the work of health care professionals and their interdependence, along with an active flow of information (communication) and participation in decision making, exerts a strong influence in health care organizations and explains why traditional management concepts fail to support their unique work. Health care providers need to continually interact with each other and in a variety of intraorganizational and extraorganizational functions to actually provide patient services and solve problems associated with the delivery of services. As such, these knowledge workers continuously exchange information and do not work through managers using a hierarchic information-sharing and decision-making process. Relations between professional workers and managers are often characterized by shared or participative decision making for many organizational functions. Health care professionals are highly independent in the management of their day-to-day work and in decision making related to the provision of health care services. In addition, they are active planners and problem-solvers related to the organization and delivery of services.

The Evolution of Organizational Architecture

Organizations (health care and other industries) typically created organizational structures to support the organization's strategy. According to Bartlett and Ghoshal (1994):

> Structure follows strategy. And systems support structure. Few aphorisms have penetrated Western business thinking as deeply as these two. Not only do they influence the architecture of today's largest corporations but they also define the role that top corporate mangers play.

They go on to say that this philosophy supported organizational growth and change as varied as integrated horizontal growth in the 1950s, diversification in the 1960s, and global markets in the 1970s and 1980s. In the 1990s, however, technology, competition, and market changes have eroded the success of the strategy-structure-systems approach. The elaborate bureaucratic systems developed to support the work of organizations in the 1970s and 1980s are identified with impeding work when rapid change and innovation is needed (i.e., under conditions of uncertainty and competition).

From Strategy, Structure, and Systems to Purpose, Process, and People

Through the 1980s, corporate size and diversification increased and organizations embraced increasingly more complex strategies, structures, reporting, and planning systems to organize and keep track of work and to control production (service delivery) processes. As a result, the day-to-day work of employees became increasingly more fragmented and standardized. When organizations needed to change quickly to become more service oriented, efficient, and innovative, large bureaucratic systems failed them. As a result, implementation of such prescriptive practices as inverting the organizational pyramid, focusing on strategic intent, corporate reengineering, and employee empowerment were widely adopted. According to Barlett and Ghoshal (1994), these corporate interventions merely treat the symptoms of the problem (symptoms associated with treating people in organizations as "replaceable parts"). They contended that there was a need for a fundamental change in how organizations were managed. "Senior managers of today's large enterprises must move beyond strategy, structure, and systems to a framework built on purpose, process, and people." (Barlett & Ghoshal, 1994, p. 79). They go on to say (1995, p. 142):

> . . .the implications for top-level managers are profound. If frontline employees are vital strategic resources instead of mere factors of production, corporate executives can no longer afford to be isolated from the people in their organizations. Furthermore, roles and responsibilities of managers must be reallocated, with those deeper in the organization taking on many of the tasks formerly reserved for those at the top.

It is this perspective that is shaping 'new age' organizations.

■ TRENDS IN HEALTH CARE

In contemporary health care organizations, the following trends are associated with changes in the way health care organizations are managing cost and quality and are redesigning work and changing organizational structure, processes, and working relationships to better fit the nature of health care service delivery (Blouin & Crabtree Tonges, 1996):

1. Organizations are becoming smaller—employing fewer people (i.e., downsizing).
2. Traditional hierarchies are being replaced by a variety of matrix-like structures, resembling shared-governance and self-managed work teams (cross-functional work teams).

3. Knowledge workers (such as nurses) are key to organizational adaptation (change), given the complexity of service functions and the interdependence on a variety of health care professionals.
4. Classical (vertical) division of labor is changing to horizontal, flat responsibility and decision structures (i.e., shared governance).
5. An economic shift has occurred, from creating products to managing services, reinforcing the importance of the relational aspects of health service delivery to customers and consumers.

These changes are consistent with trends from other industries related to how organizations are shifting from strategy, structure, and systems and moving to meet the organization's goals though purpose, process, and people.

■ CHANGING VIEWS ON WORK, LEADERSHIP, AND ORGANIZATIONS

According to Blouin and Crabtree Tonges (1996), the movement to redesign the structure of nurses' work and health care organizations began in the mid-1980s. As hospitals faced pressures to increase the quality of care while decreasing the cost of delivering services, they began to reengineer the processes of care delivery and thus restructure and redesign service delivery models. Clinical systems incorporating care and case management have been implemented, along with new decision-making structures such as shared governance. The nursing management literature reflects considerable activity related to redesigning care delivery systems and in some cases the governance structure of nursing (Jenkins, 1991; Zander, 1994). Service delivery models are becoming increasingly multidisciplinary, extending beyond the hospital to encompass a broader continuum of care. This has created new demands on health care organizations related to the technical and social aspects of work and on information management and

decision making related to service delivery. Designers of such systems face the challenge of blending consistency with flexibility in the delivery of services (to accommodate different needs), while building links to connect services and facilities and share information across the health care continuum. High-performing health care organizations create organizational designs that effectively meet both organizational and individual motivations and needs (Nadler et al., 1992).

Nurses interested in preparing themselves for successful leadership roles in a variety of capacities (practitioners, clinical specialists, educators) need to possess a wide variety of skills and abilities once thought to be relevant only for those in formal management positions. In today's knowledge-based organizations, the structure of organizations and the nature of organizational work is changing from rigid role- and department-defined responsibilities to cross-functional and team-based work. The new focus of management is to develop the organization's human resource capacity. Replacing the focus on strategy, structure, and systems, organizations are developing people who will manage work processes (individually and as members of cross-functional teams). Porter-O'Grady's view of "new age" process leadership (1997) predicts that it will replace "industrial age" management practices. Table 17-1 summarizes differences in "industrial age" and "new age" management principles. The contrasted differences between industrial and new age principles are explained in terms of organizational factors related to work, relationships, structures, and advancement.

Traditional hierarchic supervision is not needed when large numbers of highly educated knowledge workers comprise the staff of an organization. Knowledge-based workers (health care providers), with their interdependent responsibilities, and the complexity of the work it-

TABLE 17-1		
Changing Work Structures		
Organizational Elements	Industrial Age	New Age
Work	Defined by job; fixed, finite and functional	Defined by role; fluid, flexible, and focused
Relationships	Vertical, hierarchical, highly prescribed, and ordered	Horizontal, relational fluid, negotiated, changeable
Structures	Compartmentalized, authority based, command and control, highly functional	Decentralized, point-of-service designed, intersecting, loosely defined, and continuum supported
Advancement	Promotion	Mobility

From Porter-O'Grady, T. (1997). Process leadership and the death of management. *Nursing Economics, 15*(6), 287.

self are factors well suited to shared decision-making arrangements (Lawler, 1988). Shared governance provides the mechanism for information from front-line service providers to influence relevant operational decisions. Many organizations are replacing traditional hierarchically oriented authority structures with shared authority arrangements. Staff members closest to the patient are recognized as being in the best position to evaluate the effects of organizational decisions on the efficiency and effectiveness of the delivery of health care services. The performance of employees (especially those working at the point of service) is considered to be *the most* important and strategic organizational resource.

Managing at the Point of Service

Organizations expect that nurses will be able to offer cost-effective quality care, advocate for patients, coordinate the continuum of care, solve problems, and identify and remove obstacles to quality that occur at the point of service. Nurses also are frequently recognized as the link between the system and the patient—as a critical factor in determining the patient's overall satisfaction with the health care experience. An im-

portant and growing trend is for organizations to use nurses as outcome managers, team coordinators, and guardians of continuity of care for a continuum of services. Many organizations are hoping that nurses with substantial leadership skills will create 'added value' for the organization. The added value would be created by enabling nurses to meet patient expectations while problem solving or resolving barriers to faster, more caring, and more efficient delivery of services. In other words, organizations are counting on these individuals to take the attitude that "the buck stops with me" to ensure quality at the point of service. Nurses working at the point of service need to be able to manage people and resources in the entire system to meet patient needs seamlessly and efficiently. Now that we know what demands are being placed on nurses in contemporary health care organizations, let us examine the competencies needed.

Organizations expect that nurses possess the knowledge and ability to be leaders in problem solving, service delivery, productivity management, successful team work, and the management and improvement of clinical quality. In preparing nurses for such work, Krejci and

Malin (1997) studied perceptions of leadership competencies (perception of understanding and ability to carry out each competency) before and after participation in a leadership development program. The following leadership competency subjects were identified as important:

- Change
- Communication
- Conflict
- Health care environment
- Group dynamics
- Leadership nursing
- Oppressed group behaviors
- Power
- Problem setting/diagnosis
- Reframing
- Systems thinking.

As complexity increases in organizations, those who work at the point of service must increase their ability to handle expanded organizational expectations related to managing quality and effectiveness. In the Krejci and Malin (1997) study, these categories were identified as important leadership competencies for professional nurses in today's health care organiza-tions. A more detailed listing of leadership competencies is displayed in Box 17-3.

Haas and Hackbarth (1997) studied nurse managers in ambulatory care and identified the following competencies as dimensions of the future nursing management role:

- Allocating and developing human resources
- Strategic planning and controlling
- Managing human resources
- Interacting with multiple stakeholders
- Enhancing quality
- Promoting research and outcome measurement

In a case study involving redesigning the nurse manager role, Litwin, Beauchesne, and Rabinowitz (1997) reported on an organization's redesigned manager responsibilities. The scope and vision of the redesigned manager role were based on the following assumptions, related to the operation of the health care organization:

That unit-based, self-directed teams provide care to clients; the managerial role is administrative (not clinical); the staff nurse role is a care manager (managing the care of the patient on a variety of

---

B O X   1 7 - 3

Leadership Competencies

Effective Communication (understanding and ability)

Effective Conflict Resolution (understanding and ability)

Accurate Problem Diagnosis/Problem Setting (understanding and ability)

Systems Thinking (understanding and ability)

Personal Power (understanding and ability to utilize)

Effective Group Dynamics (understanding and ability)

Change Agency (understanding and ability)

Oppressed Group Behaviors (understanding and ability)

Decision Making/Reframing (understanding and ability)

Nursing's Contribution to Patient Outcomes (understanding and ability to articulate and act)

Health Care Environment (Understanding and ability to impact)

Leadership: Influence on Patient and Organizational Outcomes (understanding and ability)

From Krejci, J.W., Malin, S. (1997). Impact of leadership development on competencies. *Nursing Economics, 15*(5), 237.

levels, delegating activities to other caregivers and support personnel, and the care manager is accountable for the care of the patient and evaluation of the performance and competence of team members).

The scope and vision of the nurse manager's responsibilities were as follows (Litwin et al., 1997):

- Educated, articulate strategic planners and program developers
- Coach, mentor, motivator of staff and self-directed teams
- Challenger of status quo and facilitator of change
- Communicator and collaborator with all members of the health care team (internal and external)
- Champion for medical center's values, vision, and direction
- Standard-setter for excellence and quality improvement
- Developer and manager of fiscal resources
- Manager of human resources, with help of RN and other professional caregivers

Box 17-4 summarizes competencies identified in the Litwin et al. study.

Some of the most provocative thoughts on management and leadership are reflected in the writings of authors who call for or predict the death of traditional hierarchic management (Ackoff, 1994; Blouin & Crabtree Tonges, 1996; Drucker, 1995, 1997; Porter-O'Grady, 1997). According to Porter-O'Grady, it is not useful or feasible for managers to try to control all of the service provision processes in health care. Not only do traditional industrial model managers not have all of the necessary information, they do not have the investment and ownership of the work that the individuals who do the work have (i.e., health care providers). This means that a new management paradigm—one that invests in knowledge workers and empowers them as stakeholders in the mission and outcomes of the system—is necessary. Moving the locus of control into the hands of the knowledge worker will profoundly change the organization in terms of the conditions and circumstances of work and structures and relationships within the organization. Better decisions can be made more quickly, and increased flexibility is to be expected.

Among the many change implications of the new age paradigm is a change in the locus of control for decision making that gives rise to the need for two types of managers: manager of the system and process leader (Porter-O'Grady, 1997). Responsibility is shifted away from the manager role and toward empowered process leadership roles at the point of service. The change also calls for a stronger support, service, and system role for managers. The expectations for "new age" managers and process leaders are listed in full in Box 17-5.

A closer look at the competencies and expectations of leader managers, as identified in Table 17-1 and Boxes 17-4 and 17-5, supports the notion that the same trends identified by the *Harvard Business Review* (changes in the focus of managers) are apparent in health care. Although there is wide variance in health care setting and nursing management competency terms, these figures illustrate a common trend (managing by purpose, process, and people).

The management of people and human relations is critically important in service-based organizations, as is the need to ensure quality and efficiency. Data management (financial and clinical) that supports planning and decision making for a wide variety of purposes is also important. Once the use of data for planning and evaluation purposes was considered the purview of managers only. Use of financial and other administrative data as well as clinical data related to organizational performance and outcomes is now considered important to support decision making and evaluation at the point of service. Delegation and supervision of work per-

Dimensions of the Future Ambulatory Nurse Manager Role

Allocating and Developing Human Resources

Adjust staffing
Supervise care provided
Support staff advocacy of clients
Evaluate nursing staff performance
Facilitate staff continuing education
Participate in formulation/implementation of administrative policies and procedures

Strategic Planning and Controlling

Participate in formulation of philosophy, goals
Represent nursing on policy-making boards/committees
Participate in identifying and resolving ethical dilemmas
Monitor budget
Collaborate with risk manager

Managing Human Resources

Plan staffing
Participate in recruitment, retention, promotion, and discharge of staff
Assure resources availability for systematic orientation of nursing personnel
Initiate and follow through with disciplinary mechanisms
Participate in formulation of job descriptions

Interacting with Multiple Stakeholders

Provide input in organization marketing plans
Negotiate with vendors, third-party payers, community organizations

Enhancing Quality

Participate in interdisciplinary QI teams
Participate in preparation of QI plan
Use QI plan in practice
Implement professional standards
Collect and analyze QI data
Participate in off-site continuing education

Promoting Research and Outcome Measurement

Develop expected client outcomes
Participate in research of others
Facilitate and encourage research
Identify researchable questions
Follow guidelines to protect human subjects
Evaluate nursing research findings
Serve as a member of a research review board
Conduct own research
Utilize client classification system

From Litwin, R., Beauchesne, K., & Rabinowitz, B. (1997). Redesigning the nurse manager role: A case study. *Nursing Economics, 15*(1), 201.

formed and the monitoring of resources mobilized at the point of service to reach quality and efficiency goals now fall within the domain of process leaders, not just system managers. Inasmuch as both system managers and process leaders are concerned with ensuring quality, efficient health care services, individuals in both roles require the knowledge and competence to work with such data for planning and evaluative purposes.

"New age" leadership and management roles may not be evident in all health care organizations today; however, trends associated with the increased responsibility of professional nurses at the point of service are stimulating the need for change in the traditional authority and decision paradigms in organizations. Furthermore, as organizations desire to work smarter, faster, and more flexibly, traditional bureaucratic arrangements are actually impeding organiza-

New Age Role Expectations for Managers and Process Leaders

Manager's Role
Expectations

planning
organizing
directing
implementing
controlling
evaluating
disciplining

Orientation

institution
department
function
process
individual

Role

directing processes
managing information
managing budget and variance
manipulating information components
evaluating individual performance
conflict resolution
solving compartmental problems
meeting departmental objectives

Process Leader's Role
Expectations

coordinating
integrating
facilitating
creating access
team building
linking
sustaining

Orientation

point-of-service
fit
outcomes
team

Role

facilitating relationships
generating information
linking system support
improving information infrastructure
team relationship/performance building
coaching/learning method development
coupling system support with service
fitting system strategy to service goals

From Porter-O'Grady, T. (1997). Process leadership and the death of management. *Nursing Economics, 15*(6), 292.

tional efficiency and flexibility. Leadership skills that support the lowest level of decision making in the organization and the ability to meet the organization's goals (purpose) by way of managing work processes and working relationships are critical for all professional nurses.

Health care organizations in the 1990s and beyond are designing cross-functional, team-based work and changing organizational structure and working relationships to be able to support greater flexibility, efficiency, and quality in providing health care services.

As such, a new paradigm for the management and leadership skills necessary to support the work of the health care organization is called for. The following key points reflect the current thinking about contemporary leadership and nursing management skills.

■ KEY POINTS

- Health care organizations comprise large numbers of knowledge workers.
- The need for communication and decision making is highly decentralized in health care

organizations to support the high level of interaction and interdependence among health care professionals to provide patient care services.

- Health care organizations are similar to other non-health-related organizations in observing changes in management trends and organizational design.

- Organizations are moving away from a concentration on strategy, structure, and systems to ensure the organization's successful performance, by pursuing a focus on purpose, process, and people.

- Nurses working at the point of service require knowledge and competence in a wide array of skills once thought to fall only within the purview of formal managers.

- A fine line differentiates leadership and management, and successful leaders and managers cross between leading and managing depending on the situation.

- Nursing management is the coordination and integration of nursing resources by applying the management process to accomplish nursing care and service goals and objectives.

■ CRITICAL THINKING QUESTIONS

1. Interview two people who have roles within a health care organization that are considered to be managerial roles. Observe their behavior for a period of time. Evaluate their management type. Ask them to each describe their style/method of management.
    A. Is their analysis consistent with yours?
    B. Is either or both using classical management theories to form their behavior?
    C. Is either or both using contemporary management theories to form their behavior?
2. Consider a clinical situation in which you were recently a participant and in which management functions were implemented. Use the management functions and process of organizing, planning, leading, controlling,

and staffing to evaluate the steps of management that were actually taken in the situation you observed. What worked well? What could have been improved? What recommendations do you have?

3. Briefly describe the clinical area with which you are most familiar. Who are the knowledge workers in that setting? Do you think they see themselves as knowledge workers? Do you think that others see them as knowledge workers? What changes could be made to make this a more effectively managed unit?

4. Develop a list of what you consider to be essential skills for an effective manager. Which ones will be most difficult for you to carry out? Which skills will be seen as your strengths? What steps can you take to be able to fully implement the managerial role?

■ REFERENCES

Ackoff, R. (1994). *The democratic corporation.* New York: Oxford University Press.

Aroian, J., Merservey, P.M., & Crockett, J.G. (1996). Developing nurse leaders for today and tomorrow. Part I: Foundations of leadership in practice. *Journal of Nursing Administration, 26*(9), 18-26.

Bartlett, C., & Ghoshal, S. (1994). Changing the role of top management: Beyond strategy to purpose. *Harvard Business Review, 72*(6), 79-88.

Bartlett, C., & Ghoshal, S. (1995). Changing the role of top management: Beyond systems to people. *Harvard Business Review, 73*(3), 133-142.

Blouin, A.S., & Crabtree Tonges, M. (1996). The content/context imperative: Integration of emerging design for the practice of management of nursing. *Journal of Nursing Administration, 26*(3), 38-46.

Burns, J.M. (1978). *Leadership.* New York: Harper & Row.

Drucker, P. (1995). *Managing in a time of great change.* New York: Truman Tally Books/Dutton Publishers.

Drucker, P. (1997). *Management.* New York: Truman Tally Books/Dutton Publishers.

Edwards, P.A., & Roemer, L. (1996). Are nurse managers ready for the current challenges of healthcare? *Journal of Nursing Administration, 26*(9), 11-17.

Fayol, H. (1925). *General and Industrial Management.* London: Pittman and Sons.

Haas, S.A., & Hackbarth, D.P. (1997). The role of the nurse manager in ambulatory care: Results of a national survey. *Nursing Economics, 15*(4), 191-203.

Hanston, R., & Washburn, M. (1996). Why don't nurses delegate? *Journal of Nursing Administration, 26*(12), 24-28.

Jenkins, J.E. (1991). Professional governance: The missing link. *Nursing Management, 22*(8), 26-30.

Johnson, L.J. (1990). The influence of assumptions on effective decision-making. *Journal of Nursing Administration, 20*(4), 35.

Krejci, J.W., & Malin, S. (1997). Impact of leadership development on competencies. *Nursing Economics, 15*(5), 235-241.

Lawler, E.E. (1988). Substitutes for hierarchy. *Organizational Dynamics, 17*(1), 4-15.

Litwin, R., Beauchesne, K., & Rabinowitz, B. (1997). Redesigning the nurse manager role: A case study. *Nursing Economics, 15*(1), 191-203.

Marquis B.L., & Huston, C.J. (1996). *Leadership roles and management functions in nursing: Theory and application* (2nd ed.). Philadelphia: Lippincott-Raven.

Mayo, E. (1933). *The human problems of an industrial civilization.* Reprinted 1960. New York: Viking.

McGregor, D. (1960). *The human side of enterprise.* New York: McGraw-Hill.

Mintzberg, H. (1973). *The nature of managerial work.* New York: Harper & Row.

Nadler, D., Gerstein, M., & Shaw, R. (1992). *Organizational architecture.* San Francisco: Jossey-Bass.

Porter-O'Grady, T. (1997). Process leadership and the death of management. *Nursing Economics, 15*(6), 286-293.

Scott, W.R. (1982). Managing professional work: Three models of control for health organizations. *Health Services Research, 17*(3), 213-240.

Senge, P. (Ed.). (1994). *The fifth discipline: The art and practice of the learning organization.* New York: Currency/Doubleday.

Sibbet, D. (1997). Seventy-five years of management ideas and practice: 1922-1997. *Harvard Business Review, 75*(Suppl., Reprint No. 97500).

Spitzer-Lehmann, R. (1996). Roxanne Spitzer-Lehmann envisions the differences between leadership and management. In D. Huber (Ed.). *Leadership and nursing care management* (p. 80). Philadelphia: Saunders.

Strasen, L. (1994). Reengineering hospitals using the "function follows form" model. *Journal of Nursing Administration, 24*(12), 59-63.

Taylor, F.W. (1911). *The principles of scientific management,* New York: Harper & Row.

Weber, M. (1947). *The theory of social and economic organization.* New York: Oxford University Press.

Zander, K. (1994). Responsive restructuring. Part IV: Care management and case management. *New Definition, 9*(2), 1-2.

Managing Care Through Advanced Practice Nursing

Sharon Williams Utz and Pamela A. Kulbok

INTRODUCTION

In the environment in which we find ourselves today, the whole notion of planning takes on a different character. Strong, inflexible systems are exactly what are not needed. We need instead systems that are deeply rooted in common values and objectives, but whose constituent parts are able to adapt quickly to unanticipated developments. We need systems that are like reeds that bend in the winds of change, but are not uprooted.

Gordon Davies

Gordon Davies made this comment in the context of a discussion about the tremendous changes influencing systems of higher education both in Virginia and in the nation. The same transformed environment catalyzes the current demand for rethinking, redirection, and change in health care delivery. The rapidly changing health care system of the 1990s and beyond presents many unknowns for nurses. The future of nursing is integrally related to the systems in which nurses will practice and the common values and objectives guiding those systems. In an extensive analysis of evolving integrated health care systems, Conrad and Shortell (1997) noted that one of the key factors for successful change in the health care system is an ability to *manage the change*. The skill of managing change is one of several valued capabilities that advanced practice nurses have to offer. As discussed in Chapter 1, to thrive in this new environment as change managers, nurses must first "reinvent themselves" to make certain they have the requisite skills to fulfill evolving roles of practice in the world of managed care. One of the most important emerging roles for advanced practice nurses is that of care manager. Although all nurses will be involved in elements of care management in various settings, this chapter clarifies the context in which the role of care manager is developing, delineates the process of care management, and describes this new role for advanced practice nurses. The focus is on the knowledge and skills needed by the care manager and strategies necessary to prepare for the role.

This chapter describes the context and processes of managing care in rapidly evolving health systems at the local, regional, and national levels. *Managing care* encompasses many concepts and terms that apply to health systems organized both to achieve desirable health outcomes and to promote continuity across disconnected segments of health care delivery (Kelly,

433

Key terms	
Term	**Definition**
Care coordination	The process of interdisciplinary collaboration to facilitate the provision of immediate and long-term health services across disconnected segments of the health care system
Care management	Holistic and humanistic process of managing the care of patients, families, and/or communities to ensure desirable health outcomes and continuity of care
Continuity of care	One outcome of a system of managing care that strives to connect patients to appropriate and necessary health care providers and services in an efficient and timely manner
Managed care	Health care delivery system designed to link providers with patients to manage access, cost, and quality

1993). The language of managing care includes (but is not limited to) the following terms: *continuity of care, care coordination, care management, case management, continuum of care,* and *managed care.* Selected concepts and terms are defined throughout the chapter. However, in this critical review and analysis of the role of professional nurses in changing systems of managing care, the terms *care management* and *care manager* are used. These terms encompass key elements of care coordination and other strategies designed to ensure the quality and continuity of care. The rationale for using these two terms is based, in part, on Kelly's (1993) description of increasing public demands for a system of managing care that embraces quality management, care coordination across existing boundaries, and the controlled use of health resources. In addition, the terms *care management* and *care manager* reflect the authors' belief that the concept of *caring* is vital. *Care* and *caring* embody the holistic and humanistic essence of professional nursing practice. Throughout the chapter the terms *case management* and *case manager* also are used in an attempt to accurately reflect the writings, definitions, and positions of prominent authors in this expanding area of role specialization.

OBJECTIVES

After reading this chapter, you will be able to:

1. Analyze the evolving context of care management
2. Differentiate among managed costs, managed care, and managed health

3. Examine the essential components and processes of nursing care management
4. Compare and contrast selected terms related to systems of managing care
5. Explore strategies for learning the advanced practice role of care manager

■ THE PAST AND PRESENT CONTEXT FOR NURSING CARE MANAGEMENT
The Evolution and Essence of Nursing Practice

Case management has been practiced by many health-related disciplines since the early 1970s (Lamb, 1995). According to Lamb, target populations for case management were varied, including the chronically mentally or physically ill, technology-dependent children and adults, and individuals with complex conditions such as cancer or AIDS. In the past decade, nursing scholars have made significant contributions to the literature on care management. Existing literature provides an historical account of different types of nursing practice in the hospital setting in an effort to identify precursors to modern care management (Cohen & Cesta, 1997; Lee, 1993). In addition, several authors have acknowledged the rich contributions of public health and visiting nurses in the United States as originators of strategies that underlie care management. For example, in the preface to Bower's (1992, p. v) classic monograph on *Case Management by Nurses,* Cronenwett asserted that nursing can rightly lay claim to the practice of ". . . case management since the days of providing service coordination in public health during the turn of the century."

In the late nineteenth century, Lillian Wald and visiting nurses in organizations such as the Henry Street Settlement were pioneers who demonstrated that nurses were coordinators of services to a region. Through their interrelations with patients, neighborhoods, and social service agencies and groups, these nurses worked for improvement in health and "social betterment" of individual workers, child workers, and families with ill members in their homes (Heinrich, 1983; Sullivan & Friedman, 1984).

In the early twentieth century, another form of nursing practice and a forerunner of modern nursing care management was implemented in the cities of New York and Boston. Visiting nurses made home visits to patients recently discharged from the hospital. By 1911 more than 40 hospitals nationwide had developed social service departments and were using nurses to follow discharged patients in their homes in an effort to identify and address unmet needs (Sullivan & Friedman, 1984). The focus on care management by visiting nurses soon expanded from follow-up illness care for the sick person in the home to anticipatory care that promoted health and prevented disease for the whole family.

In 1925 Mary Breckenridge organized the first nursing center of the Frontier Nursing Service (FNS) in the mountains of Kentucky. The FNS was truly a pioneering model of managing and delivering care to disadvantaged rural populations (Lancaster, 1996). Between 1927 and 1930, six outpost nursing centers and the FNS hospital in Hyden, Kentucky were built. Public health nurses provided services from one of the rural outposts and often visited families in their homes, traveling by horseback. Mary Breckenridge was committed to improving rural populations' access to health care, and the FNS continues to deliver services today. The formative principles and practices implemented by these pioneering public health and visiting nurses, including coordination of community services, providing continuity of care, and health promotion/disease prevention, are guideposts for managing care into the twenty-first century (Box 18-1).

Writers discussing the development of nursing case management often focus on the evolution of nursing care practice models within the walls of the hospital setting (Cohen & Cesta, 1997; Lee, 1993). This approach traces the precursors of nursing case management through the progressive stages of the case method, functional nursing, team nursing, and primary nursing (Box 18-2).

At the turn of the century, the *case method* involved providing complete patient-centered care to one or more patients, predominantly in the patient's home (Lee, 1993). During the 1920s the hospitals were staffed most often by student nurses, whereas registered nurses provided complete care to patients at home (Sullivan & Decker, 1997). As a patient-centered approach, the case method was considered a precursor to primary nursing. However, the case method came to be regarded as an inefficient and costly method of care (Cohen & Cesta, 1997).

Functional nursing was practiced in U.S. hospitals from the late nineteenth century through World War II (Lee, 1993). The functional method was a task-oriented approach in which the needs of patients were broken down into discrete tasks and assigned to the appropriate caregivers, (i.e., RNs, LPNs, or unlicensed assistive personnel [UAP]) (Sullivan & Decker, 1997). Functional nursing used personnel efficiently; however, it fragmented the delivery of care to patients. Moreover, functional nursing did not allow for continuous, comprehensive, patient-centered care (Cohen & Cesta, 1997). For example, in functional nursing, one nurse might give all patients on a unit their medications and one unlicensed person might bathe a certain number of patients.

Team nursing, implemented in the 1950s, was a practical response to the RN shortage and the need to use ancillary health care personnel (Lee, 1993). In team nursing, nursing personnel were divided into teams that were responsible for providing care to groups of patients (Sullivan & Decker, 1997); nursing actions were delineated in nursing care plans, which began on admission and included plans for discharge. The nursing care plan soon became an evaluative measure for nursing practice and a tool for nursing education. Although the nurse's responsibility for patient outcomes was clearly specified in the team method, the focus on complex pro-

---

B O X   1 8 - 1

Public Health Principles: A Basis for Managing Care

- Coordination of community services
- Continuity of care across episodes and settings
- Health promotion and disease prevention

B O X   1 8 - 2

Method of Nursing Care Practice

Evolving Methods of Nursing Care Practice: From "Beyond-the-Walls" to "Within-the-Walls" and Back Again

Late 1800s	Public health and visiting nursing to provide home care
Late 1800s to early 1900s	Case method or private duty nursing
Late 1800s to 1950	Functional nursing
1950s to early 1970s	Team nursing
1970s to 1980s	Primary care nursing
1985 to present	Nursing case management

Data from Bartling, A. (1995). *Healthcare Executive, 10*(2), 7-11; Flarey, D.L., & Blancett, S.S. (1996). Case management: Delivering care in the age of managed care. In D.L. Flarey & S.S. Blancett (Eds.). *Handbook of nursing care management: Health care in a world of managed care.* Gaithersburg, Md: Aspen.

cesses and roles and the lack of fit with existing practice systems limited its effectiveness (Cohen & Cesta, 1997).

Primary nursing started in the 1970s in an effort to revive the patient-centered approach to care. Patients were consistently cared for by one primary nurse and one or more associate nurses (Lee, 1993). Primary nursing also used nursing care plans. This method promoted a more systematic approach to accountability, autonomy, and continuity of care than the earlier practice modalities of case method, functional nursing, and team nursing. However, primary nursing required considerable clerical and ancillary health care support structures in order to be effective. Ultimately, given increasing demands on existing health care systems such as budgetary constraints, increasing patient acuity, and pressures to decrease length of stay, nursing administrators found this approach to be both costly and inefficient (Cohen & Cesta, 1997).

Case management was heralded as the new nursing care method of the 1980s. According to Lee (1993, p. 29), ". . . nursing case management identifies a specific nurse to be accountable for clinical outcomes of designated patients." In this system, improved clinical and financial outcomes are the direct result of ". . . skillful application of the nursing process, timely referrals, and careful coordination."

This overview of nursing practice models, both "beyond the walls" and "within the walls" of hospitals, reveals that traditional nursing care principles and practices form a flexible basis for the evolution of strategies for managing care. From this perspective, the contention that nursing care management is a "new" nursing practice modality is debatable. What is more important is to recognize that nursing care must respond to demands for better management of care, better use of resources, and improved quality and continuity of care. The next section reviews the broad context of forces and trends driving change in the health care system and systems of managing nursing care.

Understanding the Basics: Managed Care and Managed Health Systems

As discussed in Chapters 2, 9, and 11, there is general agreement among health care consumers, providers, and policy makers that health care delivery in the United States is in the throes of a major transformation. Forecasters of health care system change suggest that we are on the path toward a revolutionary system of *managed health* (Conrad & Shortell, 1997; Shortell et al., 1995) (Figure 18-1).

The term *managed care* has several accepted uses and meanings. *Managed care* is often used to describe restructured health care organiza-

Key terms	
Term	**Definition**
Managed health	Conception of health care directed toward health promotion, disease prevention, and health maintenance of customers and populations across the full continuum of care (Conrad & Shortell, 1997)
Integrated health system	A health system organized around clinical, financial, and management processes to serve the multiple needs of populations and communities; patients receive the *right care*, at the *right time*, by the *right provider*, in the *right place*, at the *right price* (Conrad & Shortell, 1997)

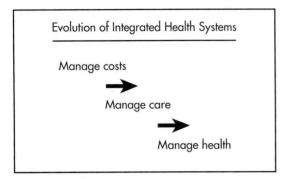

Figure 18-1 ■ Evolution of integrated health systems.

tions, such as HMOs, which were designed to control costs on behalf of purchasers of care by employing measures including insurance benefit limitations or exclusions, prepaid health plans, prospective payment methods, and/or fee schedules (Williams & Torrens, 1993). *Managed care,* or *managed health care,* as it is sometimes called, has also come to represent a broad system-oriented approach that attempts to control costs, assure quality, and improve access to health care (Powell, 1996). However, the dominant characteristic of managed care is the use of financial incentives and management controls designed to direct patients to efficient providers of appropriate care in cost-effective treatment settings (Lee, 1993). Managed care in the 1990s is viewed as a prescription to cure the ills of ". . . waste and expanding, expensive technology" in the health care system (Powell, 1996, p. 3).

Managed health is a futuristic conception of health care in integrated health systems that ". . . are learning to move from managing costs to managing care to managing health" (Conrad & Shortell, 1997, p. 36). *Managed health* is directed toward health promotion, disease prevention, and health maintenance of customers and populations across the full continuum of care (Conrad & Shortell, 1997) and is easily transferable to the practice of care man-

agement. In reality, this conception of integrated health systems is one that requires a revitalized partnership between the public and private sectors of the American health care enterprise (Baker et al., 1994). The core functions of public health, assessment, policy development, and assurance have historically been directed toward the public health mission to protect the health of the entire community. Unfortunately, ". . . vitality of the public health system has been undermined in the last two decades by escalating pressures on state and local governments to provide medical care for the poor and underinsured" (Baker et al., 1994, p. 16). At its core, public health is a population-based practice, which uses the science of epidemiology and the philosophic principles of social justice in applying scientific knowledge to improve the health of the public. Successful transformation of health care delivery from a medical model to a health system depends on the integration of the guiding principles of public health with evolving financial and clinical management systems.

As discussed in Chapters 2, 9, and 11, the transformation of the American health care enterprise is being shaped by several major structural and process-oriented trends (Bartling, 1995; Flarey & Blancett, 1996). (Box 18-3). The success of ventures directed toward managing health will depend on the integration of hospitals and public/private sector health care providers into networks of organized, community-oriented health care and social service delivery systems. The ultimate goal is to establish an entire continuum of care from health promotion to hospice care and to maximize effective outcomes across episodes of illness and pathways to wellness (Shortell et al., 1995). According to Conrad and Shortell (1997, p. 3), the maximum potential of integrated health systems would be realized only when these systems accept ". . . explicit accountability for meeting the needs of their local communities. The tran-

Major Trends in the American Health Care Enterprise

Capitation	A fixed amount of reimbursement per enrollee (per month or per year), received by providers regardless of the services provided
Carve-outs	Subcontracting for health care services, which fosters entrepreneurial opportunities for nurses as independent care managers
Insurance company ownership	Increasing ownership of managed care networks or provider groups by insurance entities (also more hospital- or physician-owned groups)
Increased decentralization	Increased efforts to move closer to patients through outreach and community-based services
Management information systems	Complex, comprehensive data bases to ensure controlled, efficient use and reporting of services
Medicare/Medicaid increases	Many states and the federal government are requiring managed care networks for their respective Medicaid or Medicare recipients
Physician control	Managed care gatekeepers; commitment and leadership by physician and nurse providers are essential to success

From: Bartling, A. (1995). Trends in managed care. *Healthcare Executive, 10*(2), 7-11; Flarey, D.L., & Blancett, S.S. (1996). Case management. Delivering care in the age of managed care. In D.L. Flarey & S.S. Blancett (Eds.). *Handbook of nursing care management: Health care in a world of managed care.* Gaithersburg, Md.: Aspen.

sition from 'covered lives' to accountability for the community population is crucial."

Disease prevention, health promotion, and accountability for meeting the needs of the community are not new models of care for professional nurses. These are essential concepts in baccalaureate and master's level nursing curricula (AACN, 1995; ACHNE, 1992). The Pew Health Professions Commission (1993) has reinforced the overarching importance of knowledge and skill in the areas of health promotion and community- or population-oriented care for all health care practitioners. Nurses have the skills and are positioned to take a leadership role in managed health systems.

In summary, nurses need to understand the historical development of models of nursing practice and the economic, political, and social forces driving the transformation of health

systems. In addition, they need to recognize the values and goals shared by professional nursing and their colleagues in other disciplines that have shaped the past, present, and future models of managed costs, managed care, and managed health. In the next section, the process of care management is described and critically examined. Knowledge of both the context and process of care management provides a strong foundation for further examination of nursing roles in systems of managing care.

■ THE PROCESS OF CARE MANAGEMENT

The role of care manager, a relatively new role in the health care delivery system, is described by Powell (1996, p. 309) as, ". . .in its adolescence, complete with identity crisis, and a growing, awkward form." As with all other roles for advanced practice nursing (e.g., clinical nurse specialist, nurse practitioner), the care manager role is complex and fraught with ambiguity. Like other advanced practice roles, nurse care managers need to have extensive knowledge about the role itself and clinical expertise relevant to the patient population to be served. (Note that, as above, the term *care manager* is used as a broader term encompassing key elements of nursing, whereas the term *case manager* is used to accurately reflect the literature cited.)

In recent years, numerous clinicians, nursing leaders, and educators have sought to define the role of care manager or case manager. The American Nurses Association issued a publication in 1988, updated in 1992, in which case management was described as a "paradoxically simple, yet complex concept" (Bower, 1992, p. 3). The ANA document presented case management as having a fundamental focus on integrating, coordinating, and advocating "for individuals, families and groups requiring extensive services" (Bower, 1992, p. 3).

Another helpful definition for nurse case managers is found in the *Standards of Practice for Case Management* (1995), published by the Case Management Society of America. This defi-

nition, which is not limited to the discipline of nursing, defines case management as follows (CMSA, 1995, p. 8):

> Case management is the collaborative process which assesses, plans, implements, coordinates, monitors and evaluates options and services to meet an individual's health needs through communication and available resources to promote quality cost effective outcomes.

Although these two definitions by the ANA and CMSA are often cited as the "official definitions" of case management, the following is a more comprehensive definition (Bower & Falk, 1996, p. 164):

> Case management is a clinical system that focuses on the accountability of an individual or group for coordinating a patient's care (or group of patients) across an *episode or continuum* of care; ensuring and facilitating the achievement of quality, clinical and financial outcomes; *negotiating, procuring, and coordinating services and resources needed by the patient and family;* intervening at key points (or significant variances from the anticipated plan of care) for individual patients; addressing and resolving consistent issues that have negative quality or cost impact; and creating opportunities and systems to enhance outcomes.

Key terms	
Term	**Definition**
Care management process	A systematic process expanding on the nursing process across episodes of illness and across multiple settings; the steps include case finding and screening, comprehensive assessment, interdisciplinary diagnosis and planning, outcome projection, implementation, planning for resource allocation, final evaluation, and follow-up
Advanced practice nursing	Nursing that is characterized as: "specialized, in terms of focus and population served; expanded, in terms of knowledge and skills; complex, in terms of clinical challenges and clinical judgment; and independent, in terms of decision-making" (Styles, 1996)

Upon reflection, there is a clear relationship between each of these definitions and the nursing process taught to all nurses as a foundation for clinical decision making. In fact, Bower (1992) notes that case management can be viewed as a process that expands on the nursing process, adding a broader view across an episode of illness and across multiple settings. Although clearly there are links to the generic nursing process, there are also differences that reveal the new skills needed by advanced practice nurse care managers (Cary, 1996; Birmingham, 1996). Within these differences lies the key to understanding the new role and becoming a skillful manager of care. An overview of the case management process is shown in Box 18-4. A description of each of the components of the case management process follows, with particular emphasis on its differences from the generic nursing process and new skills to be added by the nurse care manager.

Case Finding, Screening, and Assessment

The assessment component of the care management process has several subcomponents, each specifically focused. Assessment includes broad-based processes of analyzing an entire population of potential patients and focusing on those for whom intervention by health care professionals is needed. For the community health nurse this is a familiar approach, but for those advanced practice nurses, who are more oriented to care of individuals and groups in the acute care setting for short episodes, the broader analysis of a population will require adding new knowledge and skills. The population of interest may be a group of patients (and their families) undergoing a surgical procedure, or it may be the population of all patients living in a particular region who come to a medical center for treatment of acute and chronic illness. Knowledge of epidemiology and skill in gathering and analyzing data to identify health care needs of the population are essential to the case manager responsible for planning a comprehensive program of care for any population group. In addition, the case manager should be involved in developing links with the target population to enhance case finding.

It has been said that everyone deserves to have his or her care well managed, but not everyone needs a case manager. A well-designed screening process will identify target groups who need differing levels of intensity of care. Selecting those target groups who need care managers is a crucial step toward enhancing quality and appropriate use of resources. Target

BOX 1 8 - 4

Comparison of the Nursing Process and Case Management Process

Nursing Process	Care Management Process
Assessment	Case finding, screening, and assessment
Diagnosis	Interdisciplinary diagnosis
Planning	Planning and outcome projection
Implementation	Implementation, service planning, and resource allocation
Evaluation	Final evaluation and follow-up
Documentation and data collection	Documentation for clinical records, utilization management, and outcomes

groups who often need care managers include the following:

- Those with frequent or recent hospital admissions
- The elderly
- Those who live alone
- Those who have limited finances
- Those who have a high-need medical diagnosis or DRG (diagnostic-related group)
- Substance abusers
- Those who have complex chronic illnesses, mental illness, or dementia
- Those who are unable to follow a prescribed regimen

This list will not surprise advanced practice nurses who have experience dealing with patients with complex care needs. However, these examples also demonstrate the need for case managers to have a biopsychosocial approach and extensive knowledge and skill in all aspects of health care.

One example of a well-developed screening tool that may be used within a target group is "PraPlus" (Pacala & Boult, 1997), a screening tool for older populations, recommended by the HMO Workgroup on Chronic Care (1996). The tool is a 17-question screening device intended for use by managed care providers of Medicare populations. The tool has been tested for predictive validity and has been shown to distinguish accurately between elderly individuals at high or low risk for health problems. Trained interviewers can use such a tool to screen those who need to be seen by a care manager for more thorough health assessment, thus enhancing the efficiency of the system and the rapid referral of those with existing or potential problems.

Once an individual and family have been identified as needing a care manager, a comprehensive and focused assessment is necessary. As with all nursing assessment, the initial data collection will depend on the status of the patient and his or her environment. The assessment must be thorough and accurate, thoughtful and concise. Powell (1996, p. 242) describes the case manager assessment as the "critical pivot around which the nursing case management revolves." Typically, the case manager collects information about health and medical history and current medical status that may direct the clinician to use an established clinical pathway, protocol, or other guidelines, such as Miliman and Robertson Healthcare Management Guidelines (Powell, 1996). Central to the process is determining the patient's health goals and self-care capabilities. Information about demographic factors, health care coverage, and financial status is also needed to guide care decisions.

In summary, the first phase of the care management process requires a well-designed and comprehensive set of steps that will accurately screen individuals into groups according to levels of service needed so that appropriate service is offered. Those at high risk for health problems are identified as candidates for care management and subsequently receive intervention at the earliest possible point.

Interdisciplinary Diagnosis

Diagnosis within the care management process is a combination of medical and nursing diagnoses within an interdisciplinary team context. Although various providers from many disciplines work together to deliver care, each is individually accountable to patients and families. Legal regulations (e.g., state practice acts) and ethical standards (e.g., the American Nurses Association Code for Nursing [1985]) maintain individual accountability for each health professional to identify and address patient problems or diagnoses. In the current systems of care, patients are grouped most often by the medical diagnoses (e.g., diabetes, fractured hip), yet nursing diagnoses capture a large percentage of what constitutes patient care and thus benefits the entire team because of the broad focus on physiologic, functional, and psychosocial needs (Maas, 1997). Computer software packages incorporate the medical diagnostic categories (i.e., DRGs, ICD-9, DSM-IV). Similarly, software programs are available that contain listings and background information about the nursing diagnosis categories, such as those developed by the North American Nursing Diagnosis Association (NANDA) and the Omaha Classification System/Problem List (Martin & Scheet, 1992). Box 18-5 contains a brief summary of the two diagnostic classification systems for nursing.

A computer software package with both medical and nursing diagnostic categories al-

lows all members of the health care team to record specific and precise patient problems to be addressed. Patients often have coexisting medical diagnoses (e.g., chronic obstructive pulmonary disease) and nursing diagnoses (e.g., sleep pattern disturbance). Tracking both types of problems results in better quality care for patients and families and better data collection for analysis of the patient population.

Finally, it should be noted that multidisciplinary diagnosis in the care management process also results in identifying problem areas that are *not* addressed by the nurse or other members of the health care team. It is important that explicit decisions include recognition of the autonomy of the patient and family in the identification of problems and who will be primarily responsible in each area of care.

Planning and Outcome Projection

As in other aspects of the nursing process, planning within the care management process presumes well-developed clinical decision-making skills that allow the care manager to prioritize problems and anticipate the probable trajectory of recovery to deal with both immediate and long-term needs of patients and families. Cary (1996) emphasizes the need to validate and prioritize problems with the recipients of care and other members of the health care team. At the earliest possible point, care managers identify options with patients and families to help them make choices consistent with their values and life goals. Care managers often use "tools" in the planning of care, such as clinical pathways, protocols, or generic plans of care, which can be individualized to each patient. Guidelines may include national clinical guidelines such as those published by the Agency for Health Care Policy and Research (AHCPR), or agency clinical protocols, and standards of care from national or agency sources. Individually tailored guidelines should include specific actions to be taken by

---

B O X   1 8 - 5

Classification Systems for Nursing Diagnoses

NANDA (North American Nursing Diagnosis Association)

Defines nursing diagnosis as "a clinical judgment about individual, family, or community responses to actual or potential health problems/life processes. Nursing diagnosis provides the basis for selection of nursing interventions to achieve outcomes for which the nurse is accountable."*

Consists of 138 categories of diagnoses, organized by human response patterns.

Omaha Classification System/Problem List

A taxonomy of 44 problems commonly encountered by home care nurses. Consists of four domains: environmental, psychosocial, physiological and health-related behaviors. Knowledge, behavior and status are scored on a 5-point ordinal scale.†

---

*From Carpentino, L.J. (1997). *Nursing diagnosis: Applications to clinical practice* (p. 4). Philadelphia: Lippincott.
†From Martin, K., & Scheet, N. (1992). *The Omaha system: Applications for community health nursing.* Philadelphia: Saunders.

the patient and family as well as by health care providers, creating a "contract" for care that is understood by all parties. The care manager must often use a creative and flexible approach to design the best plan for each individual patient to achieve the best quality and most cost-effective care. This is the "art" of case management. Powell (1996) notes that the ultimate gift given by the case manager is a plan that promotes optimal self-care and control over one's life.

Projecting outcomes is a new skill for many advanced practice nurses and a crucial aspect of developing effective care management. Flarey and Blancett (1996, p. 9) state the following:

> To be effective, all case management systems must be outcome driven. They must be designed to move the patient through the process of care delivery toward the attainment of defined outcomes. Outcomes must be clearly defined and measurable.

The delineation of *appropriate* outcomes is one of the most challenging areas of nursing and, indeed, of the health care system as a whole.

In the past, outcomes that were automatically collected within the system of care included only disease types (according to ICD categories), number of other medical problems (i.e., comorbidities), and the results of treatment (e.g., the number of recoveries for surgical procedures or deaths). As managed care has revolutionized the health care system, other outcomes have gained importance, including costs of care, functional level, and patient satisfaction. Increasingly, managed care organizations are realizing that the kinds of outcomes that provide the best information include such factors as functional level, self-care capabilities, and health perception (Flarey & Blancett, 1996). Outcomes such as these are precisely the kind that nurses have focused on from the beginning of the profession. Research that emerged from the Medical Outcomes Trust, including the well-known tool entitled Medical Outcomes Study Short-Form 36 (SF-36) (Ware & Sherbourne, 1992), exemplifies an increasing awareness of the need for outcomes that reflect overall health status and functioning rather than outcomes of diseases or mortality levels.

Of increasing importance are developments in determining which outcomes are relevant to which populations of patients. Outcomes for the health care system as a whole as well as for nursing practice can be categorized in several ways. Flarey and Blancett (1996) provide a comprehensive list of categories (Box 18-6). This list includes outcomes that could be characterized as both macrolevel and microlevel outcomes. Macrolevel outcomes are those that address many of the larger system aspects and goals that are desirable for society as a whole. Examples of macrolevel outcomes shown in Box 18-6 are cost effectiveness, social responsiveness, and collaboration. Microlevel outcomes are those that are typically at the clinical level. Examples of microlevel outcomes shown in Box 18-6 are improvement in health status, patient knowledge, psychologic equilibrium, responsibility, prevention, provider knowledge, and death with dignity.

Another way of classifying outcomes on a clinical or microlevel is the Nursing Outcome Classification (NOC) system, developed by the Iowa Outcomes Project (Johnson & Maas, 1997). This list of outcomes is particularly "nurse-sensitive," although the developers emphasize that it may also describe outcomes of care by other providers. The current list of 190 outcomes includes taxonomy and Likert-type scales for each outcome to allow for precision in measuring and documenting outcomes. Examples from the NOC include Immune Status (scaled from #1, "extremely compromised," to #5, "not compromised"); Mobility Level (scaled

Macrolevel and Microlevel Outcomes

Outcomes for Case Management

Cost effectiveness

The case management model is a cost-effective vehicle for the delivery of health care services. Costs are controlled, spending is reduced, and quality care is provided in a capitated reimbursement system.

Improvement in health status

Patients leave the case management system in a healthier state than in which they entered, or the patient with a chronic disease process leaves the system with the knowledge, resources, and support needed to care for himself or herself.

Social responsiveness

The entire community becomes involved in the care of the patient receiving services through case management. Community resources are used and maximized for the benefit of the patient and family. Community agencies participate in the overall care of the patient.

Patient knowledge

Patients and families leave the case management system with a good working knowledge of the disease process and health care needs and the strategies and interventions needed to maintain health and prevent relapse.

Collaboration

The case management system facilitates total collaboration in the care of populations. All disciplines are intricately involved in the delivery of services, and each discipline supports the others in the quest for the delivery of quality cost-effective care.

Psychologic equilibrium

Patients, families, and care givers experience a sense of psychologic well-being after experiencing health care delivery through case management. There is acceptance of the disease state and the plan of care.

Responsibility

Patients emerge from the case management system with a good sense of responsibility for their overall health and life-style. Patients accept and participate in fiscal responsibility for their care.

Prevention

Patients have a greater sense of the need for preventive health care practices and begin to incorporate prevention into their daily living. This prevention practice results in healthier people and communities.

Provider knowledge

Everyone involved with the case management system becomes knowledgeable of the system's potential and effectiveness. Research of goals and outcomes provides the knowledge needed to redesign the system toward greater efficiency and effectiveness.

Death with dignity

Patients in the case management system with life-threatening, incurable disease receive full multidisciplinary support and experience death with dignity.

Modified from Flarey, D.L., & Blancett, S.S. (1996). Case management: Delivering care in the age of managed care. In D.L. Flarey & S.S. Blancett (Eds.). *Handbook of nursing case management: Health care in a world of managed care.* Gaithersburg, Md: Aspen.

from #1, "dependent, does not participate," to #5, "completely independent"); Social Support (scaled from #1, "none," to #5, "extensive" (Johnson & Maas, 1997). These are but a few examples of the nearly 200 outcomes developed through an extensive team research effort to name specific outcomes of patient care. These outcomes provide a way to measure the results of care, particularly the kind of care provided by nurses and by physical or occupational therapists. The NOC is easily computerized through brief phrases and an established coding system. Of particular value is the measurement scale (from 1 to 5) provided for each of the outcomes, which makes quantification and more sensitive measurement possible when tracking outcomes of care that change over time. Such a concise outcome list also makes it possible to examine links between diagnoses, interventions, and outcomes. Linking outcomes with other aspects of the case management process is a crucial step in measuring the success of case management for individual patients, for populations of patients, and for the health care system as a whole.

In summary, the phase of planning and projecting outcomes requires extensive clinical knowledge and the use of specific clinical guidelines tailored to the individual patient. The ability to project outcomes is enhanced by the use of outcomes at both the macrolevel, or system level, and the microlevel, or clinical level. Outcome classification systems, such as the Nursing Outcome Classification (NOC), are useful in selecting nurse-sensitive outcomes, particularly at the clinical level.

Implementation, Service Planning, and Resource Allocation

Once all parties agree on the goals and the plan for a particular patient, the care manager is then responsible for ensuring that the best care is provided using appropriate and cost-effective resources. Depending on the setting in which

the care manager works, aspects of this phase may require providing direct care or directing others in care giving. Both direct and indirect nursing care can be described and documented effectively and efficiently by the use of the Nursing Intervention Classification (NIC) system developed by the Iowa Intervention Project (McCloskey & Bulechek, 1996). Box 18-7 summarizes the NIC.

Examples of direct care for a person with heart failure could include interventions listed in NIC such as Fluid/Electrolyte Management or Teaching Prescribed Medication. In the acute care setting the care manager often works closely with direct care providers during the acute phase of (for example) heart failure. In outpatient or home care situations, nursing interventions selected from NIC might include examples such as Teaching Prescribed Activity/ Exercise, or Health System Guidance. An advantage of using the NIC system in documentation is that it provides standard language that is recognized nationally and easily computerized, using the coding system already devel-

---

B O X   1 8 - 7

Classification System for Nursing Interventions (NIC)

Definition of nursing intervention: "any treatment based upon clinical judgment and knowledge, that a nurse performs to enhance patient/client outcomes" (p. xvii).
NIC consists of 433 interventions organized by:
• Six domains
• Classes
• [Interventions]
• Nursing activities
• References

From McCloskey, J., & Bulechek, G. (Eds.). (1996). Nursing interventions classification (NIC) (2nd ed.). St. Louis: Mosby.

oped. Case managers can thus collect data about common needs and approaches to care for groups or populations of patients, while documenting care of individuals using the NIC system. The computerized system that allows ease of individual documentation must also allow care managers to aggregate data for analysis and reports.

Care managers are often responsible for negotiating and coordinating a variety of services and costs for their patients. This task requires the nurse to be well informed about financial systems and resources in the community at large—from the local to the national level. To accomplish this component of the care management process, care managers must be "system savvy" at many different levels and able to collect information from many different sources, including written, computerized, and oral. Multiple nursing interventions described in the NIC taxonomy address elements of this process in the domain of the health system, defined as providing "care that supports effective use of the health care delivery system" (McCloskey & Bulechek, 1996, p. 68). Examples of the many interventions within this domain are cultural brokerage, patient rights protection, staff supervision, multidisciplinary care conference, and telephone consultation. Once again, these categories of nursing interventions are well described, clearly defined and labeled, and easily coded into part of the database for documentation and analysis.

The implementation phase of care management requires continuous, appropriately timed monitoring and collecting of data to ascertain that the plan is going well. Skillful care managers always have a Plan A and a Plan B at their fingertips to deal with the inevitable and unpredictable problems that occur in everyday life. For example, a patient with a "simple" joint replacement surgery may do extremely well postoperatively but suddenly is unable to return home as previously planned because his or her spouse develops an acute illness. In this situation, Plan B would mean having good relationships within the network of care centers and the ability to work with subacute facilities where the patient may begin rehabilitation in a more appropriate and less costly setting.

The implementation phase is another period during which clinicians typically use protocols and clinical pathways to guide expectations about how a patient with a given health condition should progress according to the activities and time frame prescribed. Progress that differs from expectations is a *variance* and must be addressed. Variance may have a number of causes. The following are some examples:

- Environment or setting (e.g., special diagnostic test not readily available)
- Caregivers or family (e.g., caregiver not able to help patient to irrigate his or her colostomy)
- Patient (e.g., developed a fever postoperatively that slowed progress)
- Community (e.g., no rehabilitation center available for person needing care)

Although categories of variance are diverse (Frink & Strassner, 1996), it is appropriate that they be tailored to the situation so that the care manager may collect useful data about factors that may inhibit best quality and cost-effective care.

In summary, the implementation phase of the care management process is one in which the care is delivered, balancing the goal of quality care with the services and resources available. The Nursing Intervention Classification (NIC) provides a taxonomy and description of interventions or specific therapies often delivered by nurses, and is useful in describing and documenting care. Care managers need to have a foundation of expert clinical knowledge on which to base decisions and to have extensive knowledge of resources to match patient needs to appropriate services.

Key terms	
Term	**Definition**
Documentation	Written record of key information demonstrating nursing data collected, actions taken, and results; information from the patient record that provides legal information and data for researcher and/or reports
Variance	Deviations from normal quality care; anything that is not attained within the predetermined timeframe for the care plan (Tahan & Cesta, 1996).

Final Evaluation and Follow-Up

In the final phase of the care management process, the evaluation and follow-up depend very much on the setting and the role of the care manager. Increasingly, care managers are able to follow patients and families outside of traditional boundaries of the hospital or ambulatory care setting to enhance the continuity and comprehensiveness of care. Care managers in the acute care setting follow patients through a particular episode of care, for example from the preoperative stage of joint replacement surgery to the final recovery and return to routine function. Care managers who work with patients with complex chronic illnesses such as renal failure may follow them across inpatient and outpatient settings until they change providers, leave the region, or die. Other care managers in community-based settings, such as nurse-run clinics in public housing, may follow patients and families across the life span, focusing not only on daily health needs, but also on larger community level needs to address complex financial and psychosocial problems.

Elements of the evaluation and follow-up phase include comparing projected outcomes with actual outcomes of care, examining the patients' needs against services provided, comparing projected and actual costs, and analyzing the satisfaction of everyone in the system of care—patient, family, caregivers, and payers (Powell, 1996; Cary, 1996).

Documentation and Data Collection

Although documentation and collection of data occur throughout the case management process, this aspect is listed here as a separate step to call attention to its importance. Throughout all phases of the process, the care manager is recording information for several purposes. The most fundamental and essential purpose for written documentation is to enhance accurate and continuous clinical care by documenting problem areas, therapeutic approaches, and results of care. As described above, there are now well-developed taxonomies for nursing diagnoses, interventions, and outcomes that are useful in providing the standardized language for documentation of patient care.

A second purpose for documentation within the care management process is to promote accurate collection of data, which can be combined and analyzed. (See Key Terms above.) Aggregated data are useful at many levels—for clinicians, administrators, and health policy decision-makers. Continuous quality management requires accurate data to identify areas for improvement. Increasingly, health care organizations and systems are required to collect standardized sets of data for accreditation and reporting to governing bodies. Reports of this kind are referred to as *report cards,* or *panel reports* and are the basis for setting national standards or benchmarks for quality care (Flarey & Blancett, 1996). Here again, standardized nomenclature and taxonomies are essential because the most useful analyses are produced when similar language is used to describe similar phenomena across agency, system, national, and even global boundaries.

A crucial new skill for many care managers in all phases of the care management process is that of computer literacy. Care managers must be able to use computers to efficiently document data from individual patients at the point of service delivery. The computer system must enhance analysis of data about the entire group of patients to be managed. In this realm, care managers must be involved in selecting computer hardware (e.g., laptop style, which enables collection of data at the bedside, whether inpatient or outpatient settings, across the continuum) and software that promotes efficient collection of relevant data for quality care. Computerized systems are needed that allow for analysis across the street and around the world to enhance knowledge for care management. This remains one of the areas most in need of development if health care is to become seamless for individual recipients and manageable for care providers seeking access to crucial information.

■ KNOWLEDGE AND SKILLS NEEDED BY CARE MANAGERS

The above descriptions of the care manager role and the process of care management reveal the extensive demands placed on care managers in the current system of care delivery. It should be noted that advanced practice nurses make ideal care managers because their education and experience provide both high-level clinical knowledge and leadership ability. Connors (1993) examined the literature regarding the subcomponents and competencies of the case manager, and concluded that master's prepared nurses are ideally suited to fill these complex roles. More recently, Mahn and Spross (1996)

analyzed competencies of advanced practice nurses (APNs) and found a clear linkage between nursing case management functions and the knowledge and skill of APNs. The major limitation in having sufficient APN care managers has been the lack of availability and inappropriate use of advanced practice nurses in such roles. Flarey & Blancett (1996, p. 13) predict that advanced practice nurses will increasingly move into case manager roles because their quality and cost effectiveness have been documented and because the public accepts and welcomes them.

As with any role, individuals who become care managers will enter the role with varied levels of clinical and leadership expertise. Research on the development of expertise by nurses has clearly shown that education, mentoring, and experience contribute to development over time from novice to expert functioning (Benner et al., 1996). To prepare for the complex and demanding role of care manager, nurses should seek education through formal and informal mechanisms (e.g., degree programs and continuing education), mentoring, and experience with the clinical population to be served. Networking through organized groups of advanced practice nurses and case management specialists will enhance the ongoing development of knowledge and abilities for the role.

■ CONCLUSION

The *promise* of managed care is that the system will shift from simply reacting to individual episodes of illness to proactive planning of comprehensive health promotion programs that prevent late-stage, costly care as it is now typically delivered. As yet, this is an unrealized promise because of turbulence in the health care delivery system and the lack of effectively managed care for large segments of the population. Nurses can help to create a system more attuned to health promotion by developing the skills of care management and by applying them in the great variety of settings in which nurses are found. Lee (1993, p. 21) reminded us of the historic significance of "knowing how to manage care" by pointing out the words of Nightingale from *Notes on Nursing:* "All the results of good nursing . . . may be spoiled . . . by one defect, by not knowing how to manage what you do when you are there, [and by not knowing how to manage what] shall be done when you are not there"(1860, 1969, p. 35).

■ KEY POINTS

- Historically, nurses, particularly in public health, have been care managers focusing on health promotion across communities.
- Nurses can help to move managed care systems from simply *managing costs* to *managing health.*
- The care management process adds new elements to the nursing process and requires new skills for an evolving variety of roles.
- The pervasive demand for documentation of both individual care and population data requires nurses to use standardized nursing language and computerized documentation systems.
- To prepare for the complex and demanding roles of care managers, nurses need a foundation of clinical knowledge, advanced education, and skills for life-long learning.

■ CRITICAL THINKING QUESTIONS

1. Compare and contrast the current goals of managed care to the goals of public health, both past and present.
2. Analyze similarities and differences of the current model of delivering patient care using both nurses and patient care assistants in comparison to previous models such as functional nursing and team nursing.
3. Describe the role of a care manager in one or all of the following settings: acute care hospital, rehabilitation setting, insurance company, health maintenance organization, community mental health clinic, home health agency, community-based nursing clinic.
4. What are the advantages and disadvantages of using standardized nursing language to document nursing care?
5. Given the reality of "for profit" health care in the United States, what are some ethical problems that arise for nurses?
6. If you could design an ideal "integrated health system," what would it look like? What would the components be, and how would they work together?

■ REFERENCES

American Association of Colleges of Nursing (AACN). (1995). *The essentials of master's education for advanced practice nursing.* In Report from the Task Force on Essentials of Master's Education for Advanced Practice Nursing. Washington, D.C.: AACN Publication.

Association of Community Health Nurse Educators (ACHNE). (1992). *Essentials of master's level community health nursing education for advanced practice.* Louisville, Ky.: Author.

American Nurses Association. (1985). *Code for nursing with interpretative statements.* Kansas City, Mo.: American Nurses Association.

Baker, E.L., Melton, R.J., Stange, P.V., Fields, M.L., Koplan, J.P., Guerra, F.A., & Satcher, D. (1994). Health reform and the health of the public: Forging community health partnerships. *Journal of the American Medical Association, 272*(16), 1276-1282.

Bartling, A. (1995). Trends in managed care. *Healthcare Executive, 10*(2), 7-11.

Benner, P., Tanner, C., & Chesla, C. (1996). *Expertise in nursing practice: Caring, clinical judgment and ethics.* New York: Springer.

Birmingham, J. (1996). How to apply CMSA's Standards of Practice for Case Management in a capitated environment. *The Journal of Care Management, 2*(5), 9-22.

Bower, K.A. (1992). *Case management by nurses.* Kansas City, Mo.: American Nurses Publishing Company.

Bower, K.A., & Falk, C.D. (1996). Case management as a response to quality, cost, and access imperatives. In E. Cohen (Ed.). *Nursing case management in the 21ˢᵗ century* (pp. 161-167). St. Louis: Mosby.

Carey, A.H. (1996). Case management. In M. Stanhope & J. Lancaster (Eds.). *Community health nursing* (4th ed.)(pp. 357-374). St. Louis: Mosby.

Carpenito, L.J. (1997). *Nursing diagnosis: Application to clinical practice.* Philadelphia: Lippincott.

Case Management Society of America (CMSA). (1995). *Standards of practice*. Little Rock, Ark.: CMSA.

Cohen, E. (Ed.). (1996). *Nurse case management in the 21st century*. St. Louis: Mosby.

Cohen, E., & Cesta, T.G. (1997). *Nursing case management: From concept to evaluation* (2nd ed.). St. Louis: Mosby.

Conrad, D.A., & Shortell, S.M. (1997). Integrated health systems: Promise and performance. *Frontiers of Health Services Management, 13*(1), 3-40.

Connors, H.R. (1993). Impact of care management modalities on curricula. In K. Kelly & M. Maas. *Series on Nursing Administration: Vol. 5. Managing nursing care*. St. Louis: Mosby.

Davies, G. (1997). *Twenty years of higher education in Virginia*. Unpublished.

Dieckmann, J.L. (1994). Home health administration: An overview. In M.H. Harris (Ed.). *Handbook of home health care administration* (pp. 3-13). Gaithersburg, Md.: Aspen.

Ellwood, P.M. (1988). Outcomes management: A technology of patient experience. *New England Journal of Medicine, 318*(June), 1549-1556.

Flarey, D.L., & Blancett, S.S. (1996). Case management: Delivering care in the age of managed care. In D.L. Flarey & S.S. Blancett (Eds.). *Handbook of nursing case management: Health care in a world of managed care*. Gaithersburg, Md.: Aspen.

Frink, B.B., & Strassner, L. (1996). Variance analysis. In D. Flarey & S. Blancett (Eds.). *Handbook of nursing case management: Health care in a world of managed care* (pp. 194-223). Gaithersburg, MD: Aspen.

Heinrich, J. (1983). Historical perspective on public health nursing. *Nursing Outlook, 31*(6), 317-320.

HMO Workgroup on Care Management. (1996). Chronic care initiatives in HMOs—Identifying high-risk Medicare members: A report from the HMO Workgroup on Care Management. Washington, D.C.: American Association of Health Plans.

HMO Workgroup on Care Management. (1996). *Identifying high-risk Medicare HMO members*. Washington, D.C.: American Association of Health Plans.

Johnson, M., & Maas, M. (Eds.). (1997). *Nursing outcome classification (NOC): Iowa Outcomes Project*. St. Louis: Mosby.

Kelly, K. (1993). Introduction. In K. Kelly (Ed.) & M. Maas (Chair of the Board). Managing nursing care: Promise and pitfalls. *Series on Nursing Administration, 5,* xiv-xv.

Lamb, G.S. (1995). Case management. In J.J. Fitzpatrick & J.S. Stevenson (Eds.). *Annual Review of Nursing Research, 13,* 117-136.

Lancaster, J. (1996). History of community health and community health nursing. In M. Stanhope & J. Lancaster (Eds.). *Community health nursing: Process and practice for promoting health* (4th ed.). St. Louis: Mosby.

Lee, J.L. (1993). A history of care modalities in nursing. In K. Kelly (Ed.) & M. Maas (Chair of the Board). Managing nursing care: Promise and pitfalls. *Series on Nursing Administration, 5,* 20-38.

Maas, M. (1997). Personal communication via electronic mail.

Mahn, V.A., & Spross, J.A. (1996). Nurse case management as an advanced practice role. In A. Hamric, J. Spross, & C. Hanson (Eds.). *Advanced nursing practice: An integrative approach*. Philadelphia: Saunders.

Martin, K., & Scheet, N. (1992). *The Omaha system: Applications for community health nursing*. Philadelphia: Saunders.

McCloskey, J., & Bulechek, G. (Eds.). (1996). *Nursing intervention classification (NIC)* (2nd ed.). St. Louis: Mosby.

Nightingale, F. (1860, 1969, p. 35). *Notes on nursing: What it is and what it is not*. New York: Dover.

Pacala, J.T., & Boult, C. (1997). *PraPlus screening of older populations*. University of Minnesota Medical School: Department of Family Practice and Community Health.

Pew Health Professions Commission. (1993). *Health professions education for the future: Schools in service to the nation—A report of the Pew Health Professions Commission*. San Francisco: Pew Memorial Trust.

Powell, S.K. (1996). *Nursing case management: A practical guide to success in managed care*. Philadelphia: Lippincott-Raven.

Ritter-Teitel, J. (1996). New challenges and opportunities in integrated health care systems. In D.L. Flarey, & S.S. Blancett (Eds.). *Handbook of nursing case management*. Gaithersburg, Md.: Aspen.

Shortell, S.M., Gillies, R.R., & Devers, K.J. (1995). Reinventing the American hospital. *The Milbank Quarterly, 73*(2), 131-160.

Stanhope, M., & Lancaster, J. (1991). Toward a healthy tomorrow. *Family & Community Health Nursing, 14*(1), 1-7.

Styles, M.M. (1996). Conceptualizations of advanced nursing practice. In A. Hamric, J. Spross, & C. Hanson (Eds.). *Advanced nursing practice: An integrative approach* (pp. 24-41). Philadelphia: Saunders.

Sullivan, E.J., & Decker, P.J. (1997). *Effective leadership and management in nursing* (4th ed.). Menlo Park, Calif.: Addison Wesley Longman.

Sullivan, J.A., & Friedman, M. (1984). History of nursing in the community: From the beginning. In J.A. Sullivan (Ed.). *Directions in community health nursing* (pp. 3-43). Boston: Blackwell Scientific Publications.

Tahan, H.A., & Cesta, T.G. (1996). Evaluating the effectiveness of case management plans. In D.L. Flarey & S.S. Blancett. *Handbook of nursing case management* (pp. 184-193). Gaithersburg, Md.: Aspen.

Ware, J.E., & Sherbourne, C.D. (1992). The MOS 36-item short form health survey (SF36). *Medical Care, 30*(6), 473-480.

Williams, S.J., & Torrens, P.R. (1993). *Introduction to health services*. New York: Delmar.

Quality Management in Nursing Practice

P.J. Maddox

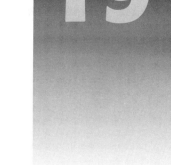

INTRODUCTION

Public expectations and perceptions of health care and health providers are changing. Among health care providers, expectations and perceptions of the health systems are changing as well. Nurses find themselves concerned with decisions about what health care should be provided, by whom, how, and at what cost. Society and the health care industry share concerns about health care access, cost, and quality (McGlynn, 1997). The techniques, tools, and approaches of quality management are useful to health care providers and managers in making tough decisions about reducing costs while managing or improving access and quality. The structured scientific process and quantitative tools used in quality improvement efforts make data-driven decision making a ready asset throughout the organization. The purpose of this chapter is to assist nurses to understand the function and use of data-driven decision making and selected quality management concepts to actively participate in quality improvement projects and serve as consultants and leaders in Total Quality Organizations.

OBJECTIVES

After reading this chapter, you will be able to:

1. Describe the history of the quality management movement and of its use in the health care industry
2. Outline the steps and tools of process improvement
3. Explain customer focus as it relates to quality in health care
4. Analyze quality improvement trends in outcomes assessment and management
5. Explain benchmarking as a quality tool in health care organizations
6. Synthesize factors related to the effectiveness of quality improvement teams

- History and evolution of quality management
- Quality management in health care: sociopolitical context
- Explanation of quality improvement (concepts, principles, and tools)
- Organizational assessment and outcomes management
- Leadership for team-based (quality) organizations

Each section is presented in a question and answer format.

■ HISTORY AND EVOLUTION OF QUALITY MANAGEMENT

Where did the concept of quality management begin?

The concept of quality management evolved in response to developments in management thought. Because managers worried about how to make their organizations better and more profitable, they explored ideas about how man-tions to improve organizational performance. Quality improvement evolved into total quality management as efforts to improve organizational performance were incorporated into management thinking.

Five significant milestones explain the development and use of quality management in industry and in the U.S. health care system. Table 19-1 illustrates these quality management milestones.

What are the developmental milestones that reflect the evolution of quality management and its adoption by the health care industry?

Milestone 1: Postmanufacturing Quality Inspection

The first milestone in the development of quality management is attributed to Frederick Taylor, who introduced the notion of quality in his *theory of scientific management* (Taylor, 1911). Taylor called for managers to plan and direct the activities of workers and to inspect the

---

TABLE 19-1

Milestones in the Evolution of Quality Management

Milestone	Year	Credited Party
I. Postproduction quality inspection	1911	Taylor
II. Use of probability and statistics to use random samples and explain variability	1931	Shewhart
III. Conceptualize/systematize approaches to quality management		
Japanese lecture series	1950	Crosby
Developed organization-wide quality approach	1951	Feigenbaum
Published handbook on quality control	1951	Juran
IV. United States recognition of quality management		
Published best-selling book	1979	Crosby
NBC documentary on quality management "If Japan can do it . . ."	1980	NBC on Deming
V. Adoption of QI/QM in health care		
National demonstration project on quality in health care	1987	Hartford Foundation (21 sites)
JCAHO accreditation standards require CQI	1992	JCAHO

quality of work/goods produced. Concepts of mass production and postmanufacturing quality inspection developed by Taylor were widely adopted by the U.S. manufacturing industry. Ironically, in more recent times, scientific management has been criticized for producing worker alienation in organizations and for failing to integrate quality into the production process (Gehani, 1993).

Milestone 2: Postproduction Sampling

A second milestone in the development of quality management is attributed to Walter A. Shewhart. Shewhart was an employee of Bell Telephone Laboratories, responsible for investigating quality problems. He discovered that the incidence of quality variations could be predicted by using probability and statistics. He and his colleagues developed sampling formulas that enabled them to inspect a small number of production items and *generalize* the results to the *entire* production output (Shewhart, 1931).

Milestone 3: Organization-wide Use of Quality Improvement Methods

The third milestone was a shift in organizational thinking about the focus and scope of quality improvement. This shift changed the focus from checking postproduction product samples for acceptable quality to developing organization-wide processes to ensure that quality is produced the first time. Three individuals are credited with contributions in the development and use of quality control processes and methods organization wide—Deming, Juran, and Feigenbaum. Their independent efforts helped to institutionalize quality improvement methods. A discussion of the unique contributions of each follows.

In 1950 Edward Deming was invited by the Union of Japanese Scientists and Engineers to deliver a series of lectures on *quality improvement meth-*

ods. He later consulted extensively with Japanese Industry in the use of quality improvement methods to improve manufacturing quality and productivity.

In 1951 Joseph Juran also lectured in Japan and published the first comprehensive reference on the use of *scientific quality methods in industry.*

Juran detailed the use of organization-wide quality management methods, including management functions (Juran, 1951). The Juran *Quality Control Handbook* explained methods for the implementation and use of statistical quality tools and techniques through the Juran Trilogy. Updated versions of the reference are widely used today (Juran & Gyrna, 1988). It is important to note that although quality management methods were adopted enthusiastically in Japan after World War II, they were not adopted by industry in the United States until some 20 years later.

Armand Feigenbaum originated the concept of *total quality control* in organizations (Feigenbaum, 1983). While an MIT graduate student, Feigenbaum identified the importance and use of quality control methods on activities throughout the entire organization. Later, he advocated the wide use of quality engineers to ensure that products were planned, developed, and produced in conformance with quality standards

Milestone 4: Adoption of Quality Management in the United States

The fourth set of milestones in the evolution of quality management was its recognition and adoption in the United States. Recognition began in 1979 with the publication of a best-selling management text entitled *Quality Is Free* (Crosby, 1979). The text discussed the impact of quality management in creating superior quality and productivity in Japanese industry. A year later, NBC produced a special documentary program about Deming's influence in Japan entitled "If Japan Can Do It, Why Can't We?" Crosby's text together with the television coverage brought Deming and the use of quality management methods to the attention of U.S. industry.

BOX 19-1

The Quality Gurus' Approaches

Phillip Crosby & Associates	W. Edwards Deming	Juran Institute, Inc
14-Step Quality Improvement Process	**14 Points of Management**	1. Quality trilogy: • Quality planning (meeting customer needs) • Quality control (measurement) • Quality improvement (change) 2. Broad operational/ perspective 3. Focus on external and internal customers expectations, targets 4. Institution-wide planning/ strategy development 5. Employee involvement 6. Group problem solving
1. Management commitment 2. Improvement teams 3. Quality measurement 4. Cost of quality evaluation 5. Quality awareness 6. Corrective action 7. Zero-defects planning committee 8. Supervisory training 9. Zero-defects day 10. Goal setting 11. Error/cause removal 12. Recognition 13. Quality council 14. Do it all over again	1. Constancy of purpose (vision) 2. Adopt new philosophy 3. Cease dependence on inspection 4. Award business contracts on various factors (not just price) 5. Improve continuously 6. On-the-job training 7. Leadership for system improvement 8. Drive out fear 9. Break down department/ program barriers 10. Eliminate arbitrary quotas and slogans without resources 11. Cease numerical quotas 12. Remove barriers to "pride of workmanship" 13. Education for everyone 14. Transforms all jobs and the organization	

Called the *Quality Gurus,* Deming, Juran, and Crosby each embraced a quality approach aimed at developing an *integrated total quality system* in organizations. There are many similarities in how each pursues organization-wide quality (Box 19-1). A summary of the unique features and differences of each guru's approach appears in Box 19-2).

Milestone 5: Adoption of Quality Management in Health Care

The fifth milestone is the adoption of quality management by the health care industry. That adoption was signaled by the National Demonstration Project on Quality Improvement in Health Care (1987) and the Joint Commission on Accreditation of Healthcare Organizations Accreditation Standards Revision (1991).

In 1987 the John Hartford Foundation sponsored the National Demonstration Project on quality improvement in health care. The project involved the pairing of 21 U.S. Health Care Organizations with quality experts from industry, to demonstrate the impact of using quality improvement methods in health care organizations. In 1992, JCAHO changed its accreditation standards, replacing

Quality Management Gurus (Concept Differences)

Definition and Measurement of Quality

Deming: definition of quality deals with predictable uniformity of the product (conformance to standards) that is largely established by use of statistical process control methods. He incorporates customers through the concept of extended process. He calls for deriving the dollar value of concerns such as customer dissatisfaction.

Crosby: definition of quality is based on conformance to customer need-based requirements. He specifies a "zero defects" standard in meeting these set requirements every time. He measures quality by way of costing "unquality."

Juran: defines quality by the fitness of the service for its intended use in meeting customer expectations. His is the most explicitly customer-focused approach to quality. He also calls for incorporating the quantification of "reducing production costs" in delivering service and "increasing revenue."

Management Commitment Differences

Deming: his first and second points (creating a constancy of purpose and adopting the new philosophy) define the tasks of management. Indeed, all of articulated points are aimed at management, implying the necessity for its undivided attention to create a total quality system.

Crosby: within his 14-step process, Point 1 deals explicitly with management commitment. He stresses the importance of communicating understanding and commitment; he is the most focused on creation of a "quality culture."

Juran: as specified in his trilogy, the quality planning, control, and improvement process seeks management support at all levels. A project approach to improvement activities is used that assigns management involvement and responsibility.

Continuous System

Deming: establishes the continuity of the quality system by repeating the 14 steps. He advocates use of the PDCA *(Plan Do Check Act)* cycle to sustain the process.

Crosby: recommends repetition of the cycle of quality planning, control, and improvement.

Juran: use of the trilogy concepts requires continuous assessment and subsequent never-ending organizational response.

Human Resource Capacity

Deming: discusses the training of all employees in his sixth point and the need for retraining to keep pace with changing customer needs in his thirteenth point.

Crosby: his eighth step specifically deals with quality education; however, his emphasis on developing a quality culture also implies a commitment to developing capacity.

Juran: does not explicitly address education or training. It is implicitly contained in the execution of the trilogy, in that knowledge is required by employees on a project-by-project basis to diagnose defects and determine remedies.

Problem Cause Elimination

Deming: uses statistical techniques to identify special causes or chance causes. He identifies variation that falls outside of control limits as special cause variation. Workers are responsible to eliminate these. Variation that falls within control limits (common causes) is the responsibility of management to eliminate.

Juran: differentiates common from special cause, and categorizes error sources. Operator error is categorized as inadvertent, willful, or resulting from improper/inadequate training or improper technique. He provides specifics for achieving the performance standard of zero defects.

Crosby: also uses the zero defects standard. His eleventh step addresses a course of action for error cause removal.

Continued

Quality Management Gurus (Concept Differences)—cont'd

Quality Goals

Deming: advocates the identification of long-term quality goals, the identification of which is built into the PDCA cycle. He believes that numerical goals (i.e., productivity goals) without regard to quality are unacceptable.

Juran: calls for the setting of customer-oriented goals as part of the annual quality improvement plan. He believes goals are important in determining the success of a quality project.

Crosby: advocates the development and use of long- and short-term goals in his tenth quality point.

Organizational Plan for Quality

Deming: the 14-point plan for quality improvement emphasizes using statistical tools at all levels. He sequentially directs the management response as a bottom-up approach.

Juran: emphasizes quality improvement through a project-by-project approach (especially relevant for middle management).

Crosby: uses a top-down approach, emphasizes a change in management culture with development of plans for its transitional management.

---

quality assurance requirements with quality assessment and improvement requirements. This change effectively ensured that U.S. hospitals would adopt continuous quality improvement over quality assurance efforts.

Quality Management and Health Care: Sociopolitical Context

Why is quality management so beneficial to the health care industry?

Four seemingly unrelated factors explain the sociopolitical environment in which health care organizations operate. First, hospital experiences with quality assurance monitoring produced a mindset that a certain number of problems or complications were *expected* and thus *accepted* as part of the health care process. This resulted in a belief that defects (errors and complications) were assumed to be a part of the care delivery process. Patient care errors, infection rates, and mortality rates, for example, were monitored, reported, and analyzed as expected phenomena that might be reduced (not eliminated). From the perspective of defining quality, such a mindset is problematic. Taken literally,

this produces a goal orientation of being "acceptable" or "pretty good," but not "perfect" or "the best."

Second, changes in the financing of health care have profoundly changed the incentives for providing health services in recent years. Before 1984 (when prospective payment by diagnosis-related groups was adopted), providers were reimbursed by the volume of services they provided (do more/get paid more). With prospective payment, financial incentives reward efficiency in the delivery of services (not volume of services delivered). In managing the cost of delivering care to fit fixed reimbursement levels, providers are encouraged to do less and use fewer resources while providing care. To the degree that unnecessary services are being provided and can be reduced, this incentive structure is desirable from a quality perspective. To the degree that important and essential services and resources are not provided and quality is adversely affected, this incentive structure is not desirable.

Third, the American public has high expectations of health care providers and the health care system, believing it to be the best in the world. They expect relatively easy access to health care and hospitals that are equipped with the latest technology and diagnostic and treatment capabilities. The public expects that their health care providers are well educated and actively using the latest battery of vaccines, pharmaceuticals, and medical devices available.

Last, this same public thinks that health care costs too much and is demanding that the health system find ways to contain and reduce costs (do more with less). At the same time, it expects the quality of health care services to stay the same or improve. Although it seems incongruous to many health care providers, our elected officials are demanding that health care professionals and health care organizations find ways to manage health care services at reduced cost while preserving or increasing quality.

So compelling are these concerns and the myriad system reactions and responses to them that countless oversight and monitoring initiatives have been created. Regulatory and accrediting bodies (private and public) have adopted review standards and criteria that reflect concerns about quality of care, given these sociopolitical factors. Currently, the first Presidential Commission on Health Care Quality is studying the state of the health care system and its efforts in providing quality health services in the United States.

The reason quality management is so important to the health care industry is that the goal of quality management is to give organizations the tools and decision methods to deliver quality service in a cost-effective and efficient manner. Quality improvement tools can help providers and managers in exploring options and making the difficult decisions associated with changing the delivery of health care (improving what we do and how we do it). The remainder of this chapter focuses on the use of quality improvement methods in health care organizations. The

necessary (but not easiest) place to begin in understanding how quality management works is with a discussion of *what quality is* and *how it is managed* in health care organizations.

■ QUALITY IMPROVEMENT: CONCEPTS, PRINCIPLES, METHODS, AND TOOLS
Quality Improvement Concepts
What is quality? And how is it managed?

Although we regularly use *quality* as a descriptive term (selectively employing a range of indicators that evidence it), the concept and definition of *quality* remain ambiguous. In fact, lack of a universal definition of *quality* in health care and other industries is perpetuated because of differences in individual perceptions and values about quality. Among those who have wrestled with the issue, it is recognized that quality has to be defined based on the product or service of interest. Harvard researcher David Garvin (1988) describes five types of quality: transcendent, product based, user based, manufacturing based, and value based. The five types of quality are defined in the Key Term box that follows.

Each type of quality can be found in health care, depending on the service or product being considered. Not only are there different types of quality, there are also different perspectives. Quality defined by the recipient of services may be very different from quality defined by the provider of services. Administrative and business services are substantively different from patient care services, as are their delivery processes. Quality is defined, in part, by *what* is being examined, depending on the expectations of providers and recipients. Both providers and recipients of service make determinations about the quality of service they receive through experience and education.

Among health care providers, notions of quality are shaped by discipline-based education and professional organizations that expect conform-

Key terms	
Term	**Definition**
Transcendent quality	Innate excellence; implies that quality is a simple property that cannot be analyzed, but is universally recognized through experience
Product-based quality	A precise and measurable variable; differences are reflected in the quantity of desired attributes of the product or service
User-based quality	Satisfaction of individual consumer preferences (vary with individuals wants and needs)
Manufacturing-based quality	Conformance to design or specifications, i.e., the degree to which the product or service meets established standards
Value-based quality	Performance of the product or service based on expectations of price or cost

ance to standards. The quality focus of professional standards promulgated by licensing and accrediting bodies, such as state boards of nursing and the American Nurses Association, has been concerned predominantly with the qualifications of providers. Professional societies and accrediting bodies have only recently introduced quality standards that focus on the processes and outcomes of service/care delivery (JCAHO, 1996; Warzynski, 1996). A discussion of outcome-based quality assessments appears later in this chapter.

Among providers of health care, our exposure to professional standards and notions of quality have evolved largely from individual professional education, through professional associations, and through work-related experiences associated with quality assurance.

What is the relationship of quality assurance to total quality management? Why are there so many quality management names?

Quality assurance identifies problems to solve them. Continuous quality improvement (CQI) builds upon traditional quality assurance concepts by employing scientific process analysis methods to examine the organization (its work systems and processes) and identify opportunities for improvement (Whetsell, 1991). Total quality management (TQM) is a structured, systematic process for organizational planning and implementation of continuous quality improvement.

The most widely recognized framework for quality assurance (the Quality Tripod) identifies the parameters of health care quality as structure, process, and outcome (Donabedian, 1986). Within a quality assurance approach to ensuring quality, health professionals make determinations about quality being achieved (or not) based on the degree to which providers have the necessary knowledge and skills for giving care (are qualified); whether the processes of care employed the appropriate therapeutic procedures (the right stuff was done at the right time); and whether the expected results or goals of care were reached.

One of the many criticisms of quality assurance is that it focuses too much on the structure and process of health service delivery and not enough on its outcomes. Donabedian contends that structure, process, and outcome are inextricably linked to quality, with no one factor superior to the other (Donabedian, 1994). The impact and limitations of QA in an organization is both a function of methods used and how they are implemented in health care organizations.

QA programs and activities are usually centralized (department or individual) and removed

BOX 19-3

Summary of Differences Between QA and CQI

Quality Assurance

1. Uses external determinants
2. Detects errors/deficiencies
3. Fixes blame/responsibility
4. Uses postevent investigation
5. QA department responsible
6. Inspires fear

Continuous Quality Improvement

1. Uses internal determinants
2. Determines requirements/expectations
3. Identifies process improvement opportunities
4. Focuses on prevention
5. All members in organization responsible
6. Inspires hope

From Fainter, J. (1991). Quality assurance; not quality improvement. *Journal of Quality Assurance* (Jan.-Feb.), *8*(9), 36.

from the day-to-day work of the organization. As such, QA observations and recommendations about problems and their solutions may never be widely seen or adopted. Perhaps the biggest criticism of quality assurance, however, is that it is usually seen as focusing on what is wrong and finding who is responsible. According to Berwick, this is an overly simplistic and punitive approach guaranteed to produce a defensive response and a rejection or rationalization of the findings (Berwick, 1989).

The *reaction* to QA may be more limiting than the *methods*. Indeed, some of the steps used in CQI may be similar to QA, but the management of the improvement process is different.

CQI and QA can be differentiated from each other. In CQI, the focus of analysis is on system-wide processes (not individuals) and is based on organization-wide responses to customers and process analysis data. It systematically analyzes characteristics of processes targeted for improvement. The premise is that by understanding why, how, and when a process fails, the organization can take action to redesign the process and improve results. QA identifies a set of criteria and determines a numerical rating of compliance with criteria. The result is that monitoring is a process of looking for "failure"

in complying with established criteria. This results in focusing on individuals and their performance to fix blame. Box 19-3 summarizes several differences between QA and CQI. Readers interested in a more extensive discussion of the similarities and differences between QA and CQI are referred to articles by Berwick (1990) and Fainter (1991).

Total quality management (TQM) is a management system to achieve organizational quality. It begins with the premise that quality is everyone's responsibility. Management is explicitly responsible for creating and managing the organization (infrastructure, resources, culture, and goals) to achieve quality. In TQM, a quality organization is evidenced by satisfied customers, empowered employees, lower costs, and higher revenues. The focus of improvement efforts are both administrative, or business processes and operations, and clinical. Further, in TQM, quality improvement is built into every phase of the organization's work beginning with planning.

In summary, whereas differences in customers, goals, focus, objectives, measures, action, and involvement may characterize differences between QA and CQI, the important take-home message is that TQM and CQI build upon QA to expand the organizational use and impact of

Key terms	
Term	**Definition**
Quality	Services that are free from deficiencies and meet customer needs
Quality assurance (QA)	Monitoring of care provided through measurement of indicators (level and incidence) to identify improvement necessary
Continuous quality improvement (CQI)	Builds upon quality assurance methods by emphasizing the organization; focuses on processes (not individuals); is customer focused; and requires that analysis and decisions be data driven
Total quality management (TQM)	Management system to achieve total quality as evidenced by satisfied customers, empowered employees, reduced costs, and higher revenues

quality improvement. A review of key terms related to quality management follows.

What are the principles of quality management?

Quality management programs in health care organizations are built on three major principles:

- Patient/customer focus: demands that health care organizations be responsive to patients as the most important customers.
- Improvement process: is use of a structured scientific process to reduce system deficiencies.
- Employee empowerment: involves efforts to use the knowledge and capabilities of all staff in the design, provision, and evaluation of services.

Why are "customers" so important in quality management? How does the concept of "customer" work in health care?

Customers and data about their expectations are pivotal to implementing the rigorous scientific methods that support the improvement process. Currently, a wide range of opinions and caveats about the importance and value of customer expectations exists. It is important for nurse leaders to understand the controversies and anticipated benefits of developing a customer focus in health care organizations.

One of the most important constructs in quality management is that the entire organization is

challenged to be "customer driven." Customers become the focus of the process of service delivery, and quality is (to a large degree) determined based on the ability of the health care provider or organization to meet or exceed customer expectations. A discussion below and in Chapter 23 about customers in health care adds to the understanding of the importance and complexity of using structured process analysis in making determinations about the quality of service delivery processes in health care organizations (patient care in particular).

In TQM, the definition of customer is broad, encompassing anyone who gets the results of another's work. Customers are of two types—those internal to the organization and those external. External customers are payers (insurance companies, HMOs, and employers), regulators, accrediting bodies, and stakeholders (the community at large).

Internal customers include employees (departments or work units), nurses, physicians, administrators, patients, and their families. Box 19-4 lists examples of internal and external customers.

For each customer, the drivers and determinants of quality will vary. Among payers, customer quality is assessed largely via statistics that reflect value. As such, quality is determined based on the level of service given the cost.

B O X   1 9 - 4

Internal and External Customers

Internal Customers	External Customers
Departments/work units	Payers (insurance companies, HMOs, employers)
Employees	Regulators
Nurses	Accreditation bodies
Physicians	Community-at-large
Patients and families	

Key terms	
Term	**Definition**
Customer	A personal beneficiary of any service/work
Customer/ supplier	One who gives a product or service to another (individual or department) in order to receive a product or service

For regulators, quality is determined by compliance with established performance criteria or standards.

Among internal customers, quality is *perceived,* based on personal experience associated with receiving service. Quality is judged based on both the characteristics of the product/service and how it is received. Among internal customers (employees and professionals), the work relationship is reciprocal, creating the "customer-supplier" relationship. For example, nurses supply information (orders) to laboratory personnel and receive products or services as a result (patients' laboratory results). Customer perceptions of quality are formed by the characteristics of the process and content of the service as it is delivered. Employees mutually depend on one another in the production of services in health care organizations. *What* is

said and done is important, as well as *how* the message or service is delivered.

Why is patient satisfaction so important?

TQM identifies patients as the most important customers of health care services and challenges organizations to design and provide services to meet or exceed their expectations and needs. Health care professionals are often skeptical and resist the notion that patient expectations and perceptions of quality should drive the health care process. Typically, professionals question how knowledgeable and objective patients can be about the technical aspects of health care services. They often think of patients as incapable of making an informed judgment on the quality of care. The patient perspective can be viewed as inaccurate because patients lack the requisite knowledge for judging technical competence (Vuori, 1987). In fact, because the technical or professional aspects of care are difficult for patients to evaluate, patients assess the quality of health care services they receive by their perceptions of the characteristics of service delivery and the professionalism and competence displayed by care providers (Lanning & O'Connors, 1990). Market research has identified detailed conceptualizations of health care quality from the customer's perspective (Berry et al., 1985; Parasuraman et al., 1986). Box 19-5 lists 10 dimensions that influence customer satisfaction in the delivery of services. Some of these factors are more important than others. The personal relationship between care provider and patient is probably the most important factor in influencing patients' perceptions of service quality (Bitran & Hoech, 1990). Nursing personnel play an especially important role in this regard because of the amount of time spent with patients (Shweikhart et al., 1993).

In a 1994 survey of managed care organizations, more than half of the respondents ranked patient satisfaction as being as important as price in determining the organization's future success in the marketplace (Stratton, 1994). Futurist Regina E. Herzlinger places in-

creasing importance on the role and financial impact of patients as consumers of health care (Herzlinger, 1997). Health care organizations that implement TQM must have mechanisms to assess patient expectations and perceptions of quality to monitor the organization's overall effectiveness. Patient focus groups, surveys (telephone and written), and response cards are widely used mechanisms for collecting feedback and data about what patients expect or want and how well the organization meets expectations.

Data related to patient satisfaction is collected primarily to improve the management of

---

B O X   1 9 - 5

Customer Determinants of Service Satisfaction

Tangibles	Facility attractiveness
	Employee appearance
	Characteristics of other customers
Reliability	Dependability
	Consistency of service delivery
Responsiveness	Employee willingness
	Promptness in service delivery
Competence	Employee knowledge
Understanding the customer	Effort to learn customer needs
	Individualized attention
Access	Distance to facility
	Waiting time
	Hours of operation
Courtesy	Staff politeness and mannerisms
Communication	Ability of employees to explain material in an understandable way
	Openness to questions
Credibility	Trustworthiness of staff
Security	Physical safety
	Confidentiality

customer relations and to assess the quality of care and service delivered, which are internally manageable factors. Such data may also be used to manage factors external to the organization, such as market positioning and competitiveness (Jones & Sasser, 1995). Outcomes management and organizational benchmarking that supports the management of external factors (i.e., competitiveness) are discussed later in this chapter.

In TQM, information (data) about customer expectations is intended to be available and used throughout the organization by all levels of personnel to plan and improve patient care services (Shweikart & Strasser, 1994). Such information is useful for improving the quality of internal and external organizational processes.

Quality Improvement Tools

What is process improvement? How is it done?

The second major principle of TQM is process improvement. Quality management requires that a structured (scientific) process be used by a team (project team) focused on a particular problem, responding to an opportunity or designing a new process. Within process improvement are embedded two important elements—use of project teams and the scientific method known as the *PDCA cycle* (Deming, 1982). The scientific method used by project teams is the PDCA cycle (also called the *Deming cycle* or *Shewhart cycle*). *PDCA* is an acronym that stands for *Plan-Do-Check-Act.*

A number of quality improvement project models are available for use in organizing and managing project teams. No one model is ideal for all organizations and settings. In adopting a project model, it is important to realize that the model itself does not bring about improvement nor does it define the teams work or methods. Some widely recognized models include Hospital Corporation of America's FOCUS-PDCA model, the Juran Project model, Florida Power and Light's Qualtec model, and the Process Design Model (Plsek, 1993). All of these models

share a common goal—the establishment of a project improvement team with the necessary skills, resources, and organizational support to get the process improvement job done.

What do project improvement teams do? What makes a team effective?

A working knowledge of what teams deal with and how they conduct their work is useful. A discussion of project team responsibilities and the steps and tools involved in a team-based quality improvement project follows.

Step 1: Defining the Problem and Establishing the Team As the first step to initiating a quality improvement project, top management and/or a quality council decides which concerns, issues, or opportunities will be targeted for improvement. Decisions are usually based on the organization's priorities and the gains expected from a given improvement project. Once decided, management or the quality council appoints a quality improvement project team. Teams usually represent a cross-section of organization members, each of whom has had some training in quality management techniques (Scholtes, 1995). For health care organizations, members consist of managers, staff members (clinical, technical, administrative—both professional and nonprofessional), and physicians.

Step 2: Documentation of the Problem Rather than rushing to action about the cause(s) of a problem, the quality improvement project team must develop a clear understanding of the process failure or opportunity for improvement. To accomplish this, QI teams employ the scientific process (PDCA cycle) and use specific statistical and analytic tools (Schroeder, 1992). The following seven tools are commonly used by improvement teams to pinpoint and document a problem and its root cause(s):

- Cause-and-effect (fish bone) diagrams
- Flow charts
- Pareto charts
- Frequency distributions (histograms)

- Scatter diagrams
- Run charts
- Control charts

Although it is beyond the scope of this chapter to explain in detail the rationale and techniques for the use of each tool, a brief explanation appears in the Key Terms box that follows. To demonstrate the knowledge and discipline required by a project team in using these tools, Figure 19-1 gives an explanation of one of the most commonly used tools (flow charts), and examples of the other tools are given in Figures 19-2 through 19-8. During an improvement project, several process analysis tools are used

by a project team, depending on the nature of the process being studied and the phase of the project.

The application of process analysis tools is the same whether the process is of a clinical or administrative nature. Reported uses of process analysis methods within the full cycle of an improvement project are found in the nursing literature. Two such examples, Patton (1993) and Dansky and Brannon (1996), have reported experiences in applying quality improvement methods to administrative and clinical processes.

Step 3: Measurement and Analysis The next step in the quality improvement process is

Key terms	
Term	**Definition**
Flow charts/diagrams	A graphic method for depicting the steps in a process and identifying who is affected; it documents all of the sequential activities involved in a process
Cause-and-effect diagram (fish bone diagram)	Also called an *Ishikawa* diagram (for its originator), a diagram for listing theories of causes; it supports a brainstorming process identifying causes of a problem by asking "why"? Four categories of possible causes are examined: people, methods, materials, and equipment
Pareto charts	Displays the frequency of problem causes in descending order (most to least), using a bar chart; based on the Pareto economic principle, that 20% of the causes account for 80% of the occurrences of the problem; it depicts the few contributors that account for most of the problem
Histograms (frequency distributions)	Graphic representation of the mathematical relationship between the value of a variable and the relative frequency with which it occurs; it documents the range of performance levels by segmenting the data by factor
Scatter diagrams	Displays the relationship between two or more variables (types of data); a simple form of correlation; useful in identifying the cause of problems
Run charts	Displays the results of a process in the order they are produced; each result is plotted in sequence and then connected to form a line graph; the graph is useful in highlighting trends
Control charts	Also called *Shewhart's* chart, for continuing test of statistical significance; displays upper and lower statistical limits; useful in assessing whether observed variation is reasonable; upper and lower limits are calculated from actual process measurements

Flow charts are one of the most basic and commonly used tools of total quality management. They are used to diagram the sequential steps of the process being examined and to help team members visualize how work processes actually take place through and across all organizational contacts/departments. Flow charts/diagrams serve four specific functions. First, they identify the essential participants (i.e., internal and external customers) of the process. Second, they define the process and help make obvious what the current process is. Third, they are useful in identifying inefficient, unnecessary, and redundant steps in the process. Fourth, they help establish agreement on how to measure the efficiency and effectiveness of actions. This facilitates the team reaching consensus about process problems: breakdowns, delays, redundancies, and bottlenecks.

To use a flow chart/diagram, the team must first understand how it is constructed. The team or a consultant must have a working knowledge of flow charting symbols; each represents the different types of steps, activities, decision points, feedback loops, and outputs possible in a process. Second, the team must apply such symbols to graphically construct a chart representing every aspect (every single step, progression of steps in sequence, decision branch and initial, and final outputs) of the process under review.

Flow diagram symbols:

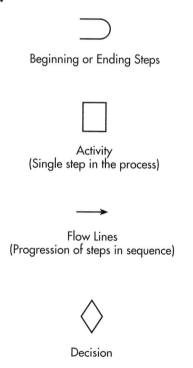

Beginning or Ending Steps

Activity
(Single step in the process)

Flow Lines
(Progression of steps in sequence)

Decision

Figure 19-1 ■ Use of flow charts in the quality improvement process.

Possible Causes of Increased UTIs in Patients With Indwelling Urinary Catheters

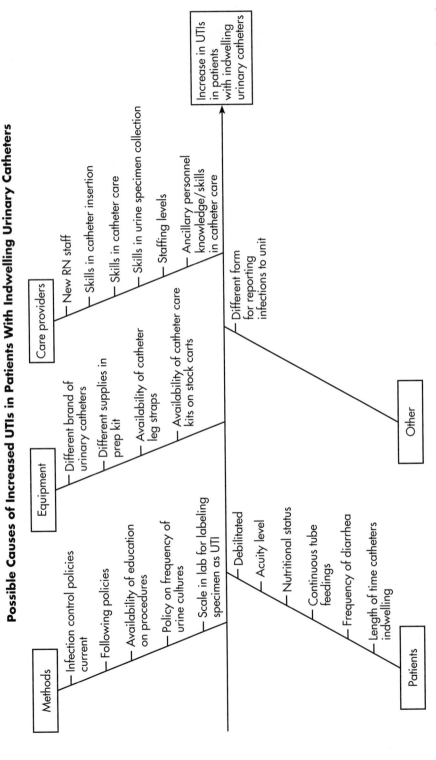

Figure 19-2 ■ Fish-bone diagram. Application examples of process analysis tools. (From Schroeder, P. [1992]. Improving quality and performance: Tools and techniques. In Schroeder, P. [Ed.]. *Improving quality and performance: Concepts, programs, and techniques* [p. 37]. St. Louis: Mosby.)

the measurement and analysis of the problem. This step usually begins with examining immediately available data (i.e., data that identify the discrepancy between customer expectations and actual service delivery). The visible signs of a problem may indicate only the symptoms of the problem, not the root cause. To improve a process, the root cause of problems must be known. To identify root causes, teams must understand the concept of variation. This is one of the most important aspects of scientific process analysis.

Identification of Root Cause(s) Every process contains variation: variation in the production/service delivery process, materials employed, time of performance, etc. In health care, the quality of service and response to service (outcome) may vary, even when delivery processes are standardized. This makes identification of root cause(s) difficult. A good example of this are outcome variations for patients. Even with rigorous standardization of care interventions and materials, patient outcomes vary. One of the strengths of QI is that it makes use of strict process control methods and statistical analyses to assess the significance of variation observed. The goal of analysis is to identify the type of process variation (causes) in order to differentiate controllable from uncontrollable. One of the reasons this is so important to the health care industry is that when variation is reduced, delays and waste due to poor quality are reduced, as are costs (Whetzell, 1991).

Control charts are used by QI teams to identify two types of variation: variations that fall inside the control limits of the process (common causes) and those that fall outside the control limits of the process (special cause). This is important information in that common cause variation can be reduced by altering the process. Special causes are produced by factors independent of the process and can be reduced only by eliminating those factors. When common and special cause variation is known, the improvement

team is able to focus its efforts on identifying what in the delivery process might reduce or eliminate common cause variation.

Summary of the Improvement Process

Regardless of the improvement project model employed, a project team acquires the appropriate data in the *Plan* phase of the PDCA cycle. An analysis of the data is conducted, and the results are used to identify hypotheses about the underlying causes of the problem. Using an experimental approach, the team tests each hypothesis to identify the root cause. In selecting a solution to address the underlying problem, both the technical and the human aspects of change are considered. The optimal process improvement solution is implemented in the *Do* phase of the PDCA cycle. Postimplementation assessment is done in the *Check* phase, and results achieved are tracked to ensure that expected gains are made. Finally, in the *Act* phase, if expected improvement gains are made, changes in the delivery process are permanently and widely adopted (as appropriate). If gains do not meet expectations, further analysis and intervention are undertaken by the project improvement team (Schroeder, 1992).

■ ORGANIZATIONAL ASSESSMENT AND OUTCOMES MANAGEMENT

How is outcomes management used in quality improvement?

As quality organizations have become data driven, they have found it useful to be able to compare quality data among organizations. The subject matter of such data may be patient related (attributable to a given patient population), or it may be related to administrative and business processes. Data comparisons among organizations for quality management purposes are referred to as *benchmarking* (Aspling & Lagoe, 1996). A *benchmark* is the overall performance of an organization or individual that is judged to

Text continued on p. 476.

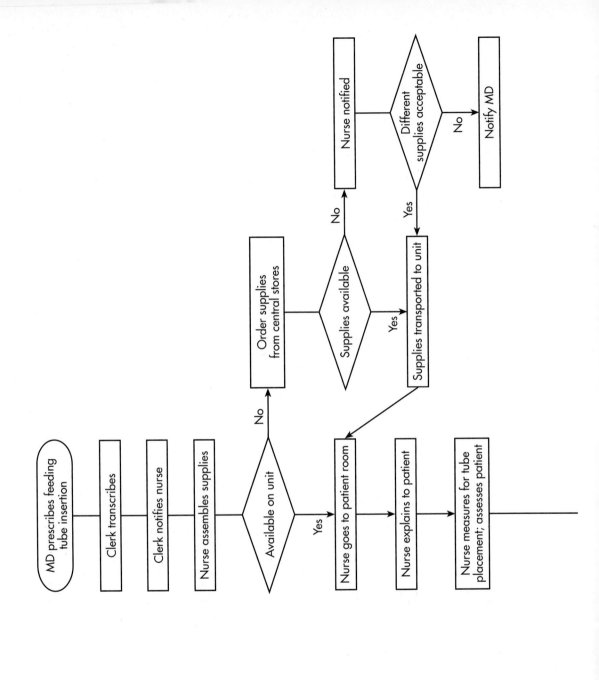

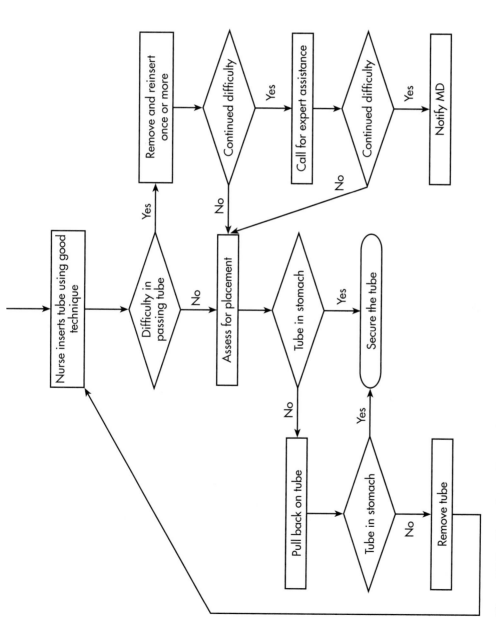

Figure 19-3 ■ Flow chart. (From Schroeder, P. [1992]. Improving quality and performance: Tools and techniques. In Schroeder, P. [Ed.]. *Improving quality and performance: Concepts, programs, and techniques* [p. 40]. St. Louis: Mosby.)

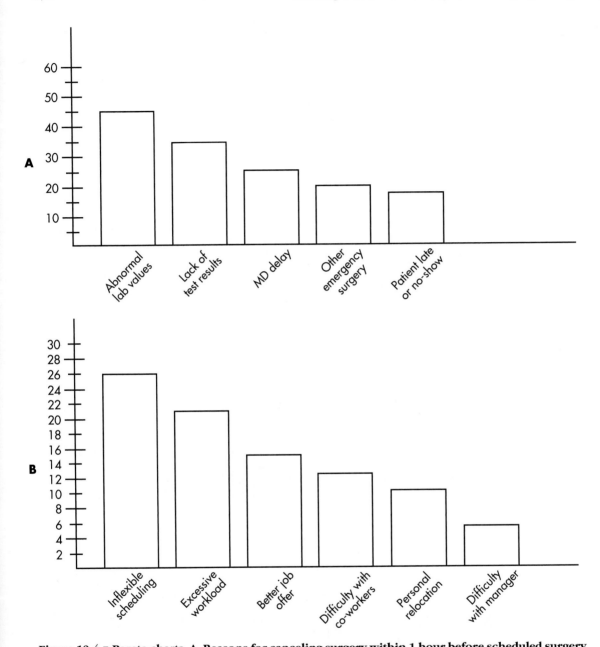

Figure 19-4 ■ Pareto charts. A, Reasons for canceling surgery within 1 hour before scheduled surgery time. B, Nurses' reported reasons for leaving hospital employment. (From Schroeder, P. [1992]. Improving quality and performance: Tools and techniques. In Schroeder, P. [Ed.]. *Improving quality and performance: Concepts, programs, and techniques* [p. 36]. St. Louis: Mosby.)

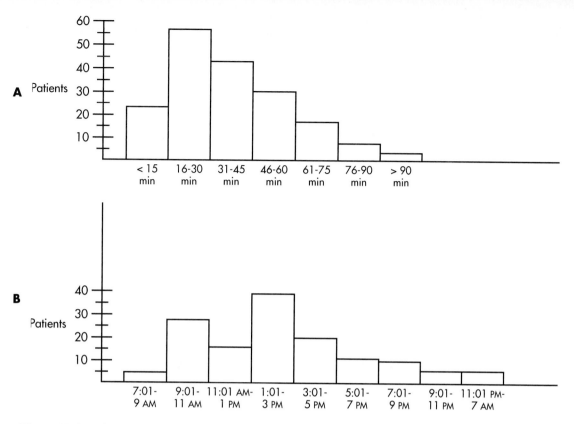

Figure 19-5 ■ Histogram. A, Waiting time in clinic. B, Time of day of patient admissions to unit during 2 weeks of the month. (From Schroeder, P. [1992]. Improving quality and performance: Tools and techniques. In Schroeder, P. [Ed.]. *Improving quality and performance: Concepts, programs, and techniques* [p. 35]. St. Louis: Mosby.)

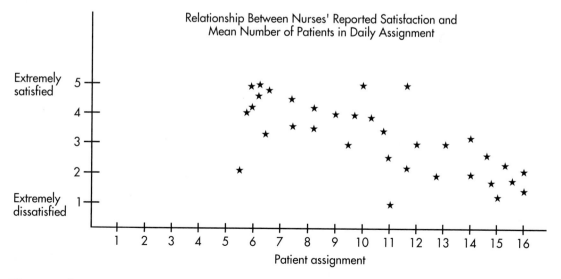

Figure 19-6 ■ Scatter diagram. (From Schroeder, P. [1992]. Improving quality and performance: Tools and techniques. In Schroeder, P. [Ed.]. *Improving quality and performance: Concepts, programs, and techniques* [p. 41]. St. Louis: Mosby.)

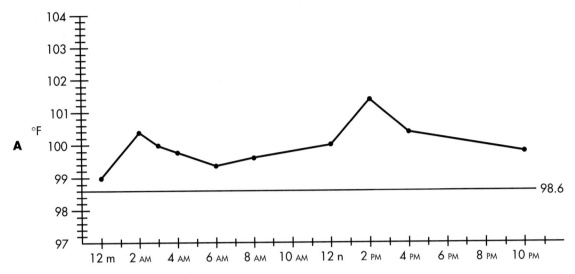

Note: In this instance, normal temperature replaces the mean.

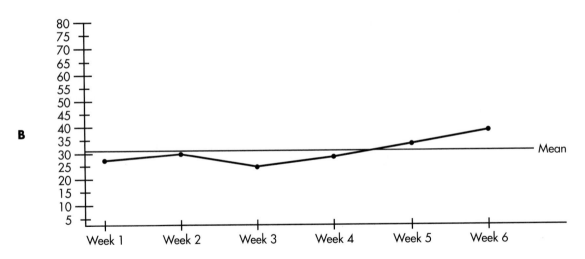

Figure 19-7 ■ Run charts. A, Temperature chart. B, Number of infiltrated peripheral IVs requiring re-starts. (From Schroeder, P. [1992]. Improving quality and performance: Tools and techniques. In Schroeder, P. [Ed.]. *Improving quality and performance: Concepts, programs, and techniques* [p. 32]. St. Louis: Mosby.)

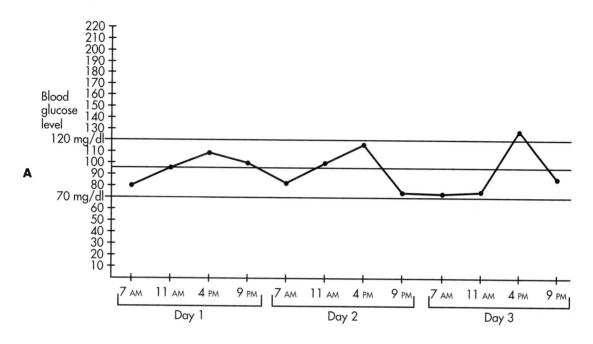

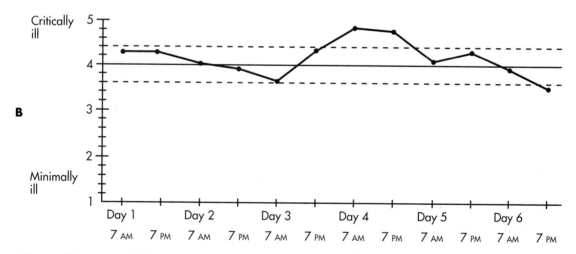

Figure 19-8 ■ Control chart. A, Blood glucose control chart for person with diabetes. B, Acuity level of patients cared for on unit. (From Schroeder, P. [1992]. Improving quality and performance: Tools and techniques. In Schroeder, P. [Ed.]. *Improving quality and performance: Concepts, programs, and techniques* [p. 34]. St. Louis: Mosby.)

represent the best achievable standard for a product or service. Benchmark comparisons are used to help determine what the goals or targets for specific organizational improvement should be. The process of benchmarking involves surveying the competition or industry leaders to obtain data on their products, services, and practices and to compare one's own organization to these data. Data derived from health care or non-health-care organizations may be included in such comparisons. This represents two types of benchmarking practices: world-class (outside the industry) and competitive (inside the industry).

It is important to distinguish the concept and use of critical paths from benchmarks. Critical paths are optimal sequencing and time plans for interventions by care providers in managing a given diagnosis, procedure, or population. They are designed to minimize delays, reduce resource utilization, and thus reduce costs while improving quality. Critical paths are used by health care providers and case managers in organizing and planning the delivery of care to individual patients.

In addition to being able to distinguish between benchmarks and critical paths, it is also important for nurses in leadership positions to understand the difference between critical paths and clinical practice guidelines. Although practice guidelines have many names (e.g., practice parameters, clinical protocols), they are not the same as critical paths. Practice guidelines are systematically developed statements to assist provider and patient decisions about appropriate health care for specific clinical circumstances (Field & Lohr, 1990). According to the Institute of Medicine (IOM) (1990), good guidelines must meet the test of validity, reliability, and reproducibility; applicability and flexibility; clarity and documentation; and scheduled review and modification. Many clinical guidelines that meet the IOM's criteria are available from the Federal Agency for Health Care Policy and Research located in Rockville, Md.

The benchmarking process involves a systematic approach to gaining information: planning for data collection, obtaining the data, and analyzing data to identify improvement opportunities. These steps are self-explanatory. What is not obvious is the considerable time and effort that must be spent on planning. In planning for the collection of data, the services, processes, and activities relevant to the benchmark

Key terms	
Term	**Definition**
Benchmark	Overall performance of an individual or organization that is judged to represent the best achievable standard for a product or service
World-class benchmark	Comparisons derived from outside the health care industry; particularly applicable for administrative and business processes
Competitive benchmark	Comparisons derived from organizations within the health care industry
Critical path	Based on a particular diagnosis or patient population, the ideal course of treatment (procedures, optimal sequencing and timing of clinical interventions)
Clinical practice guidelines	A scientifically determined set of specifications for the provision of clinical services to patients by diagnosis or population; also called *practice parameters* or *practice protocols*

are identified, along with internal and external benchmark partners. In addition, the necessary type of data (kind and level or unit of measurement) is identified, along with measurement and collection methods and possible sources. The organization also identifies databases and their suitability, as a source of comparative data (Patrick & Alba, 1994).

Because recent interest and focus have shifted to outcomes management, a number of sources of organizational data are available. A number of organizations, including JCAHO and even the Health Care Financing Administration (HCFA), have developed outcomes based on report-card measurements with some form of case mix adjustment. More than 40 states publish severity-adjusted morbidity and mortality information about inpatient performance. Currently, state agencies and a number of state hospital associations, the American Hospital Association, and the Health Care Financial Management Association maintain performance databases. This is despite the fact that HCFA has stopped publishing comparability data. The American Nurses Association recently sponsored the Nursing Quality Report Card Study, the results of which are available (Warzynski, 1996).

A very large study is underway by the American Quality Foundation. Under their auspices, the International Quality Study is seeking to understand the best management practices in three industries in addition to health care: banking, automotive, and computer. More than 250 hospitals are participating. Data collection consists of a survey (IQS) that contains 125 items in five benchmark categories:

- Business organization
- Service development
- Delivery process and customer satisfaction
- Quality and strategic positioning
- Culture

Finally, no discussion of benchmarking would be complete without mentioning the Malcolm Baldridge Award for Quality. This national award came into being when President Reagan signed the 1987 Malcolm Baldridge National Quality Improvement Act. It was established to increase U.S. managers' awareness of the importance of quality and to provide a framework for measuring the effect of TQM efforts. Two awards are given annually in each of three categories: manufacturing, service, and small business. To determine award winners, a seven-category 1000-point scoring system has been established; criteria are refined annually. The benchmark categories for the award are leadership; information and analysis; strategic quality planning; human resource utilization; management of process quality; quality and operational results; and customer focus satisfaction (Barber, 1996).

Although the concept of benchmarking in health care is just developing, several databases currently contain within-industry data (predominantly on hospitals) on financial and clinical outcomes. However, there is criticism and controversy about such databases, especially related to the uniformity and accuracy of the clinical performance data that has been collected. Such criticism is profoundly significant, because it casts doubt on the utility of data for quality management and public decision-making purposes. Nevertheless, the use and development of benchmarking is predicted to expand in health care and other industries (Patrick & Alba, 1994; Warzynski, 1996).

■ LEADERSHIP FOR TEAM-BASED (QUALITY) ORGANIZATIONS

Why is total quality management not just a technical process? Why is the concept of employee empowerment so important in TQM?

The total quality management approach is more than a set of rigorous, scientifically prescribed, problem-solving techniques. The TQM approach provides health care organizations with the values necessary to deliver quality service (Maddox, 1992). Presumably, the patient-focused orientation in quality-focused organizations demands that employees be given more responsibility to anticipate, prevent, and problem-solve customer expectations in their everyday work. In terms of staff/management relations, traditional authoritarian styles of management based on policy (rigidity) and management control are not compatible with a TQM environment. Neither are bureaucratic and redundant (hierarchic) decision structures. These practices and structures are being discarded. Decentralization of decision making to the lowest level and in the least bureaucratic form is replacing them. This degree of decentralization requires that employees be empowered to accept greater responsibility for the quality of care and service they and the organization provide.

Delegation is an important factor in the benefit and success of employee empowerment. Although selected work functions and decisions may be delegated, managers retain the responsibility for overseeing the completion of tasks and for setting expectations for performance. Delegation allows employees to participate and ex-ercise independent judgment in matters that are outside of their usual work scope. The reverse side of this opportunity for employees is that they must accept responsibility for their participation and for their own and the entire organization's performance. Such expectations require that employees be well educated and prepared to work in teams. The success of interdisciplinary team-based work is one of the most important factors predicting the success of total quality management in health care organizations. It is important to understand that QI teams are not the same as committees; thus their leadership and management are not the same (Box 19-6). According to Parisi (1994), a team is composed of individuals who are involved or affected by a problem or quality issue and who work together to solve a common problem. Specifically, the team should consist of a small number of people with useful knowledge and skills who are committed to a common purpose or goal for which they hold themselves mutually accountable. They report to the organizational authority that appointed them (Katz & Green, 1992).

B O X   1 9 - 6

Differences Between Teams and Committees

Team	Committee
Shares leadership roles	Strong, clearly-focused leader
Limited members (5-6)	Unlimited members
Members have a range of authority in the organization	Members are at similar levels in the organization
Designed for short terms of work	Ongoing
Has defined goals	Has changing goals
Uses a scientific approach for process improvement	Sometimes uses CQI tools and techniques
Recommends permanent solutions	Recommends quick fixes
Measures performance directly by assessing collective work by-products	Measures effectiveness indirectly by its influence on others

From Parisi, L.L. (1994). Process improvement. Committee or team. *Nursing Quality Connection, 4*(2), 5.

Managers are responsible for ensuring that employees have the resources, knowledge, skills, and abilities to do their work. A number of resources are available to accomplish this goal: coaching, mentorship, and education (provided or sponsored by the organization) are particularly important.

The roles and skills of managers and leaders in quality organizations have moved away from the old norms—exercising power to demand conformity—to sharing authority with empowered employees. Managers and leaders in this context serve as coaches and developers of others (Zalenik, 1992). Increased employee participation in the matters that affect employees is encouraged. Decision making extends beyond an employee's individual work and sphere of influence to employee participation in determining organizational policies and directions. At another level it extends to team and peer relations in managing the work and working relationships that teams create. This means that leadership competency among employees of all levels, involving delegation, motivation, and working in and for self-led teams, is essential.

■ KEY POINTS

- Quality management evolved as a new management construct beginning in the early 1930s, gaining substance in the 1950s and momentum in the 1980s. Public pressures to increase the quality of and access to health services while reducing costs mean that total quality management uses in the health care industry are likely to make the 1990s the decade of quality.
- Three major principles characterize quality management programs in health care:
  - Patient/customer focus: Health care organizations are responsive to patients as the most important customers.
  - Improvement process: Use of a structured scientific process and statistical measurement methods to reduce system deficiencies.
  - Employee empowerment: Active involvement of staff at all levels to use their knowledge and capabilities in the design, provision, and evaluation of services.
- Critical paths are optimal sequencing and time plans for interventions by care providers in managing a given diagnosis, procedure, or population. They are designed to minimize delays, reduce resource utilization, and thus reduce costs while improving quality.
- A benchmark is the overall performance of an organization or individual that is judged to represent the best achievable standard for a product or service. Benchmark comparisons are used to help determine what the goals or targets for specific organizational improvement should be.
- Successful implementation of total quality management in health care organizations requires nurse leaders (managers and team members) to have a working knowledge of scientific, data-oriented statistical methods; new human and technical skills; and an appreciation for and ability to work effectively in teams. Skills associated with motivation and coaching are essential leadership skills for clinicians and managers alike.
- To be able to work effectively as team members and leaders in health care organizations, nurses need a working knowledge of the tools and techniques of quality improvement and total quality management.

■ CRITICAL THINKING QUESTIONS

1. Identify a clinical problem on a unit where you have experience. Given the problem identified, what method(s) would a QI team use to identify and analyze the process?
2. Identify at least three reasons nurses do use quality improvement techniques to measure the effectiveness of their work. Rank these in

order of their importance in actually determining the level of quality nursing care.

3. Not all health care organizations regularly employ quality improvement strategies to evaluate their activities. What are the most likely reasons why quality improvement is not used to its fullest?

4. Identify all the customers in a clinical area with which you are familiar. Evaluate to what extent each group of customers are typically treated as though they are valued by the unit. If not all customers are treated as you believe they might be, list what could be done to change these patterns of behavior. Rank the actions in order of priority.

5. Consider a clinical problem that you have observed. If you were to put together a quality improvement team to deal with this problem, who would be on it? What would their first priority be?

■ REFERENCES

Aspling D.L., & Lagoe, R.J. (1996). Benchmarking for clinical pathways in hospitals: A summary of sources. *Nursing Economics, 14*(2), 92-97.

Barber, N. (1996). *Quality assessment for healthcare: A Baldridge-based handbook*. Milwaukee, Wis.: American Society for Quality Control.

Berry, L.L., Zeithaml, V.A, & Parasuraman, P. (1985). Quality counts in service, too. *Business Horizons, 28*(3), 44-52.

Berwick, D.M. (1989). Continuous improvement as an ideal in health care. *The New England Journal of Medicine, 320*(1), 53-56.

Berwick, D.M. (1990). Peer review and quality management: Are they compatible? *Quality Review Bulletin, 16,* 246-251.

Bitran, G.R., & Hoech, J. (1990, Winter). The humanization of service: Respect at the moment of truth. *Sloan Management Review,* 89-96.

Crosby, P.B. (1979). *Quality is free: The art of making quality free,* New York: New American Library.

Dansky, K., & Brannon, D. (1996). Using TQM to improve management of home health aides. *Journal of Nursing Administration, 26*(12), 43-49.

Deming, W.E. (1982). *Quality, productivity, and competitive position*. Cambridge, Mass.: Center for Advanced Engineering Study, Massachusetts Institute of Technology.

Donabedian, A. (1986). Standards for quality assessment and monitoring. *Quality Research Bulletin, 12,* 99-108.

Donabedian, A. (1994). The epidemiology of quality, *Inquiry, 22,* 292.

Fainter, J. (1991, January-February). Quality assurance, not quality improvement. *Journal of Quality Assurance, 8*(9), 36.

Feigenbaum, A.V. (1983). *Total quality control* (3rd ed.). New York: McGraw-Hill.

Field, M, & Lohr, K. (Eds.). (1990). *Clinical practice guidelines: Directions for a new program,* Washington, D.C.: National Academy Press.

Garvin, D.A. (1988). *Managing quality: The strategic and competitive edge*. New York: The Free Press.

Gehani, R.R. (1993). Quality value-chain: A meta-synthesis of frontiers of quality movement. *Academy of Management Executive, 7*(2), 29-42.

Herzlinger, R.E. (1997). *Market-driven health care: Who wins, who loses in the transformation of America's largest service industry.* Reading, Mass.: Addison-Wesley.

Institute of Medicine. (1990). *Clinical practice guidelines: Directions for a new program.* Washington, D.C.: National Academy Press.

Joint Commission on Accreditation of Healthcare Organizations. (1991). *Transitions: from QA to QI: Using CQI approaches to monitor, evaluate and improve quality.* Oakbrook Terrace, Ill.: The Joint Commission.

Joint Commission on Accreditation of Healthcare Organizations. (1996). *Accreditation manual for hospitals.* Oakbrook Terrace, Ill.: The Joint Commission.

Jones, T.O, & Sasser W.E. (1995, November-December). Why satisfied customers defect. *Harvard Business Review,* pp. 88-99.

Juran, J.M. (1951). *Quality control handbook,* New York: McGraw-Hill.

Juran, J. & Gryna, R. (1988). *Juran's quality control handbook.* (4th ed.). New York: McGraw-Hill.

Katz, J., & Green, E. (1992). *Managing quality: A guide to monitoring and evaluating nursing services.* St. Louis: Mosby.

Lanning, J.A., & O'Connors, S.J. (1990). The healthcare quality quagmire: Some signposts. *Hospitals and Health Services Administration, 35*(1), 39-54.

Maddox, P.J. (1992). Successful implementation of a CQI process. In J. Dienemann (Ed.). *Continuous quality improvement in nursing.* Washington, D.C.: American Nurses Publications.

McGlynn, E.A. (1997). Six challenges in measuring the quality of health care. *Health Affairs, 16*(3), 7-21.

Parasuraman, P., Zeithaml, V.A., & Berry, L.L. (1986). *SERVQUAL: A multiple item scale for measuring customer perceptions of service quality.* Cambridge, Mass.: Marketing Science Institute.

Parisi, L.L. (1994). Process improvement: Committee or team. *Nursing Quality Connection, 4*(2), 5.

Patrick, M., & Alba, T. (1994). Health care benchmarking: A team approach. *Quality Management in Health Care, 2*(2), 38-47.

Patton, M.D. (1993). Action research and the process of continual quality improvement in a cancer center. *Oncology Nursing Forum, 20*(5), 751-755.

Plsek, P.E. (1993). Tutorial: Quality improvement project models. *Quality Management in Health Care, 1*(2), 69-81.

Scholtes, P.R. (1995). Teams in the age of systems. *Quality Progress, 28*(12), 51-59.

Schroeder, P. (1992). *Improving quality and performance: Concepts, programs, and techniques.* St. Louis: Mosby.

Shewhart, W. (1980 [1931]). *Economic control of quality of manufactured product.* Milwaukee, Wis. American Society of Quality Control.

Shweikart, S.B., & Strasser, S. (1994). The effective use of patient satisfaction data. *Topics in Health Information Management, 15*(2), 49-60.

Shweikart, S.B., Strasser, S., & Kennedy, M.R. (1993). Service recovery in health service organizations. *Hospital & Health Services Research, 38*(2), 3-20.

Stratton, B. (1994). Do customers know what they want? *Quality Progress, 27*(4), 6.

Taylor, F.W. (1911). *The principles of scientific thought.* New York: Harper.

Vuori, H. (1987). Patient satisfaction: An attribute or indicator of the quality of care? *Quality Review Bulletin, 13,* 106-108.

Warzynski, D. (1996). Nursing's quality report card outcomes project. *STAT Bulletin,* July.

Whetzell, G. (1991). Total quality management. *Topics in Healthcare Financing, 18*(2), 12-20.

Zalenik, A. (1992, March-April). Managers and leaders: Are they different? *Harvard Business Review,* 126-135.

Zeithaml, V.A., Berry, L.L., & Parasuraman, P. (1990). *Delivering quality service: Balancing customer perceptions and expectations.* New York: The Free Press.

CHAPTER 20

Program and Project Management

Doris F. Glick and Karen MacDonald Thompson

INTRODUCTION

The health care system is changing at an unprecedented rate. Future directions are set through the development of innovative programs and projects, and successful program development is based on judgments about the future. Thus successful creation of health programs is grounded in effective decisions and strategies for long-term survival and success.

Programs are the building blocks of the constantly evolving health care system, and planning and development are the tools that build the system. If nursing is to play a vital and dynamic role in the emerging health care arena, indeed if nursing is going to survive as a professional discipline, nurses need to be proactive. They need to know how to effectively design, create, and manage innovative programs and organizations that successfully deliver health services in a changing health care environment. A systematic and logical approach to the development of programs increases the probability of successful implementation and outcomes.

Program management involves the process of assessing, planning, implementing, and evaluating programs. This chapter describes the process and selected models for planning programs that effectively meet assessed health care needs of designated groups or populations. Program implementation is discussed with a focus on care management that makes optimal use of existing resources. Program evaluation addresses issues associated with measuring and using health outcome data.

The development of new programs in today's health care environment calls for taking initiative, and some risk, to create innovative new designs that effectively address health care problems. Effective programs are those that address relevant problems, are consistent with the mission of the parent organization, and have long-term sustainability (Pollack, 1994).

OBJECTIVES

After reading this chapter, you will be able to:

1. Summarize the history of health planning efforts in the United States
2. Compare and contrast selected models for health program planning
3. Analyze the relevance and process of needs assessment for program development
4. Identify issues related to obtaining funding for health programs
5. Examine the process of evaluation of program outcomes

■ HISTORICAL PERSPECTIVES OF PROGRAM PLANNING

Interest in health planning and evaluation has grown along with the growth of the health care industry in this century. Coordinated regional planning for health services, however, was not established nationwide until after World War II. Efforts at health planning before that time were scattered.

In the 1920s the American Public Health Association Committee on Administrative Practice and Evaluation addressed the haphazard development of public health programs by encouraging health officers across the country to engage in program planning. At the same time, the Committee on Costs of Medical Care addressed the social and economic dimensions of health services. This committee cited the increasing costs and unequitable distribution of health services nationwide that resulted from the lack of comprehensive health planning. Following this report, several states began to coordinate medical services for their citizens (Stanhope, 1996).

In 1944 the American Hospital Association set up its Committee on Postwar Planning. At this time, also, government and other third-party payer financing of health care services became widely established, and public demand for health services grew. Recognizing a need for additional health care facilities and hospital beds, Congress enacted the first federal attempt to legislate health planning in 1946: the Hospital Survey and Construction Act, also known as the *Hill-Burton Act.* This act provided funding to assess the need for hospitals, and if needed, to plan and construct hospitals and public health facilities (Lancaster, 1988). Consequently, the number and variety of health care agencies began to increase and interest in evaluation of program effectiveness and accountability grew.

In the 1960s the Great Society programs of President Lyndon Johnson were grounded in the conviction that the federal government had a responsibility to meet the health, social, and economic needs of citizens and that the federal government could efficiently deliver such services. Legislation such as the Community Mental Health Centers Act of 1963 (P.L. 88-464) provided authority for state governments to plan mental health programs. This act specifically defined, for all future health planning legislation, the mutual roles of consumers and health professionals to work together as advisors for the planning process. The Regional Medical Program legislation of 1965 (P.L. 89-239) improved the quality of tertiary health care services. This act also mandated that consumers and health care professionals collaborate to address major health problems such as heart disease, cancer, kidney disease, and cerebrovascular accidents (Stanhope, 1996).

During this era the Office of Health Planning was established in the former Department of Health, Education and Welfare (DHEW, the predecessor of the Department of Health and Human Services, DHHS). This office had no direct authority for health planning until 1966 when the Comprehensive Health Planning Act of 1966 and the Public Health Service amendments (P.L. 89-749) were enacted by Congress. This legislation was intended to develop a national system for health planning and provided grants for planning, development, and implementation of a range of public health services. Among the outcomes of this act were development of a method for organized planning within states; compilation of data on existing needs and resources; establishment of protocols for review of facilities; and the development of a process for cooperation among health care agencies and government (Stanhope, 1996).

Subsequently, the Comprehensive Health Planning Act was extended when the National Health Planning and Resources Development Act of 1974 (P.L. 93-641) was enacted. Together these landmark pieces of legislation provided structure, process, and function for a national health planning system. They aimed to facilitate community control over local health services through coordinated health planning efforts. Included in this law was the mandate that consumer participation on decision-making groups be at least 51% (Archer et al., 1984).

The National Health Planning and Resources Development Act of 1974 provided more structure for and authority over federal program funds than the legislation of 1966. Nevertheless, government continued to lack the power to realize significant steps in improving the health of the population; increasing accessibility and quality of services; controlling costs; and preventing duplication of services. The government continued to have no control over the private health care sector (Stanhope, 1996).

Early in the 1980s a deregulatory philosophy pervaded at the federal level. This era of "new federalism" brought cost shifting, cost reduction

and more competition to the health care system. President Reagan wanted to end the federal government's role in health planning, and the National Health Planning and Resources Development Act was repealed through the budgetary process. Funding was so drastically reduced that it became impossible for health planning to continue in most areas of the country, and health system agencies were deleted from the federal government's regulatory agencies.

Today the national health planning system has ended, although many states have retained certificate-of-need (CON) laws. CON was the primary regulatory mechanism used by the federal health system agencies (Rohrer, 1996). CON regulations mandate that the need for additional health services at the community level be documented before new programs are developed or existing programs are expanded significantly. For example, CON may be required before a nursing home can add beds or before a home health agency may be established. The absence of federal authority allows local communities or groups to address their own needs without government support or sanction. However, it also sets up a competitive climate in which the most effective communities or groups get what they can at the expense of other communities or groups (Archer et al., 1984; Stanhope, 1996).

In 1993 President Clinton proposed a major reform of the health care system. At that time it was decided that the federal government would no longer have a role in health planning. Instead, by setting limits on health insurance and overall health care costs, it is anticipated that the government will influence planning decisions of private providers and health care agencies (Kropf, 1995).

Health planning today is not coordinated; it is controlled, instead, by the various interests of the health care industry. Hospitals, physicians, pharmaceutical companies, health maintenance

Key terms	
Term	**Definition**
Hill Burton Act	Enacted by Congress in 1946, this was the first federal attempt to legislate health planning; provided federal funds to assess need and to plan and construct hospitals and public health centers (Lancaster, 1988)
Comprehensive Health Planning Act of 1966 and Public Health Service amendments (P.L. 89-749)	Legislation to develop a national system for health planning; provided grants for planning, development, and implementation of a range of public health services
Certificate of Need	Primary regulatory mechanism used by the federal health system agencies (Rohrer, 1996); Certificate of need regulations mandate that the need for additional health services at the community level be documented before new programs are developed or existing programs are expanded
Needs assessment	Systematic appraisal of type, depth, and extent of health problems and needs as perceived by patients, health providers, or other key informants (Stanhope, 1996); information provided by needs assessments is a basis for decisions on fund allocation (Soriano, 1995)
Assessment process	Consists of data collection, data analysis, and diagnosis or conclusions (Finnegan & Ervin, 1989); most models provide a format for analysis of the people, the environment including resources, and health problems or concerns
Planning	Process of selecting and carrying out a sequence of actions designed to achieve a stated goal (Stanhope, 1996)
Strategic planning	Broad-range determination of overall purpose and direction of an organization; systematic and continuous process designed to identify and define a problem, formulate strategies, and implement solutions (Jaeger, 1995)
Tactical planning	Short-range determination of specific details of broader goals (Huber, 1996)

organizations, and insurance companies all influence the direction of the health care system (Kropf, 1995). Tomorrow's health care system will be shaped by such decisions about how, where, by whom, and for whom health care will be delivered. If nurses are to play an effective role in overall health planning, it is imperative for them to take a proactive role in various organizations and in communities where many major decisions about the delivery of health care now are made.

■ THE PROCESS OF PROGRAM PLANNING

Health organizations and professions exist for the purpose of providing services to meet the health needs of designated groups or populations. Strategic planning is the process that enables organizations and professions to effectively anticipate and respond to changes in health needs. Effectiveness is measured by the extent to which service delivery results in specific outcomes that improve the health status of those served (Jaeger, 1995).

A program is an organized response intended to meet the identified needs of individuals, families, groups, or communities by reducing or eliminating one or more health problems. Program planning is the process of selecting and carrying out a sequence of actions designed to achieve a stated goal (Stanhope, 1996). It is deciding what will be done, when it will be done, who will do it, and how it will be done. Planning, therefore, is deciding how to accomplish preconceived goals. A successful program begins with an idea that must be carefully developed and molded into a feasible plan. Such planning is closely connected to change, because implicit in the outcome of most plans is the decision to change or not to change (Archer et al., 1984).

Planning is frequently categorized as either strategic planning or tactical planning. Strategic planning is broad-range planning that determines the overall purpose and direction of an organization. It is a systematic and continuous process consisting of a sequence of steps designed to identify and define a problem, formulate strategies, and implement solutions. Strategic planning is an ongoing process in which the end (evaluation) of one planning cycle becomes part of the beginning (assessment) of the next cycle (Jaeger, 1995). In contrast, tactical planning is a more short-range determination of specific details of broader goals (Huber, 1996).

Flaws in planning can result from three errors within the planning process that have been identified by Levenstein (1985) and are described in Box 20-1. Such errors in planning are likely to result in difficulties in implementing the program and diminish the probability of achieving the desired outcomes.

B O X   2 0 - 1

Potential Errors in Planning

1. Errors in fact: the plan is based on faulty information.
2. Errors in assumption: the plan is based on false assumptions.
3. Errors of logic: the plan is based on incorrect reasoning.

From Levenstein, A. (1985). Planning. *Nursing Management, 16*(9), 54-55.

Most of these errors can be avoided if the plan is grounded in factual information, correct assumptions, and sound reasoning. The more complete and accurate the information that is available to the planners, the more accurate the predictions and logic can be. Effective strategies to develop programs to meet tomorrow's health care needs and make optimal use of existing services must be grounded in a comprehensive understanding of currently existing needs and resources. The first step to developing a successful program, then, is a thorough and well-documented needs assessment. As Witkin and Altschuld (1995, p. xv) wrote:

> The central decision for all organizations is, What is the best way to portion out the available resources, including time, money, and organizational efforts, to meet all the demands—the needs—that compete for them?
>
> Such decisions may be based on intuition, political pressures, past practices, or personal preferences, and they may be made by boards or managers. But the most effective way to decide such issues is to make needs assessment the first stage of planning.

■ NEEDS ASSESSMENT

The most important step in successful problem solving is identifying and defining the problem.

Disease patterns, health needs, and resources change over time; therefore successful health planning is cyclic and requires a constant updating of assessment data to ensure that program efforts address real problems and priorities. Moreover, to convince funding agencies to support a project, documentation of a need for the planned service is essential.

Contemporary changes in the health care system have resulted in a significant movement from the institution as the site of health care delivery to the community as the site of service. In planning programs that will be based in institutions or in communities, it is imperative that program planners understand the existing needs, resources, and culture of a designated community before planning new programs and services. All patients are part of a larger community. They are influenced by the environment of that community and rely on its resources to meet their health needs.

Needs assessment provides basic information about the health problems, health risks, behaviors, and attitudes of various groups of potential patients. It analyzes the use, or possible misuse, of existing health services and identifies duplication, gaps, and inequities in those services. A well-done assessment provides clues and suggests strategies for appropriate interventions.

Adequate needs assessment for health programs not only addresses problems, issues, and resources within the target population for whom the program is intended, it also examines the organization that implements the program and the community in which the program will be located. An important initial consideration in planning programs is to decide what people, organizations (or divisions of organizations), or communities will be involved. The question "Who should benefit from this program?" is critical in the early stages of program planning. Assessment then examines the health needs of target groups to determine who could be helped by the anticipated program. Assessment determines gaps or duplication of needed services (availability), examines the quality of existing resources to meet the identified needs (adequacy), and identifies barriers to the use of existing resources (acceptability).

The assessment process has three components: data collection, data analysis, and diagnosis or conclusions (Finnegan & Ervin, 1989). Many good multivariate models have been developed to guide the needs assessment process. The amount of data gathered for a needs assessment can be voluminous. Therefore use of a conceptual model can provide a framework for organizing data in a logical way so that valid inferences and conclusions can be drawn. In general, most models provide a format for examination of the people, the environment, and the health problems.

Different data collection methods provide different kinds of information about health needs of target populations. Schultz and Magilvy (1988), for example, compared three different needs assessment strategies. They concluded that census and survey data provide a global picture of a population, whereas ethnographic methods provide more details about health beliefs and experiences. Ultimately the choice of models and methods for a needs assessment depends on the needs of the program and the time, resources, and knowledge available to carry out the process (Soriano, 1995).

A thorough needs assessment includes the data outlined in Box 20-2. This data includes an assessment of the demographic and health parameters of the target population, exploration of prevailing health values and attitudes, examination of existing resources in the community, and assessment of relevant political, environmental, and legal issues. Attention also should be directed to the availability of support and re-

B O X 2 0 - 2

Components of a Needs Assessment

- *Examination of previous programs* similar to the program under consideration. Planners can learn and benefit from the success or failure of similar projects
- *Morbidity and mortality data:* Provide insights about the kinds of health problems from which people suffer and help to identify which groups of people are the most vulnerable; program planning can then be directed at those groups who are most at risk for specific health problems
- *Demographic data:* Population size is the most useful predictor of future needs and use of health resources*; other relevant demographic variables that affect patterns of health status include age, race, sex, ethnicity, family structure, education, occupation, income, and health insurance status
- *Examination of existing programs/resources:* To avoid duplication or gaps in needed services; in assessing the need for health care programs,

the following aspects of existing resources should be considered†:
quality of care
accessibility and availability of resources
continuity of care
effectiveness of care
efficiency of care
acceptability of care
- *Community perceptions:* To ensure program acceptability, use, and success, program planning must address the prevailing culture and attitudes among those who will be affected by or involved in the program's implementation
- *Legal constraints:* Regarding professional practice (licensing and certification), federal regulations (issues such as affirmative action and accessibility for the handicapped), reimbursement issues, and local ordinances that may be related to the planned program
- *Environmental issues and political climate:* Issues and trends likely to have an impact on the success or failure of the project

*From MacStravic, R.E.S. (1984). Performance auditing for health care supervisors for planning, evaluating, and managing departmental activities. *Health Care Supervisor, 2*(2), 67-77.
†From Clement, D.E., Wan, T.T.H., & Stegall, M.H. (1995). Evaluating health care programs and systems: An epidemiologic perspective. In D.M. Oleske (Ed.). *Epidemiology and the delivery of health care service.* New York Plenum.

sources from the organization that will be responsible for the planned program. Useful sources of needs assessment data are listed in Box 20-3.

The trend today is for many health services, even those provided by hospitals, to be delivered in communities. For community-based services to be successful, citizen participation and a sense of ownership are essential. When members of a community participate in planning new programs and are empowered to take responsibility for their own health, it is more likely that planned services will be used appro-

priately and outcomes will be positive. Conversely, if the target population does not recognize a need for the intended program, the program is likely to fail.

Community development is "the process of working in collaboration with community members to assess the collective needs and desires for healthful change and to address these priority needs through problem solving, use of local talent, resource development, and management" (Lassiter, 1992, p. 10). When a community development approach is used in health planning, community members (representatives of the tar-

B O X   2 0 - 3

Sources of Data for a Needs Assessment

- Census data for demographic parameters
- Morbidity and mortality reports for patterns of health and disease
- Local and state health departments
- Community planning agencies
- Phone books for lists of existing resources
- Newspapers
- Surveys of potential program clients for information, beliefs, and values
- Interviews with key informants who are knowledgeable about the target population
- Focus groups with potential beneficiaries and/or key stakeholders
- Local, state, and federal policies and legislation for legal parameters and constraints

get population) participate in assessment, planning, and delivery of health services. Community development theory is closely related to the concept of empowerment. When individuals and groups are empowered through participation in assessment of their own needs and in planning and delivery of their own health care, they are enabled to be more effective in controlling and participating in transforming their lives and environment (Glick et al., 1996).

Community development theory applied to the management of health programs means that the program planner (change agent) is regarded as a partner with members of the target population rather than as an authority. Local people have firsthand knowledge about the health problems that they experience and they know what preventive measures and treatments are compatible with their culture, life-styles, and community norms. By working through members of a community, planners can acquire greater knowledge and insights about the popu-

lation and gain access to established links in the community.

Development of a successful community-based program should include members of the involved community at every step of program planning and management. The first essential step in working with a population in the community is to establish rapport and gain trust. This may be done as the needs assessment process is carried out. Participation of community members in the needs assessment process may involve a survey of all members of the community or focus groups with key members of the community. These inquiries should include questions about perceptions of one's own health needs and different questions about the health needs of other members of the neighborhood. If program planning is to be successful, it is important to explore which health services in the community are currently used by the target population, which are not used, and why.

Community members may be involved in delivery of services, either as volunteers to augment funded services or as paid staff of the program. In addition, community residents should be included on advisory boards and should participate in program evaluation. The more community members participate in the development of a program, the greater will be their sense of "ownership" of that program and, consequently, the greater the likelihood that the program will achieve its objectives and result in positive changes in health status. The following case study is an example of community involvement.

■ PLANNING MODELS AND TECHNIQUES
Precede-Proceed

The Precede-Proceed model is a comprehensive approach useful for planning, implementing, and evaluating large multidisciplinary projects. *Precede* (predisposing, reinforcing, and enabling forces in educational diagnosis and evaluation) and *Proceed* (policy, regulatory, and or-

Needs Assessment for a Community Nursing Center

Faculty of the School of Nursing at the University of Virginia wanted to establish a community nursing center that would serve residents of two public housing settings. The project began with a comprehensive needs assessment of the target population. Demographic data revealed that residents of one apartment building were primarily elderly, whereas residents of the other apartment complex were mostly women and children (50% under age 18). Both areas had a large minority (African-American) population. Epidemiologic data revealed a high infant mortality rate among minorities and a prevalence of hypertension and diabetes. Using a community development paradigm, nursing students interviewed residents and key informants. They found that residents were concerned about problems such as drug and alcohol abuse and the need for better parenting skills. Focus groups were conducted with residents to expand understanding of the problems; these groups also served to inform community members about the intended program, to begin to establish trust and rapport, and to initiate citizen participation in the project (Glick et al., 1996).

ganizational constructs for educational and environmental development) used together provide a continuum of steps for developing and evaluating programs. The title refers to the actions of patients and is meant to highlight the importance of emphasizing what causes precede specific health behaviors and what behaviors precede specified health benefits (Schust, 1996).

The Precede part of the model for planning strongly emphasizes diagnosis of the problem to ensure that a program will focus on the right issues. The first two phases of this model provide for problem identification through epidemio-

logic and social diagnosis. These steps examine and prioritize health problems and identify factors that have adversely affected quality of life. The third phase diagnoses behaviors that contribute to health problems. Identified behaviors then become the objective for change and the focus for program outcomes.

The fourth phase of Precede describes the causes of the behaviors identified in phase three and categorizes these causes into three groups:

- Factors that predispose or motivate people to want to engage in certain behaviors
- Factors that enable people to take appropriate health-related actions
- Factors that reinforce specific behavior

The intent is that if the planned project reinforces behavior that people are motivated and enabled to do, the desired outcomes of the project are likely to be attained.

Phase five of Precede is the planning of strategies for resources, time, and interventions to achieve the identified program outcomes. And phase six is the actual development and implementation of the program.

The Proceed part of the model provides for an assessment of resources (financial and staff) needed to implement the program; an examination of potential barriers to the program; and an assessment of policies that support or inhibit the program. This part of the model provides for the development of a timetable to carry out the project, development of a budget, assignment of staff, and designation of specific responsibilities (Schust, 1996).

The Precede-Proceed model is a comprehensive and helpful framework to assist planners to identify essential elements for the development of larger projects. It may be especially suitable for interdisciplinary projects that require interorganizational cooperation and that rely on the behavior of patients to achieve desired outcomes. Indeed, in today's health care environment, such programs may be the norm.

PERT

One technique used by planners to plan, schedule, and monitor large projects is the Program Evaluation and Review Technique (PERT). This method was created in the 1950s for a collaborative project among Lockheed Aircraft Corporation, the United States Navy, and Booz-Allen & Hamilton, Inc. The technique was developed to assist with planning and managing activities required to develop the Polaris missile (Stanhope, 1996).

A successful program begins through a carefully planned process that shapes and elaborates on an idea. Careful consideration must be given to who should participate, when the optimal time to plan is, what data and information is needed, what resistance can be anticipated, and what factors will enhance the success of the project (Schust, 1996).

PERT provides an organized method with which to list sequentially all of the individual steps required to achieve a goal. A timetable is established for each task, with attention to which tasks are prerequisite to the completion of other tasks. A target date for program implementation is established. Information about time and tasks is charted on a flow plan so that all of the interrelated activities can be viewed and progress can be monitored (Hermann et al., 1992; Schust, 1996).

An example of a typical PERT chart is shown in Figure 20-1. Boxes represent individual events or tasks, and arrows connect dependent tasks so that interrelationships can be visualized. Numbers above the arrows indicate the estimated time necessary to complete a task.

Critical Path Method

Critical Path Method (CPM) is a network programming method that focuses on the optimal use of time, activities, and resources to complete activities. Similar to PERT, this method sequences necessary program activities and provides a technique for estimating the time a project will take from beginning to completion. CPM uses the longest estimated time required to complete a task, as judged by those experienced with the activity. Planners can then determine which tasks are likely to require the greatest amount of time to complete. It is thus possible to identify the amount of resources needed to complete activities at various points along the program's "critical path."

Use of CPM allows planners to monitor progress and to identify problems early in the process so that corrective action can be taken. In addition, it provides a structure for evaluating the amount of time and resources being used by the project. In this way resources can be increased or decreased as needed, and deviations from initial estimates can be identified.

CPM is most useful for detailed planning purposes. The critical path technique has been adapted for case management purposes by hospital nursing services and home health agencies. Through use of CPM techniques, critical paths are used to plan, monitor, and evaluate patient outcomes. Using this method, required activities of each staff member are listed on a daily basis and the amount of time required by an individual patient from admission to discharge can be estimated. Deviations from the expected course of activities and outcomes can be identified early in the process, and goals and plans can be adjusted to most efficiently meet the patient's needs for care (Stanhope, 1996; Hermann et al., 1992; Zander, 1988).

■ PROPOSAL DEVELOPMENT

The first step in developing a proposal for a project is to identify appropriate sources of funding. This is an essential step as well as a major challenge. Many sources of public and private funding provide money only for projects that fall within a very specific area of interest. Block grants, in contrast, are federal funds with-

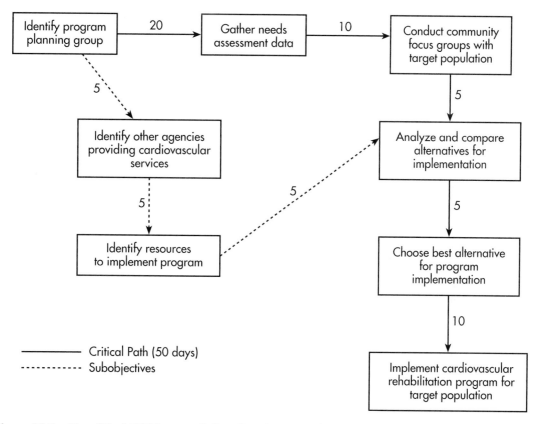

Figure 20-1 ■ **Simplified PERT network for planning a cardiovascular rehabilitation program. Numbers represent days needed to complete activities.** (Modified from Stanhope, M. [1996]. Program management. In M. Stanhope & M. & J. Lancaster [Eds.]. *Community health nursing: Promoting health of aggregates, families, and individuals* [4th ed.]. St. Louis: Mosby.)

out specific conditions attached given to state or local governments to be used for a general purpose (Stanhope, 1996). Federal money in the form of block grants may be spent in different ways in each state and may result in inconsistency from state to state in the benefits available to vulnerable populations. Various sources of funding are more or less appropriate for a given project depending on the focus of the program to be developed and the nature of the organization that will receive the funding. It is critical to find a good "match" for a project before pursu-

ing a funding source. A single program may be funded by more than one source. Major funding sources for health-related projects are listed in Box 20-4.

Development of a proposal for a program is guided by a statement about the mission of the project. A mission statement broadly sets forth the purpose and focus for the existence of an organization or a program. It provides a basis for expectations about all functions to be carried out (Andrews, 1990). A mission statement describes the values and beliefs of a venture. The

Key terms

Term	Definition
Program	Organized response intended to meet identified needs of individuals, families, groups, or communities by reducing or eliminating one or more health problems (Stanhope, 1996, p. 394); may also be considered to be projects, services, or ventures
Block grants	Federal funds given to state or local governments for a general purpose; no specific conditions attached (Stanhope, 1996); block grants allow federal money to be used in diverse ways in different places
Precede-Proceed model	Comprehensive approach for planning, implementing, and evaluating large multidisciplinary projects; title refers to the actions of clients and is meant to highlight the importance of identifying what causes Precede-specific health behaviors and what behaviors Precede-specified health benefits (Schust, 1996)
Target population	Group of individuals who have one or more health problems or risk factors in common and for whom a program is intended
Program Evaluation and Review Technique (PERT)	Planning technique using an organized method to list steps required to achieve a goal; information about time and tasks is charted on a task flow plan with attention to which tasks are prerequisite to the completion of other tasks so that all of the interrelated activities can be viewed and progress can be monitored (Hermann et al, 1992; Schust, 1996)
Critical Path Method (CPM)	Network programming method similar to PERT; uses the longest estimated time required to complete a task, as judged by those experienced with the activity, so that planners can identify the amount of time and resources needed to complete the process
Mission statement	Broadly describes the purpose and focus for the existence of an organization or a program; describes values and beliefs of a venture, and provides a basis for expectations about all functions to be carried out (Andrews, 1990)
Goals	General statement of a desired future state or condition; goal statement should be broad, attainable, and long range (Schust, 1996)
Objectives	Clearly written statements about specific activities necessary to accomplish a goal; they are short-term, directly measurable action statements that have a specific time frame and describe what will be done, who will do it, when it will be done, and what outcomes are expected
Program implementation	Process of putting the plan into action; includes the management and actual delivery of services to carry out the planned strategies and accomplish the desired objectives of a program

mission statement for a successful program should be compatible with the mission of the parent organization within which it will function. A useful mission statement is well written and clearly specifies who will be served, what will be accomplished, why this service is provided, and how it will be known that the service has been provided (Pollack, 1994). A mission statement provides a context for the development of goals and objectives for a program.

Major Sources of Funding

- *Grants* Funding; usually from the federal or state governments, awarded for projects that are experimental, demonstration, or research in focus; usually awarded to not-for-profit organizations*
- *Contracts* Agreements in which money is given in exchange for the provision of a specific and designated service; have very definite expectations and allow very little flexibility*
- *Public funds* Tax revenue spent to provide services for the public that are administered by federal, state, or local government agencies
- *Private foundations* Money for special new or experimental projects provided by grants through private foundations; most foundations have specific funding guidelines and support only certain kinds of projects
- *Fee for service* Money paid to an organization or an individual, retrospectively, in exchange for a specific service
- *Gifts* Money provided to organizations or individuals with the understanding that it will be used for a specific purpose; local philanthropic organizations and small foundations can be an excellent source of "seed money"

*From Schust, C.S. (Ed.). (1996). *Community health: education and promotion manual.* Gaithersburg, Md.: Aspen.

Goals are statements about where you want to go—a long-term hope or aspiration. In planning a health program or project, a goal is a general statement of a desired future state or condition. A goal statement should be broad, attainable, and long range (Schust, 1996).

Objectives are clearly written statements about a series of specific activities that are necessary to accomplish a goal. They are short term and directly measurable and have a specific time frame. Objectives are specific, measurable statements about what will be done, who will do it,

when it will be done, and what outcomes are expected. They are action oriented and usually begin with a verb. Well-written objectives for a project facilitate evaluation. If the objectives are measurable, it follows that measuring the objectives is a prime determinant of whether a project has attained its desired outcomes.

Healthy People 2000: National Health Promotion and Disease Prevention Objectives (USDHHS, 1991) is a useful reference for developing objectives for specific target populations. This document focuses on health promotion and disease prevention to limit unnecessary human suffering and on financial costs of prevalent preventable diseases and functional impairments. Organized by age category, these objectives focus on preventing the major causes of disease and disability in this country: heart disease, cancer, stroke, injuries, HIV infection, drug and alcohol abuse, and low-birth-weight infants. This document can provide planners with useful benchmarks for identifying and quantifying objectives and lends credibility to written proposals for health programs.

A budget translates operational objectives of the program into a financial plan. It is a useful tool for both planning and evaluating program management. It may also become a "political document" useful for negotiating adequate funding to implement the desired program (Huber, 1996). For purposes of developing a proposal for a program, a budget is a plan that specifies the amount of money necessary to carry out the designated project and describes how the funds will be spent. It lists all of the costs or prices of supplies, equipment, space, and personnel needed to accomplish the stated objectives.

■ PROGRAM IMPLEMENTATION

Program implementation is the process of putting the plan into action. It includes the management and actual delivery of services to carry out the planned strategies and accomplish the ob-

---

C A S E   S T U D Y

Planning for a Community Nursing Center

The development of a proposal to establish a community nursing center was based on data compiled by the needs assessment process. Documentation about the need for health services by the target population and about existing resources in the community provided sound justification for planning the program. The mission for the nursing center program is to provide services for vulnerable residents of the community, to establish settings for clinical practice for education of nursing students, and to provide for faculty and graduate student research. This focus is consistent with the mission of the University (parent organization) to engage in education, research, and service. Goals and objectives address the concerns expressed by the target population in the assessment phase and incorporate conceptual paradigms of community development, care management, and faculty practice. The Community Nursing Center has received several grants from private foundations and has been funded for 5 years by a grant from the Division of Nursing, USPHS.

C A S E   S T U D Y

Implementation of a Community Nursing Center Project

The Community Nursing Center is a collaborative project between the School of Nursing and the local housing authority. Construction of the two nursing clinic facilities was managed by the housing authority, with close adherence to HUD requirements for handicapped accessibility. The program coordinates with the Health Department, the Board for Aging, the local mental health agencies, the Free Clinic, and hospitals and physicians. A case-management model is used for providing services for patients. A School of Nursing faculty member directs the nurse-managed services and has overall accountability for the project. Each of the clinics is managed by an advanced practice nurse who is a School of Nursing faculty member (faculty practice model) and serves as instructor for students who practice at the clinics. Secretaries and receptionists are public housing residents who have been hired by the project in keeping with the community development model. A data management system is being developed to enhance management of clinical, administrative, and research data.

---

jectives of a program. Change theory is useful in helping to develop support for the program by funding agencies, administrators, program recipients, and other health and social service providers.

Implementation of a new program requires strategies for the following:

- Recruiting, hiring, and supervising staff
- Obtaining and equipping facilities
- Marketing the program
- Managing financial resources and budget
- Collaborating with relevant health and social service agencies and providers to implement case management strategies to ensure that patients receive appropriate care and to optimize use of existing resources

- Managing information for clinical, administrative, and research purposes
- Seeking funding to ensure sustainability of the project

■ PROGRAM EVALUATION

Program evaluation generates information about the relevance, progress, effectiveness, impact, and efficiency of a program (Kaluzny & Veney, 1993). In evaluation, the terms *formative* and *summative* are used to indicate different purposes for the use of this information. These respective purposes are (1) to make programmatic changes for program improvement (formative evaluation), and (2) to draw conclusions regarding the program (summative evaluation)

Key terms	
Term	**Definition**
Program evaluation	Form of disciplined inquiry to produce information to assist in making informed judgments about a program
Formative evaluation	Ongoing program evaluation that provides information regarding program structure and process to enhance programmatic changes that will maximize attainment of program goals
Summative evaluation	Program evaluation conducted at the end of a program to draw conclusions regarding attainment of program goals and desired outcomes
Program relevance	Degree to which the program is needed and appropriate to meeting the identified need
Program progress	Extent to which the program implements activities that will result in attainment of program goals
Health outcomes	Change in health resulting from implemented actions
Program effectiveness	Ability of the program activities to bring about change or produce a desired outcome in program participants
Program impact	Extent to which the program produces outcomes as compared with alternative programs
Program efficiency	Program cost per outcome as compared with alternative programs

(Patton, 1986). The type of evaluation to be conducted on any program depends on its purpose and the audience, or consumers, of its findings.

Evaluation Purpose and Objectives

The purpose of the evaluation should guide the development of the evaluation plan and the execution of that plan. Therefore clear objectives for the evaluation should be determined before the evaluation plan is developed. Once objectives for the evaluation are determined, an evaluation plan can be developed that is consistent with those objectives and will provide relevant information. For example, a comprehensive evaluation is unnecessary if the evaluation objective is only to determine the annual progress of a program.

Consumers of Program Evaluations

The program evaluation process should be conducted in collaboration with the consu-

mers of the evaluation. The more involved consumers are in the planning of the evaluation, the more likely they will be to trust the evaluation. That is, if the objectives of the evaluation are consistent with the consumers' objectives, the more likely the consumers are to value and use the findings of the evaluation (Patton, 1986). The benefit of getting the consumers "vested" in the evaluation becomes more important when the findings of the evaluation indicate that these individuals should make programmatic adjustments or changes. Resistance to change can be minimized by involving the decision makers in the evaluation process.

Consumers of program evaluations are often numerous and can vary considerably with regard to their relationship to the program and whether they are interested in using the evaluation formatively or summatively. Potential consumers include program directors, program funders, providers of similar services, potential developers of similar programs, and program recipients or their advocates.

Program directors would be most likely to use evaluation information for formative purposes. Because program directors are responsible for administering the program and ultimately for the program's success, directors would be interested in using evaluation information as feedback for making future decisions regarding program improvement and as documentation to pursue ongoing funding to ensure sustainability of the program (Rossi & Freeman, 1989). Alternatively, program funders would be most likely to use evaluation information for summative purposes. Funders of programs ultimately want to know whether the program worked. Future or even current funding of programs is often contingent on evidence that the program is effective.

Providers of similar services and potential developers of similar programs may use program evaluation information both summatively and formatively. Providers of similar services would use the evaluation information in a summative manner as conclusions or evidence on which to base their practice or provision of services. If, however, those providers were also involved in a similar program or considering establishing such a program, they might use the information in a formative manner. Using the information as feedback for decision making might prevent similar pitfalls or problems. Lessons learned from one program might be useful for improvement in other similar programs.

Program recipients and their advocates would use evaluation information summatively, since they would be interested in whether a program works. For example, parents of children with diabetes would be interested in knowing what benefits to expect from sending their children to a diabetes camp before they pay for the program. Recipients and their advocates are interested in evidence regarding program effects.

Types of Evaluation

Historically, health care evaluation has followed Donabedian's (1982) model for medical care evaluation. Within this model, evaluation of care falls under the three categories of structure, process, and outcome. Structure evaluations determine if the setting, materials, equipment, qualifications of staff, and organizational structure are appropriate to meet program objectives. Evaluations of program process focus on the care and services delivered with regard to type, quantity, and quality. Outcome evaluations look at the outcomes or results of the care and services. In other words, did the program make a difference? This model has evolved into different conceptualizations and classifications of types of program and health care evaluation. For example, Kaluzny and Veney (1993) include relevance, progress, effectiveness, impact, and efficiency as components of program evaluation.

Evaluation of program relevance is a component of both program evaluation and program planning. The likelihood that the program activities will meet the needs identified in the needs assessment is increased by using a conceptual framework appropriate to the program. Although development and implementation of a theory-based program plan increases the probability of program success, evaluation of program relevance may reveal irrelevancies related to the population or subpopulations (i.e., what worked with one gender or ethnicity may be inappropriate for other groups), the timing of program activities, or flaws in the conceptual framework.

The evaluation of program progress includes monitoring program activities to determine if the program is in fact being implemented as planned (i.e., avoid deviating from the plan by going off on a tangential aspect). This type of ongoing formative evaluation allows programmatic changes to be made during the course of the program, thus promoting quality assurance and staying on course (Rossi & Freeman, 1989; Royse, 1992). Examples of activities to be monitored through progress evaluation include the number and type of services provided, hours of operation, and number of patients seen.

Effectiveness evaluation deals with determining if the program activities result in the desired patient outcomes (i.e., Does the program work? Did the program do what was intended?). Effectiveness evaluation determines whether the program met its intended objectives and is, therefore, summative by nature. Impact evaluation is similar to effectiveness evaluation in that it is involved with looking at patient outcomes. The distinction, however, is that in impact evaluation, the outcome is compared with either no program or an alternative program (Schalock, 1995). Efficiency evaluation, too, is a form of outcomes evaluation and is focused on the incremental cost per unit of patient outcome produced by a program as compared with an alternative program.

Although a comprehensive program evaluation that incorporates all aspects of the program is ideal, program evaluation is time consuming and costly. Because it is rarely practical to conduct a comprehensive program evaluation in light of these time and dollar requirements, the development of the evaluation plan should be guided by the evaluation, purpose, and objectives, focusing on the priority aspects.

The Evaluation Process

Similar to the research process, the evaluation process includes a series of steps that, guided by the evaluation questions, systematically move the evaluator to the answers. Steps in the evaluation process are outlined in Box 20-5.

Formulation of the evaluation questions should be directed by the purpose and objectives of the program evaluation. The nature of the questions will guide the type of evaluation

---

BOX 20-5

The Evaluation Process

Determine evaluation purpose/objectives
Formulate the evaluation questions
Formulate the evaluation design (determine methodology)
Identify information requirements (define data)
Identify data sources and formulate data collection strategy
Collect data
Process data
Analyze data
Interpret findings
Disseminate findings
Utilize findings

Data from DiLima, S.N., & Schust, C.S. (1996). Program evaluation. In *Community health: Education and promotion manual.* Gaithersburg, Md.: Aspen.

---

to be conducted and the subsequent methodology used. Guided by and congruent with the evaluation questions, the information or data requirements must be identified. The identification of conceptually meaningful measures is critical to the evaluation validity (i.e., Does the measure accurately reflect the construct of interest?). Next, the sources of data and the means of data collection must be determined. Data collection, processing, and management, which may include recoding, data transformation techniques, and handling of missing data, must enable prescribed data analysis. Data analysis will be determined by the evaluation question, the evaluation methodology employed, and the level of data collected.

On completion of data analysis, the findings are interpreted. Any conclusions drawn from the evaluation should be explicitly justified by the data. The consumers receive a written report of the findings of the evaluation. Different versions of the report should be formatted to meet the level of sophistication of the various consumers. For example, evaluation terminology and clinical jargon should be avoided when preparing reports for program recipients.

The evaluation process ends with use of the evaluation findings. The use of evaluative information for program improvement or adjustments, however, is an ongoing process in which the end (the evaluation findings) becomes the beginning (updated assessment data on which to base program planning and implementation).

Data Sources

Data for program evaluations must not only exist but also be accessible to evaluators. Establishing access to requisite data can often be political and time consuming. Involving the data gatekeeper early in the evaluation planning may facilitate access during data collection. Sources of data include but are not limited to program records and documentation, including clinical, financial, and administrative records; interviews with program participants, and surveys and observations of program participants; and community health indexes such as mortality and morbidity data (Stanhope, 1996).

Evaluation Methods

Methods for program evaluation generally fall into one of two categories: qualitative and quantitative. *Qualitative analyses,* which allow for in-depth, detailed evaluations on a small number of people or cases, include naturalistic inquiries and case studies (Patton, 1986). Data for qualitative analyses include narrative descriptions from individuals about their experiences, feelings, attitudes, and thoughts related to a program. Qualitative methods are appropriate when the topic of interest deals with patients' experiences and feelings or when the topic is so poorly understood that reliable and valid measurement tools are unavailable. Narrative data from qualitative inquiries can often provide the

building blocks on which to base the development of a more structured questionnaire.

Quantitative analyses, on the other hand, use standardized instruments for the purpose of quantifying (i.e., assigning a numerical value to a phenomenon) to simplify and make sense of a large amount of data. Quantitative analyses include descriptive surveys with cross-sectional or longitudinal designs, correlational designs, and quasiexperimental designs. This section on evaluation methods focuses on methodologies for the various types of *outcomes* evaluations—specifically, effectiveness, impact, and cost-effectiveness evaluations. Methodologic details are beyond the scope of this chapter. However, numerous manuals and texts are available that outline these and other evaluation methods.

Effectiveness Evaluation Effectiveness evaluation determines the extent to which program activities brought about the desired change or outcome in program recipients. Therefore a comparison measure must be made using program as own comparison with either pre-post change comparisons or longitudinal status comparisons (Schalock, 1995). The outcome of interest must be operationalized and measured at appropriate time intervals specific to the anticipated program effects. Such outcomes may include health status, functional status, patient satisfaction, knowledge, pain, health behavior, or quality-adjusted years of life. Specific statistical tests and tests of significance must be appropriate for the level of measurement.

Impact Evaluation As opposed to effectiveness evaluations, where pre-post measures determine program effects on program participants, impact analyses determine program impacts compared with either no program or an alternative program. Thus impact analyses use either a matched-pairs design or an experimental/control design (Schalock, 1995). The program impact is quantified as the statistically significant difference between the program outcomes and the comparison outcomes.

Efficiency Evaluation Efficiency evaluation involves determining the program costs in relation to program outcomes, usually for comparison with alternative programs. There are several methods for efficiency evaluation, including cost-benefit analysis, cost-minimization analysis, and cost-consequence analysis. However, cost-effectiveness analysis has become the most popular of these techniques and the focus of an effort by the U.S. Public Health Service to standardize efficiency methodology (Gold et al., 1996). Cost-effectiveness analysis involves computing a cost-effectiveness ratio for two alternative programs: the program under study and either "the usual" program, another program, or no program. The cost-effectiveness ratio is the difference in the costs of the alternative programs divided by the difference in the outcomes of the alternative programs. In other words, the cost-effectiveness ratio is the "incremental price of obtaining a unit health effect" from a given program when compared with an alternative (Gold et al., 1996, p. 27). If a program is both more effective and less costly, there is no need to calculate the cost-effectiveness ratio, since this is obviously the more preferable program. Often, though, programs under study are both more effective and more costly, and cost-effectiveness ratios can provide valuable information regarding the relationship and trade-offs between costs and outcome that assist in program decision making. "Interventions that have a relatively low cost-effectiveness ratio are 'good buys' and would have high priority for resources" (Gold et al., 1996, p. 27).

One prerequisite for any cost or efficiency analysis is the establishment and/or existence of cost-accounting systems for each alternative program. To determine the cost effectiveness of

a program compared with an alternate program, data related to the costs and effectiveness of both programs must exist and be accessible.

Significance of Program Evaluation

Rising costs of health care require programs that have been demonstrated to be effective and efficient. Initiatives of the Agency for Health Care Policy and Research support the determination and implementation of "evidenced-based" programs and practices. No longer can the U.S.

C A S E S T U D Y

Evaluation of a Community Nursing Center

The evaluation plan of the Primary Care Nursing Center is being developed. It will be a comprehensive evaluation in that it will include process evaluation, outcomes evaluation, and a cost-effectiveness analysis. Currently, process evaluation is conducted annually to determine if the program is meeting its process goals of (1) providing case management for residents of public housing; (2) providing clinical teaching sites to graduate and nurse practitioner students and to 40% of undergraduate nursing students; and (3) providing a clinical practice site for faculty advanced practice. Documentation from the PCNC clinics and the School of Nursing provide the data necessary to determine if these goals are achieved. This information is used formatively to make program adjustments where appropriate. To determine patient outcomes, data regarding patient satisfaction are being collected. In addition, plans are being formulated to incorporate the collection of nursing-sensitive patient outcomes using the Nursing Outcomes Classification (Maas et al., 1996). To determine cost effectiveness of the PCNC, a cost-accounting system is being developed so that clinic costs can be compared with that of comparable care in other settings.

health care budget sustain expenditures for in-effective and inefficient care. Only through evaluation of programs and services can effectiveness and efficiency be determined. Summative program evaluation provides evidence of program effectiveness and efficiency. Formative program evaluation, through program monitoring, evaluates the progress of a program and provides information for decision-making regarding program changes. Formative evaluation is the basis for quality assurance/improvement and provides evidence-based rationale for programmatic changes. This cyclic process of planning-implementing-evaluating-changing promotes the likelihood of attainment of program goals and outcomes.

■ KEY POINTS

- Program planning, management, and evaluation are essential skills for nursing leaders to ensure efficient and effective programs that meet the health care needs of relevant populations.
- A program is an organized response intended to meet the identified needs of individuals, families, groups, or communities through targeted activities that enhance health status and/or reduce or eliminate one or more health problems.
- Coordinated regional planning for health services peaked between the years after World War II and the early 1980s. Since that time, systematic government involvement in health planning has diminished; private providers and agencies within the health care industry now control the decisions that shape the health care system.
- The most important step in successful program development is identifying and defining the problem to be addressed. A needs assessment provides basic information for developing strategies for appropriate interventions.

- When a community development approach is used in health planning, community members (representatives of the target population) participate in assessment, planning, delivery, and evaluation of health services. Such an approach promotes a greater sense of "ownership" of the program by the members of the target population and, consequently, fosters the likelihood that the program will achieve its objectives and result in positive changes in health status.
- Program models and techniques, such as the Precede-Proceed model, PERT, and CPM, provide tools to systematically organize the program plan.
- Program evaluations provide information on program structure, process, and outcomes to assist in making informed judgments about a program. Program evaluations may be used to make program changes to improve program structure or process or to draw conclusions about the outcomes of a program.
- Rising costs of health care require programs that have been demonstrated to be effective and efficient. The cyclic process of assessing-planning-implementing-evaluating-changing promotes the likelihood of attaining such outcomes.

■ CRITICAL THINKING QUESTIONS

1. Consider one of your clinical experiences, and identify a program that you might develop that would positively effect a need that you saw in the clinical area. Begin with a needs assessment and answer these questions:
   A. What needs exist?
   B. What resources are available or could be acquired?
   C. In what ways does the prevailing culture in the institution, among the people involved, and in the community influence

the program planning process in this instance?

2. Using the program that you identified in No.1, make a creative and comprehensive list of where you would get the data to answer the questions about the existing needs and the available or potential resources, e.g., if you conducted a focus group, who would you invite? Using Box 20-2, list the specific sources of information in your community.

3. Now follow a similar process using an entire community. That is, identify a community need that really interests you. What information will you need for a community assessment? Where, specifically, will you get it? What possible barriers might you encounter?

4. Read a local newspaper and identify a community need that might lend itself to a program planning activity. Using the material in this chapter, how would you go about dealing with the need? Use either the Precede-Procede model or PERT to guide your thinking about how to set forth a plan.

5. Take either your clinical assessment and plan or your community assessment and plan and identify, roughly, the amount of funds you would need. Where would you go to seek funds? What potential obstacles might you encounter? How would you try to overcome the obstacles? Who might be your allies? Your critics and resisters?

■ REFERENCES

Andrews, M.M. (1990). Strategic planning: Preparing for the twenty-first century. *Journal of Professional Nursing, 6*(2), 103-112.

Archer, S.E., Kelly, C.D., & Bisch, S.A. (1984). *Implementing change in communities: A collaborative process.* St. Louis: Mosby.

Clement, D.G., Wan, T.T.H., & Stegall, M.H. (1995). Evaluating health care programs and systems: An epidemiologic perspective. In D.M. Oleske (Ed.). *Epidemiology and the delivery of health care services.* New York: Plenum.

DiLima, S.N., & Schust, C.S. (1996). Program evaluation. In *Community health: Education and promotion manual.* Gaithersburg, Md: Aspen.

Donabedian, A. (1982). *Explorations in quality assessment and monitoring, Vol. 2, The criteria and standards of quality.* Ann Arbor: Health Administration Press.

Finnegan, L., & Ervin, N. (1989). An epidemiological approach to community assessment. *Public Health Nursing, 6*(3), 147-151.

Glick, D.F., Hale, P.J., Kulbok, P.A., & Shettig, J. (1996). Community development theory: Planning a community nursing center. *Journal of Nursing Administration, 26*(7/8), 44-50.

Gold, M.R., Siegel, J.E., Russell, L.B., & Weinstein, M.C. (1996). *Cost-effectiveness in health and medicine.* New York: Oxford University Press.

Hermann, M.K., Alexander, J.S., & Kiely, J.T. (1992). Leadership and project management. In P.J. Decker & E.J. Sullivan (Eds.). *Nursing administration: A micro/macro approach for effective nurse executives,* Norwalk, Conn.: Appleton & Lange.

Huber, D. (1996). *Leadership and nursing care management.* Philadelphia: Saunders.

Jaeger, F.J. (1995). Strategic planning, an essential management tool for health care organizations, and its epidemiologic basis. In D.M. Oleske (Ed.). *Epidemiology and the delivery of health care service.* New York: Plenum.

Kaluzny, A., & Veney, J. (1993). Evaluating health care programs and services. In S. Williams & P. Torrens (Eds.). *Introduction to health services.* New York: Wiley.

Kropf, R. (1995). Planning for health services. In A. Kovner (Ed.) *Jonas's health care delivery in the United States* (5th ed.). New York: Springer.

Lancaster, J. (1988). History of community health and community health nursing. In M. Stanhope & M. & J. Lancaster (Eds.). *Community health nursing: Promoting health of aggregates, families, and individuals,* (2nd ed.). St. Louis: Mosby.

Lassiter, P.G. (1992). A community development perspective for rural nursing. *Family & Community Health, 14*(4), 29-39.

Levenstein, A. (1985). Planning. *Nursing Management, 16*(9), 54-55.

Maas, M.L., Johnson, M., & Moorhead, S. (1996). Classifying nursing-sensitive patient outcomes. *Image, 28*(4), 295-301.

MacStravic, R.E.S. (1984). Performance auditing for health care supervisors for planning, evaluating and managing departmental activities. *Health Care Supervisor, 2*(2), 67-77.

Patton, M.Q. (1986). *Utilization-focused evaluation* (2nd ed.). Newbury Park: Sage.

Pollack, C.D. (1994). Planning for success: The first steps in new program development. *Journal of School Nursing, 10*(3), 11-15.

Rohrer, J.E. (1996). *Planning for community-oriented health systems.* Washington, D.C.: American Public Health Association.

Rossi, P.H., & Freeman, H.E. (1989). *Evaluation: A systematic approach* (4th ed.). Newbury Park: Sage.

Royse, D. (1992). *Program evaluation: An introduction.* Chicago: Nelson-Hall.

Schalock, R.L. (1995). *Outcome-based evaluation.* New York: Plenum.

Schultz, P.R., & Magilvy, J.K. (1988). Assessing community health needs of elderly populations: Comparison of three strategies. *Journal of Advanced Nursing, 2*(13), 193-202.

Schust, C.S. (Ed.). (1996). *Community health: Education and promotion manual.* Gaithersburg, Md.: Aspen.

Soriano, F.I. (1995). *Conducting needs assessments: A multidisciplinary approach.* Thousand Oaks, Calif.: Sage.

Stanhope, M. (1996). Program management. In M. Stanhope & M. & J. Lancaster (Eds.). *Community health nursing: Promoting health of aggregates, families, and individuals,* (4th ed.). St. Louis: Mosby.

U.S. Department of Health and Human Services. (1991). *Healthy people 2000: National Health Promotion and Disease Prevention Objectives* (USDHHS Publication No. [PHS] 91-50213). Washington, D.C.: U.S. Government Printing Office.

Witkin, B.R., & Altschuld, J.W. (1995). *Planning and conducting needs assessments: A practical guide.* Thousand Oaks, Calif.: Sage.

Zander, K. (1988). Nursing case management, *Journal of Nursing Administration, 18*(5), 23.

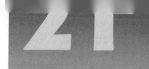

Managing Resources

Juliann G. Sebastian and Marcia Stanhope

INTRODUCTION

Nurses must be expert clinicians in the current health care environment and also manage the resources required to provide clinical care in a thoughtful way (Dreisbach, 1994). This places both clinical and managerial responsibilities on all nurses, including those in staff positions in every environment—acute care, subacute care, ambulatory, community-based, public health, home health, or occupational health. Because the nursing profession regards patients as the center of attention, nurses have not always thought that managing resources was within their set of responsibilities. However, in today's environment, clinicians are more aware than ever of resource limitations and are being held accountable as stewards of the resources within their areas of control. This chapter focuses on the issue of resource management in a rapidly changing, cost-conscious environment and on strategies for using resources for clinical care judiciously.

OBJECTIVES

After reading this chapter, you will be able to:

1. Explain the importance of managing resources to promote clinical quality in times of change
2. Forecast resource needs for clinical care
3. Construct and monitor a basic budget for a clinical service
4. Explain why people are the most important resources in health care
5. Delineate strategies for investment in human resources
6. Analyze the clinical implications of new strategies for acquiring and managing information

■ RESOURCE MANAGEMENT CHALLENGES IN A HYPERTURBULENT MANAGED CARE ENVIRONMENT

Controlling the rising cost of health care remains a challenge for policy makers, administrators, and clinicians. Three primary approaches have been used to achieve this goal (Hackey, 1993). First, the way health care is organized has changed from a "cottage industry" dominated by individual providers to a heavy managed care saturation in which clinical, administrative, and fiscal functions are integrated. Second, health planning efforts at local and statewide system levels and review bodies focusing on professional standards have been implemented to "rationalize" health care spending (Hackey, 1993). Finally, strategies for health care reimbursement continue to evolve, creating new incentives for clinicians to evaluate and change their practice patterns.

Changes in health care reimbursement have influenced health professionals' awareness of their responsibilities to manage resources wisely. As discussed in Chapter 3, before 1983 health care was reimbursed on a retrospective, cost basis. Clinicians had little need to be concerned about the cost of care, since whatever was billed for was paid for by third-party payers as long as the services were covered by the plan. That changed in 1983 when the federal Tax Equity and Fiscal Responsibility Act of 1983 was passed. At that time the Health Care Financing Administration put into place a prospective payment system for health services based on diagnosis-related groups (DRGs). Under a prospective payment system for inpatient care, hospitals stood to lose money if patient care cost more to provide than would be recovered in reimbursement. This change created strong awareness of cost control issues at the hospital level.

Managed care, and in particular capitated managed care, has created strong incentives at the level of individual clinicians to manage resources wisely. In a fully capitated environment, providers receive a fixed amount of money per enrollee each month to manage the care of each enrollee. No matter what care clinicians think is necessary for the enrollees in their panel, the revenue does not change. In fact, the funds do

Key terms	
Term	**Definition**
Resource management	Judicious stewardship over the resources under one's area of responsibility
Patient classification systems	Method for predicting the amount of nursing resources needed by the case mix of patients at a given time; includes attention to the ability of patients to provide care for themselves as well as the amount of therapeutic or diagnostic work needed
Risk adjustment	Systems that focus on the risk of patient mortality and identify key demographic and clinical variables thought to make the risk of mortality higher for some patients than for others
Flexible budgeting	A budget that is developed for a certain period (usually a fiscal year) and modified throughout the year (usually on a quarterly basis) as service volume changes
Zero-based budgeting	Starts each year at ground zero without using the budget of an earlier year as a basis for the new budget

not really represent reimbursement in the traditional sense at all. They are paid prospectively, or *before* receiving clinical services, rather than retrospectively. If providers spend more on the care of patients than has already been paid in capitation, the providers lose those funds. On the other hand, if providers spend less on clinical care than the capitated amount, they may keep the savings. Capitated payment systems create strong incentives at the level of individual providers to manage resources wisely.

Of course, these incentives create critical ethical dilemmas for providers as well. All health professionals are bound by codes of ethics to act in their patients' best interest and to do no harm (nonmaleficence). Capitated payment systems create incentives to provide as little service as possible. It is unethical to withhold clinical care needed by a patient in order to maximize revenue savings.

In times of great change, resource management is a particular challenge. The current health care environment is characterized as *hyperturbulent,* meaning that changes are occurring with tremendous speed and that the changes themselves are dramatic. Incremental changes build one upon the other and are continuous. The nature of change today is discontinuous; that is, one change may contradict or have little relationship to those preceding it. Three key resource management challenges face nurses and other health care providers in this environment.

First, thoughtfully managing resources requires time and energy. Both are difficult to marshal when change is hyperturbulent. Second, actions needed to manage resources under one set of circumstances may be the opposite of actions needed to manage resources under a new set of circumstances. In a hyperturbulent environment, apparently contradictory resource management needs may be present. For example, in communities that are only moderately saturated

with managed care, and in those in which some reimbursement is capitated, whereas other reimbursement is on a fee-for-service basis, providers need to generate revenue from providing only those services that are absolutely necessary (incentive under capitation) and simultaneously generate revenue from providing services generously (incentive under fee for service). Third, in hyperturbulent times, organizations must introduce innovations more quickly to adapt to environmental pressures. Service innovations require intense start-up resources, thereby creating a drain on the total pool of resources. Each of these pressures creates unique challenges to resource management in times of change.

What Is Resource Management?

Resource management refers to exercising judicious stewardship over the resources under one's area of responsibility. The kinds of resources used to provide clinical care are financial, human, information, space, materials, and services. It would be easy to think of resource management only in terms of the charges for services. However, this perspective would be much too limited, since it ignores all of the many inputs required to produce services. Each of these inputs has value and because of that must be used thoughtfully. Nurses and other clinicians should weigh the benefits of using certain resources in providing clinical care against the cost of those resources to determine if the value added by using them outweighs the cost.

For example, a home health nurse who provides wound care for a quadriplegic patient with a large decubitus ulcer will plan the dressing changes in advance to minimize use of unnecessary supplies such as gauze pads. A staff nurse in a hospital will ensure that all charge tickets for supplies are recorded for the correct patient so that the hospital can track its costs accurately. A nurse case manager in a managed care company who participates in an interdisciplinary team that sets utilization review criteria will question what is to be gained by various procedures and tests.

The purpose of resource management is not to limit the use of resources, but to focus attention on identifying those resources that are necessary in particular situations. In some cases, this may mean that more costly resources are used than may have been customary. Resource management involves ongoing attention to the value to be gained by using resources.

Figure 21-1 illustrates the relationship between resources, clinical care, and outcomes. It also shows how resource management relates to Donabedian's (1966) model of quality, which is still used today. According to this model, quality is multidimensional and includes the *structure* of inputs used to deliver care, the actual care delivery *processes,* and the *outcomes* of care. Resource management focuses on thoughtful use of the inputs to care.

■ FINANCIAL RESOURCES

Most resources used in providing clinical care can be "monetized," or converted to some monetary value. Staff time, for example, can be monetized by calculating the total value of the wages and fringe benefits associated with that time. Clinicians may be tempted to believe that if no new supplies or equipment are purchased for care, the care is free to the institution. Of course this is not the case if any resources are used, such as staff time, because most resources have a financial value. Exceptions are nonmonetary resources, such as energy. Even some resources that may seem nonmonetary can be monetized. For example, the reputation of a physician practice can be assigned a dollar value as "goodwill" on the asset side of a balance sheet.

Four activities are important in managing financial resources. First, nurses must predict which resources are necessary to provide clinical care. Second, all nurses should understand

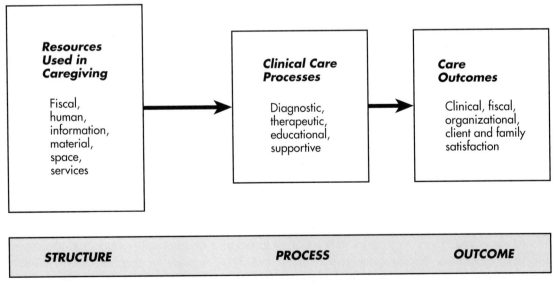

Figure 21-1 ■ Relationship between resources, clinical care, and outcomes. (From Donabedian, A. [1966]. Evaluating the quality of medical care. *Milbank Memorial Fund Quarterly, 44*[3], 166-206).

how budgets are used as tools to plan and manage clinical activities, particularly in times of change (Dreisbach, 1994). Third, it is critical for nurses to know how to control costs while retaining excellent clinical quality. Finally, nurses need to have the skills to evaluate the cost effectiveness of the care they provide and to help continually improve the cost effectiveness of care.

Forecasting Resources Needed for Clinical Care

Before one can determine the value of resources that are needed to provide care, one must identify which resources are needed. At the level of a unit, program, or department, this is accomplished primarily by using patient classification systems to forecast the need for registered nurses. Such classification systems have a number of limitations. One limitation is that they do not help predict how many different types of nurses are needed for patient care. For example, a patient classification system will not offer help in determining how many baccalaureate-prepared or masters-prepared nurses are needed, nor will such systems differentiate between the types of specialization needed to care for certain patient populations (e.g., one could not predict whether it would be preferable to employ an adult clinical nurse specialist or an adult nurse practitioner based on data from a patient classification system).

Another limitation of patient classification systems is that not all systems have been subjected to rigorous psychometric testing. This means that the reliability and validity of the instruments has not been established through testing their use under controlled circumstances. Why is this a problem? Nurses must be able to depend on these systems to accurately forecast staffing needs and to do so in a predictable manner every time the system is used. If the system is not reliable and valid, the predictions that re-

sult cannot be counted on to be accurate. Although some patient classification systems are being developed for ambulatory care (Androwich & Haas, 1996) and home care (Stanhope, 1997), the majority focus on inpatient care. Finally, many patient classification systems are in use today, which makes it impossible to compare staffing needs or the clinical outcomes associated with varying levels of staffing from one institution to another.

Patient Classification Systems These systems usually predict needs for nursing resources based on tasks needed by the case mix at a particular point in time, on the level of involvement patients can have in their own self-care, or by the types of therapeutic or diagnostic work being done with patients. For example, nurses working on a specific shift may rate how many patients have intravenous lines, whether patients require total or partial care, or how many are receiving chemotherapy or are scheduled for surgery. Although acuity is implied by these measures, the emphasis is on time required for tasks.

Risk Adjustment Mechanism Risk adjustment mechanism is a critical adjunct to patient classification systems. Whereas patient classification systems purport to adjust for the intensity of nursing resources needed by those patients, they often do not adequately capture the variations in risk across patients. Most risk adjustment systems today focus on the risk of mortality and identify key demographic and clinical variables thought to make the risk of mortality higher for some individuals than for others. For example, patient age is often associated with a higher risk of mortality. Gender is sometimes a risk factor that must be accounted for, as is presence of multiple illnesses (comorbidities). Certain physiologic parameters may be incorporated into risk adjustment, such as blood pressure, respiratory rate, or blood oxygen levels. The Acute Physiology and Chronic Health Evaluation (APACHE III) is an example of a tool used for patient classification of acutely ill patients that incorporates a risk adjustment system (Rogy et al., 1996).

Finally, activity charts and job analyses help predict resources needed for new services. Activity charts are sometimes called *GANTT* charts (Mariner-Tomey, 1994) and are matrices that list all activities required for a project and the relevant timeframe. Figure 21-2 illustrates a sample activity chart for a new employee health service. Job analyses (Fottler et al., 1994) are structured examinations of the work that needs to be accomplished to meet the goals of a service. The endpoint of a job analysis is development of a job description. Job analyses help planners determine both the types of personnel needed and the number of each type. This information is critical in building a budget for a service.

Budgets as Tools for Planning and Evaluating Change

Budgets are important tools for planning, monitoring, and evaluating changes in nursing services.

Estimating Resource Needs Budgets provide a structured way of estimating resource needs. The Employee Wellness Program at ABC

------- FY 98-99 -------

Program Components	1st qtr.	2nd qtr.	3rd qtr.	4th qtr.
Hire exercise physiologist and secretary	X			
Complete exercise protocols	X	X		
Program start-up	X	X	X	X
Internal marketing	X	X	X	X
Outcomes measurement		X		X
Evaluation		X		X

Figure 21-2 ■ Activity plan employee wellness program.

Company in Box 21-1 illustrates a typical budget. In this example, the nurses who are developing the program have estimated the revenues for the program for fiscal year 1998-1999, including the amount allocated to the program by ABC Company and the amounts they estimate will be received from patients paying privately for services. They also estimated the expenses associated with operating the program for this same period. These expenses include the number of full-time equivalent (FTE) staff needed to implement the program. The budget page should be accompanied by a written justi-

BOX 21-1

Budget for the Employee Wellness Program, ABC Company, Fiscal Year 1998-1999

Revenues

Departmental allocation	226,000
Private pay	$10,000
TOTAL	$236,000

Expenses

Direct expenses
  Salaries

1 FTE nurse @ $40,000	$100,000
1 FTE exercise therapist @ $35,000	
1 FTE staff assistant @ $25,000	
Fringe benefits @ 20%	20,000
Supplies (office supplies, disposable program supplies)	10,000
Equipment and maintenance (exercise equipment and computers)	75,000

Indirect expenses

Administration	$12,000
Utilities	$6,000
Environmental services	$3,000
TOTAL	$226,000
Excess of revenues over expenses	$10,000

fication, indicating why each item on the list of expenses is necessary. For example, staff expenses might be justified in this way:

> One FTE nurse is needed to do program planning and ongoing evaluation and provide health education on wellness topics including nutrition, stress reduction, smoking cessation, and exercise. One FTE exercise physiologist is needed to prescribe exercise regimens in collaboration with employees' physicians, to coach employees during exercise sessions, and to plan and monitor the exercise program. One FTE staff assistant is needed to maintain program records, make appointments, order equipment and supplies, and coordinate billing with third-party insurers.

Different types of budgets meet different needs (Finkler & Kovner, 1993). The Employee Wellness Program budget is an *operating budget*. It lists the expenses associated with operating the program for a year. *Capital budgets* outline expenses associated with major investments in physical facilities or equipment and permit the long-range financial planning necessary to make those investments. *Cash budgets* focus on the unit or organization's cash needs over specified time periods. These budgets assist with ensuring that cash is available when necessary. Organizations must have cash available at specific times to pay employee salaries, to make utility and debt payments, and to pay bills for equipment and supplies.

A number of different budgeting processes may be used. The two processes that are most commonly discussed today are *flexible budgeting* and *zero-based budgeting* (Finkler & Kovner, 1993). A static approach to budgeting involves developing a budget for the fiscal year and providing units with monthly or quarterly reports on their progress on staying within the projections of the budget. When it is time to prepare the next year's budget, the original budget is used as a starting point and a certain percentage increase is added to revenues and expenses, based on projections of market conditions (demand for services and availability and cost of inputs such as personnel, supplies, and equipment). For example, in developing a budget for the next year of the Employee Wellness Program's operation, the nurse manager might add a 5% increment to all costs.

With flexible budgeting, a budget is developed for a certain period of time (usually a fiscal year) and modified throughout the year (usually on a quarterly basis) as service volume changes. Changes in service volume modify the needs for resources such as personnel and supplies required to meet the demand. Because of this, it is helpful to measure the progress of a unit or department against what should be spent in providing the resources for the volume of service that was actually provided, rather than against estimations of service demand that may have already changed dramatically. This is a particularly useful approach to budgeting in times of rapid change.

Zero-based budgeting involves beginning budget preparation each year from "ground zero" or without using the budget from the prior year as a starting point (Feltau, 1993). In preparing a zero-based budget, one must include a justification (or rationale) of all costs, because zero-based budgets assume that no program or unit will automatically continue in the next year. Another important element of zero-based budgeting is that one must prepare budget projections for more than one alternative level and type of service. These different budget projections with their accompanying justifications are called *decision packages* and make it possible to make decisions each year about the best expenditure of scarce resources. A major disadvantage to zero-based budgeting is the time required to prepare the decision packages. Whether organizations choose to use this budgeting process is based on their estimation of the value to be gained by the additional time and expense of preparing decision packages.

Greer and Wanamaker (1996) point out that when planning future services, the only costs that are important to consider are those that are relevant to the proposed new services. Agencies that have cost accounting information systems in place are better able to identify relevant costs than those without such systems. Cost accounting information systems make it possible to separate the costs of providing service into variable, fixed, and mixed costs. Variable costs change in direct proportion to the amount of service provided, such as the cost of dressing supplies for a home care patient requiring wound care. Fixed costs do not change with the amount of service provided, but are "sunk" (Greer & Wanamaker, 1996, p. 60) costs, such as the cost of leasing the building in which the home care agency is housed. Mixed costs contain some elements that are variable and some that are fixed (Box 21-2).

This is important because fixed costs are often not relevant to making decisions about accepting new contracts or providing new services. As a result, some new services that may not appear to be financially viable when analyzing total costs may actually generate more revenues than the expenses required to support them once the fixed costs have been disregarded.

In the Employee Wellness Program example (Box 21-1), the costs of staff time are fixed, because those staff will be employed on an annual, salaried basis. Costs of supplies and equipment maintenance that are directly related to the number of patients served are variable costs. Costs of utilities are mixed, because some utilities will be used no matter how many patients are served, although some increase in utility usage will occur as more patients are served (e.g., water, electricity). If ABC Company receives an offer to contract with another branch, for example, DEF Company, to allow DEF's employees to use the wellness program, the only costs

---

B O X   2 1 - 2

Budget for Healthy Living Home Care Program, Fiscal Year 1998-1999

Revenues

Private pay	$100,000
Third party reimbursement	775,000
Local government grant	125,000
Charitable contributions	50,000
TOTAL	$1,050,000

Expenses

Direct expenses	
Salaries	$500,000
Fringe benefits	10,000
Supplies	75,000
Equipment and maintenance	80,000
Travel	20,000
Office lease	80,000
Indirect expenses	
Administration	55,000
Utilities	50,000
Environmental services	30,000
TOTAL	900,000
Excess of revenues over expenses	$150,000

---

that need to be taken into account when pricing the service are those that are variable. This is because the fixed costs have already been covered by the original funding and will not change.

Variance Analysis This is a strategy for monitoring resource consumption that complements the budgeting process. Because budgets are used both for planning and for monitoring, it is important to use a systematic approach to achieve both goals. Analyzing variations of actual resource use from planned resource use is a component of monitoring the budget. It is simple to review a variance report, such as the example in Table 21-1, and identify areas where resource use is above or below that which was

TABLE 21-1

Variance Report for the Employee Wellness Program, ABC Company, First Quarter, 1998-1999

Item	Actual	Budget	Variance
Salaries	27,250	25,000	(1,250)
Fringe Benefits	5,450	5,000	(450)
Supplies	3,000	2,500	(500)
Equipment	10,000	18,750	8,750
Administration	2,750	3,000	250
Utilities	1,450	1,500	50
Environmental	1,000	750	(250)
TOTAL	40,900	46,450	6,600

predicted. It is more difficult, however, to determine why that occurred and whether the variation represents a problem that should be corrected. For example, Table 21-1 shows that the variance in *actual* expenditures from *planned* expenditures for the months of July, August, and September (assuming a July 1 to June 30 fiscal year) was $6600 below budget for the Employee Wellness Program. This is determined by adding the positive (below budget) and negative (over budget) variations noted in the last column. Negative variances are indicated by parentheses. At first glance, this might appear to be excellent management of resources. However, note the parts of the budget that varied from what was planned.

Less money was spent on equipment than expected. This may have occurred because a new piece of equipment, such as a computerized exercise machine, had not yet been purchased. If this piece of equipment was a key part of a new exercise program, spending less than intended in this category of the budget may not be an indication of quality service. On the other hand, more was spent on salaries and fringe benefits than intended. This may have been because service volume was up and staff worked overtime

to manage the volume. Rather than being an indication of poor resource management, it may represent prudent allocation of resources in line with service volume.

When analyzing budget variances, nurses should be aware of three general causes of variation: wage rate (or price) variances; use (or quantity) variances; and volume variances (Finkler & Kovner, 1993). Wage rate (or price) variances occur because the cost of raw materials used in providing a service or producing goods was higher than expected. For example, the wages paid to staff may have been higher than expected at the beginning of the budget cycle because a shortage developed in the local labor market. The prices of supplies may also have risen related to market conditions. Staff may have been scheduled for overtime, resulting in variation from the originally planned use of that "raw material." More supplies may have been used than planned, which represents a quantity variation from what was planned for use of that particular raw material. If negative variances in either of these areas occurred because of faulty forecasting or inefficiency, action should be taken to improve the situation. On the other hand, if variations occurred because of labor market conditions outside of a manager's control, it may be difficult to correct the situation unless a totally new approach is taken, such as job redesign.

If service volume variance was above or below predictions, different responses are appropriate. In a fee-for-service environment, service volume higher than predicted is usually desirable and suggests that the budget should be adjusted to reflect the increase. In a capitated environment, service volume that is higher than predicted may not be desirable, although many different factors must be considered when analyzing the situation. Higher-than-predicted service volume in a health promotion program such as the Employee Wellness Program in this example is likely to be viewed positively even in a capitated environment because of the desired reduction in expenditures for sick time and lost productivity. The key to variance analysis is analyzing which factors may be causing budget variances, whether any corrective actions should be taken, or whether budget variances suggest that program design should be reevaluated.

Cost Management

Clinical Issues Cost management in times of rapid change and uncertainty can lead to difficult clinical issues. A focus on cost control as a first priority can reduce clinical quality. Nurses should emphasize the provision of high quality care in a fiscally prudent manner, rather than emphasize only cost control. There are two reasons for this: (1) it is unethical to allow quality to deteriorate simply for the sake of cost control; and (2) if quality deteriorates, the agency will not be able to compete in a managed care environment. A major clinical issue is that it is often difficult to determine what costs are associated with providing particular nursing services and what factors influence those costs. Without this information, efforts to manage costs will be ineffective. This section proposes strategies for dealing with both of these clinical issues.

Administrative changes can facilitate cost management while promoting quality clinical care. Lowe (1996, p. 17) notes "as we strive to improve quality with fewer resources, attention must be directed to the processes of care and the systems that support the providers" (Sovie, 1995). St. Joseph Healthcare System in Albuquerque, New Mexico (Lowe, 1996) initiated a series of changes in a nursing organization designed to reduce unplanned variations in the processes of care. Seven strategies were implemented:

1. Establishing shared governance across the nursing services in all four hospitals in the system
2. "Layering patient care" (Lowe, 1996, p. 15) by acuity levels
3. Establishing core clinical competencies for nursing staff and unique competencies for selected patient populations
4. Developing clinical pathways for common problems and clinical protocols for more complex chronic health problems
5. Reengineering patient care to a modified team approach, including multiskilled technicians and allied health therapists on the teams (e.g., physical therapists, dietitians, respiratory therapists)
6. Developing multiple patient education strategies to foster self-care, including use of booklets and videos
7. Including physician concerns and preferences in clinical pathways and improvements in administrative efficiencies.

Although most of these strategies have been described elsewhere (e.g., see Chapter 5 for a description of shared governance), the concept of layered patient care was a unique approach to planning for nursing resources. This approach is highly patient-centered, involving organization of patient care units around needs for care. Box 21-3 illustrates the layers and examples of clinical areas included within each layer. Nurse staffing requirements were based on patient acuity.

Fiscal strategies can complement modifications in processes of care. A new approach to accounting can be used to help manage costs of clinical care by more accurately identifying those factors responsible for inefficiencies. This makes it possible to change processes of care to enhance efficiency.

Activity-based Cost Management This type of management (McKeon, 1996; Storfjell & Jessup, 1996) focuses on determining the costs of specific services based on the factors that drive service processes to be more or less efficient. Knowing the factors that drive costs or improve clinical outcomes is the first step toward prudent cost management. The framework for activity-based costing is depicted in Figure 21-3.

In this framework, the vertical axis indicates the steps involved in cost finding, whereas the horizontal axis indicates cost management strategies (McKeon, 1996). The first step in cost finding is to pool the resources associated with a particular function or department, such as nursing service. These resources may include people, space, or equipment (Storfjell & Jessup, 1996). For example, if the cost of the nursing staff in a school health clinic is $120,000, that amount would go into the resource pool.

The next step is to identify the major factors that increase or decrease use of that particular resource. These factors are called *resource drivers*. The major resource drivers for the use of nursing staff are time spent with or on behalf of patients, wage rate, and number of patients (Storfjell & Jessup, 1996). Next, one identifies the primary activities involved in providing services within that unit, program, or department. In the case of a school clinic, one major activity is obtaining parental permission to treat the children.

Factors that cause the cost of that activity to vary include preparation of letters of permission and follow-up to nonrespondents. These factors are referred to as *activity drivers*. Time involved in preparation of letters of permission varies by the language and educational level of the parents. Time involved in follow-up to nonrespondents varies by whether the school has an accurate address for the family or whether the family has a permanent address (compared with living temporarily with friends or in migrant camps or shelters). The activity drivers influence the final cost objective, which in this case would be the total cost of providing care to children in the school health clinic. Once these total costs have been determined, it is possible to identify those factors that drive the costs of individual activities higher and to design strategies to manage the costs of the activities. In a school health clinic,

B O X   2 1 - 3

Layered Patient Care at St. Joseph Healthcare System

Layers of Care	Examples of Clinical Areas Included
Intensive care	Intensive care units
Monitored care	Critical care, telemetry
Diagnostic care	Short stay (72 hr medical/surgical)
Transitional care	Skilled nursing
Subacute care	Rehabilitation, geropsychiatric care
Ambulatory care	Home health, emergency, ambulatory clinics

Modified from Lowe, A. (1996). Reducing variation in patient care: Nursing responds to capitation. *Journal of Nursing Administration, 26*(1), 16.

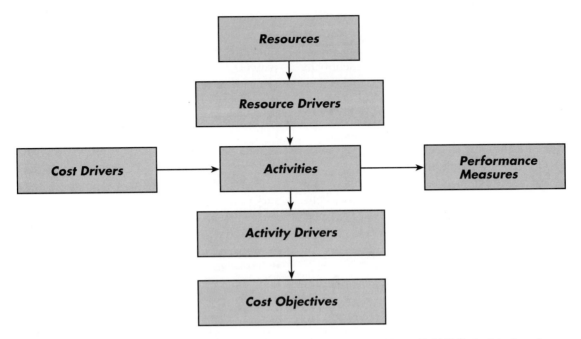

Figure 21-3 ■ **Conceptual framework for an ABCM system.** (From McKeon, T. [1996]. Activity-based management: A tool to complement and quantify continuous quality improvement efforts. *Journal of Nursing Care Quality, 10*[2], 18.)

there will be many activities. Other activities include providing care to faculty, staff, and families, outreach and case finding, and providing health education and group screening programs.

The horizontal axis in Figure 21-3 illustrates the cost management aspect of ABCM. Cost drivers are those factors that "caused the activity to take place" (McKeon, 1996, p. 21). In the example of obtaining parental permission to treat, one cost driver would be new children enrolling in the school. An additional cost driver would be the presence of an emergency health problem in a child without a previously signed permission slip. Performance measures may be financial or nonfinancial and reflect outputs (rather than outcomes) of the particular activity. Examples might be the rate of completed permission slips (whether permission is granted or

not) or the proportion of respondents who grant permission to treat their children. Using ABCM, nurses would work with an interdisciplinary team to determine the relevant performance measures and then identify the cost drivers and activity drivers that could be improved upon. This forms the framework for cost management and for changing processes of care to enhance efficiency.

Nurses Controlling Costs Nurses can help control costs by being cost conscious when using resources and by streamlining processes of nursing care to maximize inclusion of the latest research findings into models of evidence-based practice. For example, home health nurses might work with their patients to plan dressing changes carefully to conserve resources. If a family pet habitually ruins a sterile field, advance planning can manage this problem. The home health nurse can also draw upon research findings indicating when sterile technique is unnecessary and clean technique is appropriate, thereby reducing the need for more expensive supplies.

Cost Effectiveness

Cost-Effectiveness Analysis This refers to comparing the costs and outcomes of a service or program with the costs and outcomes of an alternative program designed to achieve the same goals (Stanhope, 1996). Essentially, one is trying to find the least-cost alternative to achieving desired goals. Often, people speak of cost-effectiveness analysis as if the goal were simply to reduce costs. This is not the case: "the objective of a cost-effectiveness analysis is to rank alternative treatments on the basis of cost per unit of output or outcome" (Jacobs, 1997, p. 371). Cost-efficiency analysis, by comparison, is used to compare program costs only (Stanhope, 1996). Cost effectiveness can be expressed by the following ratio (Jacobs, 1997, p. 371):

$$\frac{(EC_2 - EC_1)}{(EQ_2 - EQ_1)}$$

In this ratio, the numbers *1* and *2* refer to two alternative treatments or programatic approaches to achieving the same goals. *EC* is the expected cost, and *EQ* is the expected quantity of output (e.g., numbers of patients served) or outcome (e.g., the proportion of patients who quit smoking for at least 3 months). Each number in the ratio reflects the probability of a particular cost or outcome and therefore varies from *0* to *1.0.*

Budgets in Cost-Effectiveness Analysis Budgets are critical tools for cost-effectiveness analysis because they contain lists of all expenditures and can be used to formulate the numerator in the equation. Program or service goals are used to develop the denominator.

■ HUMAN RESOURCES
Human Capital Theory

Human capital is an economic theory that purports that employees are assets of an organization, like other resources (money, supplies, facilities) because they have a high economic value. Employees' assets are the knowledge and skills that they bring to the work environment. As with any other asset, the employee asset deteriorates over time as new technology emerges. To enhance the asset of the employee, retooling, retraining, or updating must occur as organizational environmental changes occur. "Human capital economics is a system of 'inputs,' 'processes,' 'outputs,' and 'adjustments'. . . made to increase the potential and performance . . . human resources contribute to . . . employers and self" (Odiorne, 1984, p. 25; Swansburg, 1996, pp. 35-37).

When nurses join an organization, they bring to the work force an *asset portfolio* that is added to the *human capital portfolio* of the organization. The asset portfolio includes the "inputs" of the nurse: education, experience, certifications, skills. The employer provides for a "process" to involve the nurse with the organization and to enhance the nurse's knowledge and skills, such as orientation and continuing education. The nurse then provides "outputs" to the organization, such as competent or expert practice (Swansburg, 1996).

In recruiting and employing a nurse, the organization considers the human capital portfolio and how the nurse's asset portfolio fits with the mission and goals of the organization. The organization's goals include establishing a productive and stable work force who will provide the skills needed to meet the goals of the organization in the long term (Swansburg, 1996).

Human Resources as Catalysts for Change

Change is ever present in the current environment, especially in the work environment where human resources are essential to making change happen. Change often results in disagreement, confusion, inaccurate perceptions, uncertainty, resistance, frustration, threatened self-interest, anger, and stress for individual employees. Such responses in individual employees (human resources) create additional responsibilities for nurse leaders. Initially, change results in apathy and lack of motivation; therefore the nurse leader should accept the challenge to motivate other staff for action (Greene, 1997; Hein & Nicholson, 1986).

Greene (1997) suggests that a leader can motivate others to action by exhibiting energy and enthusiasm for the change and by directly talking with employees. She suggests the leaders complete a self-assessment to first determine their own level of motivation for change by the following:

- Assessing what it is that stimulates them to complete a task
- Assessing their self-leadership capabilities
- Analyzing their level of tolerance for change
- Analyzing their level of patience with others during the change process
- Analyzing their ability to control their own emotions

The nurse leader who conveys enthusiasm for change can challenge other employees to use their abilities to create the change. To effect change, nurses should be risk takers and committed to the change, and they must be competent nurses as well as leaders (Hein & Nicholson, 1986).

Figure 21-4 depicts a model for planned change that outlines a process to be used to assist all employees to become catalysts for change. It is evident in this model that anyone within an organization can recognize a need for change. The nurse who sees the need for change analyzes the need and assists all who are to be involved in the change to understand the need (target groups). If the target group is willing to assist in making the change, plans must also be made for evaluating the change. If the target group resists, new plans must be developed for reintroducing the needed change (Hein & Nicholson, 1986).

Investment in Human Capital

One of the largest investments an organization makes is in its human resources. This investment can be measured in terms of dollar value. A change in the value of the employee can be measured over time by (1) the number of dollars spent to recruit, pay, orient, and develop the employee through staff development, continuing education, or formal education and (2) the employee's output in performance. Nursing leadership can increase the value of nurses by creating a market demand for nurses with differing cognitive as well as technical skill levels through such practices as differentiated practice models, participative management, career development, and job enrichment programs for nurses. An effective organization will work toward attaining a highly productive work force based on recruiting, retraining, and developing nurses who can assist the organization in meeting its future needs (Swansburg, 1996).

A number of approaches are used by organizations to recruit staff, including advertising, career days, open houses, professional recruiters, and employee referrals. The most effective forms of recruitment are employee referral and other informal methods such as self-referral and rehire of former employees. These informal methods provide the organization with employees who tend to remain with the organization the longest (Gillies, 1994; Swansburg, 1996; Harris, 1994; Kongstvedt, 1989; Sullivan & Decker, 1988).

In selecting persons for a job the nurse leader will want to match the job with the individual's asset portfolio. Today, an organization's human resource department (or personnel department) is involved in recruiting and hiring of staff. However, the nurse leader will want to be involved in the selection process because a personal commitment to the new employee develops if the nurse leader chooses the applicant to "fit" the job. It also gives applicants an opportunity to ask specific job-related questions and assess the environment in which they will be working.

The most important tool used in the recruiting process is the interview. The interview is a reciprocal interaction between the nurse leader (hiring nurse) and the applicant (candidate). The nurse leader uses the interview to create a positive image of the work setting and to assess the applicant's ideas, accomplishments, knowledge, and skills. Conversely the applicant is as-

sessing the interviewer's abilities as a leader (Gillies, 1994). Box 21-4 gives an overview of the applicant's and the nurse leader's approach to the interview (Swansburg, 1996).

Retention and *development* of staff are critical aspects of managing human resources. The first 6 to 12 months are critical for both the employer and the nurse because each is involved in establishing a mutually satisfactory working relationship. The following provide an environment in which the new employee may achieve satisfaction with the work environment (Harris, 1994):

• Adequate orientation with participation by senior staff
• Training in new skills and abilities required for the job

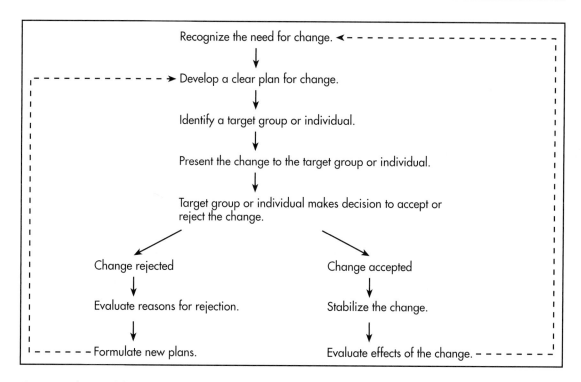

Figure 21-4 ▪ Model for the introduction of planned change. (From Hein, E., & Nicholson, M. [1986]. *Contemporary leadership behavior: Selected readings.* Boston: Little, Brown.

BOX 21-4

The Interview Interaction

The Hiring Nurse	The Candidate
1. Gives information about job and institution.	1. Gives information about self.
2. Assesses competencies the candidate possesses in relation to job opening.	2. Assesses opportunity for developing and using competencies.
3. Evaluates candidate's personal characteristics in relation to staff members with whom candidate will work (fit to staff).	3. Assesses ability to relate to employees with whom candidate will work.
4. Assesses candidate's potential to move organization toward its goals.	4. Assesses potential for achieving personal career goals.
5. Assesses candidate's enthusiasm and state of health.	5. Assesses institution's climate and employee morale.
6. Forms impressions about candidate—behavior, appearance, ability to communicate, confidence, intelligence, personality.	6. Assesses opportunities for promotion and success.
7. Assesses candidate's ability to do job.	7. Assesses own ability to do the job.
8. Determines facts about candidate.	8. Determines facts about organization and working conditions.

From Swansburg, R. (1996). *Management and leadership for nurse managers* (2nd ed). Sudbury, Mass.: Jones & Bartlett, p. 130.

- Assignment of a mentor who can provide support and answer questions
- On-going discussion between the nurse leader and the employee
- Continuous encouragement and support by the leader and fellow employees

The leading cause of turnover in an organization is job dissatisfaction resulting from money concerns, recognition, scheduling responsibility, and stress. Turnover is expensive for the organization, costing up to $50,000 per year for the costs of hiring, orientation, salary, temporary employees, overtime, lost revenue from low productivity of new employees, and staff morale. Thus it is less costly to put into place a program that will encourage new and continuing employees to stay in the work environment as productive members.

Retention is enhanced by the following (Harris, 1994; Swansburg, 1996):

- Offering advancement opportunities within the workplace
- Providing fair and equitable salaries for similar jobs
- Training and development opportunities
- Recognizing the contributions of employees
- Participative management
- Employee counseling
- Open discussions
- Offering extended benefits to families, such as childcare, eldercare

To increase the human capital portfolio of the organization, to enhance the asset portfolio of the nurse, and to retain a quality work force, the employer and the nurse will want to work together to provide for the continuing develop-

Key terms

Term	Definition
Variance analysis	Strategy for monitoring resource consumption that complements the budgeting process; analyzes variations between resources used and the planned use of resources
Activity-based cost management	Way to determine the costs of specific services based on factors that drive service processes to be more or less efficient; includes cost finding and cost management
Human capital	Economic theory that says employees are assets of an organization just like any other resource, e.g., money, supplies, facilities, because they have high economic value
Clinical ladder	Horizontal development system in health care whereby professionals can be promoted without moving out of their clinical roles
Career ladder	Vertical development system that offers nurses career advancement opportunities in management, administration, teaching, and research
Compensation	Comes in many forms including salary, benefits including health and disability insurance, retirement funds, bonuses, employee stock options, childcare, and eldercare

ment of the nurse throughout the nurse's career. A planned organizational program of employee development may include orientation, internships, career mobility ladders, inservice education, management development, mentoring, continuing education, and formal education options (Gillies, 1994; Sullivan & Decker, 1988; Swansburg, 1996).

The orientation as previously discussed is to assist new employees in getting involved immediately in their jobs and to ensure that new employees are safe and competent in practice. The content of the orientation depends on the job requirements and includes a review of the strengths, the policies and procedures of the organization, and familiarizing the employee with the facility and other staff. Nurse internships are becoming more popular and in some states are required before the new graduate or a nurse changing to a new specialty may practice autonomously (Texas, 1997). The internship is a period of closely supervised assessment to ensure safe and effective nursing practice. The internship may be for a defined period of time or until such time as the nurse leader has assessed the nurse to be ready for autonomous practice (Gillies, 1994; Sullivan & Decker, 1988; Swansburg, 1996).

Career or clinical ladders offer the nurse an opportunity to attain promotions within clinical nursing. The clinical ladder is described as a "horizontal development system" with specific criteria for evaluating nurses' performance while allowing them to remain in the clinical setting. The career ladder is a "vertical system" that offers the nurse opportunities other than in the clinical area, such as management, administrative, teaching, and research. A clinical ladder improves nursing care and motivates nurses to pursue educational goals and develop career goals and rewards them with money, benefits, recognition, and job satisfaction. The clinical ladder may begin at a level of *beginner* or *novice* and advance through several stages (levels) to *expert* nurse, with well-defined experience and education, skills and knowledge, and supervision requirements at each level (Gillies, 1994; Sullivan & Decker, 1988; Swansburg, 1996).

Inservice education differs from continuing education and is a common development activity within organizations. Inservice programs are designed to inform nurses about new procedures, new treatment techniques, the operation of new equipment, new organizational services, and any changes in organizational structure and job functions (Gillies, 1994; Sullivan & Decker, 1988; Swansburg, 1996).

Management development is an educational activity designed to assist nurse managers in developing new skills and to assist them in accurately assessing and evaluating, making quality decisions, taking effective action, and confronting and solving real problems. Management development can be a vertical system approach for providing upward mobility to nurses within an organization (Gillies, 1994; Sullivan & Decker, 1988; Swansburg, 1996).

Mentoring is a process by which a new staff nurse and a senior staff nurse are paired together to promote the professional achievement of the new nurse. Mentoring is only successful when there is a suitable match between the mentor's style and the new nurse's needs. Both individuals benefit from the mentoring relationship. The mentor teaches, guides, advocates, counsels, promotes self-confidence, serves as role model, seeks opportunities, and recommends the new nurse to others. As the nurse progresses in a career, the nurse then rewards the mentor by recommending him or her to others for honors and awards, promoting the mentor's ideas, and promoting the mentor as consultant or speaker (Gillies, 1994; Sullivan & Decker, 1988; Swansburg, 1996).

Continuing education is a system external to the organization that is designed to assist the nurse to meet career goals for life-long learning. Unlike inservice, or *staff development* as it is often called, the employer's needs are secondary and the nurse's needs are the primary reason for participating in classes, workshops, institutes, or individualized instruction. Organizations may offer continuing education programs within their facilities or may send the nurse to offerings outside the organization. Because continuing education is primarily for the nurse, the organization may or may not pay for this type of development. However, as with formal education, which may lead to additional educational degrees, these two forms of education add to the nurse's asset portfolio, thus making the nurse a valuable member of the organization. Because of this, some employers provide for tuition/registration reimbursement for these activities. A plan for career development within an organization includes a combination of the above activities and strategies for personnel to be promoted horizontally or vertically within the organization (Gillies, 1994; Sullivan & Decker, 1988; Swansburg, 1996).

A career planning and development program that includes an assessment of how the individual nurse functions best is essential to the nurse's *motivation* to perform at a high level. The nurse leader, who is familiar with motivation theories, can use such information to negotiate with the nurse to act; however, it is the nurses' choice to help meet the organization's goals. Some nurses are motivated by extrinsic rewards, such as recognition, benefits, money, awards, and group "norm" behaviors, whereas others are intrinsically motivated by goal achievement, perceptions of their work environment, attitudes, and equality of treatment.

Integrity, energy, the ability to negotiate, and sensitivity provide for an environment of self-motivation. Motivation is said to involve the emotions rather than logic; therefore it is important to assess the nurse's feelings, wants, desires, and personal expectations as well as skills and abilities that he or she brings to the job. With this information the nurse leader can establish a motivating environment for the nurse by the following (Gillies, 1994; Swansburg, 1996; Harris, 1994):

- Building a career development program with the nurse
- Sharing information about the organization
- Encouraging teamwork
- Sharing appreciation and respect for the nurse's work
- Recognizing the work of others
- Assisting the nurse to meet career goals
- Providing for job enrichment
- Providing rewards for teamwork, innovations, and creativity
- Involving the nurse in the development of the mission and goals of the organization

Compensation for quality performance comes in many forms: salary, benefits such as eldercare or childcare, employee stock options (ESOPS), bonuses, and retirement funds. The system of compensation is one of financial rewards based on measured levels of productivity that benefit the organization in increased capacity to deliver services or in cost savings, both of which are important to managed care systems. A well-planned system of compensation will establish productivity measures, including persons' hours to provide care, number of encounters, or patients seen, cost of supplies used, and the length of the encounter (number of days in hospital, number of visits). Savings to the system results in bonuses or other benefits for the nurse. Such a plan can motivate nurses to a high level of productivity as long as they feel that the compensation is related to preparation and responsibility and is comparable with others in a similar job category. Inequity in these factors causes dissatisfaction, lack of motivation, and turnover.

Competency Issues: Retooling the Work Force for the Future

To assess competence effectively one must be able to define that which is incompetent. The National Commission for Health Care Certifying Agencies (1991) has suggested that incompetencies are demonstrated through repeatedly improper acts, rather than examination failures or lack of continuing education. The competent professional performs work accurately, makes correct judgments, and interacts with other professionals effectively. Competence is demonstrated and maintained through one's practicing life. Competence is the application of knowledge and the interpersonal decision-making and psychomotor skills expected for the practice role. It is characterized fundamentally as judgment and wise action in complex and uncertain situations with conflicting values and ethical stances. In addition to knowledge, skills, and abilities, one is competent when one can reflect and make critical decisions through decision-making analysis. It is the obligation of licensed practitioners such as nurses to commit to the educational and professional qualifications for practice initially and, as continuing clinicians, to practice competently and safely throughout their career.

Continuing competency is placed in the context of risk management and having mechanisms in place in an organization to reduce the risk of harm to patients. The assurance of competency is a partnership between individual practitioners and the employer. Initially individuals have the burden of proof, showing that they have met entry-level requirements for nursing through the educational process. In continuing competency the burden shifts to those who conduct the approval process to show why individuals have or no longer desire the approval previously granted. Competency is initially evaluated through licensure. In continuing competency a number of factors go into evaluation, including additional educational degrees, certification, and employer evaluation.

All nurses must meet generalist core competencies for professional entry and a set of specialized core competencies as they continue in practice, especially if they are moving vertically on the career ladder. The health care system currently has two models for assuring nurses' competency: a proactive model and a reactive model. The proactive model provides nurses a number of options by which to maintain and to assess their competency. All options become a part of a professional portfolio, which in this chapter is referred to as the nurse's *asset portfolio*. First, nurses can engage in self-assessment to identify self-strengths and weaknesses. The self-assessment includes a reflective statement, critically evaluating the nurse's own practice. In addition, the professional portfolio may include on-the-job clinical competency evaluations, skill evaluations, a resumé to show career progress, certifications for specialty areas of practice, publications, and research activities. Also included in the portfolio will be agency evaluations of performance, productivity, and peer evaluations. The formal learning process and continuing education are part of the activities that nurses engage in to assure continued competency. As in the career development plan, continuing education and university courses should be directed toward clinically relevant practice. Finally, the professional portfolio may include a competence improvement plan, which includes stated goals and objectives of the nurse for future development, activities to meet the goals and objectives, and how the nurse would like the activities to be evaluated to determine whether the goals and objectives of the plan have been met. The nurse may engage in such activities as computer-simulated reviews, evaluation of clinical practice, or review of charts by peers and managers for appropriate documentation and outcomes related to the nurse's plan of care for the patient (Citizens Advocacy Center, 1996).

The reactive model of evaluation of competency is currently in place and involves interventions based on evidence of a nurse's incompetence. This model relies on evaluation of the nurse's clinical practice by peers, managers, and patients. Continuing education is usually a requirement of this model. In many states there is a required reporting relationship between boards of nursing and clinical organizations, as well as a voluntary reporting relationship between boards of nursing and certifying organizations. The current system provides discipline based on errors made by the nurse in a practice. Discipline is given either by the organization or by the board of nursing in the state in which the nurse is licensed (Citizens Advocacy Center, 1996).

Competency assessment is mandated by boards of nursing, certifying bodies, and voluntary credentialing organizations such as the Joint Commission on Accreditation of HealthCare Organizations. In establishing a competency assessment system for a nurse, the nurse's rights must be balanced with the rights of the patient for protection from incompetent practice. The nurse has the right to know what is expected in the job situation. If incompetent practice seems to be occurring, the nurse has the right to a full, fair hearing and due process and a usable and credible training program to correct the problem. Conversely, the patient has the right to a speedy process and review to protect him or her from harm or incompetent practice. Organizations that undertake continuing competency assessments must recognize their own liability and responsibility for the validity and reliability of the assessment. They must be able to defend the point that an individual is deemed competent or incompetent. In the validity evaluation they must be able to identify the weaknesses in knowledge, skills, abilities, and performance that seriously impair a nurse's functioning. In assessing reliability the organization must consistently evaluate all nurses in the same manner, with minimal variation in the methods.

A goal for competency evaluation must be established within an organization. If the goal is remediation, a professional portfolio will assist in establishing the strengths and weaknesses of the work force and in the design of a program to fit the needs of individuals to enhance their competency within their job situation. If the goal is removal, the pattern of behavior of the nurse must be established over time and reported to the appropriate administrator of the organization or to the appropriate regulatory body. It is essential that nurses have a commitment to continued competency. If nurses follow a career development program, they will be professionally mobile throughout their career and will be able to move from one position to another and from one state to another. This involves keeping up with current knowledge and skills and practicing state-of-the-art nursing. It has been noted by the Pew Foundation Health Professions Commission that the needs of health care delivery are changing. Although the nursing profession has a solid tradition in expanding its responsibilities to meet the needs of the health care delivery system and patients, nurses of the future need to be trained in diagnostic and therapeutic technology, information management, patient demand management, and community-based practice to meet the needs of the general population. Nurses also need to be aware of cost-effective and consumer-responsive care. Nursing will increasingly focus on the skills of collaboration, effective communication, and team work as they learn to work in multidisciplinary groups and differentiate nursing practice roles in order to emphasize evaluating the impact on patients.

It is essential that organizations do more focused planning to project the needs for a future workplace and to provide education, training, and appropriate distribution within the health care system. This will require the establishment of work force guidance, determining the appropriate numbers and kinds of nursing personnel needed and offering short-term programs for retooling nurses, as services within the health care delivery system change. In addition, such a program should include monitoring and evaluating the short-term and long-term effectiveness of the policies and the changing work force needs.

To implement a work force plan the organization will want to consider incentive programming such as loan repayments, scholarships, tuition reimbursement, and work release so that nurses will be retrained for the positions most needed in an organization.

Employee Relations in Times of Change

The organizational climate and the behavior of the nurse leader will make a difference when changes occur within an organization. The nurse leader can assist employees find change stimulating by providing an awards system for employees for creative, innovative ideas even when the intended results may not be as they were originally planned. A nurse leader can encourage employees and reward independent actions and critical thinking and problem solving. When an organization's goals and objectives are behaviorally defined and quantified and activities clearly outlined to meet the objectives, nurse leaders can monitor performance based on known expectations from outlined goals, objectives, and activities. Employee assignments can be designed so they fit with the work plan and behavioral expectations will be known by the worker.

Change does not occur spontaneously but is suggested by someone or some environmental force inside or outside a system. Therefore employees can be involved in the development for change, resulting in a less negative response to such change. Through involvement, staff and managers can define their roles within the organization and adjust their behaviors based on the total system needs for change. Reactions to change and resistance are natural processes and are proportional to the employee's investment in the current system. For example, if the employee was hired into an agency with a specific organizational structure and management style, the employee may be satisfied with how the system works and therefore may attempt to block any changes. In addition, if a proposed change seems to be directed at bringing in a new philosophic approach, for example, moving from team nursing to primary nursing, the new approach may be misunderstood and therefore staff resist the change. Detailed information regarding the new approach is essential to get the staff to buy into such a change. Any change that threatens the viability of an employee group within the organization is subject to resistance. Such groups provide informal power to employees, and they may feel they are being blamed for belonging to a group. A change in a group as a result of organization change may be seen as punishment from administration. A threat to group membership based on relationships of common beliefs and values is a threat to the self-interest of the employee.

Overt behavior of personnel within a change situation may involve open hostility, silence, or false acceptance. Reactions to change are often related to the depth of the change within the organization. For example, total agency structure change may result in a major resistance to such change. Employee acceptance to change may be gained through the following:

- Starting the change process with top executives
- Engaging in exciting strategies for implementing change
- Providing information in advance to all employees, especially those affected
- Involving all employees in the planning and implementation

- Providing feedback when problems occur in the change process
- Making adjustments as needed to affect smooth change
- Protecting the autonomy of the individual employee

■ INFORMATION MANAGEMENT

As discussed in Chapter 22, today's health care delivery system requires a mechanism for handling large information data bases for controlling operations within the system, as well as within subsystems, such as nursing. These information systems are usually referred to as *information management systems.* These are computerized processes whereby conversations or written materials can be added regularly regarding patient, financial, or personnel information, as well as management decisions. Such a system allows for transmission of information more reliably and efficiently than through the multiple unlinked computer systems usually found within an organization. There are several purposes for such a system (Gillies, 1994; Swansburg, 1996):

- To make relevant patient data available in a usable form so patient care problems can be solved
- To process information to support management functions such as receiving data from departments and supplying data to departments to make policy decisions, operating decisions, as well as patient care decisions
- To provide a comprehensive automated information processing system for all phases of the nursing process
- To develop a care plan for families and patients

Forecasting Information Needs

Management information systems (MIS) have been found to rapidly and accurately manipulate large quantities of data, thereby saving time for the nurse, who can then be deployed to provide direct care services. In multiple studies nurses have been shown to spend about 40% of their time in some form of indirect care including communication and information processing. In a nursing organization a computerized system would be helpful in a number of arenas: to collect, transmit, analyze, and report patient-related, employee-related, and process-related information among the managers, nurses, and families. Such a system could also be used for projecting workload needs, summarizing patient classification data, projecting personnel recruitment, hiring and scheduling, evaluating nursing resource use by patients, monitoring supplies, budgeting, recording payroll, and analyzing quality of care data (Gillies, 1994; Swansburg, 1996).

In addition, computerized systems at the bedside may be used in direct patient care for measuring vital signs, evaluating blood chemistry values, analyzing fluid and nutrient needs, controlling drug infusion therapy, monitoring medication administration, providing nursing care plans, providing a simple method of documentation, and monitoring quality indicators. In addition to those just mentioned, physician's orders may be added to the computerized patient record and then implemented and evaluated by the nurse. A nursing comprehensive system as described above, and usually referred to as *NIS,* may be accessed by voice activation, by writing on the computer screen, or by use of the keyboard (Gillies, 1994; Swansburg, 1996).

In the management information system as a whole, in which the NIS is usually a subsystem, the nurse manager can prepare business letters and memos, develop and refine nursing policies and procedures, analyze data from the NIS system for reports of productivity, prepare staffing schedules and inpatient acuity reports for each day or shift, and analyze cost of nursing care for units of service, depending on the acuity of patients in the various units (Gillies, 1994; Swansburg, 1996).

In addition, the management information system has multiple other uses: forecasting personnel use; tracking outcomes of care; maintaining equipment and supplies inventories; tracking the personnel through their career development programs; establishing, monitoring, and evaluating a recruitment program; and evaluating a human capital portfolio for the organization. Also, GANTT charts may be computerized for implementing new services or for monitoring the progress of activities of programs as described earlier in the chapter (Gillies, 1994; Swansburg, 1996).

Another part of the management information system is that commonly referred to as the *Hospital Information System,* or *HIS,* which processes data related to all patient care services and transmits information to appropriate departments such as nursing, medicine, laboratory, x-ray, dietary, and administration so that multiple efforts can be coordinated for more effective patient care (Gillies, 1994; Swansburg, 1996).

Finally, the module on human resource management is an important part of the overall MIS, integrating personnel payroll as well as cafeteria-style benefits offered to and accepted by the employees (Gillies, 1994; Swansburg, 1996).

To forecast information needs for an organization, representatives from all departments or units of an organization should be represented on the planning committee, including managerial and staff level personnel. To prepare for a MIS the committee should review the agency's current system for types of information and methods for recording and transmitting data to determine what is available and what is lacking in the current system. While determining what is available and needed, the committee should also plan for information storage, processing, and retrieval and select software to meet the identified needs. The three areas that the committee should have available in the overall management information system are hospital or health care agency information system, nursing information system, and human resources management system, as well as software that will assist in identifying areas or collecting data on areas previously described for each of the three systems.

Few nurses have had experience with management information systems. The following tips are offered in the development of a new system (Gillies 1994; Swansburg, 1996):

- Choose software first
- Request software information from several vendors
- Provide vendor with pertinent information about size of agency, number of departments, type of departments, numbers of patients
- Provide information about the capabilities of the system users
- Provide information about other computerized systems within the organization
- Have the planning committee make a site visit to an organization where the selected software has been used
- Observe use of software in a similar organization
- Have vendor install, maintain, and duplicate system information and train personnel
- Have vendor phase out former system

Future Trends in Information Management

Management information systems are growing and developing rapidly, as organizations move on to the information highway. Trends for future automation include automated medical records, artificial intelligence, use of optical disks, and robotics.

The automated medical record and voice interaction for data input were discussed earlier. Use of artificial intelligence would assist in enhancing the process of clinical decision making. Such a system creates a model of reality based

problem-solving, analyzing all the factors that are input about a patient; describes the risks and uncertainties related to alternative interventions; selects a course of action to meet a specific objective; and suggests implementation of selected actions and evaluates the effect of the action. This system model provides a template for nurses to use to structure decision-making problems. As such, NIS provides assessment information about the problem and the computer analyzes the characteristics of the problem and presents possible decision alternatives with advantages and disadvantages of the alternatives. From this information the nurse can then select the best decision for the patient.

Robotics is already being used in surgery for positioning surgical instruments, in laboratories for transporting and placing samples, and in nursing for delivery of supplies and medications. "User friendly" is another trend that is making information technology more accessible and easier to use. Problems are usually solvable with the menu-driven software and help menu. It has become much easier to design self-made programs within hours or days rather than months. These are but a few of the trends that nurses will want to be aware of in preparation for system changes within health care delivery (Gillies, 1994; Swansburg, 1996).

Human Technology Interface: Issues in Adjustment to Information Intensive Systems

Information management systems is a futuristic concept in nursing and health care delivery, and although we can use such systems for a number of work-related activities, systems cannot provide everything. The computer has become a necessary information tool within nursing and health care delivery. It is a necessity in management. Being computer literate is no longer an option but a must for nurses, nursing educational curricula, and in nursing practice. One major concern to all in this age of computers is the accidental or intentional access by persons without right to specific information. Restrictions and security precautions, especially related to patient information, are essential. Essential information can be inadvertently communicated to health care workers, to insurance companies, and to others and used to the detriment of the patient. Likewise, employees' vitaes, health information, academic information, performance evaluations, or disciplinary procedures could be communicated to peers, other managers, and external agency sources who have no right to or responsibility for the information. In making decisions about a management information system, one should think carefully about access to information. What information should be included within the system? How should it be classified so that access can or cannot be limited as is necessary? (Gillies, 1994; Swansburg, 1996).

Computers have changed the way work is done. The pace of work has increased because of the processing of data, and expectations of staff productivity have grown commensurately. Although the expectation is that work and decisions will be error free, this may not always be true. Therefore the nurse must have the expert knowledge to judge whether a decision that is suggested by a computer program, such as an artificial intelligence program, is accurate. Also, communication through e-mail has taken away the human element of interactions. Humans may begin to view each other as inanimate objects and less valued sources of information. Therefore the computer should not be viewed as something that will replace one-on-one human interaction. Interaction is important and provides more flexibility in decision making when working on creative projects and in case conferences in which patient problems are discussed and suggestions regarding resolution of

patient problems are handled. The human interactive process can result in a consensus on the best decision for a patient intervention. As in the use of any knowledge, skill, or ability, there must be a balance (Gillies, 1994; Harris, 1994; Swansburg, 1996).

■ KEY POINTS

- Fiscal resources, human resources, and information resources are the basic building blocks of health services and must be managed prudently to achieve the best outcomes for all stakeholders at the lowest cost.
- Because all resource allocations represent an opportunity cost (i.e., if funds are spent in a particular way or if one's time is invested in a certain manner, funds and time are not available for other investments), professional and advanced practice nurses must evaluate which resource allocations are most likely to yield benefits for patient, family, and community health outcomes.
- A planned and thoughtful approach to resource management is especially important in a hyperturbulent managed care environment.
- Budgets, one method for estimating resource needs, are used to plan, monitor, and evaluate changes in a unit or agency.
- Cost management is more than keeping costs low; rather, it includes strategies to provide quality care in a cost-effective manner that looks at processes and systems of care.
- Employees are one of the richest assets of any organization, and from an economic perspective they are considered human capital.
- Turnover in any organization is expensive, and thus employers try to establish programs that allow their employees to continue to grow and develop and to remain in the organization.
- The use of management information systems is a way to manipulate large amounts of data with the goal of saving nursing time.

■ CRITICAL THINKING QUESTIONS

1. Explain the impact that managed care has had on clinicians' incentives to manage resources wisely.

2. Explain how resource management relates to Donabedian's model of quality.

3. Identify a key activity within your clinical area and, using Figure 21-2, analyze resource drivers, activity drivers, and cost drivers. Determine how a better understanding of these drivers can help improve the efficiency of the particular activity you have identified.

4. Analyze strategies that nurses can use to continue to develop their skills and knowledge bases during times of rapid and unprecedented change. Work together with your classmates to develop a plan for nurses in the midst of organizational restructuring to maintain their sense of energy, vitality, and quest for lifelong learning.

5. Interview the director of clinical information systems at one of your local health care agencies about the key challenges in building, maintaining, and using clinical information systems today. Ask him or her whether the information system incorporates nursing languages for health diagnoses, nursing interventions, and nursing outcomes.

■ REFERENCES

Androwich, I., & Haas, S.A. (1996). Nursing-sensitive outcomes in ambulatory care. *Series on Nursing Administration: Outcomes of effective management practices, 8,* 54-70.

Citizens Advocacy Center. (1996). *Continuing professional competence: What's your vision? A policy development conference.* Washington, D.C.: Author.

Donabedian, A. (1966). Evaluating the quality of medical care. *Milbank Memorial Fund Quarterly, 44*(3), 166-206.

Dreisbach, A.M. (1994). A structured approach to expert financial management: A financial development plan for nurse managers. *Nursing Economics, 12*(3), 131-139.

Felteau, A.L. (1993). Tools and techniques to effect budget neutrality. *Nursing Administration Quarterly, 17*(4), 59-64.

Finkler, S.A., & Kovner, C.T. (1993). *Financial management for nurse managers and executives.* Philadelphia: Saunders.

Fottler, M.D., Hernandez, S.R., & Joiner, C.L. (1994). *Strategic management of human resources* (2nd ed.). Albany, N.Y.: Delmar.

Gillies, D. (1994). *Nursing management: A systems approach.* Philadelphia: Saunders.

Greene, I. (1997). Increasing performance and motivating staff for middle management. *Home Health Care Management & Practice, 9*(4), 31-35.

Greer, O.L., & Wanamaker, J.E. (1996). Cost accounting: Toward a measure of truth. *CARING, Dec.,* 56-62.

Hackey, R.B. (1993). Regulatory regimes and state cost containment programs. *Journal of Health Politics, Policy, and Law, 18*(2), 491-502.

Harris, M. (1994). *Handbook of home health care administration.* Gaithersburg, Md.: Aspen.

Hein, E., & Nicholson, M. (1986). *Contemporary leadership behavior: Selected readings.* Boston: Little, Brown.

Jacobs, P. (1997). *The economics of health and medical care* (4th ed.). Gaithersburg, Md.: Aspen.

Kongstvedt, P. (1989). *The managed health care handbook.* Gaithersburg, Md.: Aspen.

Lowe, A. (1996). Reducing variations in patient care: Nursing responds to capitation. *Journal of Nursing Administration, 26*(1), 14-20.

Marriner-Tomey, A. (1994). *Nursing management.* St. Louis: Mosby.

McKeon, T. (1996). Activity-based management: A tool to complement and quantify continuous quality improvement efforts. *Journal of Nursing Care Quality, 10*(2), 17-24.

Odiorne, G. (1984). *Strategic management of human resources.* San Francisco: Jossey-Bass.

Rogy, M.A., Oldenburg, H.S., Coyle, S., Trousdale, R., Moldawer, L.L., & Lowry, S.F. (1996). Correlation between acute physiology and chronic health evaluation (APACHE) III score and immunological parameters in critically ill patients with sepsis. *British Journal of Surgery, 83*(3), 396-400.

Sovie, M. (1995). Tailoring hospitals for managed care and integrated health systems. *Nursing Economics, 13*(2), 72-83.

Stanhope, M. (1996). Program management. In M. Stanhope & J. Lancaster (Eds.). *Community health nursing: Processes in promoting health of individuals, families, and aggregates* (4th ed.). St. Louis: Mosby.

Stanhope, M. (1997, June). Presentation made at the International Congress of Nursing meeting, Vancouver, B.C., Canada.

Storfjell, J.L., & Jessup, S. (1996). Bridging the gap between finance and clinical operations with activity-based cost management. *Journal of Nursing Administration, 26*(12), 12-17.

Sullivan, E., & Decker, T. (1988). *Effective management in nursing.* Menlo Park, Calif.: Addison Wesley.

Swansburg, R. (1996). *Management and leadership for nurse managers* (2nd ed.). Sudbury, Mass.: Jones & Bartlett.

Texas Board of Nursing administrative regulations, 1997.

USDHHS. (1981). *To assure continuing competence: A report of the National Commission for Health Care Certifying Agencies.* Publication No. HRA81-5. Washington, D.C.: U.S. Government Printing Office.

Nursing Informatics: A Means for Change

Margaret R. Grier and Russell C. McGuire

INTRODUCTION

Nursing informatics is the collection, storage, retrieval, and communication of clinical data. These data form information for nurses to use in patient care, which in turn becomes knowledge for building nursing science and improving health care. Computers and other technologies are useful for acquiring, processing, transforming, and communicating data, information, and knowledge. Because of the focus on managing and processing data to form information and to build knowledge, nursing informatics is essential for making the changes in nursing practice required for the rapidly evolving system of health care in the United States and elsewhere.

> Nursing informatics is a combination of computer science, information science, and nursing science designed to assist in the management and processing of nursing data, information, and knowledge (Graves & Corcoran, 1989, p. 227).

> Nursing informatics is the use of information technologies in relation to those functions within the purview of nursing. . . . Therefore, any use of information technologies by nurses . . . is considered nursing informatics (Hannah et al., 1994, p. 3).

This chapter gives an overview of nursing informatics as an instrument for making changes. This is followed by a description of computer systems for managing, processing, and communicating clinical information. Approaches to computerizing nursing records are presented, and the usefulness of standardizing nursing language is discussed. The chapter ends with brief descriptions of innovative nursing systems. After reading this chapter, you will appreciate the value of nursing informatics and can help change clinical practices with your use of its principles.

1. Analyze the value of nursing informatics in a changing health care environment
2. Describe computerized information systems and how they evolved in health care
3. Develop guides for selecting electronic information systems
4. Design tools for making changes in nursing practice
5. Evaluate strategies for introducing innovations and making organizational changes

■ OVERVIEW

Health care is delivered in dynamic, complex, and ever-changing environments. Changes in medical treatments, regulations for federal and state reimbursement, and public knowledge about making individual and collective health care choices create growing demands for information. Evidenced-based decision making, outcome-focused care, and cost effectiveness depend on information. To respond proactively to these changes and the growing demands for clinical information, computer systems (with varying degrees of success) are being devised to collect, store, retrieve, analyze, and communicate health status and health care information. Manual systems of information have been used for these purposes for years, with distinct disadvantages. Aggregating and analyzing the data in these written records are inefficient and difficult, if not impossible, procedures. These paper-and-pencil records produce the well-known phenomenon of notes in nurses' pockets rather than in patient records, and an over-reliance on the memories of nurses and other care providers. Information technology can aid in collecting, storing, retrieving, and

Key terms	
Term	**Definition**
Nursing data	Particular and distinct units or facts about patients observed, perceived, or gathered by nurses doing patient assessments and seeking patient information
Nursing information	Patient data organized to derive meaning and make diagnostic, care planning, and administrative decisions
Nursing knowledge	Patient information synthesized and tested to identify relationships and to explain and predict outcomes of nursing actions
Nursing database	Collection of patient data arranged to facilitate managing, processing, storing, and retrieving information and knowledge and for managing and evaluating nursing care
Managing data	Documenting, aggregating, organizing, manipulating, and presenting patient information
Processing data	Procedures used to make informed clinical decisions, and to transform nursing data into information and information into knowledge

analyzing patient care data when the systems are based on concepts from informatics. Appropriately designed and deployed computerized systems of information can transform patient care data into clinically relevant and useful information and knowledge.

Health care is information intensive—30% to 40% of nursing time is spent on collecting data and processing information (Jydstrup & Gross, 1966). The time and effort nurses devote to information management show the necessity of making changes in the ways clinical data are acquired, processed, and communicated. Nursing is an information-intensive activity. In an environment of cost containment, data gathering and processing must be focused and efficient. Nurses make many varied and complex decisions. They need to be efficiently and effectively informed if quality care is to be delivered at low cost. New ways for managing information must be devised and developed to support the many clinical, operational, and strategic choices required in nursing practice.

> The computer can significantly increase critical care nursing productivity by reducing the volume of this work (information collection and processing) and by changing the way information flows through the system (McHugh, 1986, p. 294)

New paradigms for managing information are a challenge for the emerging health care industry as a whole, and nursing in particular. Nursing informatics is concerned with organizing and managing data, information, and knowledge (Figure 22-1). The field blends knowledge from a variety of disciplines and is a combination of computer science, information science, and nursing science (Frisse, 1992; Graves & Corcoran, 1989). Informatics has four major functions (Lorenzi et al., 1995) that can help meet the need for more effective and efficient managing of patient care information:

1. Developing methods for the acquisition and presentation of data

2. Structuring representations of data, information, and knowledge
3. Managing changes to optimize the use of information
4. Integrating information from diverse sources (e.g., homes, hospitals, libraries)

■ COMPUTERIZED INFORMATION SYSTEMS

Computerized health care information systems range from very simple, stand-alone personal computers to complex, integrated systems using several remotely connected data processors for data collection and subsequent analysis. No matter how simple or how complex, computerized information systems have several elementary components in common: *hardware* (input devices, central processing units, output devices) and *software* (word processors, spreadsheets, databases, multimedia applications, communication programs, operating system software, and specialized applications). In addition, there are *networks* of computers for use across widely distributed sites.

Computer Hardware

Input Devices The computer operator uses input devices to transfer data and operating instructions from the outside world to the central processing unit of the computer. The following are typical input devices associated with the computer:

- Keyboard
- Terminal
- Video display monitor
- Mouse
- Touch screen and light pen
- Voice recognition device
- Floppy and hard disk drives
- Compact disk drive

These devices electronically transfer data in the form of binary digits (0 and 1) to the central processing unit for mathematical manipulation and

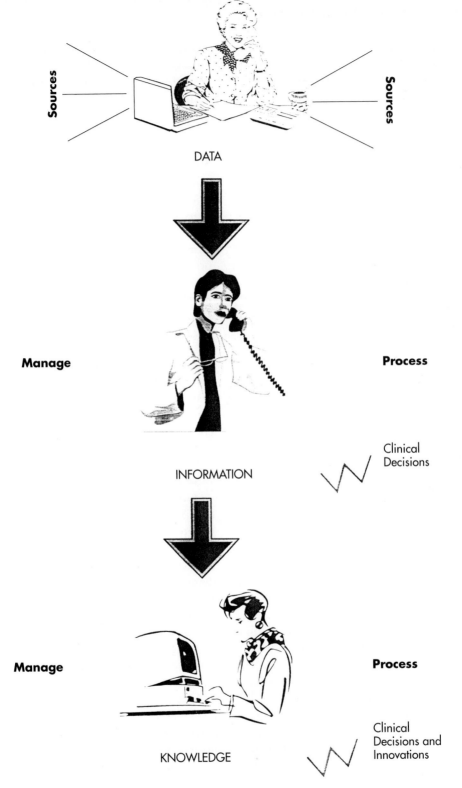

Figure 22-1 ■ For legend see p. 537.

Figure 22-1 ■ Nursing informatics focuses on clinical data, information, and knowledge. Nurses gather clinical data from a variety of sources, including machines. These data are managed and processed using electronic devices and mental processes to produce information for making clinical decisions. The information is transformed into knowledge for making new discoveries about nursing practice as well as for making clinical decisions.

Key terms	
Term	**Definition**
Hardware	Physical devices that provide handling function such as input, processing, storage, or output of computer data
Software	Series of programming statements that perform a specific computer-related application; categories include systems, operating, application, and programming
Network	Devices and software applications that provide communication and data transfer between two or more computer systems
Health care information system	Computer and communication system used by health care providers to collect, process, store, and analyze data

transformation into a form compatible with the user's needs.

Central Processing Unit All processing functions involved in executing a computer's applications are controlled by the central processing unit (CPU). The CPU consists of the control unit, arithmetic logic section, and main memory unit. The control unit monitors and controls all the main functions of the computer through software known as the *operating system.* Examples of operating system software for personal computers include Microsoft's DOS (MS-DOS), Microsoft's Windows, and Apple's MacIntosh Operating System. The CPU controls and coordinates the computer system's operating instructions to provide a smooth flow of binary data within the hardware and associated applications by using soft-

ware programs. The arithmetic logic unit, in coordination with the control unit and the operating system software, performs the necessary mathematical and logic routines for the computer system.

The main memory unit of the CPU is the working memory of the computer. Two types of memory are associated with a computer: the READ-ONLY MEMORY (ROM) and RANDOM-ACCESS MEMORY (RAM). The ROM is the permanent memory of the computer and stores the software used by the CPU to coordinate the internal activities of the computer. This memory cannot be manipulated by the user and usually is set by the computer manufacturer. RAM is the memory associated with running computer application programs (software). This memory can be manipulated by the user and resides in the computer in a way that allows users to run computer programs efficiently. The size of the memory unit varies with the computer type. Typical personal-computer-based information systems have memory sizes ranging from 16 to 64 megabytes (MBs). The complexity of the typical software application to be used is considered when memory size is chosen. With the complexity of operating systems such as Windows 95 and 98, and the capability of personal computers for multitasking several software applications simultaneously (e.g., having the word processor and spreadsheet applications open at the same time), memory size should be at least 32 MBs, with 64 MBs preferred.

Output Devices After data are manipulated within the CPU of a computer, they can be displayed in various forms. Output devices include the following:

- Video display monitors
- Printers, either black/white or color laser, ink jet, and dot matrix
- Graphic image displays
- Magnetic media
- Voice devices

Software

The functionality of a computer is in the application programs or software used to perform tasks. Thousands of software programs and packages are available to the health care professional using a computer. Software programs can be placed in several distinct categories: operating software, word processors, electronic spreadsheets, databases, multimedia-media applications, communication packages, and specialized applications.

Operating System Software This software is critical for the smooth operation of the computer hardware and ancillary peripherals (i.e., input, output, and communication devices). Operating system software uses the hardware to control and coordinate the application software.

The operating system software is responsible for transforming application software code into machine operations that are meaningful to the user. It also is responsible for control of input and output devices such as the keyboard and printer.

The computer uses the operating system and application software to generate data. Often these data are generated in a format for storage and re-use at a later time. To accomplish the task of storing for later retrieval and use, storage devices are used. These devices range in configuration from the floppy disk, usually 3.5 inches and holding 1.44 MBs, to storage devices storing data in the terabyte (TB) range (1 TB = 1 trillion bytes). Typically, storage devices include floppy disks, magnetic tapes, hard disk drives (generally in the gigabyte [GB] range in personal computers to TB sizes in large, multimedia-tasking, corporate information systems), and compact disks.

Word Processors Word processors are software packages used to manipulate written text. Examples of word processing packages include Corel's WordPerfect® and Microsoft's Word®. These applications allow the computer user to enter, manipulate, edit, store, retrieve, and print text. Word processing software controls font size, formats pages and paragraphs, and embeds objects such as artwork into the text of a document.

Electronic Spreadsheets Spreadsheets, such as Lotus 1-2-3® and Microsoft's Excel,® are used to perform mathematical calculations. The numbers are manipulated and the calculations made by user-defined formulas. Electronic spreadsheets were first used as accounting tools (budget monitoring and formulation, financial modeling and forecasting). Spreadsheets are used as decision support tools for health care executives. The size of a particular spreadsheet is determined by the user and limited only by the software manufacturer's construction. The size can range from 120 to 130 columns and 2,000 to 10,000 rows. The intersection of a column and row is known as a *cell*. The cell is the area within the spreadsheet where numbers and formulas are entered and edited and results are calculated. Output from a spreadsheet can be stored for future use, transported to other software applications, displayed on a terminal, displayed in numeric and graphic form, and printed.

Databases Databases are used to organize, store, and manipulate records and files. The records and files consist of user-defined elements that have particular meaning for the user. For example, a database could consist of patient care information, patient demographics, past medical history, and initial nursing assessment. Saba and McCormick (1996) described four database structures:

1. Hierarchic—Data files are arranged in a particular order or ranking; all the data files are linked to each other, having a common base or root.

2. Network—Data files are linked together through a pointer that has a central relationship among the records; this linkage has a commonality, in that each file is linked to another file through a common data element (e.g., patient name, Social Security number, health record number).

3. Relational—Two or more files are linked to one another by attributes in a particular file; this type of database generally consists of rows and columns, corresponding to individual records in the database and to fields in the database respectively.

4. Object oriented—This is a higher level of data management than the foregoing structures; in this type of database structure, ideas or concepts are reflected, not just relationships among the data elements and files. The data objects have a defined set of characteristics and are placed in defined classes or categories.

Multimedia Applications Information can be presented in many different ways using computer technology. Drawing from the business sector, health care professionals are now using multimedia software packages to disseminate their research and ideas to the general and health care publics. Software such a Harvard Graphics® and Microsoft's Power Point® help the nurse construct and organize presentations. These software applications help the computer user choose presentation background (colors and texture), select letter fonts and sizes, and add audio and visual enhancements in the forms of sound and animation. For patient teaching the nurse can develop traditional slide presentations, make hand-out notes, or generate real-time presentations with screens of moving objects and sounds.

Communication Programs Communications software generally can be categorized as telecommunication applications that allow for transfers of voice, image, and data from one computer to another or to several computers at one time. Health care professionals are using a combination of voice, image, and data in the form of modem transmission over *plain old telephone lines* (POTS) and teleconferencing such as Microsoft's Net Meeting® for interaction and electronic mail (e-mail, Microsoft's Windows Messaging®). These software applications allow the user to communicate and interact in real-time with other computer users close by and around the world. The information also can be stored and forwarded at a later time. For example, a nurse in a rural area can photograph a particularly troublesome wound, place the photo with documentation on e-mail, and acquire the guidance of a wound expert elsewhere in the state.

There is growing evidence to suggest that electronic resources, both e-mail and Web-based self-help documents, will result in substantial cost savings to clinics (Kane & Sands, 1998, p. 109).

Specialized Software Applications

Health care environments present the clinician with many challenges in collecting and analyzing patient data. Specialized software has been developed in two major categories: health care finances and clinical patient management. Specialized software can be found in just about every aspect of health care service delivery. This includes delivery across the continuum from acute care (e.g., medical/surgical, preoperative, obstetrics, pediatrics, psychiatric care) to community health services (e.g., home health, hospice). Health information system vendors have been designing and enhancing financial and reimbursement information system software since the late 1960s. With the advent of diagnosis-related groups (DRGs) in the early 1980s, vendors focused their research and design efforts on clinical data collection and outcome measurement applications. Health care system planners, health care administrators, and information system departments are moving toward the integration of financial and clinical systems to support the continuum of cost-effective care.

Networks

The basic units of an information system generally are considered to be the hardware associated with the computer terminal (terminal, keyboard, video display, and printer). Because of the complex nature of modern health care delivery, computer hardware used in isolation (stand-alone) is becoming rare as distributed systems of computers become the norm. Networks of computers continually are being designed and enhanced for use in health care. Stallings and Van Slyke (1998) described three types of networks: wide-area, local-area, and wireless.

1. Wide-area networks (WAN) are links to the outside world. They connect computer users to other users and systems through the telephone company's communication infrastructure. Wide-area networks support voice, data, and image transmissions.

2. Local-area networks (LAN) are used to connect users within a local, somewhat defined, geographic area such as a building or closely grouped set of buildings.

3. Wireless networks connect information system users to computer and communication hardware using wireless transmissions of data. Examples of a wireless network are the electrocardiogram and cellular phone.

Health Care Systems

Information system designers and vendors developed hardware and software configurations around the early needs of health care providers. In the 1970s through the early 1980s the major issues faced by health care providers were of a financial and reimbursement nature. Changes in Medicare reimbursement methods (DRGs) forced information system developers to focus their designs on the collection and analysis of clinical data. Health care facility planners, administrators, and information system departments moved toward an integration of financial data with patient and service delivery data. This evolution continues along distinct developmental levels: mainframe to distributed data processing, financial to clinical data acquisition, and centralized data storage and retrieval to client-server technology and user-defined data manipulation.

Health care information systems traditionally have been oriented toward the finances of service delivery. Trends in health care reimbursement, however, necessitated the integration of financial data with clinically relevant data. In the past, most health care information systems were mainframe in architecture and designed around the concept of centralized data processing (centralized hardware, data manipulation, data storage, and user support). Access for the end user to this centralized unit was provided through a terminal wired to the mainframe computer. Data manipulation by the end user was accomplished by accessing the mainframe's applications software and data storage. Major considerations for implementing a centralized data processing system are control and security of data, centralization of information user support, and economies of scale. This latter consideration refers to providing access for many users of the system at a reasonable cost. Centralized data processing systems usually require a large expenditure in expensive mainframe computer equipment. These systems are viewed as somewhat rigid when a request for specialized programming is made by the end-user.

The expense of running a centralized mainframed information system is cost prohibitive when many users are associated with an organization. This led developers to explore less expensive alternatives for processing massive amounts of health care data. Costs associated with personal computers, linked through a network, steadily declined over the 1980s. These lower computer costs led to a system design known as *distributed data processing* (Figure 22-2). Stallings and Van Slyke (1998, p. 33) described a distributed processing facility as "one in which computers, usually smaller computers, are dispersed throughout an organization. The objective of such dispersion is to process information in a way that is most effective based upon operational, economic, and/or geographic considerations, or all three." Each computer within a distributed processing design is connected to the system through a network. Often the computer user has a powerful personal computer at his or her desk and an avenue to shared resources such as laser and color printers and a variety of software applications. Client-server architecture provides the system user with access to application programming, third-party software applications, file servers, e-mail servers, and Internet access in a cost-effective manner.

However, this wider accessibility to health care information increases the concerns about data security. A fundamental right of patients is that information about their health state, care, and treatment is valid and confidential. Concerns about the confidentiality of patient information have been exacerbated by the ease with which data can be accessed electronically and the growing demand for electronic transmission of patient data, particularly communications over the Internet. "The most common threat to confidentiality (of patient information) is the inappropriate accessing of information by authorized providers" (Patient Confidentiality Must Be Safeguarded, 1997, p. 14). The long-standing problem of nurses breaching patient confidentiality through informal conversations on an elevator or in a lunch room is well known. Reinforcement of standards of professional conduct and protection of the integrity and confidentiality of patient data are mandatory with the use of electronic information systems because of the ease with which widespread data can be accessed. Limiting data access and auditing the identities of nurses and other individuals accessing information are valuable policies to enforce. Passwords authenticate users, and these codes should be secured and changed frequently. Electronic patient data can be automatically verified and checked for errors to help ensure data integrity. Policies and technologies therefore exist for protecting the security and integrity of patient information in an electronic form, perhaps better than information contained in a paper format (Rind et al., 1997; Safran et al., 1995).

Health information systems combine computer technology and communications technology to acquire and integrate financial and clinical data. This integration of financial and clinical data gives health care providers access to information for making patient care decisions from the perspectives of both clinical efficacy and clinical cost effectiveness. The components of a health care information system allow for clinical and health management decision making and provide for input of information from the clinical sciences (medicine, pharmacy, dentistry, nursing, allied health, rehabilitation) as well as

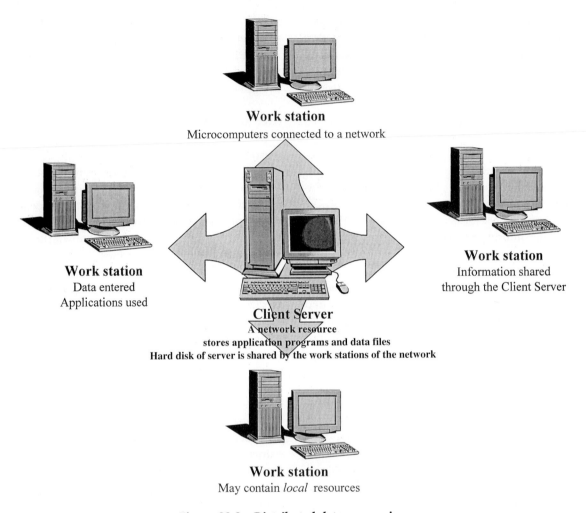

Work station
Microcomputers connected to a network

Work station
Data entered
Applications used

Work station
Information shared
through the Client Server

Client Server
A network resource
stores application programs and data files
Hard disk of server is shared by the work stations of the network

Work station
May contain *local* resources

Figure 22-2 ■ Distributed data processing.

from the management, behavioral, information, and communication sciences.

■ COMPUTERIZING NURSING RECORDS

Major efforts in nursing informatics focus on organizing, structuring, and automating health care information systems to address the demands of nursing practice. Systematizing and automating clinical data for use in nursing practice results in direct increases in nursing pro-

ductivity because information becomes more readily accessible to more people; data are electronically aggregated and organized; computing, tracking, and reminding are automatic; errors are decreased; and records are easier to read. The results of one study (Minda & Brundage, 1994) showed that computerized nursing documentation took half the time of handwritten documentation and almost twice as many observations were noted in the computerized systems compared with the manual system. The seconds per rotation were 3.5 for the computerized documentation, compared with 7.6 seconds for the handwritten documentation.

Changing from manual documentation to an automated information system is difficult. Integrating computer-based information systems into nursing practice, regardless of setting, introduces innovations and changes the organization. The success of the integration depends on how well the people and the organization are managed, making expertise in nursing informatics a critical component of the change process. Various approaches using concepts from informatics have been employed to change the ways information is managed and processed in nursing practice. Addressed here are *selection* of a computer system, *redesign* of manual systems of information, use of a *continuous quality improvement* framework, alteration of the focus to *outcomes relative to resource use,* and *other innovative strategies.* Many benefits can result from the computerization of nursing data, but nurses must assume responsibility for preparation in the area of informatics.

System Selection

Selection of a health care information system begins with choosing a system design, hardware and software vendor, and implementation team. However, these choices cannot be made in isolation. First, the mission, purpose, and goals of the organization must be determined; then the needs and goals for data gathering and information dissemination must be identified. Experts, facilities, staff, and other resources cannot be identified nor hardware and software selected until the information needs and goals have been clearly specified. The choices are best made in a collaborative process with clinical, administration, system, and informatics experts. Administrative planning is necessary and should be derived from the strategic plan for the par-

ticular health care organization. External influences such as reimbursement projections, competition, and business sector changes (i.e., willingness to pay for health care services) are analyzed for the cost impact of the implementation project. The next step in the selection process is to analyze the organization's information needs from both clinical and financial perspectives. A request for proposal (RFP) of a computer system is developed and sent to prospective computer system vendors for responses. The RFP is written to elicit responses from vendors as to how their particular products will meet the needs of the organization. The vendors' proposals are collected and analyzed for a match with the organizational information needs, followed by choosing a vendor and awarding a contract for implementation.

The system vendor, in conjunction with an expert in informatics and the information system department, begins to plan the organization's information systems design. The plan should include the following:
• System development
• System construction
• User education
• Implementation time lines
• Information system evaluation
• System enhancements and upgrades
Development of a health care information system by an organization is a continuous process as well as an evolving endeavor. The effectiveness in meeting the various technical and complex needs of the health care provider (the end-user of any system) must match the expertise of the information and communication system designers and developers.

Redesign

Two approaches to computerizing nursing records are (1) directly converting an existing manual documentation system to an electronic system and (2) redesigning the existing manual system of documentation for computerization (McHugh, 1986). In other words, the paper forms used to document nursing care manually can be placed on a computer for nurses to key in electronically rather than in writing. Or the manual system of documentation can be reviewed, revised, and restructured to take full advantage of the automation capabilities of a computer. Neither approach is as straightforward as it seems; both require extensive iterative planning and evaluation of multiple strategies. The first approach requires less change by staff, creates less stress and resistance, and requires less training, but results in few improvements over the paper system. Major problems with computerizing an existing manual system are that the inefficiencies in paper-and-pencil documentation remain and the difficulties in aggregating data for analyses of clinical performance and resource use continue. With the redesign approach, a complete review of the forms and charting procedures is required, with checklists, codes, standardized terms, and forms developed for use in a computer system.

According to McHugh (1994), changes in how patient care is documented must be made if the anticipated benefits from the computerized patient record are to be realized. The old approach to charting focused on narrative documentation, organized around clinical services, with inefficient and difficult information retrieval. The new approach focuses on patients' problems, the related care requirements, and health status changes. Highly structured forms with coding of data are used, avoiding charting by exceptions and providing the nurse with memory supports. The computerized documentation guides care as well as documents it by using detailed and coded flow sheets of nursing activities. The documentation of home health care was changed to benefit from computerization. The federal government required Form 485, the plan of care, for patients receiving

home care. This document was used for recording data manually over time and one or more visits, and the data contained therein were included in agency reports. An electronic version of Form 485 was created that incorporated health assessment items, physician orders, and functional status measures. These data are recorded on a computer at the point-of-care in the home, and become automatically available for repetitive use and reports immediately and at a later time elsewhere in the organization.

Even though redesigning a documentation system for automation is a more costly and stressful change, it is the preferred approach because more efficient use is made of computer capabilities and greater gains are realized in nurse productivity. At Michael Reese Hospital in Chicago the paperwork time was reduced by more than 2 hours per nurse on a 12-hour shift with redesign of the documentation for an automated nursing record system (McHugh, 1986).

Continuous Quality Improvement

As described in Chapter 19, another approach to changing a documentation system is through continuous quality improvement (CQI) (Henry et al., 1994; Hlusko et al., 1994; Romano, 1994). According to Romano, CQI requires administrative involvement, a definition of quality, continuous examination and improvement in major processes, and teamwork. All of these requirements are necessary for redesigning information systems, and they provide a useful framework for electronic automation of nursing documentation.

Using CQI to change from a manual to an electronic system for managing the finances in one nursing department reduced the labor consumed from 52% ($45,542) of the department resources to 6% (Hlusko et al., 1994). Henry et al. (1994) used CQI principles to design a system for managing telephone triage in a community clinic for AIDS patients. Data were missing from the patient records, and the triage nurses had difficulty accessing the relevant data that were available. The new system improved the triage process by providing more timely access to data, tailoring the data entry, and using automated reminders to both physicians and nurses. Romano (1994) said that integrating the implementation of innovative technologies within a CQI program facilitates adoption and enhances the evaluation of the resulting improvements in patient care. She described changes made in the 15-year-old Hospital Information System at the Clinical Center of the National Institutes of Health using CQI techniques (automation of advance directives, blood administration, patient allergy information, infection controls, medication administration, and continuity of care).

Outcomes and Resources

Another area in which nursing informatics is helping change health care is patient classification or acuity systems (Finnigan et al., 1993). Despite the fact that patient classification systems were the foundation of the integrated financial and clinical data systems mentioned earlier in this chapter, they are now obsolete. These systems are being replaced by outcome-focused, resource-monitoring systems. To remain competitive within the rapidly changing environment of managed health care, both finances and quality must be measured to ascertain that the care provided has value equal to its cost.

Nursing must have a "specific plan designed to achieve predetermined outcomes" (Finnigan et al., 1993, p. 65). Critical pathways tracking patient outcomes, providers' time, and organizational resources are being introduced to achieve these goals (Chu & Thom, 1994; DiJerome, 1992; Ireson & Grier, 1998). The critical pathway is used to monitor the timed progression of interventions and resulting patient outcomes; there is a variance if a patient does not respond

as expected. The parameters for these pathways, and the variances from them, are more easily identified, tracked, and analyzed with the use of computerized systems of information. Electronic systems generate warnings when variations in pathways occur, allowing for early management of problems. In addition, the systems generate reports, for example, on resource consumption, differences between nurses in interventions used, and probabilities of outcomes in a defined population of patients.

Other Strategies

The development and implementation of a computerized system of nursing data must be planned, as well as the resulting organizational changes. Establishment of a committee or task force with all levels of nursing staff represented is mandatory. Such a group is needed to plan the change and serve as resource personnel for implementing the new system. A nurse with expertise in informatics is an invaluable resource for managing both the technologic changes and the organizational changes occurring with a new information system. For instance, if the paperwork for patient admission and discharge is automated, the timespan for admitting and discharging patients is shortened. The nursing and housekeeping services for discharging patients and then admitting new patients also must be accelerated to realize benefits from system use. An informatics person familiar with models of change (as discussed in Chapter 6) anticipates problems from the introduction of information technology and knows techniques for managing the effects on people and their work within an organization (Lorenzi et al., 1997).

A useful starting point for planning the system is something already in place (e.g., goals of patient care). Administration should be involved in planning for the change and should support the development of the system before and after implementation. A committee consisting of administrators, clinicians, system analysts, and informatic experts is valuable. During and after implementation of the system, these committee members should meet with unit managers to discuss problems and clarify issues. All interested parties, inside and outside the institution, should be informed of the developments and the anticipated and actual benefits from deployment of the redesigned information system. Some techniques for introducing innovations and making organizational changes are listed in Box 22-1.

Benefits

By improving information managing and processing, the health care industry can provide higher quality care and operate more efficiently, thus lowering the costs of operations. Information technology can be applied to improve these processes and as a result generate more revenue and streamline operations. These goals can be accomplished by using information technology to increase patient throughput, support data collection at patients' bedsides and other points of care, schedule critical paths for outcome achievement, replenish supplies at time of use, speed reimbursements via computer interfaces with third-party payers, and lower transport costs with electronic communications among and between patients and care providers (Chu & Thom, 1994).

Nursing informatics provides valuable tools for making changes that can lead to improved quality of care and cost savings for patients as well as organizations. To fully realize these benefits, nurses must seek continuing education in nursing informatics (Cassey & Savalle-Dunn, 1994). Becoming computer literate teaches nurses how the machines organize and facilitate nursing tasks. Developing word-processing skills helps nurses communicate and move between computer screens. Learning about databases aids understanding of the relational fields in the computerized health care record. Using spreadsheets prepares nurses for managing budgets and schedules. Interacting with computer networks and electronic mail opens global interfaces to other systems.

■ NURSING LANGUAGE

Clark and Lang (1992, p. 61) said: "If we cannot name it, we cannot control it, finance it, teach it, research it, or put it into public policy." If we do not have terms that are used consistently to identify and describe elements of nursing practice in diverse settings, we cannot make the changes necessary for providing high-quality care at the least cost. In an article about picking fights, Gebbie (1997) said the development of national health care data sets that included nursing variables was worth fighting for. Data sets with nurse-sensitive and nurse-specific elements are needed to both aggregate and compare nursing diagnoses, actions, outcomes, and resource use across patient units and organizations at the state, national, and international levels.

B O X   2 2 - 1

Innovation and Change Techniques

Educate	Communicate	Negotiate	Cooperate
Coerce	Mobilize resources	Time events	Anticipate resistance
Emphasize benefits	Video inservices	Use mock charts	Audit charts
Evaluate	Motivate	Empower	Involve

A uniform language for documenting nursing care is a prerequisite to a computerized health-care record, inclusion of nursing information in financial and policy-making databases, and studies of patient outcomes. For more than 25 years nurses have been working to identify, standardize, and code names for the elements of nursing practice (Gordon, 1985). These labels have been categorized to form taxonomies or classifications of nursing elements. Thus there are the beginnings of nomenclatures in nursing that are being organized into taxonomies, forming the start of a standardized nursing language. Efforts are underway to test and validate these schemes so that standard terms are used to describe nursing practice. Arguments against standardizing the language nurses use in the provision of patient care are that the terms are inflexible and not clinically useful (McCloskey & Bulechek, 1994). But classifications of language are tools just as maps are tools that help one reach a destination; they make it easier to select a nursing diagnosis, intervention, and desired outcome. As McCloskey and Bulechek observed (1994, p. 60): "A map is a tool that makes it easier to get to the desired destination, but when one arrives at the destination . . . then one should put down the map and appreciate the scenery."

Nursing Taxonomies

The North American Nursing Diagnoses Association (NANDA) This Association has classified more than 104 nursing diagnoses, or labels for patient problems, which are amenable to treatment by nursing actions (Gordon, 1985; Kim et al., 1989). The classification itself is known as *NANDA*. Examples of the diagnostic labels are *impaired mobility, fluid volume deficit,* and *ineffective coping*. Each diagnosis is accompanied by a list of defining characteristics. NANDA is not inclusive of the terms used and patient problems encountered by nurses, nor do other classification schemes include all the NANDA concepts (Zielstorff et al., 1992). Even so, this is the oldest nursing taxonomy, and it is in increasingly wide use. NANDA provides a base for describing and comparing the actions nurses take for specific patient problems and the outcomes to expect for those problems and at what costs. From such data, the needed changes in nursing practice can be identified, planned, initiated, and reimbursed.

The Nursing Interventions Classification (NIC) NIC is a comprehensive categorization of nursing interventions (McCloskey & Bulechek, 1996); examples are *anxiety reduction, shock management,* and *fall prevention*. Each intervention is labeled, defined, and accompanied by a set of nursing actions. The taxonomy is organized into domains with classes of 433 interventions performed across specialties and settings. The interventions are coded and linked to the diagnostic labels in NANDA, the classification of nursing outcomes (NOC), and the patient problems in the Omaha System. Using NIC, nurses can identify the interventions used to achieve certain outcomes for patient problems, thus facilitating reimbursement.

The Nursing Outcomes Classification (NOC) NOC contains categories of patient outcomes that are sensitive to nursing interventions (Johnson & Maas, 1997; Maas et al., 1996). Examples of nursing outcomes are *caregiver emotional health, mobility level,* and *nutritional status*. Each of the 190 outcomes is labeled and defined and has an associated group of indicators and measures for determining achievement. NIC will allow comparisons of nursing outcomes across a variety of aggregates, such as settings, diagnoses, and age-groups.

The Home Health Care Classification System (HCCS) Included in this taxonomy (Saba, 1992) are 147 nursing diagnoses, four classes *(assess, care, teach, manage)* of 166 interventions, and discharge status *(improved, stabilized, deteriorated)*. Examples of the 20 home health care components used to organize the HCCS are *self-care, activity,* and *metabolic.*

The Omaha Community Health System

This taxonomy consists of nursing diagnoses, interventions, and outcome ratings for patient problems (Martin & Scheet, 1992). Included in the Omaha System are 40 patient problems, four categories of 62 intervention targets, and three outcome measures *(knowledge, behavior, patient status).* This system was used to describe the patients of four diverse home-care agencies, the nursing services they received, and the outcomes of that care (Martin et al., 1993). The median age of the patients was almost 70 years; 70% of the home visits were by nurses, who identified more than 9,000 patient problems and provided more than 96,000 interventions. The patients improved an average of .52 (on a 5-point scale) on each of the three outcome ratings.

A Minimum Set of Nursing Data

An important vehicle for change in nursing practice is the Nursing Minimum Data Set, or NMDS (Ryan & Delaney, 1995; Werley & Lang, 1988). The NMDS is a system for uniformly collecting the least amount of data that are absolutely necessary for describing a nurse-patient encounter. The purposes for establishing a core of essential nursing data were to be able to do the following:

- Describe the nursing care of patients in a variety of settings
- Compare nursing data across settings
- Project trends in nursing care
- Stimulate research
- Influence health policy

The NMDS is critical for making changes in nursing practice because it includes variables essential for ascertaining the quality and costs of nursing care. Such minimum sets of nursing data are nationally mandated in Australia (Glidden & Weaver, 1994) and Belgium (Sermeus & Delesie, 1994).

B O X   2 2 - 2

NMDS Elements

Nursing Care

Nursing diagnosis
Nursing intervention
Nursing outcome
Nursing care intensity

Patient Demographics

Personal identification
Date of birth
Sex
Race and ethnicity
Residence

Service Elements

Agency number
Health record number
Number of nurse
Admission or encounter date
Discharge or termination date
Disposition of patient
Expected payer

From Werley, H.H., & Lang, N.M. (1988). *Identification of the nursing minimum data set.* New York: Springer.

The system is a set of 16 categorized items, with definitions, which provides the information needed by multiple users (Box 22-2). The NMDS contains three categories of data: *nursing* (four elements); *demographic* (five elements); and *service* (seven elements). Ten of the demographic and service elements are collected on all hospitalized Medicare patients as part of the data required for the Uniform Hospital Data Discharge. Although standardizing the vocabulary, measures, and codes for the NMDS elements is a challenge, the ability to describe and cost out nursing services and then be reimbursed for those services makes the effort worthwhile.

Evaluations of the NMDS across settings (Ryan & Delaney, 1995) showed that the data are available in patient records and can be retrieved and linked from one element to the other. The four nursing elements were available in 40% to 100% of patient records; great variation existed in the availability of the demographic and service elements, with the unique provider identification number not available. (A code for identifying health providers is not used in the United States, but is used in other countries.) The costs for collecting the NMDS data elements ranged from $20 to $80 manually, and 5¢ to 50¢ by computer. A computer system facilitated documentation of the NMDS and the retrieval of the data collected. Use of the nursing taxonomies (NANDA, NIC, NOC) described previously can help standardize the data collected for the nursing elements in the NMDS, whereas the use of multiple other language systems will lead to data that cannot be compared across aggregated groupings. The nursing element *intensity of care* is the most problematic of the four elements within this category. It is unlikely that one item of data will adequately account for the costs of nursing care.

Future Challenges

Although there is not, as yet, an internationally accepted nursing classification system, efforts are underway to establish a system for describing patient problems, nursing actions, and patient outcomes. As observed by Ozbolt (1996, p. 62): "Assessing the effectiveness of care requires standardized data aggregated in databases for comparisons across time, conditions, and institution." The American Nurses Association, the European Union, and the International Council of Nursing are collaborating on the development and acceptance of a standardized taxonomy to describe nursing care worldwide (McCormick et al., 1994). The International Council of Nurses, in collaboration with the World Health Organization, is working to establish an international set of minimum nursing

data comprising *problems/diagnoses, interventions,* and *outcomes.* Once endorsed by nursing organizations around the world, the classification scheme will be submitted to the World Health Organization for approval and inclusion in the International Classifications of Disease.

A shortcoming of the nursing taxonomies created to date is that they lack multidisciplinary perspectives. This problem is being addressed by linking the nursing classifications with schemes from other health care disciplines. The Institute of Medicine (1991) said health care vocabularies must be standardized for the patient record and recommended collaborative efforts in developing a clinical data dictionary. The National Library of Medicine is establishing a Unified Medical Language System (Humphreys & Lindberg, 1989) that maps terms from different taxonomies, including NANDA, NIC, NOC, HCCS, and the Omaha System. The Systematized Nomenclature of Medicine III (better known as *SNOMED III*) includes NANDA and will add NIC and NOC. The value of a uniform language for describing and comparing nursing practices across settings cannot be overestimated. Standardizing nursing language will facilitate selection of the most appropriate and cost-effective nursing interventions, define and predict patient outcomes from nursing care, help interprofessional and intraprofessional communication, assist in staff and other resource allocations, promote reimbursement for nursing services, contribute to the development of computerized systems of health care information, convey the nature of nursing to the public, address policy issues critical to the profession, and aid the development of nursing knowledge and the teaching of nursing practices.

■ INNOVATIVE INFORMATION SYSTEMS

Given evidence (Henry, 1995) that the greater the nurse's knowledge and experience, the higher the quality of patient assessments, nursing diagnoses, and care plans, information systems become imperative. Structured forms, linkages to knowledge bases and taxonomies, systematic analyses and comparisons of nursing interventions and treatment strategies, increase nursing knowledge and expand clinical experiences. The linkage of nursing diagnoses to processes of care and patient outcomes enables the evaluation of nursing care in terms of both quality and cost. Whether documentation is manual or electronic, more nursing data are collected when the documentation is structured in some manner (Zielstorff et al., 1993). The number of innovative information systems being developed and implemented therefore is not surprising. "The true megachanges for the next decade will center around gathering, managing, and using clinical information (Lorenzi et al., 1995, p. 391). The following are brief descriptions of a very few of these systems:

- A system (EmSTAT) at Hennepin County Medical Center in Minneapolis, Minnesota, improves communication, facilitates continuity of care, and decreases redundancy in documentation. A client-server architecture and Oracle database are used to automate the tracking, triaging, and registering of patients seen in the emergency department. An automated patient-locator board, which is globally accessible, uses abbreviations, symbols, colors, lights, and icons to present compacted information logically and legibly for use in real time and for retrospective analyses. Patient assessments (quick or full) can be done by physiologic systems or by chief complaint using lists, buttons, and toggles for quick input. Patient data are entered into the tracking and triaging system on entry to the emergency department, and a registration slip is generated for the patient. The authors describing this system noted the advances made in automated real-time documentation by nurses, the difficulties of human-machine interfaces, the need

for multiple interfaces with other systems, and the necessity of planning for upgrades of hardware (Zimmerman & Clinton, 1995).

- The Nursing Case Management Computerized System is an interactive computer program that enhanced team planning of individualized care, decreased paperwork, aided the development of team care plans, and facilitated improvements in the quality of patient care. This system was developed at the New England Medical Center Hospital for use with HIV and AIDS inpatients and outpatients using a 16 MX/1.44/2 personal computer. The computerized care plan for use by nurses, allied health workers, and physicians is menu driven with columns for nursing diagnoses, patient outcomes, care goals, and interventions. The patient outcomes are time limited and generate optional interventions for selection by the care provider. A critical path form is produced and used by the nurse case manager to monitor the interventions and patient responses. Any variances and their causes are noted by the nurse case manager, and the team then revises the plan of care as needed (DiJerome, 1992).

- In northwestern Kansas, nurses provide health care to elderly patients in their homes using telemedicine. The Interactive Home Health Care systems provide for audio and video interactions over local cable systems, as well as patient monitoring and data input and retrieval by the nurse. Two units are used—a base station used by the nurse and a home unit attached to a television used by the patient. The nurses electronically visit patients at regularly scheduled times each week. When a real home visit is necessary, the nurse makes the visit or assigns a home health nurse to make the visit. The average home visit by a nurse to provide skilled care costs $60; the estimated cost of in-home care using telemedicine is $30. The early results from demonstration of this system indicated the need for high-quality sound, particularly for elderly patients. The collection of computerized data by the nurses is being refined, and difficulties the nurses had adapting to the new mode of care delivery are being addressed (Lindberg, 1997).

- NurseLink was an electronic bulletin board operated by the School of Nursing at the University of Colorado Health Sciences Center in Denver. The electronic bulletin board was designed originally for communication of research findings to nurses in local clinical agencies but then was redesigned into the Denver Free-Net, a community computing system for consumers to access information, particularly about health and human services. Using a personal computer, modem, and telecommunications software, the citizens of Colorado can access information contained in the system via dial-in telephone lines or Internet. Skiba and Mirque (1994) conceptualized the system as an electronic city, where users select from a menu the buildings (e.g., Science, Art) they would like to enter. The Health Care Building contains numerous areas, one of which focuses on health promotion materials such as consumer tips and an interactive question-answer section. Among other areas in the Health Care Building is a database of more than 600 support groups and on-line publications for health care professionals.

- An expert system has been developed to assess pregnant women's risk of preterm birth. Normal gestation is 40 weeks, but 8% to 12% of the births in the United States occur before 37 weeks' gestation. The knowledge base of 520 rules for the expert system was developed using machine learning, statistical, and validation techniques. The expert system accurately predicted preterm or full-term deliveries for 53% to 89% of 9419 cases. In comparison, traditional screening methods result in accurate predictions for only 17% to 38% of cases (Woolery & Grzymala-Busse, 1994).

■ **KEY POINTS**

- Computerized health care information systems range from simple, stand-alone personal computers to complex, integrated systems using several data processors remotely connected for data collection and analysis. These systems have revolutionized the way information is gathered, handled, and made available in the clinical area.

- To use health information systems it is important to have some understanding of the hardware that is needed, including input devices, central processing units, and output devices, as well as the software that is the standard at the institution.

- Complex health care information systems have been developed that are expensive in both software and hardware. However, the greatest expense generally comes in training the staff to use the system.

- A key aspect in the change of medical documentation from a paper system to a computerized information system comes in the selection of the best system to meet the needs of the institution. Even when the best system is chosen, it is not uncommon for some aspects to need redesigning and adaptation to serve the data needs of the specific organization.

- A uniform language for documenting nursing care is a prerequisite for a computerized health record-keeping system. Classification of nursing language is like designing a road map, in that the record-keeping system is a tool to help those using it reach their destination.

- Some of the more common nursing languages or taxonomies are the North American Nursing Diagnoses Association (NANDA), the Nursing Interventions Classification (NIC), the Nursing Outcomes Classification (NOC), the Home Health Care Classification System (HCCS), and the Omaha Community Health System.

- The Nursing Minimum Data Set (NMDS) is a system for uniformly collecting the least amount of data that are absolutely necessary for describing a nurse-patient encounter.

■ CRITICAL THINKING QUESTIONS

1. Determine which nursing information system is used in one of the agencies in which you practice. From your own experience, how useful is it? What do you see as its limitations? Interview at least two members of the nursing staff to determine their evaluation of the system. What changes would they recommend?

2. What is the availability of other forms of data transmission in the agency with which you are most familiar other than via computer? For example, if data are transmitted over telephone lines, or through other forms of distance technology, how effective has it been? What have been the limitations? The advantages?

3. Engage in a discussion with a group of health care professionals or students about issues regarding patient confidentiality that must be taken into account as computerized and other forms of telemedicine grow. Identify at least five issues, and discuss ways to counteract the negative impact.

4. Review the nursing taxonomies that are briefly described in this chapter. Which ones(s) have you had experience with? What were the limitations of the taxonomy? What were the values? What changes can you suggest?

■ REFERENCES

Cassey, M.Z., & Savalle-Dunn, J. (1994). Sketching the future: Trends influencing nursing informatics. *Journal of Gynecologic & Neonatal Nursing, 23,* 175-182.

Chu, S., & Thom, J. (1994). Information technology as a proactive strategic weapon in health care. *Journal of Nursing Administration, 24*(4), 5-7.

Clark, J., & Lang, N.M. (1992). Nursing next advance: An international classification for nursing practice. *International Nursing Review, 39,* 109-112.

DiJerome, L. (1992). The nursing case management computerized system: Meeting the challenge of health care delivery through technology. *Computers in Nursing, 10,* 250-258.

Finnigan, S.A., Abel, M., Dobler, T., Hudon, L., & Terry, B. (1993). Automated patient acuity. *Journal of Nursing Administration, 23*(5), 62-71.

Frisse, M.E. (1992). Medical informatics in academic health science centers. *Academic Medicine, 67,* 238-241.

Gebbie, K.M. (1997). Picking the right fight. *Nursing Outlook, 45,* 142-143.

Gliddon, T., & Weaver, C. (1994). The community nursing minimum data set in Australia. In S.J. Grobe & E.S.P. Pluyter-Wenting (Eds.). *Nursing informatics: An international overview for nursing in a technological era* (pp. 163-168). New York: Elsevier.

Gordon, M. (1985). Nursing diagnosis. *Annual Review of Nursing Research, 3,* 127-146.

Graves, J.R., & Corcoran, S. (1989). The study of nursing informatics. *Image, 21,* 227-231.

Hannah, K.J., Ball, M.J., & Edwards, M. (1994). *Introduction to nursing informatics.* New York: Springer-Verlag.

Henry, S.B. (1995). Nursing informatics: State of the science. *Journal of Advanced Nursing, 22,* 1182-1192.

Henry, S.B., Borchelt, D., Schreiner, J., & Musen, M.A. (1994). A computer-based approach to quality improvement for telephone triage encounters in a community AIDS clinic. *Nursing Administration Quarterly, 18*(2), 65-73.

Hlusko, D.L., Weatherly, K.S., Franklin, K.G., Wallace, S., & Williamson, S. (1994). Computerization of a nursing financial management system using continuous quality improvement as a framework. *Computers in Nursing, 12,* 193-200.

Humphreys, B., & Lindberg, D.A.B. (1989). Building the unified medical language system. In L. Kingsland (Ed.). *Proceedings of the Thirteenth Annual Symposium on Computer Applications in Medical Care* (pp. 475-480). Washington, D.C.: IEEE Computer Society Press.

Institute of Medicine. (1991). *The computer-based patient record: An essential technology for health care.* Washington, D.C.: National Academy Press.

Ireson, C.L., & Grier, M.R. (in press). Variances in patient outcomes. *Outcomes Management for Nursing Practice.*

Johnson, M., & Maas, M. (1997). *Nursing outcomes classification.* St. Louis: Mosby.

Jydstrup, R., & Gross, M. (1966). Cost of information handling in hospitals. *Health Services Research, 1,* 235-260.

Kane, B., & Sands, D.Z. (1998). Guidelines for the clinical use of electronic mail with patients. *Journal of the American Medical Informatics Association, 5,* 104-111.

Kim, M.J., McFarland, G., & McLane, A. (1989). *A pocket guide to nursing diagnosis* (3rd ed.). St. Louis: Mosby.

Lindberg, C.C.S. (1997). Implementation of in-home telemedicine in rural Kansas: Answering an elderly patient's needs. *Journal of the American Medical Informatics Association, 4,* 14-16.

Lorenzi, N.M., Gardner, R.M., Pryor, T.A., & Stead, W.W. (1995). Medical informatics: The key to an organization's place in the new health care environment. *Journal of the American Medical Informatics Association, 2,* 391-392.

Lorenzi, N.M., Riley, R.T., Blyth, A.J.C., Southon, G., & Dixon, B.J. (1997). Antecedents of the people and organizational aspects of medical informatics: Review of the literature. *Journal of the American Medical Informatics Association, 4,* 79-93.

Maas, M., Johnson, M., & Moorhead, S. (1996). Classifying nursing-sensitive patient outcomes. *Image, 28,* 295-301.

Martin, K.S., & Scheet, N.J. (1992). *The Omaha System: Applications for community health nursing.* Philadelphia: Saunders.

Martin, K.S., Scheet, N.J., & Stegman, M.R. (1993). Home health clients: Characteristics, outcomes of care, and nursing interventions. *American Journal of Public Health, 83,* 1730-1734.

McCloskey, J.C., & Bulechek, G.M. (1994). Standardizing the language for nursing treatments: An overview of the issues. *Nursing Outlook, 42,* 56.

McCloskey, J.C., & Bulechek, G.M. (Eds.). (1996). *Nursing interventions classification (NIC)* (2nd ed.). St. Louis: Mosby.

McCormick, K.A., Lang, N., Zielstorff, R., Milholland, K., Saba, V., & Jacox, A. (1994). Toward standard classification schemes for nursing language: Recommendations of the American Nurses Association Steering Committee on Databases to Support Clinical Nursing Practice. *Journal of the American Medical Informatics Association, 1,* 421-427.

McHugh, M.L. (1986). Increasing productivity through computer communications. *Dimensions of Critical Care, 5,* 294-302.

McHugh, M.L. (1994). Structuring nursing data for the computer-based patient record (CPR). In S.J. Grobe & E.S.P. Pluyter-Wenting (Eds.). *Nursing informatics: An international overview for nursing in a technological era* (pp. 302-306). New York: Elsevier.

Minda, S., & Brundage, D.J. (1994). Time differences in handwritten and computer documentation of nursing assessment. *Computers in Nursing, 12,* 277-279.

Ozbolt, J.G. (1996). From minimum data to maximum impact: Using clinical data to strengthen patient care. *Advanced Practice Nursing Quarterly, 1*(4), 62-69.

Patient confidentiality must be safeguarded before life-saving information can be transmitted via the Internet. (1997, Oct.) *AHCPR Research Activities, 209,* 14-15.

Rind, D.M., Kohane, I.S., & Szolovits, P. (1997). Maintaining the confidentiality of medical records shared over the Internet and the World Wide Web. *Annals of Internal Medicine, 127,* 138-141.

Romano, C.A. (1994). The clinical application of computer information systems to continuous quality improvement. In S.J. Grobe & E.S.P. Pluyter-Wenting (Eds.). *Nursing informatics: An international overview for nursing in a technological era* (pp. 665-669). New York: Elsevier.

Ryan, P., & Delaney, C. (1995). Nursing minimum data set. *Annual Review of Nursing Research, 13,* 169-194.

Saba, V.K. (1992). The classification of home health care nursing: Diagnoses and interventions. *Caring Magazine, 11,* 50-56.

Saba, V.K., & McCormick, K.A. (1996). *Essentials of computers for nurses* (2nd ed.). New York: McGraw-Hill.

Safran, C., Rind, D., Citroen, M., Bakker, A.R., Slack, W.V., & Bleich, H.L. (1995). Protection of confidentiality in the computer-based patient record. *MD Computing, 12,* 187-192.

Sermeus, W., & Delesie, L. (1994). The registration of a nursing minimum data set in Belgium: Six years of experience. In S.J. Grobe & E.S.P. Pluyter-Wenting (Eds.). *Nursing informatics: An international overview for nursing in a technological era* (pp. 144-149). New York: Elsevier.

Skiba, D.J., & Mirque, D.T. (1994). The electronic community: An alternative health care approach. In S.J. Grobe & E.S.P. Pluyter-Wenting (Eds.). *Nursing informatics:An international overview for nursing in a technological era* (pp. 388-392). New York: Elsevier.

Stallings, W., & Van Slyke, R. (1998). *Business data communications* (3rd ed.). Upper Saddle River, N.J.: Prentice Hall.

Werley, H.H., & Lang, N.M. (1988). *Identification of the nursing minimum data set.* New York: Springer.

Woolery, L.K., & Grzymala-Busse, J. (1994). Machine learning for an expert system to predict preterm birth. *Journal of the American Medical Informatics Association, 1,* 439-446.

Zielstorff, R.D., Cimino, C., Barnett, G.O., Hassan, L., & Blewett, D.R. (1992). Representation of nursing terminology in the UMLS Metathesaurus: A pilot study. In M. Frisse (Ed.). *Proceedings of the Fifteenth Annual Symposium on Computer Applications in Medical Care* (pp. 392-396). New York: McGraw-Hill.

Zielstorff, R.D., Hudgings, C.D., & Grobe, S.J. (1993). *Next generation information systems: Essential characteristics for professional practice.* Washington, D.C.: American Nurses Publishing.

Zimmerman, M., & Clinton, J.E. (1995). Computerized tracking, triage, and registration. *Topics in Emergency Medicine, 17*(4), 49-63.

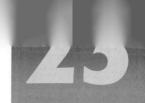

Marketing Management

Wade Lancaster

INTRODUCTION

New forms of organizations, including those in health care that are designed to respond quickly and flexibly to accelerating change in technology, competition, and consumer preferences, are replacing traditional bureaucratic hierarchic organizations. These new organizations, characterized by flexibility, specialization, and an emphasis on relationship management, have created subtle changes in the concept and practice of marketing (Webster, 1992). Marketing is usually associated with business. As consumers, most people are familiar with marketing activities, especially advertising. As a result of television, radio, and print advertising, people recognize brand names and corporate logos of businesses.

Although most people have visited shopping centers, compared prices, and evaluated and purchased a wide range of products from retailers, they less frequently deal with the marketing efforts of firms marketing to other organizations rather than to individuals. However, marketing plays an important role in contemporary society. Not-for-profit organizations, for example, advertise their need for contributions to feed hungry children; representatives from environ-

mental groups speak at colleges, soliciting new members; and health care organizations spend large sums of money on print, verbal, and billboard advertising. Effective marketing is not a peripheral activity but rather a critical determinant of organizational success. Despite the fact that most people deal regularly with some components of marketing and know something about it, there are many aspects of marketing that most people have never considered. To understand marketing more fully, it must first be defined.

This chapter introduces the basic concepts and responsibilities of marketing and explains its relevance to nursing and health care. First, the nature and scope of modern marketing is described, and then the contemporary consumer-oriented marketing philosophy is presented. Next, the role of marketing at different levels in the health care organization is introduced, outlining a corporate level strategic planning process, which is pivotal to strategic marketing planning. Finally, the discussion shifts to strategic marketing and marketing management, centering on key issues facing health care marketers.

OBJECTIVES

After reading this chapter, you will be able to:

1. Define marketing and trace its evolution
2. Describe the scope of marketing
3. Analyze the different philosophic views of marketing's role in the organization
4. Differentiate between services and products
5. Identify a health care organization's major consumer groups
6. Define the key elements of strategic planning and evaluate its importance for marketing
7. Explain the role of portfolio analysis and expansion strategy models
8. Explain how strategic marketing works
9. Explain the functions of marketing management

■ WHAT IS MARKETING?

Marketing, as a process, is as old as humanity, existing since barter, trade, or exchange began among primitive peoples. In contrast, marketing as an academic discipline is relatively new. Since its inception, the formal study of marketing has been constantly changing and the concept of marketing has undergone several conceptual as well as perceptual transitions. Currently, marketing can be viewed from several different perspectives; among them three are notable: macro, micro, and philosophy.

A *macro perspective* of marketing views it as a set of social and economic processes (Webster, 1992) that focus on the broad marketing activities that take place in the overall economy. Thus *macromarketing* refers to the process that facilitates the total flow of a nation's goods and services from producers to consumers to benefit society. This chapter does not deal with the issues related to macromarketing, but instead focuses on a micro view of marketing that is more useful in nursing and health care.

A *micro perspective* of marketing views its functions as organizational activities rather than as social or economic processes. It is a managerial approach that emphasizes problem solving, decision making, planning, implementation, and control in a competitive marketplace (Webster, 1992). Thus *micromarketing* refers to the way an individual organization plans, executes, and allocates its marketing activities to benefit its customers, which in health care are individuals, families, groups, and communities.

Traditional View: Marketing as a Business Function

For many years marketing was considered to be a business function associated with the sale of products. The formal study of marketing investigated the creation, stimulation, facilitation, and valuation of transactions between profit-seeking business firms and want-gratifying consumers. For the most part, attention was focused on the managerial problems of large consumer goods producers who catered to the needs of the mass markets. In contrast, relatively little attention was devoted to the marketing of services and this is especially true of health care services. However, as many nations became more oriented toward services, the differences between the marketing of products and services became apparent.

Services generally have four characteristics that distinguish them from products:
1. Intangibility
2. Inseparability from the service provider

BOX 23-1

Key Differences Between Services and Products

Services	**Products**
Services are often intangible. They may involve acts, deeds, performances, efforts. Many services cannot be physically possessed.	Products are tangible. They are objects, things, materials.
Services are frequently inseparable. The quality of many services cannot be separated from the people providing the services.	Products can be manufactured by one firm and marketed by another.
Services are usually perishable. Unused capacity cannot be stored or shifted from one time to another.	Products can be stored. Surpluses in one period can be applied against another.
Services may vary in quality over time. It is difficult to standardize some services because of their labor intensiveness and because of the involvement of the customer.	Products can be standardized. Mass production and quality control can be used.

3. Perishability
4. Variability in quality

Box 23-1 identifies differences between products and services. The pivotal difference is that products are *things* and services are *performances* (Berry, 1987). Products can be touched, inspected, and stored until they are needed. Services, in contrast, are *intangible*. They cannot be felt, inspected, possessed, or returned if the purchase is unsatisfactory.

Products are manufactured, sold, and consumed. In contrast, services are first sold and then produced and consumed. Provision and consumption of services often occur simultaneously. The provider delivers services directly to the consumer, with the service provider being, in effect, an inseparable part of the service. This is especially clear in nursing. For example, in home health care a person or a family contracts with an agency to deliver nursing care to the home. Services are often labor intensive. Because they are inseparable from the provider, they cannot be inventoried or saved. Thus unused capacity cannot be stored or shifted from one time to another; it is perishable.

Finally, services are, in many regards, more heterogeneous than products. Manufactured products can be regulated within rather strict standards, whereas the quality of services can vary from one provider to another. Moreover, service quality, even when given by the same provider, can vary over time, since people-based services (as opposed to machine-based services) are difficult to standardize. Therefore, it is important to recognize that although the same services may be rendered, the service may be different from what was expected or from one time to another (Zeithaml et al., 1990). The ultimate marketing goal in business is to attract and satisfy customers and generate a profit for the company in the process. Thus the marketing of services in the broadest context is consistent with the traditional view.

Broadened View: Marketing Applies to Any Organization

In 1969 Kotler and Levy's landmark article criticized the then prevailing view of marketing as "a function peculiar to business firms." They suggested that marketing is a more pervasive so-

---

Key terms

Term	Definition
Marketing	Process of planning and executing the conception, pricing, promotion, and distribution of goods and services to create exchanges that satisfy individuals and organizational goals (Marketing News, 1985, p. 1)
Macromarketing	Process that facilitates the total flow of a nation's goods and services from producers to consumers to benefit society
Micromarketing	The way an individual organization plans, executes, and allocates its marketing activities to benefit its customers
Services	Intangibles that cannot be felt, inspected, possessed, or returned if the purchase is unsatisfactory

---

cietal activity performed by different organizations in a wide variety of contexts. They observed that nonbusiness organizations have products and services, as well as customers, and use marketing tools; however, it is the business organization that has developed and used the science of effective marketing. Therefore Kotler and Levy argued that because all organizations perform marketing or at least marketing-like activities, the choice facing managers is not whether to market, for no organization can avoid marketing. The choice is whether to do it well or poorly. Kotler and Zaltman (1971) coined the term "social marketing," which they defined as the design, implementation, and control of programs calculated to influence the acceptability of social ideas and involving considerations in product planning, pricing, communication, distribution, and marketing research. Shortly thereafter, Kotler (1972) proposed that marketing is concerned with "how transactions are created, stimulated, facilitated, and valued." The focus is on transaction, which is "the exchange of values between two parties." Thus marketing takes place whenever (1) there are two social units, (2) one is seeking a specific response from another, (3) the response probability is not fixed, and, (4) one attempts to produce the desired response by creating and offering values to the market.

In its broadest sense, marketing is simply a conscious, systematic approach to the planning, implementation, and evaluation of exchange relationships. Marketing, including health care marketing, is the process of providing satisfying goods and services in exchange for value. The value may be profit, as in the traditional business definition, or it might be dollars that are used to staff a hospital and buy the latest equipment, or the value of "doing something for someone else" as perceived by a volunteer. There are two parties to the exchange, and both the buyer (user or consumer) and the seller (or provider) must receive benefits.

Marketing strategies are tailored to the organization, the community, and the specific products and services. As is shown in the next section, organizations are guided by different philosophies, which influence their approach to marketing. Some choose an intrusive, aggressive, hard-sell marketing style, whereas others select a marketing style that conforms to their traditional professional standards, avoiding advertising and hard-sell tactics.

The Focus of Production, Product, Selling, and Marketing Philosophies

Production
Product   PRODUCTION → SELLING → CONSUMPTION
Selling

Marketing   CONSUMER   INTEGRATED   CONSUMER   ACHIEVE
                 →NEEDS   →MARKETING   →SATISFY   GOALS

T A B L E   2 3 - 1

Orientations Toward Marketing

	Starting Point	Focus	Means	Goals
Production	Factory	Manufacturing	Technologic process	Utilize capacity
Product	Engineering	Product	Product design	Making quality products
Sales	Management	Selling existing products	Aggressive selling and advertising	Maximize sales volume
Marketing	Market	Fulfilling actual and potential customer needs and wants	Consumer orientation, profit orientation, integrated marketing	Profits through satisfied customers

Philosophic View: Organizational Role of Marketing

Organizations typically have a philosophy that indicates the types of activities the organization values. The role of marketing and its relative importance to an organization are often reflected by this philosophy. Four philosophies under which organizations practice marketing deserve mention: production, product, selling, and marketing (Box 23-2).

A *production orientation* is one of the oldest philosophies guiding organizations. These organizations focus their attention on running a smooth production process, often neglecting human needs to meet the production process requirements. Production orientation is based on the supposition that consumers will demand products and services that are available and affordable and therefore the organization should focus on pursuing efficiency in production and distribution (Kotler & Clarke, 1987). This philosophy is appropriate under two sets of circumstances: (1) when demand exceeds supply and the organization attempts to increase output; (2) when production costs are high and improvements in productivity are required to bring them down (Table 23-1).

Some health care organizations focus on running a smooth production process. For example, medical and dental practices using assembly-line principles are run as though they are processing objects rather than people. Large numbers of patients may spend long periods in waiting rooms, describe their problem to a

Key terms	
Term	**Definition**
Production orientation	Focuses attention on pursuing a smooth, efficient production process
Product orientation	Focuses on providing offerings that the organization thinks will be good for the public
Selling orientation	Emphasizes stimulating the interest of potential clients in the organization's existing offerings
Marketing orientation	Views the main task of the organization as determining the needs and wants of target markets and satisfying them through the creation, promotion, pricing, and delivery of appropriate and competitively viable offerings

nurse or assistant, see the medical, dental, or nursing practitioner briefly, pick up their prescription, fill out their insurance forms, pay their bills, and leave. Although this way of operating can maximize the practitioner's efficiency in seeing patients, it is often considered to be unfriendly and impersonal.

A *product orientation* assumes that the major task of the organization is to deliver the products or services it thinks would be good for the market. Managers subscribe to the belief that by "building a better mousetrap, the world will beat a path to your door." This orientation assumes that products or services offering the most quality, performance, and features will be recognized by consumers as being superior and therefore will be in demand. Many organizations love what they sell and believe strongly in its value. Organizations that never grow beyond a product orientation have marketing myopia (i.e., nearsightedness), which eventually leads to their demise. A classic example is the railroad industry; its management thought users wanted trains rather than transportation and ignored competitive offerings by the trucking industry, such as door-to-door pickup and delivery (Cooper, 1985).

A product orientation is a paternalistic approach to marketing that assumes the organization knows best what is good for the consumer. This orientation is especially prevalent in the health care field. If new equipment or technology means better patient care, it is acquired. Health care providers are often so enamored with the quality, the sophistication, and the technology of the care they deliver that they fail to recognize consumer dissatisfaction and discomfort caused by health care delivery. They focus on the number of patients seen or the number of procedures or tests administered and emphasize service delivery quality as perceived by the professional. The patients' needs receive little consideration. This, however, is changing because of managed care, in which both cost containment and consumer satisfaction must be achieved.

A *selling orientation* holds that consumers will not buy enough unless the organization stimulates their interest in its existing products and services by undertaking a large selling and promotion effort. Three basic tenets underlie this concept. One is that products and services are not bought; they are sold. The second is that consumers are plentiful; some may buy again, but others will not. In either case, there is no great concern about repeat business. The third basic tenet is that a variety of sales-stimulating devices, such as advertisements, personal selling, and promotional giveaways, can effectively convince consumers to buy (Cooper, 1985).

Although the selling orientation may not traditionally have been prevalent in health care, some organizations believe they can substantially increase the size of their market by becoming more selling oriented. Rather than modify their products or restructure their services to make them more attractive, these organizations increase their budgets for advertising, outreach, personal selling, and other forms of sales promotion. For example, some home health care agencies react to declining patient volumes by increasing the frequency of visits made by liaison nurses to referring hospitals, by increasing their public relations budgets, and by developing new agency brochures. Many hospitals are confronted with the problem of empty beds; some try "selling" their community on using the local hospital. Physicians located in major cities are finding extreme competition for patients; some of them are attempting to "sell" to patients by advertising. The focus in each of these examples is on short-term results: increasing patient volume. But their use in no way implies that the organization has moved into a marketing orientation that would generate more clients in the long run. In managed care, the marketing is done to the employer, who essentially purchases services according to a predetermined benefit schedule for all employees.

Some organizations have discovered the value of refocusing their attention away from production, products, or selling to their clients. A *marketing orientation,* also known as the *marketing concept,* recognizes that the main purpose of the organization is to create a satisfied customer (Webster, 1992). Achieving or-

Key terms	
Term	Definition
Customers	Those who buy products and services
Consumers	Those who use products and services
Clients	Either customers, consumers, or both

ganizational goals depends on determining the needs, wants, and values of target markets and satisfying them through the design, communication, pricing, and delivery of appropriate and competitively viable products and services. It begins with a well-defined market, focuses on consumer needs, integrates all consumer-affecting marketing activities, and generates profits by creating consumer satisfaction. This approach is especially suited to managed care and is based on three tenets (Cooper, 1985):

1. An active plan of marketing research is required to determine consumer wants, needs, and values. The organization must systematically study customer needs, wants, perceptions, preferences, and satisfaction, using surveys, focus groups, and other means, and must constantly act on this information to improve its offerings to better meet consumer needs.
2. All target market or consumer-related activities are integrated.
3. Successfully satisfying the consumer results in repeat business, consumer loyalty, and organizational support, all of which contribute to the satisfaction of the organization's goals.

It may be instructive at this juncture to briefly compare the production, product, selling, and marketing orientations. The marketing orientation focuses on the needs of the consumer, whereas the other orientations, collectively, focus on the needs of the organization. The production, product, and selling orientations all take an inside-out perspective. They start within the organization, focusing on what it has available to offer, and, in the case of the selling orientation, use various sales-stimulating devices to achieve profitable sales. In contrast, the marketing orientation takes an outside-in perspective. It begins with existing or potential consumer needs, plans a coordinated set of programs and services to serve those wants, needs, and values, and in return, satisfies its goals through creating satisfaction. In short, the marketing orientation is really the antithesis of the other orientations. As Peter Drucker stated (1974, p. 64), "The aim of marketing is to make selling superfluous. The aim of marketing is to know and understand the consumer so well that the product or service fits him and sells itself."

Historically, the production and product orientations have dominated the health care field. More recently, however, the trend has shifted toward the selling and, even more important, the marketing orientations. One impediment to a more rapid transition involves differentiating between needs and the perception of needs. That is, identifying and responding to consumer health needs has traditionally been accepted as the responsibility of health professionals, who have defined these needs from their profession's perspective rather than from the perspective of the consumer. The focus on the consumer to determine needs is what differentiates marketing from a client service mode of planning (Cooper, 1985). At present the consumer in a fee-for-service setting may be a patient or in managed care may be a purchaser who is often the employer of the patient.

The marketing orientation states that consumer wants and needs, as determined by consumers, must be met if the health care organization is to survive. Marketing is in part a "state of mind." It is a willingness to always think of the client or patient first, recognizing that when the client is satisfied, other organizational goals can be realized as well. The starting point for marketing is putting the consumer first. It makes little sense to spend money developing a marketing strategy to increase the patient load of a private health care provider's practice while ignoring basic "antimarketing" behavior among employees. For example, the same practitioners who are often willing to pay for marketing studies fail to see that patients are being lost every day because of the way they have been treated by the receptionist, nurse, or other care giver.

In contrast, those who realize that marketing means more than filling appointments or beds and includes providing services that consumers want have been more successful than their less-enlightened competitors. This marketing concept is true in a fee-for-service economy as well as in managed care if the purchaser considers customer satisfaction when selecting providers and at the time of contract renewal. There remains, however, a certain degree of skepticism with regard to applying the marketing concept to health care. Few object to the consumer orientation, but many object to the hard sell and similar tactics sometimes used in aggressive marketing.

Few organizations, health care or otherwise, have managed to truly adopt the philosophy of a consumer orientation. Many organizations only pay lip service to the philosophy and then wonder why marketing does not work as well as expected. A major factor underlying a marketing orientation is that resources must be invested to determine what consumers truly want. This can be time consuming and expensive. However, if marketing takes its rightful place at the center of provider decision making and focuses on the consumer, it can have a significant impact on many of the important factors affecting cost (Duda, 1990).

What Marketing Is Not

Marketing should not be equated with either advertising or selling. As Drucker notes, ". . . . selling and marketing are antithetical rather than synonymous or even complementary" (1974, p. 64). Advertising through mass media (newspapers, magazines, radio, television, billboards, direct mail) and personal selling (direct one-to-one contact) are only two of the promotional tools available to the marketer for communicating with target markets. Advertising is a small but visible part of the marketing plan. It is sometimes selected by marketers as the most efficient way to communicate with consumers about an organization's offerings. Personal selling is often used to communicate with small, narrowly defined target markets of decision makers, who influence many other consumers.

Ideally, the appropriate promotion tools are selected after the organization has determined the appropriate consumer group (target market), designed services to satisfy those consumers, priced the services at a level acceptable to both consumers and the organization, and developed a plan to make the services available to consumers.

Definition

So far, the discussion of marketing has been in general terms, characterizing it as encompassing all the activities involved in anticipating, managing, and satisfying demand via exchange. To be more precise, the American Marketing Association offers the following definition of marketing (Marketing News, 1985, p. 1):

> The process of planning and executing the conception, pricing, promotion, and distribution of ideas, goods, and services to create exchanges that satisfy individuals and organizational goals.

This broad definition takes into account all parties involved in the marketing effort: members of organizations that produce products and services, resellers of products and services, and customers or clients. Furthermore, marketing activities may be carried out by a range of organizations, including health care providers.

Three things about this definition of marketing should be noted. *First,* marketing is defined as a process that relies on planning and execution and not just haphazard actions designed to achieve satisfying goals. *Second,* marketing seeks to create exchanges that satisfy all parties involved. *Third,* marketing includes the conception, pricing, promotion, and distribution of offerings such as ideas, goods, and services. It is not limited to only one or two of its tools, such as advertising or selling, as previously mentioned.

Exchange

Marketing offers a variety of concepts and techniques that can be adapted to meet the needs of health care organizations, including its core concept of exchange (Houston & Gassenheimer, 1987). Health care organizations, like all others, depend on an exchange process between providers and consumers, and the objective of marketing is to create exchanges. An *exchange* is a process in which two or more parties voluntarily provide something of value to each other. Certain conditions are necessary before an exchange can take place. One set of conditions focuses on the qualities of humans, who are considered to be goal-seeking and goal-ranking and capable of anticipating the consequences of their acts, directing their acts toward specific consequences, and creating innovative behaviors that suit their purposes. A second set of conditions specifies at least two entities, each having something valued by the other, each being capable of communicating about the offering, and each being capable of making the offering available (Houston & Gassenheimer, 1987).

Exchanges take place within a market. In this sense, a *market* consists of individuals and orga-

Key terms	
Term	Definition
Exchange	Process in which two or more parties voluntarily provide something of value to each other
Market	Consists of individuals and organizations with the desire and ability to purchase a particular product or service
Needs	That which customers require to survive as individuals and organizations
Desires (or wants)	That which customers would like to have to make their lives more pleasant or their activities easier to carry out

nizations with the desire and ability to purchase a particular product or service. Thus a given market may consist of organizational buyers, consumers, or both.

Successful marketing is customer driven: it addresses customer needs and desires and emphasizes the building of long-term relationships. *Needs* are that which customers require to survive as individuals and organizations. *Desires* or *wants* are that which customers would like to have to make their lives more pleasant or their activities easier to carry out. Competition for customers is intense, so addressing customers' needs and desires is essential, as is developing long-term relationships. Today's new leading organizations engage in exchanges within ongoing relationships (Webster, 1992).

■ MARKETS, CONSUMERS, AND CUSTOMERS

Market Segmentation and Target Markets: Attracting New Customers

The health care market consists of a wide range of consumers, with an equally diverse array of needs and desires. Marketing's mandate is to create exchanges and develop long-term relationships, which entails a two-step process: attracting new customers or clients from among all the potential *consumers* in the market; and then keeping them. One of the problems facing health care marketers is identifying all of the di-

Key terms	
Term	Definition
Market segmentation	Dividing heterogeneous markets into a number of smaller, more homogeneous submarkets
Target market	Defined group of consumers or organizations with whom a firm wants to create marketing exchanges

verse consumer groups in the market, which includes care seekers, care providers, third-party payers, and a variety of others. When an organization identifies its consumers in global, generic terms, such as "the market" or "everyone," it is clear that its managers do not understand marketing. Eventually, every organization realizes that trying to be everything to everybody is impractical.

Health care organizations by nature have some inherent specialization such as cardiology, psychiatry, ambulatory care, long-term care, emergency medicine, or home health care services. That specialization determines the types of consumers they are capable of serving. Yet within these specialty areas are consumers with varying needs, wants, and desires. To focus on more meaningful, manageable groups of consumers, marketers engage in market segmentation by dividing heterogeneous markets into a number of smaller, more homogeneous submarkets. Then one or more of these submarkets is selected as a target market. Although several submarkets can be targeted, each one requires a unique set of marketing activities designed to achieve consumer satisfaction.

There are many ways to segment a market. The most frequently used bases are demographic characteristics of potential clients, geographic location, health needs, behavior, benefits, and utilization needs (Lancaster, 1989). An oncology practice, for example, might segment the market based on the various types of cancer that can be identified, such as leukemia, skin cancer, or lung cancer. Similarly, a specialized addiction treatment center's segments could include alcohol, food, tobacco, or gambling. And a counseling center's market might be segmented by age (i.e., children or adults).

For most health care organizations the primary consumer group consists of actual and potential care-seekers, known as *patients.* The buyer-seller relationship of traditional exchange processes must be modified in much of health care because the patient has a greater than normal professional dependency on the provider. Most people have limited knowledge of medical terminology or the complexity of medical diagnosis or care and cannot accurately evaluate the health care provided. Hence, patients are more dependent on the professional care giver. At one time, people would never have questioned their provider's choices and decisions. Today, however, patients are more prone to shop for a provider who has privileges at their preferred health care institution, if their insurer or managed care plan allows this choice.

A variety of marketing efforts have been directed toward attracting potential patients from this consumer group. For example, advertising has been used to communicate the potential benefits (satisfaction) to be derived from using the services of the health care provider. Public relations activities, such as heart transplant recipient reunions, health fairs, or baby fairs, are also used to attract new patients.

Physicians represent another important consumer group because they often refer their patients to other health care providers. Physicians are especially important for hospitals because most patients are admitted by those physicians who have staff privileges. Consequently, physicians significantly influence hospital occupancy rates. Thus hospitals often focus much of their marketing efforts on physicians.

When their patients need care that is outside their expertise, physicians use a referral system. With the abundance of specialists, physicians are learning that marketing to other physicians is also important. Because a long-term care facility is often recommended by a physician, nursing homes, rehabilitation centers, home-health care organizations, and others have targeted physicians with their marketing efforts. Typically, the patient or responsible care giver chooses a facility from the group recommended by the physician. If a health care provider is not in the suggested group, there is little chance it will be considered.

Another important consumer group is third-party payers, which includes managed care organizations, insurance companies, government, and employers. Their fundamental concern is with having health care providers control costs while efficiently providing adequate levels of treatment. As payers, insurance companies are important target markets for nursing homes, hospitals, and other health care institutions. If they are not satisfied with the quality of care or the charges for procedures, they can use their considerable financial influence to make changes.

The health care market also includes several other important consumer groups, such as contributors and volunteers. Both of these groups are especially important for not-for-profit health care organizations. It is also essential to recognize that both of these groups have their own needs that must be satisfied. Contributors want their donations to go to worthwhile organizations and to make a difference. Likewise, volunteers' needs must be satisfied if they are to continue to offer their services. Volunteerism is an important part of the not-for-profit health care organization's ability to appear less institutional and more caring and friendly. Patients appreciate the "pink ladies" and "candy stripers" who are common in many hospitals and extended-care facilities. Because of the increased number of women in the work force, the ranks of volunteers have thinned and many organizations compete for their time. Another group that should be considered is employees, both potential and current. Because the supply of health care professionals fluctuates, recruiting becomes a marketing activity aimed at satisfying the needs of potential employees.

Cultivating Existing Clients

Attracting new clients is merely the first step for a successful health care organization. Today's savvy marketers recognize that it is five times more expensive to acquire a new client than to retain one; thus cultivating clients has become a primary concern for institutions today (SHPM, 1995). According to Alvis R. Swinney, senior vice president and chief marketing officer of Baylor Health Care System in Dallas (SHPM, 1995, p. 1):

> It's economic suicide to concentrate on acquiring new customers without doing everything in your power to retain existing customers. The more you know about what keeps your current customers happy, and keeps them your customers, the better you will be at acquiring new ones.

Thus marketing is about having clients, not merely acquiring them. That means that market-

ing not only should have new client strategies that focus on creating exchanges, but should also work at making existing clients better clients by developing relationship marketing strategies.

Relationship marketing requires innovation and service and selling after clients become clients. It incorporates a client-oriented culture, a high-touch environment, in which clients are treated as individuals. Time is devoted to learning something about them, customizing the relationship, being accessible and responsive to routine and nonroutine client needs, and customizing services to meet the needs of individual clients (SHPM, 1995; Berry, 1987). It involves keeping them informed and creating an atmosphere of trust and institutional credibility. After all, clients want relationships with competent, communicative institutions (SHPM, 1995) and providers.

In addition, relationship marketing entails reselling clients on the benefits they received from the relationship. It also includes periodically thanking clients for their business and encouraging client loyalty by rewarding the best clients with price discounts, with service extras, or in other ways. Finally, marketing to existing clients involves monitoring their satisfaction levels and perceptions of service quality, and earning their loyalty by being loyal (Berry, 1987).

Marketing to Employees

Marketing has traditionally been directed toward the exchanges and relationships that occur between organizations and external markets. Yet just as important are the exchanges and relationships that occur between organizations and other constituents and within organizations. Employees, for example, are internal rather than external clients. Consumers exchange money for various goods and services, whereas employees exchange their labors for various considerations. In this context, internal marketing to employees can be viewed as attracting, motivating, and retaining qualified personnel through job products designed to satisfy their wants and needs (Berry, 1987).

Research demonstrates the effects these internal clients can have on a service organization's success. Specifically, they can make or break a service organization. Employee dissatisfaction can negatively affect quality of care, client loyalty, co-worker cooperation, and profitability. Nursing care, in particular, consistently emerges as the key determinant of patient satisfaction. A strong relationship exists between nurses' satisfaction with their employment and patients' perceptions of quality of care, measured in terms of their intent to return and their willingness to recommend a hospital or provider to friends and family (Atkins et al., 1996).

As health care organizations upgrade their capability for satisfying the wants and needs of external customers, they should first focus on satisfying the wants and needs of their internal customers, such as the nursing staff. They should place an increased emphasis on both employee and patient perceptions of satisfaction when developing strategic marketing plans. Therefore nurse managers should regularly measure employee satisfaction as one way to monitor service quality. They should also work closely with their human resources department to understand and influence employees' work environment and maintain a high level of job satisfaction.

Because there are many diverse consumer groups to be served, a coordinated effort must be directed toward the various target markets of health care institutions. Each target market requires different marketing efforts and activities to successfully satisfy it. Because health care organizations have a number of different target markets to satisfy, strategic marketing assumes an important role.

■ STRATEGIC PLANNING

During the 1980s new forms of business organizations became prominent. There was a trend toward more flexible types of networks, alliances, and partnerships (Webster, 1992). These new, sophisticated organizations turned to strategic planning as a major systematic approach for adapting to change. Strategic planning is carried out at the highest level of management to give the organization direction for long-term growth and survival. In general, strategic planning consists of all the activities focused on developing a clear organizational mission, setting measurable objectives for fulfilling the mission, and identifying strategies to meet those objectives.

As a hierarchic process, strategic planning is quite useful in providing guidance to marketing decision making. Strategic planning, in the broadest sense, seeks to match markets with products and other corporate resources to strengthen a firm's competitive stance. It provides the structure for choosing markets in which to participate and deciding what marketing action to take. Thus *strategic planning* can be defined as the managerial process of determining how to align the organization's long-term goals and resources with its changing marketing opportunities.

Sophisticated organizations comprise three levels: corporate, business, and functional. At the top, corporate level managers are concerned with issues affecting the entire organization and their decisions impact all other levels. The president, vice-presidents, and central administration at a university, for example, operate at this level. The business level of an organization consists of units that are generally managed as self-contained businesses. It is at this level that competition actually takes place. Colleges and schools, such as Nursing, are the business units at a university. Each business unit will include all the various functional areas necessary to perform its work. So the Nursing School will consist of various functions, such as teaching, research, marketing, accounting, and finance, administered by faculty, staff, and administration.

Strategic planning, as a hierarchic process, is typically performed at each organizational level. The strategic plans at higher organizational levels provide direction for the lower levels. Thus corporate strategic plans guide the development of the strategic plans at all other levels.

Strategic Planning Process

Although individual organizations may approach strategic planning differently, a general process applies to strategic planning at every level. It is presented here as a step-by-step approach to make it easier to understand. Generally, organizations are involved in different stages of the process simultaneously and do not necessarily follow such a definite, lock-step approach. In general, the strategic planning process consists of defining the organizational mission; performing a situation analysis; setting objectives; establishing strategic business units; developing strategy; implementing tactics; and monitoring results. The process is applicable for small and large firms, goods and services firms, and for-profit and not-for-profit institutions.

Organization Mission

Organization mission refers to the basic purpose of an organization. It describes the scope of the firm and the dominant emphasis and values, based on that firm's history, current management preferences, resources, and distinctive competencies. Years ago, Drucker (1974) pointed out that organizations need to answer the following questions: What is our business? Who is the customer? What is of value to the customer? What will our business be? What should our business be? Although the first question sounds simple, it is really the most profound question an organization can ask.

Situation Analysis

In situation analysis, sometimes called *SWOT analysis,* an organization identifies its internal strengths (S) and weaknesses (W), as well as external opportunities (O) and threats (T). Situation analysis seeks answers to two general questions: Where is the firm now? In what direction is the firm headed? These questions are answered by recognizing both company strengths and weaknesses relative to competitors; searching the environment for potential opportunities and threats; assessing the organization's ability to capitalize on opportunities as well as to minimize or avoid threats; and anticipating competitors' responses to company strategies.

Set Objectives

The situation analysis is designed to provide the necessary background and stimulus for managers to think about basic goals of the organization. Objectives are normally described in both quantitative terms (dollar sales, percentage profit growth, market share) and qualitative terms (image, level of innovativeness, industry leadership role).

Strategic Business Units

After defining its mission, performing a situation analysis, and setting objectives, an organization establishes strategic business units. Each strategic business unit (SBU) is a separate operating unit in an organization. It may be a self-contained division—such as a children's medical center; a product line, such as cancer treatments; or a product department, such as a fertility clinic—within an organization with a specific market focus. SBUs are the basic building blocks of a strategic plan, and each SBU has these general attributes: an individual orientation, a precise target market, its own strategy, clear-cut competitors, and a distinctive differential advantage.

Strategy Development

Overall organizational strategy is often accomplished in two stages. First, there is some form of portfolio analysis, by which an organization individually assesses and positions every business unit, product, or service and decides what to do with each. Second, the organization develops an expansion strategy; that is, it decides on the addition of new products, services, and markets.

Several systematic approaches to planning have been devised to enable organizations to develop their strategies more effectively. Two approaches to portfolio analysis and two strategy models are presented next: the Boston Consulting Group matrix, the General Electric business screen, the product/market opportunity matrix, and the Porter generic strategy model.

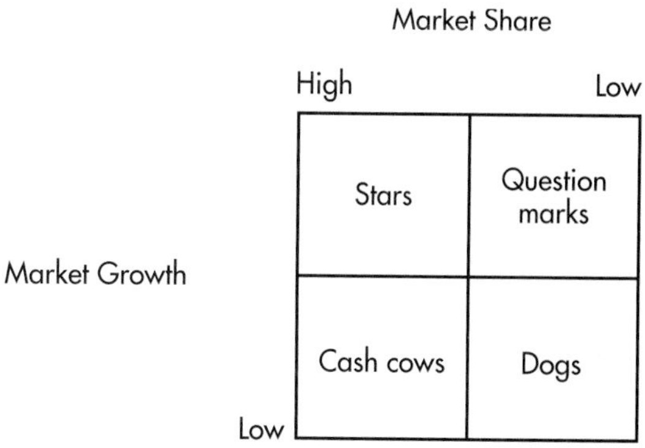

Portfolio Analysis

The first step in portfolio analysis is to identify the organization's key products and services. The organization then has to determine which of those products and services should be given increased support, maintained at the present level, phased down, or terminated. The principle is that the organization's resources should be allocated in accordance with the attractiveness of each product or service rather than equally to all. The task is to identify appropriate criteria for evaluating the attractiveness of various products and services.

Boston Consulting Group Portfolio Approach One of the earliest and most popular portfolio evaluation approaches was developed by the Boston Consulting Group, a management consulting group (Henderson, 1979). Its scheme called for rating all of an organization's products or services along two dimensions: market growth and market share.

Market growth is the annual rate of growth of the relevant market in which the product or service is sold. *Market share* is the organization's revenues as a ratio to the leading firm's revenues. By dividing market growth into high growth and low growth, and market share into

Figure 23-1 ■ The Boston Consulting Group growth-share matrix. (Modified from Henderson, B.D. [1979]. *Henderson on corporate strategy.* Cambridge, Mass.: ABT Books.)

high share and low share, four types of products, services, businesses, or programs emerge (Figure 23-1).

Stars are an organization's products or services that enjoy a high share in fast-growing markets. The organization will devote increasing resources to its stars to keep up with the market's growth and maintain its leadership share.

Cash cows are products or services that enjoy a high share in slow-growth markets. Cash cows typically yield strong cash flows to an organization, which pay the bills for other products or services that lose money. Without cash cows, an organization would need continuous subsidy.

Question marks are products or services that have only a small share in fast-growing markets. The organization needs to decide whether to increase its investment in its question mark products or services, hoping to make them stars, or to reduce or terminate its investment, on the grounds that funds could find better use elsewhere in the organization.

Dogs are products or services that have a small market share in slow-growth or declining markets. Dogs usually make little money or lose money for the organization. Organizations often consider shrinking or dropping dogs unless it is necessary to offer them for some other reason.

General Electric Portfolio Approach
General Electric has formulated another approach to portfolio evaluation that has received considerable attention (Day, 1977). They call it the *strategic business planning grid*. It uses two basic dimensions: market attractiveness and organizational strength. The best products or services to offer are those that serve attractive markets and for which the organization has high organizational strength.

Market attractiveness is a composite index made up of market size, market growth rate, profit margin, competitive intensity, cyclicality, seasonality, and scale economies. More attractive markets would tend to have large size, rapid growth rates, high profit margins, little competition, little sensitivity to macroeconomic cycles, minor seasonal patterns, and ample scale economies.

Organizational strength is also a composite index comprising relative market share, price competitiveness, service quality, knowledge of client/market, sales effectiveness, and geography. An organization could capitalize on strengths such as a strong presence in a market, low cost and fees, high-quality services, considerable market knowledge, good selling skills, and prime location.

To implement the General Electric approach, the factors making up each dimension are scaled and weighted so that each current product or service receives a number indicating its market attractiveness and organizational strength. The numbers can therefore be plotted in a grid (Figure 23-2). The grid is divided into three zones. The green zone consists of the three cells at the upper left, indicating products and services in which the organization should invest and grow. The yellow zone consists of the cells stretching diagonallly from the lower left to the upper right, indicating products and

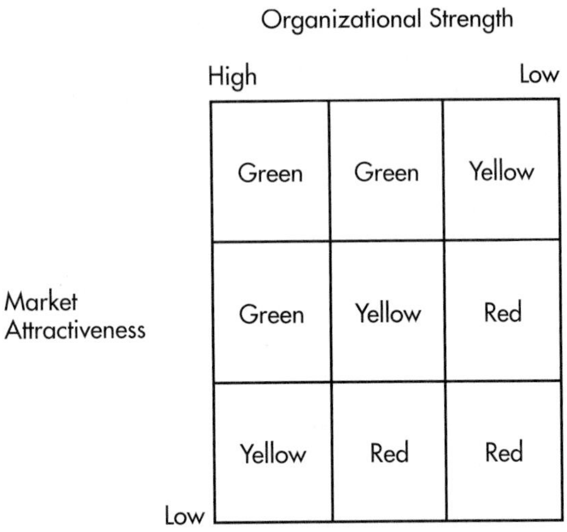

Figure 23-2 ■ **The General Electric strategic business screening grid.** (Modified from Day, G.S. [1977]. *Journal of Marketing, 41* [April], 29-38.)

services that are medium in overall investment merit. The red zone consists of the three cells in the lower right, indicating products and services that should be given serious consideration for harvesting or divesting.

Expansion Strategy Models

As a result of its portfolio evaluation, an organization might discover that too few of its products or services fall into the star, cash cow, or green zone category. Then a strategy is needed to search for new products or services and market opportunities.

Product/Market Opportunity Matrix
One useful device for doing this is known as the *product-service/market opportunity matrix* (Ansoff, 1957). As the name implies, it is a two-dimensional matrix, consisting of four cells, with products/services along the top and markets on the side (Figure 23-3). Each cell has a name.

Market penetration represents efforts to achieve an organization's growth objectives by deepening its penetration into existing markets

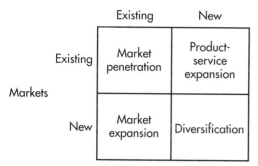

Figure 23-3 ■ The product-service/market opportunity matrix. (Modified from Ansoff, H.I. [1957]. Strategies for diversification. *Harvard Business Review, Sept.-Oct.,* 113-124.)

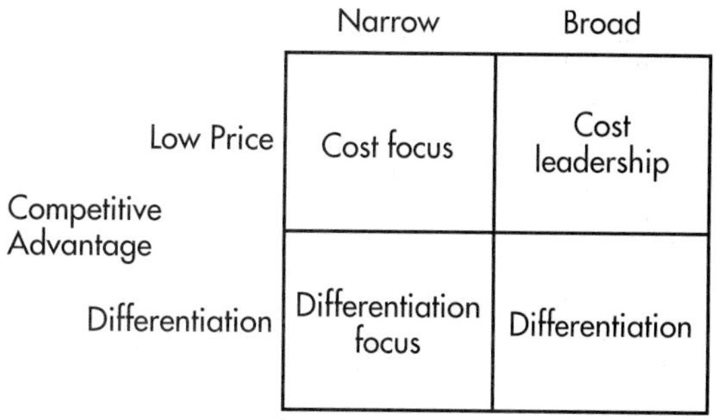

Figure 23-4 ■ The Porter generic strategy model. (Modified from Porter, M.E. [1985]. *Competitive advantage: Creating and sustaining superior performance.* New York: Free Press, pp. 11-26.)

with existing products or services. This can be done by persuading current clients to use more of the product or service or by attracting new clients. An example in health care would be a primary care group practice attempting to increase market share by directing their marketing efforts toward consumers in the area who are currently served by the practice to increase their use of existing services.

Market expansion entails offering existing products or services to new markets. This can be accomplished by either focusing on different market segments in the same geographic area and attracting new types of clients or expanding into new geographic markets with similar types of clients. For instance, a psychologist who opens a satellite office in a nearby community is attempting to grow by market expansion.

Product-service expansion involves creating new products or services to the same market. The organization wants to generate more business from its existing client base. This requires identifying unsatisfied needs that can be met by introducing new or modified products or services. Adding an AIDS clinic or a hospital wing

dedicated to adolescent addiction treatment, which introduces new services for a hospital, is an example of service expansion.

Finally, *diversification* would have the organization offering totally new products or services to new markets. This approach carries the most risk because the organization cannot build directly on its strengths in its current markets or with its current products or services. Health care organizations, as well as many others, have discovered that diversification can be expensive and full of pitfalls. Unfamiliarity with the products or services and the market has led to many business failures.

Porter Generic Strategy Model Another way to systematically approach strategic planning is suggested by the Porter (1985) model, which is based on two dimensions: market scope and competitive advantage (Figure 23-4). Market scope is viewed as either broad or narrow, and competitive advantage concentrates on either lower cost or differentiation. By combining the two dimensions, the Porter model identifies these basic strategies: cost leadership, differentiation, and focus.

Market scope refers to how broad the organization views its target market. At one extreme, it can select a broad market scope and try to appeal to most consumers in the market. The organization might consider all consumers as part of one mass market or, more likely, divide the total market into segments and target all or most of those. At the other extreme, an organization can focus on only a small portion of the market.

Competitive advantage refers to the way an organization tries to get consumers to purchase its products or services rather than those offered by competitors. Two basic strategies are again possible. It can try to compete by offering similar products and services as competitors, but at lower prices, which typically requires having a lower cost structure than competitors. An organization may also compete through differentiation, that is, offering consumers something different from and better than competitors' products or services. If differentiation is successful, prices higher than competitors can typically be charged.

With a *cost leadership* strategy, an organization appeals to a broad market and offers products or services in large quantities. Through economies of scale, the organization is able to minimize per-unit costs and offer low prices. This allows it to have better profit margins than competitors, respond better to cost increases, and attract price-conscious consumers.

With a *differential* strategy, an organization aims at a large market by offering products or services viewed as quite distinctive. The products or services have a broad appeal yet are perceived by consumers as unique by virtue of design, features, availability, and reliability. As a result, price is less important.

With a *focus* strategy, an organization seeks a narrow target segment by offering low prices or a unique product or service. It is able to control costs by concentrating efforts on a few key products or services aimed at specific consumers or by building a specialized reputation and serving a market that may be unsatisfied by competitors.

The results of the previous portfolio analysis and corporate level strategic planning for long-term growth and survival provide guidance for each strategic business unit (SBU). Given the corporate focus or vision, each business unit needs strategic plans indicating how the business unit expects to compete effectively in the marketplace. A marketing strategic plan describes how the marketing manager will execute the business strategic plan.

■ STRATEGIC MARKETING PLANNING

Marketing operates in an environment that includes a number of factors directed by top management, such as developing long-term strategies for growth and survival. Other factors are directed by the marketing department as it chooses markets in which to participate, decides on marketing programs for those markets, and allocates resources to them.

The strategic planning process is useful to coordinate these factors and provide guidance for decision making. Broadly speaking, the strategic marketing process consists of developing a market definition, delineating marketing objectives, and determining marketing strategies that will accomplish those objectives.

Market Definition

Defining the market is an important first step; it can usually be deduced from the mission statement and is central to identifying the market to be served, the competition, and the key environmental factors for determining the best strategic marketing alternatives.

Marketers use a variety of methods to arrive at a market definition. Because defining the market is important for effective strategic planning, a great deal of effort is expended on this step. Using multiple methods to identify the market helps to avoid overlooking some aspect of the organization's offering, and thereby minimizing

Key terms	
Term	**Definition**
Cash cows	Organization's products or services that enjoy a high share in slow-growth markets
Competitive advantage	How an organization tries to get consumers to purchase its products or services rather than those offered by competitors: lower cost or differentiation
Cost leadership	Strategy that appeals to a broad market and offers products or services in large quantities
Differential strategy	Aims at a large market by offering products or services viewed as distinctive
Diversification	Organization offers new products or services for new markets
Dogs	Products or services that have a small market share in slow-growth or declining markets
Focus strategy	Seeking a narrow target segment through low prices or a unique offering
Market expansion	Offering existing products or services to new markets
Market penetration	Efforts to achieve corporate growth objectives by deepening penetration into existing markets with existing products or services
Market scope	How broad or narrow the organization believes its target market to be
Organization mission	Basic purpose of an organization
Portfolio analysis	Identifying the key products and services of the organization and determining which should be given increased support, maintained at the present level, phased down, or terminated
Product-service expansion	Creating new products or services for the same market
Question marks	Products or services that have only a small share in fast-growing markets
Situation analysis (SWOT)	Identification of internal strengths (S) and weaknesses (W), as well as external opportunities (O) and threats (T)
Stars	Products or services that enjoy a high share in fast-growing markets
Strategic business units (SBUs)	Separate operating unit in an organization
Strategic planning	Managerial process of determining how to align the organization's long-term goals and resources with its changing marketing opportunities

an opportunity for others. Some health care providers, by their very nature, predefine their market. Community hospitals, regional hospitals, and county public health departments, for example, serve specific markets.

One task in defining the market suggested by the Porter model is describing the scope or segment the provider chooses to serve. More specifically, consumer groups are identified in terms of geography, demographics, or desired benefits. The services offered may be limited to specific procedures, such as open-heart surgery, or diseases, like AIDS. The geographic or service area could be defined in terms of the number of miles in a radius around a clinic, representing the distance patients would travel to see a provider. Obviously, the willingness to travel will vary from one patient to another depending on the provider's reputation, referrals, access, parking, and proximity to the patient's home or place of work. The scope could be a city, county, or regional area. Some health care providers (particularly for-profit hospitals and nursing home chains) have determined that they want to be national in scope, whereas others have set goals to be international in scope.

Demographic scope might be defined by age (children's hospitals, elderly care), gender (birthing centers, mammography clinics), religion (Catholic, Presbyterian, or other denominational hospitals), and other specific, identifiable, and quantitative characteristics of the population.

Scope defined by benefits sought must be expressed as benefits that *consumers* want, not those of health care professionals. Some patients want to use the same physician that the celebrities use. The benefit sought is prestige. Some patients want to be admitted to a specific hospital that is known to have performed the necessary procedure most frequently. The perceived benefit is risk reduction through experience. The hospital that has performed the most heart-lung transplants is considered to be the most experienced. Some patients want to be admitted to the hospital that is known for having the latest technology or the most up-to-date equipment. The benefit sought is risk reduction through advances in technology.

Market scope often has to be narrowed when resources, whether financial, natural, or human, are limited. Nursing shortages in some areas have caused hospitals to close units until the necessary number of nurses could be recruited. Market scope is easily (and often preferably) narrowed when a large enough set of consumers are satisfied by a specific benefit. Generally,

the scope is broadened with successes over time as additional resources become available and economies of scale can be achieved.

Another aspect of market definition is identifying distinctive competencies and assets. Johns Hopkins Hospital is known for its research and experimentation in bone-marrow transplants for leukemia patients. This is a *distinctive competency,* something it does better than many others. Maintaining distinctive competency is a never-ending pursuit as competitors identify, improve, and adopt new ideas, services, and benefits to better satisfy consumers.

An *asset* is something the health care provider has that is more valuable than what others possess (e.g., a clinic located in a densely populated, built-up area). Other clinics may not be able to build in that location. For either a distinctive competency or an asset to be of true value, consumers must perceive that it is beneficial. That perception is formed in connection with competitive offerings.

Marketing Objectives

Setting marketing objectives follows a hierarchic structure. After the situation analysis, a review of the organization's mission and objectives is the starting point for determining marketing objectives. If marketing objectives are achieved, they should help the organization accomplish its overall objectives. Marketing objectives typically include revenues, market share, growth, innovation, and public responsibility (Duncan et al., 1992).

Revenue objectives should be tied to another objective. Merely setting an objective for some dollar amount that should come in to the health care organization is shortsighted, because the outflow of money is also crucial. An example of a marketing revenue objective would be "to generate revenues of $12,500,000 by year's end while holding expenses to budgeted amounts."

Market share objectives are tricky because the percentages are based on the quantity and quality of competitors in the selected market. For example, a local community hospital could say that it has a 100% share of the market (town) where it is located. But the important question is, How many people leave town for their medical care? Consequently, hospitals use a variation of market share based on occupancy rates or bed census data.

Growth is usually set as a percentage over the previous year in terms of revenue, market share, or census rates. Growth for growth's sake is not always desirable, which is sometimes a difficult lesson to learn. Almost any organization can reach growth objectives, but at what cost? Often, remaining the same size and increasing profitability is a more important objective.

Innovation objectives could include new services to be offered, speeding up service delivery, or being the leader in developing or offering new technology. Public responsibility objectives are publicly mandated for most not-for-profit hospitals, nursing homes, and hospices. Many for-profit providers have also included public or social responsibility in their objectives. For example, some hospitals aim to serve a certain percent of indigent patients or to return a certain amount of money to the community in the form of health benefits.

Marketing Strategies

No leadership position lasts forever. The dynamic health care market and ever-changing technology mean that no competitive advantage can be sustained in the long run without a great deal of thought and effort. To further complicate the strategic marketing process, the long run itself is becoming shorter as the rate of change becomes increasingly rapid. There is no single, established way in which a health care organization can assure success; rather, a number of possibilities exist. To achieve a sustain-

able competitive advantage, the Porter model suggests four basic marketing strategies: differentiation, low cost, focus, and horizontal integration (Duncan et al., 1992). These marketing strategies can be accomplished in a variety of ways.

Differentiation Strategies Differentiation strategies center around the services offered but go beyond the fundamental core service. They include quality of service, faster service delivery, technologic innovation, services innovation, and reliability.

Most health care providers like to think they can differentiate their institution on the basis of the service they offer to consumers. Quality is often mentioned by health care providers, but they only partially determine quality. It is the consumer's perception of what constitutes quality that will be used to judge it. In the consumer's view, quality is achieved only when the service meets or exceeds expectations.

Realistically, quality can be perceived by the consumer only from other environmental cues, since few people have the expertise to actually judge competent medical care. Thus friendly nurses, clean and pleasant surroundings, prompt responses to patient call buzzers/lights and questions, convenient hours of operation, and so on are used to judge quality for many hospitals, long-term-care providers, and private practices.

Individual consumers are not the only health care customers to judge quality, however. Physicians and other health care professionals are more likely to judge the quality of an institution by assessing equipment, physicians who are currently on staff (or who have staff privileges), the competence of the nursing staff, and the organization and leadership provided by the nonmedical staff.

Strategies can be formulated to improve or maintain quality over time. When quality is allowed to deteriorate, whether planned or unplanned, use of the facility will eventually decline as well. A hospital's emergency room is generally a resource consumer, but it can increase admissions by 25% or more. If a community hospital's emergency room is using cash and does not lead to at least some increase in admissions, it might be neglected and allowed to deteriorate over time, and it is likely that this perception of deterioration would also carry over to the rest of the institution. To avoid this unplanned side effect, it might be better to face the issue squarely. Especially in the case of a community hospital, public meetings could be held to demonstrate to the citizens that the hospital cannot afford to provide quality emergency care and, with group consensus, decide to close the unit.

Consumers can be impatient; they value their time and will not wait for service. Horror stories about such things as long waits in the emergency room and sick patients left in wheelchairs outside the x-ray room are shared with family and friends. To avoid negative word-of-mouth communication, care givers need to think about faster service delivery. To "speed service delivery" does not mean to do things faster but to rethink why the delays occur and correct the underlying reasons. Faster responsiveness can develop into a sustainable competitive advantage.

Another way a health care organization may improve patients' or potential patients' perception that it provides quality care is to inform them about some of the special diagnostic capabilities and treatment expertise that the hospital or clinic offers. When differentiation through technologic innovation is selected, large sums of money must be available, since breakthroughs in medical equipment are costly. The price for new technology generally decreases over time, but to maintain technologic innovation as a competitive strategy, there must be money to purchase new equipment as soon

as it becomes available. Communicating information about new technology to patients is another necessary and expensive part of maintaining technologic innovation as a competitive advantage.

Being a services innovator can provide differentiation opportunities. The first hospitals to offer a physician referral service met the needs of two of their consumers—patients and physicians. The hospital that developed the referral service first could use it as a differentiating strategy. When others copy the new service with similar offerings, there is less opportunity to differentiate.

Reliability, or standardization to achieve consistent quality, is another differentiating strategy. Service reliability is a goal for most health care organizations. Services are difficult to standardize because the consumer participates in the simultaneous production and consumption of services, and as previously indicated, the human beings involved in health care delivery (patient, physician, nurse, therapist) are not capable of performing in the same way every time they might encounter the same situation. However, a prescribed routine known to all can achieve some level of consistency in admitting or new patient procedures, preoperative preparation, and discharge planning.

Many freestanding urgent-care facilities have attempted to standardize procedures and thereby provide the additional benefit of "avoiding long emergency room waiting time." However, procedures that are more unusual and do not fit the standards are often sent on to the more sophisticated hospital emergency rooms.

Some caution must be exercised in selecting any of the differentiation strategies. Differentiation will not work when the superior attribute highlighted is meaningless or unimportant to the consumer. In addition, if the health care provider has a differentiating attribute that provides benefits but consumers do not know about it, there is no advantage. For example, a new technology is used to better diagnose a patient's problem, but the patient is unconscious when the equipment is used. The patient will not perceive the benefit unless told that the hospital cares enough to purchase the wonderful, new equipment that works so much faster (or is less intrusive, or whatever the benefit may be).

Health care managers must realize that not providing quality in the delivery of health care is costly. As mentioned, lawsuits abound. In addition, there are costs associated with doing things incorrectly. Consider a hospital or nursing home billing statement that contains errors. Not only is there the cost of finding the error and redoing the statement, there is also the cost of losing a positive consumer attitude and perhaps a patient.

Cost Leadership Strategies Although cost leadership strategies are generally associated with low costs that can be translated into low prices, a high-price strategy can effectively position an organization as a quality health care provider. However, the consumer must perceive that the benefits (aesthetically pleasing surroundings, attentive care, or latest technology) are worth the higher price.

In manufacturing, being the low-cost producer in an industry can be a significant competitive advantage. It allows the firm to make many more choices about the price, quality, and profitability of its products. Cost leadership strategies include reducing overhead, controlling raw materials, reducing labor costs, redesigning the offering, automation, location, increasing government subsidy, no frills, and combining low cost and high quality (Duncan et al., 1992). Many of these cost strategies seem manufacturing-oriented, but they have important marketing implications. However, low-cost strategies must be selected carefully. Few people want to think that they are receiving "cheap" health care.

Reducing overhead is a strategy usually selected when an organization is mature. Overhead generally consists of rent, utilities, and other expenses that would occur even if there were no patients. It can also include administrative salaries, insurance, and other ongoing costs. The health care provider might have invested too much in overhead during times of growth. Many organizations are quick to add employees and facilities when times are good, but they rarely cut back when times are difficult. The result is excessive overhead. One way for a hospital to reduce overhead is to close off a wing or eliminate an infrequently used department.

Sometimes spending more money can reduce overhead, as when a physician moves to a newer building with more energy-efficient heating and cooling. Control of raw materials or factors of production can provide a competitive advantage in terms of price as well as availability. When the University of Virginia was having difficulty recruiting nurses, the administration decided to provide financial assistance to nursing students who agreed to practice nursing at the medical center after graduation. This gave the administration much more control over the hospital's major factor in service production—its nurses.

Reducing labor costs is a difficult strategy for today's health care organizations to implement. As with other service industries, health care is labor-intensive. In addition, the industry requires skilled labor. Because of the shortage of trained personnel, wages and salaries are going up rather rapidly. Moreover, certification standards for qualified personnel must be met. Thus certification standards, skilled-labor shortages, and wage inflation make it difficult to reduce labor costs. Rather than focusing on reducing the labor costs, proper scheduling, job redesign, and other forms of efficiency must be emphasized. Costs can be reduced by better matching consumer demand and labor availability.

Another cost leadership strategy is to redesign the offering to change the product offered so that it becomes less costly but no less desirable. An extended-care facility with an excellent reputation in the community for cleanliness, good food, and competent and sympathetic care givers could probably reduce the square footage in patients' rooms—and thereby reduce the cost of construction, heating/cooling, and maintenance—without harming its image.

Labor-intensive services are difficult to automate, but not impossible. Blood pressure checks have been automated. In addition, a finger stick for routine blood work could be automated by using a machine, but would the public accept a machine instead of a nurse? In another service industry, many bankers continued to believe that consumers would want to talk to a real person when cashing checks or depositing money. However, the banks that were the first to automate with teller machines have been very profitable. Can similar results be achieved in health care?

A location that is attractive because of its proximity to patients' homes and work is a valuable asset, especially if other health care providers cannot duplicate the location. Because people do not want to travel great distances for most health care, demographic studies of population are an important part of choosing a location for a facility. Satellite offices and hospital branches that are available where patients want to receive care have become increasingly important. Although satellite offices and hospitals do not typically cut costs for the organization, they do cut costs for the patient, which can lead to increased market share and improved efficiency for the health care provider.

Some hospitals find it worthwhile to establish centers in shopping malls. These centers can enhance a hospital's reputation by demonstrating its commitment to providing easily accessible outpatient health care and by increasing the hospital's visibility, which in turn can lead to increased bed census rates and economies of scale.

Mobile units, long used by the Red Cross to gain more blood donations, are another method of achieving the optimum in health care delivery. Other institutions are now using movable diagnostic equipment to be closer to patients.

A no-frills strategy eliminates all "extras" from services—a rather direct approach that tells consumers from the beginning that there will be no frills and in return they will receive a lower price. Home health offered by a hospital seems to fit this strategy. On the other hand, for many who are admitted to a large hospital ward, few "frills" are perceived. Caution has to be exercised in positioning "no frills" so that the patient perceives that only the extras have been eliminated. Otherwise the perception may be of poor care.

The combination of low cost and high quality offers higher-cost services only to consumers who prefer it. Overall costs can actually be reduced by moving along the experience curve and by achieving economies of scale (brought about by increased market share). Accurate assessment of demand, careful planning, and increased expertise (actual movement along the experience curve) are crucial to the successful implementation of this strategy.

Focus Strategies Focus strategies are often implemented when an organization has limited resources. The organization does not compete across the board, but only in selected areas. The market definition is narrowed to identify a select group to serve. Enough resources can then be devoted to that consumer group to achieve some degree of prominence or even dominance. In addition, increased specialization may lead to the development of greater understanding and satisfaction on the part of the particular group targeted, which may in turn increase usage and loyalty.

A sharply focused strategy has the benefit of being difficult for the competition to attack. Yet at the same time such a strategy often restricts the organization's ability to grow. Focus strategies include service, segment, geographic area, and low-share markets (Duncan et al., 1992).

A focused service is one part of a service line. Rather than attempting to offer a complete line of services, which usually includes some mangy dogs and underperforming cash cows, the organization offers only a part of a service line. Usually, an organization will focus on a service in which it has greater expertise and when it believes that some economies of scale may be achieved with a smaller service line. For example, a teen counseling center might select a focus strategy based on the population segment served. A nursing home that focuses on Alzheimer's patients has also selected a focus strategy.

The geographic-area strategy is used by most community hospitals. They serve a specific geographic market and are the only hospital in the area. The private practice of an individual psychologist generally uses a geographic-area focus strategy as well. As the practice develops and flourishes, a second office may be opened that extends the geography.

Low-share markets are those that are not of sufficient size to interest the larger health care providers. A hospital or physician practice that specializes in less common diseases can satisfy a smaller market extremely well and thereby capture virtually all of the patients with that disease. This strategy can be more profitable than trying to capture a small part of a larger market that includes many large and knowledgeable competitors. This strategy emphasizes profitability rather than size or growth.

Horizontal Integration Horizontal integration occurs when one competitor buys out a competitor. The competitors are deemed to be on the "same level" and thus the term *horizontal integration.* In essence, an organization is buying market share. From a marketing perspective, the concern is which competitor will best enhance the organization's strategy.

Many not-for-profit organizations do not have a choice but are told by their governing or regulating bodies that they will take over the operations of another facility (usually one that is performing poorly). For-profit organizations buy out others for a variety of reasons, including increasing market share, achieving economies of scale, gaining the other organization's experience in the market, or eliminating an aggressive competitor.

In horizontal integration, organizational issues must be considered as well as the match between the purchasing organization's marketing strategy and the purchased organization's strategy. If they are similar, the integration can be implemented smoothly. But if the strategies are different, decisions must be made about changing to be more like the purchasing organization's strategy (or vice versa) or to broaden the services offered by maintaining the strategies of both organizations. These considerations should be discussed before the acquisition to determine if there is a good strategic fit.

■ MARKETING MANAGEMENT

Once the general marketing strategy has been selected, marketing management's task is to translate the generalities of the strategy into meaningful distinctions for consumers. The selected strategy becomes the marketing strategy when a target market is selected and a marketing mix developed to meet the target market's needs.

An effective marketing program begins the process of selecting target markets by segmenting the broader market by certain demographic variables, health needs, psychologic needs, interests, or utilization functions (Lancaster, 1989). The major benefits of market segmentation are the following (Lovelock, 1985):

1. A more precise definition of consumer needs and behavior patterns
2. Improved identification of ways to provide services to population groups
3. More efficient utilization of resources through accomplishment of a better fit between products, services, and consumers

The marketing mix must be designed and coordinated to present the competitive advantage to the targeted consumers. Traditionally, the *marketing mix* has consisted of product, promotion, distribution, and price.

A *product* is anything that can be offered to a market for attention, acquisition, use, or consumption. The product in health care is often intangible and may be difficult to define and evaluate. An enlightening way of viewing health care products is in three levels: the core product, the formal product, and the augmented product.

The *core product* answers the question "What is this consumer really getting?" The product is simply the packaging of a problem-solution. For example, a woman who invests time and transportation costs in visiting a family planning clinic for counseling is not buying a clinic filled with comfortable chairs and magazines for entertainment. Instead, she is buying hope for a planned future. A man arranging his schedule to attend a smoking cessation clinic is not buying a lecture; he is buying the chance to live a longer and more productive life.

The second level, or the *formal product,* refers to the packaging of the core product. Although health care is delivered primarily in the form of a service, it may have as many as five characteristics: a quality level, features, styling, a brand name, and packaging. For example, a family planning clinic exhibits a demonstrable quality level in that the service providers have a

certain level of competence. The service of family planning has features, such as being offered at a reduced fee or at no cost to qualified recipients, as well as possibly requiring only moderate waiting before being seen. Likewise, the service has a specific styling, such as when providers are friendly, caring, and concerned for their consumers. Similarly, the service has a certain formal name, such as "Community Family Planning Clinic." Finally, the service is packaged within branch offices or within nice, comfortable, and accessible facilities.

The third level, or the *augmented product,* refers to the totality of benefits that a person receives or experiences by obtaining the formal product. The augmented product of a smoking cessation clinic, for example, includes not only the classroom lecture, but also an entire set of accompanying benefits and services, such as instruction, counseling, support, an emergency number to call if the desire to smoke becomes too strong to handle alone, and an increased feeling of self-worth for having overcome a difficult habit.

Promotion is the marketer's means of communication; it is used to make products familiar, acceptable, and even desirable to the target market. Promotion, far more than advertising, includes personal selling, public relations, various incentives, and the behavior and attitudes of employees. Often overlooked is the effect of employee attitudes when they are in contact with consumers. A sullen, irritable employee sends a negative message, whereas a pleasant, helpful employee conveys a positive image for the organization.

Distribution calls for providing an adequate delivery system. Planning in this area entails selecting or developing appropriate outlets and deciding on their number, size, and locations. In reaching target markets, multiple facilities may be required. Distribution includes more than just facility location. It refers also to the hours of operation, scheduling procedures, transportation considerations, signs and instructions directing people to the facilities, proximity to other related services, and parking facilities.

Price, the final element in the marketing mix, refers to the cost that consumers must accept to obtain the product. Pricing is multifaceted in health care and includes all that must be endured to receive services, including actual fees, transportation, waiting time, stigma attached to treatment, and the personal or impersonal nature of treatment. In addition to fees, other costs to be considered when pricing services includes opportunity, energy, and psychic costs. Opportunity costs are best described as the difference in benefits to the consumer if investment is made in some activity other than the health care service. For instance, a person may perceive a greater return on satisfaction by visiting a museum or library than attending a lecture on the hazards of poor dietary behavior. If the costs involved (farther to drive, longer time involved) are greater for the lecture than for the visit to the library, the individual will "economically" choose to go to the library. Energy costs and psychic costs should also be examined, and if they present influential factors, they should be manipulated to increase or decrease use of the health care offering.

Once the target market is identified and the marketing mix is determined, the marketing strategy should provide a sustainable comparative advantage and serve as the cornerstone for making decisions. In addition, it should be reviewed on a periodic basis to make sure the organization's competitive advantage still exists and is desired by consumers. When competitive pressure is increasing, revenue is decreasing or static in what should be a time of growth, or the excess of revenues over expenses is declining, health care managers must reassess whether the competitive advantage is still meaningful to consumers.

The market naturally works to cut the competitive advantage of a leader by technologic and environmental changes that erode protective barriers. In addition, competitors learn how to imitate the leader and negate or equalize the competitive advantage. The organization itself may not take action to protect its position. This passive reaction may occur either because the company does not perceive a threat from competitors or because the threat is dismissed as unimportant. Sometimes an organization does not respond because any action is considered to be detrimental to the organization's overall strategy.

An organization can engage in defensive moves to thwart prospective challengers. One defensive move is to signal intentions to defend a position. If a smaller hospital announces its intention to build specialized labor/delivery rooms, a larger competitor in the region could increase its advertising budget to promote its already in-place specialized maternity care. It has signaled that it will defend its position.

Others will attempt to foreclose avenues for attack, as when a large group practice adds previously uncovered specialties to provide comprehensive care. "Raising the stakes" is another way to combat competition. A hospital that purchases high-technology diagnostic equipment that no other hospital in the area can afford is raising the stakes.

Finally, a competitor can attempt to reduce the attractiveness of the market by using the mass media, which has covered health care extensively. For example, a number of articles have been written about the financial and personnel difficulties faced by home health care organizations. Potential entrants to the industry may find it less attractive if they are exposed to a number of such articles or commentary in the mass media.

The final step in implementing any strategy should be assessment or control. A marketing audit looks at all marketing activities to determine if there are areas where marketing could be improved, if the marketing effort is supporting the organization's mission, goals, and strategic objectives, and if the results of the marketing effort were as planned.

■ KEY POINTS

- Although marketing is a process that has been in effect for many years, it has only in the last two decades been used extensively in health care.
- Both products and services are marketed, and services are often quite heterogeneous.
- In health care, a marketing orientation would necessitate that the organization carefully determines the needs and wants of its target market and then satisfies these needs and wants by creating, promoting, pricing, and delivering appropriate and competitive offerings.
- Markets should be segmented so that appropriate services can be targeted to the consumers who need or want them.
- In health care, consumers are those who actually seek care, physicians, health care and other employees of the organization, and payers of the services as well as contributors and volunteers.
- Strategic planning is a process for aligning the organization's long-term goals and resources with its changing marketing opportunities.

■ CRITICAL THINKING QUESTIONS

1. What are the major differences between the traditional view and the broadened view of marketing?
2. Select a clinical setting with which you are familiar and answer these questions based on your observations:
   A. What is the unit/agency's mission?
   B. If they have segmented the market, what are the characteristics of the market segment they serve?
   C. Who is their competition?
   D. Based on what you have learned from this chapter, what advice can you give the unit/agency to increase profitability?
3. Select a community agency with which you have had experience/knowledge. Who are the current external clients? What additional clients might be attracted? How? Who are the internal customers? How satisfied do they appear? If they are not fully satisfied, what would you do to make them satisfied customers?
4. Conduct a brief SWOT analysis of a unit or agency with a group of classmates or colleagues. Then answer these questions:
   A. Where is the unit/agency now?
   B. Where it is headed?
5. Identify all marketing strategies that you recognize in one clinical agency with which you are familiar. How would you evaluate the number, type, and effectiveness of these strategies? What would you do differently?

■ REFERENCES

Ansoff, H.I. (1957). Strategies for diversification. *Harvard Business Review,* Sept.-Oct., 113-124.

Atkins, P.M., Marshall, B.S., & Javalgi, R.G. (1996). Happy employees lead to loyal patients. *Journal of Health Care Marketing, 16*(4), 15-23.

Berry, L.L. (1987). Big ideas in services marketing. *The Journal of Services Marketing, 1*(1), 5-9.

Cooper, P.D. (1985). *Health care marketing: Issues and trends.* Germantown, Md.: Aspen.

Day, G.S. (1977). Diagnosing the product portfolio. *Journal of Marketing, 41*(April), 29-38.

Drucker, P.F. (1974). *Management: Tasks, responsibilities, practices.* New York: Harper & Row.

Duda, D.F. (1990). Marketing must turn savage. *Modern Healthcare,* April 16, 50.

Duncan, W.J., Ginter, P.M., & Swayne, L.E. (1992). *Strategic management of health care organizations.* Boston: PWS-Kent.

Henderson, B.D. (1979). *Henderson on corporate strategy.* Cambridge, Mass.: ABT Books.

Houston, F.S., & Gassenheimer, J.B. (1987). Marketing and exchange. *Journal of Marketing, 51*(Oct.), 3-18.

Kotler, P. (1972). A generic concept of marketing. *Journal of Marketing, 36*(April), 46-54.

Kotler, P. & Clarke, R.N. (1987). *Marketing for health care organizations.* Englewood Cliffs, NJ: Prentice-Hall.

Kotler, P., & Levy, S.J. (1969). Broadening the concept of marketing. *Journal of Marketing, 33*(Jan.), 10-15.

Kotler, P., & Zaltman, G. (1971). Social marketing: An approach to planned social change. *Journal of Marketing, 35*(July), 3-12.

Lancaster, W. (1989). Marketing mental health services: Back to the basics. *Psychiatric Annals, 19*(8), 435-438.

Lovelock, C.H. (1985). Concepts and strategies for health marketers. In P.D. Cooper (Ed.). *Health care marketing: Issues and trends.* Germantown, Md.: Aspen, pp. 19-28.

Marketing News. (1985). AMA Board approves new definition. *Marketing News,* March 1, 1.

Porter, M.E. (1985). *Competitive advantage: Creating and sustaining superior performance.* New York: Free Press, pp. 11-26.

SHPM. (1995). Relationship marketing: More important now than ever before. *SHPM's Planning and Marketing, Nov.,* 1-6.

Webster, F.E. Jr. (1992). The changing role of marketing in the corporation. *Journal of Marketing, 56*(Oct.), 1-17.

Zaltman, G., & Vertinsky, I. (1971). Health services marketing: A suggested model. *Journal of Marketing, 35*(July), 19-27.

Zeithaml, V.A., Parasuraman, A., & Berry, L.L. (1990). *Delivering quality service.* New York: The Free Press.

Consultation as a Tool for Change

Juliann G. Sebastian and Marcia Stanhope

INTRODUCTION

This chapter examines ways in which consultation can facilitate change. Professional nurses are increasingly called on to serve as consultants both within their own employing health care organizations or schools of nursing and to a variety of organizations at local, national, and international levels (Scholz, 1996). Sometimes nurses are employed specifically as consultants, such as in educational institutions, hospitals, or home health or in state public health programs. These nurses provide consultation and technical assistance to individual and district health departments and to a variety of voluntary and not-for-profit organizations. Other nurses establish consulting firms to provide this service to a variety of groups or organizations, (e.g., legal nurse consultants). Nurses may establish consulting practices to assist individuals and families in changing health behaviors. Finally, nurses with special expertise are often asked to provide expert advice and consultation to other programs or departments within their own organizations. For example, a key aspect of the work of occupational health nurses is consulting with management about matters related to employee health, safety, and wellness.

In each of these examples of consulting, nurses' skills in interpersonal communication, partnership, assessment, critical thinking, planning, and clinical expertise make them particularly well qualified to serve as consultants. Consulting provides nurses with opportunities to engage in planned change (Tiffany & Lutjens, 1998).

In fact, consultation is an ongoing responsibility of professional nursing practice. Whenever one nurse has special expertise and other nurses, other health care professionals, or community members request that nurse's expertise, he or she has the opportunity to consult. For example, a parish nurse working with a patient anticipating a new surgical procedure calls a nursing colleague who has special expertise in caring for people who have had that procedure. This creates an opportunity for the second nurse to consult with his or her colleague on this issue.

Consultation is a core component of advanced nursing practice (Ingersoll & Jones, 1992; Patterson et al., 1995). According to an early report by the American Nurses Association (1986), consultation made up 40% to 69% of the roles of clinical nurse specialists. More recent analyses of the role continue to emphasize the importance of consultation (Naylor & Brooten, 1993). Advanced practice nurses are called on more often to serve as consultants at the organizational level. Nurses also may be called on as internal consultants to share their expertise for issues related to a particular clinical problem.

Organizations are increasingly relying on advice from external consultants. Furlow (1995, p. 13) said that:

> . . . when uncertainty abounds, consulting flourishes as people seek out experts to "show them the way." The current social, economic, and political environment within which health care is delivered is in such a state of rapid and profound change that it is a time of deep ambiguity.

Furlow goes on to speculate that the nineties may become known as the "decade of the consultants," because so many organizations have found it useful to solicit outside advice as they attempt to make changes. Consultants play a key role as change agents within society. Whether they should actually "show the way" is a question that will be addressed by examining theories of consultation.

In this chapter, the thinking from leading consultants and theorists is shared to help in considering how consultation can be used as a tool for effective change, whether through functioning in a consulting role or working in an organization that is using a consultant.

OBJECTIVES

After reading this chapter, you will be able to:

1. Define what is meant by consultation
2. Explain how consultation can be a tool for change
3. Analyze selected theories of consultation to determine strategies to facilitate productive change
4. Examine issues related to consulting during times of rapid and continuous change
5. Identify skills needed for effective consultation
6. Examine ethical and legal issues associated with consulting

■ WHAT IS CONSULTING?

Consultation is an interactive process, involving both client and consultant in problem identification, role negotiation, and problem solution. It is based on a dynamic helping relationship and does not involve simply a one-way flow of information (Marriner-Tomey, 1996). A specialized example is that of occupational health nurses. The American Association of Occupational Health Nurses explains that an occupational health nurse consultant is (AAOHN, 1986, cited in Roy, 1997, p. 10):

> a registered nurse who serves a client as an advisor for evaluating and developing employee health services. The occupational health nurse consultant can provide services in administration, education, practice and research in occupational health and safety.

This example illustrates how nurses in any setting may create change in their work environments.

The common theme in these definitions is the emphasis on an exchange between consultant and client in a way that builds the client's capacity to manage future problems or challenges. The client shares a need with the consultant, who indicates whether he or she has the necessary expertise to provide assistance. Together, they define the need as clearly as possible, and the consultant facilitates the client's ability to solve the problem. The mutuality involved in this type of problem solving is consistent with Bhola's theory of planned change, in which each party involved takes an active role in defining the problem and developing solutions (Bhola, 1994; Tiffany & Lutjens, 1998). Consultation is time-limited and based on a contractual relationship between consultant and client (Alvarez, 1993).

Consultation differs from collaboration and mentoring because the goals of each of these processes differ. Whereas the goal of consultation is to provide advice and assistance with problem solving, the goal of collaboration is to work together to jointly define and resolve issues. Collaboration is based on the premise of shared power and a balance of expertise across all participants. However, effective consultation uses collaboration as the means to achieve the goal of solving problems and developing innovations. Mentoring aims to provide assistance in the professional development of a protege. In this case, the mentor does have special expertise, but the focus of the interaction is on the protege's development rather than on solving a clinical or organizational problem.

Lippitt and Lippitt (1986) describe consulting as "an interactive process of seeking, giving, and receiving help" (cited in Patterson et al. 1995, p. 231) and outline six stages in the consulting pro-

---

B O X 2 4 - 1

Phases of Consultation

Engagement and entry
Contract formulation and establishment of a
   helping relationship
Problem identification
Goal setting and planning
Implementation
Contract completion and termination

From Lippitt, G.L., & Lippitt, R. (1986). *The consulting process in action* (2nd ed.). San Diego, Calif.: Pfeiffer.

---

cess (Box 24-1). These stages represent the development, implementation, and termination of a relationship that is problem or issue focused. "The goal of consultation is to show clients how they can empower themselves to take more responsibility, feel more secure, deal constructively with their feelings and with others in interactions, and internalize flexible and creative problem-solving skills" (Sebastian & Stanhope, 1996, p. 856).

A critical component of the consulting relationship is evaluating whether the goals of consultation have been achieved. Evaluation should occur at planned stages throughout the process to give the client the opportunity to provide feedback and to make it possible to make reasonable changes before the conclusion of the process. Informal evaluation through frequent telephone contact is also a necessary part of maintaining a positive relationship (Scott & Beare, 1993).

■ HOW CAN CONSULTING BE A TOOL FOR CHANGE?

Consultation is an action-oriented intervention that is by definition focused on change and forward movement from an existing state to a desired state. It is a tool for helping clients develop new or improved skills in areas they identify as needs. Consultants are change agents. Their roles focus specifically on change—collaborating with clients to determine problems or issues for which different approaches are needed, determining the changes that may be desirable, working together to devise strategies most likely to be successful in implementing desired changes, and developing plans for evaluating the effectiveness of the changes in resolving the original problems. Consultants may work with organizational clients interested in internal organizational changes, or they may work with policy makers devising policies that affect large numbers of people and organizations. Most often, nurse consultants with baccalaureate preparation focus their consultation efforts on the needs of individual recipients of health care and families within their agency of employment. Masters' and doctorally prepared nurse consultants are more likely to include organizations and policy makers as clients. Box 24-2 outlines a range of potential clients of nurse consultants and the nurses most likely to work with those clients.

Nurse consultants may be employed temporarily to help a particular organization. Such individuals are normally referred to as *external consultants.* Simply bringing in an outside consultant has strong symbolic value. Furlow and Higman (1995, p. 5) say that "hiring a consultant symbolizes the beginning of change." The other common approach is to call on individuals currently employed within an organization who happen to have special skills in an area of need, to function in a consulting capacity on a time-limited basis. These individuals are thought of as *internal consultants.*

What Advantages and Disadvantages Do External Versus Internal Consultants Have in Facilitating Change?

Hiring external consultants can be advantageous for an organization, since they are not already part of the organization's culture and have no vested interests. Therefore they have more freedom to suggest actions that may differ from the usual ways of working. External consultants also bring with them the value of knowing multiple ways of accomplishing changes that may be less

BOX 24-2

Clientele and Level of Preparation of Nurse Consultants

Clients	Nurse Preparation
Individual patients and their families	Baccalaureate
Staff nurses in other departments or units of the organization	Baccalaureate or masters' prepared
Managers of individual departments, service lines, or divisions of an organization	Masters' prepared
Entire organizations, including schools of nursing	Masters' or doctorally prepared
State departments of health	Masters' or doctorally prepared
Groups of organizations, such as alliances, partnerships, managed care networks	Doctorally prepared
Federal policy makers and local, national, international governments	Doctorally prepared
Professional organizations or accrediting bodies	Doctorally prepared

apparent to those who have worked inside one organization for a long period.

A common example of external consultation involves hiring a consulting firm to provide an assessment of an organization's structure. This is often initiated because the organization is faced with financial dilemmas, such as the need to reduce costs to remain competitive. The consulting firm normally assigns a team to spend time working with the organization over a period of weeks, months, or even years. This allows the consulting team to learn more about the organization's culture and to collaborate with organizational management throughout the process of assessing the need for change, recommending changes, and implementing changes. The costs of this type of consultation depend on the complexity of the project, the expertise required, the number of consultants used, and the time frame involved.

Employees may resent external consultants, because consultants do not have to live with the outcomes of the recommended changes. External consultants who recommend painful changes, such as reorganization or downsizing, do not typically see the individual or group as they struggle with implementing those changes. Neither are the external consultants usually the ones who actually must tell employees that they may lose their jobs or be moved to other positions (Furlow, 1995).

Internal consultants, on the other hand, have the advantage of knowing the organizational culture and possessing insights into the kinds of changes that can work in an organization. They understand the organizational history and the informal power structures and can recommend implementation strategies that most effectively build on the organization's strengths. However, internal consultants may be viewed with skepticism by some employees, because there may be a perception of bias or favoritism both in terms of the choice of internal consultants and the rec-

ommendations made by the consultants (Furlow, 1995).

The Hospice Consultation Team established at the Philadelphia Veterans' Affairs Medical Center (Abrahm et al., 1996) is an example of internal consultation. These teams were mandated in 1992 for all Veterans' Affairs (VA) hospitals to respond to the complex palliative care needs of veterans with cancer. The team at the Philadelphia VA was composed of a medical oncologist, a nurse coordinator with special hospice training, a hospital chaplain, and an oncology social worker. The team's purpose was to complement the care provided by other services within the VA and to focus heavily on identifying and solving problems that might not otherwise be identified. The nurse coordinator completed initial assessments on all clients referred to the team, and then individual team members worked with clients as appropriate. The team met weekly to discuss client problems, recommend solutions, and evaluate the progress made.

Team members identified problems in the areas of pain control, skin and oral care, nutritional care, side effects of medications, anxiety, depression, anger, information needs regarding financial support or community resources available to families, and spiritual concerns. The team was able to complement the services already available for veterans with cancer and, by adding a new dimension of care, created a change in the care delivery system. Their consultation efforts were directed toward staff, patients, and families and involved joint problem solving, making recommendations, and providing information through educational sessions and individual counseling (Abrahm et al., 1996).

Whether internal or external consultants are selected depends on the nature of the problem and the organization's capacity. One very real issue in making such a choice is cost. The organization may not have sufficient funds to hire an external consultant. However, administrators may think they can reallocate a particular employee's responsibilities on a temporary basis to benefit from that individual's expertise as internal consultant. Such reallocation still costs money, of course, but the funds have already been spent on that individual's salary and therefore new funds do not have to be allocated as long as it is possible for someone else to temporarily assume the internal consultant's usual job responsibilities (Roy, 1997). Key questions asked within the organization in choosing between external and internal consultants are:

- What issue are we facing?
- What skills do we need to help with this issue?
- What organizational strengths can we draw on in managing change?
- Who is the best qualified to help us with this change?
- What driving and restraining forces are present in our situation that may influence the effectiveness of an external or internal consultant?
- Given our analysis of the need and context for change, should we invest in an external or an internal consultant?
- What are our goals for the consultation?

■ HOW DO THEORIES OF CONSULTATION HELP US UNDERSTAND THE PROCESS?

Several models of consultation have been developed and can be found in practice. This chapter focuses on Edgar Schein's three classic models because they have held up over time and are consistent with the nursing process and with the values of assisting clients to empower themselves to take action. Schein's process model in particular encourages the consultant to work as a partner with the client and is consistent with the collaborative model of planned change within complex systems outlined by Bhola (1994). Bhola's theory of planned change aims to bring the planner and the adopter of change

together in a participatory relationship that is especially congruent with nursing values of client autonomy (Tiffany & Lutjens, 1998).

Schein (1969) defines *purchase-of-expertise consultation* as the purchase (hiring) of a professional helper by a client to provide expert information or service. Buyers may be individuals, groups, or organizations. In this model the client defines the need for the consultant. The need is defined as information the client seeks or an activity the client wants implemented. The advantage of this popular model is that the client does not have to spend time or energy solving the identified problem, because that is the responsibility of the "expert consultant." The disadvantage is that the client may question the quality of the consultation if the client has identified the wrong problem or does not like the consultant's solution.

Although this model often is used, it may be unsatisfactory in effectively and efficiently identifying and resolving client problems. Once the consultant has implemented steps to solve the problem, the client must live with the consequences of the changes. This model is likely to be effective by itself only when problems are simple and the client needs specific expert information (Rokwood, 1993).

Another popular consultative model identified by Schein (1969) is the *doctor-patient model,* in which the consultant is employed by the client (who may or may not actually be a patient) to diagnose the problem and prescribe solutions without assistance from the client. Again, the major advantage of this model from the client's viewpoint is that it requires limited time and energy. This model is often applied in nursing situations requiring consultative services. For example, the director of nursing at the local hospital calls in a nurse consultant from the local university. Nurse performance is poor, according to the director, and the nurse consultant is asked to diagnose what is wrong

Key terms	
Term	**Definition**
Client	Individual(s) representing self, group, organization, community, nation, or government who have a problem and need change to occur
Consultation	Interactive process involving a client and a consultant in problem identification, role negotiation, and problem solution; characterized as a helping relationship
Content consultation	Situation in which client and nurse share information about a problem and the consultant solves the problem
Process consultation	Involves nurse and client in mutual problem solving

with the department. If the problem is found to be poor management rather than poor performance by the staff, the administrator may be reluctant to accept the diagnosis. Because the client does not help diagnose the problem, the goals of consultation may not be met.

The purchase of expertise and doctor-patient models are content models of consultation, since they deal with the content (or nature) of the problem. In contrast, the major goal of the *process consultation model* is to help the client assess both the problem and the kind of help needed to resolve the problem (Schein, 1969). The process consultation model focuses on the process of problem solving and emphasizes collaboration between consultant and the client (Rokwood, 1993). Process consultation incorporates assessment of the underlying organizational culture that influences both the problem and its resolution (Schein, 1989). Both consultant and client participate in the problem-solving steps that lead to changes or to actions for problem solution. The assumptions underlying each of the three models are listed in Box 24-3.

Content and process consultation models do not need to be mutually exclusive (Rokwood, 1993; Schein, 1989). Instead, although consultants should emphasize process consultation, they should be willing to share their expertise

when appropriate. Because process consultation is collaborative, Schein (1989) recommends that the consultants be willing to offer opinions and advice at various stages of the consultation process. Thus, although the major emphasis should be on process consultation, consultants may find it effective to integrate the three models at selected points.

In the process model, the consultant is a resource person whose primary goal is to provide the client with choices for decision making. The process consultation model includes the same steps as the nursing process, that is, establishing a nurse-client interaction based on trust to assess the problem, define the problem, plan and implement actions, and evaluate the outcomes of nursing interventions. Nursing interventions may be described as direct client care or as consultation activities, depending on the goal of the intervention.

Process Consultation

Process consultation involves a temporary relationship between client and consultant for the purpose of bringing about change. Consultation may be proactive or reactive. Proactive consultation is directed toward anticipating a future problem and taking steps to prevent it. Reactive consultation is directed toward an existing prob-

Assumptions of Schein's Consultation Models

Purchase-of-Expertise Model

1. The client correctly diagnoses the problem.
2. The client correctly communicates the needs to the consultant.
3. The client correctly assesses the consultant's expertise to provide the information or perform the service.
4. The client knows the consequences of implementing the services suggested by the consultant.

Doctor-Patient Model

1. The client is willing to reveal information needed by the consultant to make an appropriate diagnosis.
2. The consultant is able to get an accurate picture of the problem through observation.
3. The client accepts the diagnosis and the prescriptions offered by the consultant.

Process Model

1. Clients often do not know what the problem is and need assistance in problem diagnosis.
2. Clients are not aware of the services a consultant may offer and need assistance in finding proper help.
3. Clients want to improve situations and need guidance in identifying appropriate methods to reach goals.
4. Clients can be more effective if they learn how to diagnose their own strengths and limitations.
5. Consultants usually cannot spend enough time learning all variables that may help or hinder suggested courses of action, so they need to work with the client who has intimate knowledge of the effects of proposed courses of action.
6. The client who learns to diagnose situation problems and who engages in decision making about alternative courses of action will be actively involved in implementing actions for problem resolution.
7. The consultant is an expert in problem diagnosis and in establishing an effective helping relationship, and passes these skills on to the client.

From Schein, E.H. (1969). *Process consultation: Its role in organizational development.* Reading, Mass.: Addison Wesley Longman.

lem through therapeutic intervention. For example, a hospital developing a home health agency contacts the nurse consultant to assist with defining the "best practice" models for home health. The board wishes to be proactive and plan for the needs of high-risk families. Conversely, the administrator of an ambulatory clinic has found that nurses are missing work for minor health problems and that health costs are skyrocketing. The nurse consultant is asked to help explore solutions to the problem. In this ex-

ample, the administrator is reacting to an existing problem requiring immediate intervention.

Once the client has been identified, the nurse must decide the best method(s) for intervening in the problem situation. Several approaches are described on the following pages.

Rosenkoetter (1997) developed a framework for consultation in international health care situations that is applicable for all consultants regardless of location, whether internal or external. This model describes the consultative process as one that involves expertise, mutual understanding, reciprocal learning, sociocultural exchange and collaboration, consensual deliberation, and progressive growth and development.

First and foremost, a nurse must be an expert in the problem area in which the consultation is to occur. Expertise is gained through a combination of education, experience, values, and beliefs. To be an effective expert consultant, a nurse should be a good communicator, effective listener, and self-starter and enjoy problem solving and creative challenges (Roy, 1997).

Mutuality is critical for effective consulting relationships (Rosenkoetter, 1997, p. 183) and requires respect on the part of the nurse and the client for the ideas of the other. On this basis an agreement is established that clarifies the outcomes expected from the relationship between the client and the nurse consultant. Such an understanding helps prevent misinterpretations, frustrations, and poor outcomes.

Reciprocal learning begins when the nurse understands the culture, values, and beliefs of the client. At the same time the client will want to be certain there is a "fit" between the client's needs and the consultant's expertise. Does the consultant have similar values and beliefs? Is the consultant flexible and willing to listen, observe, and exchange ideas? (Furlow & Higman, 1995)

Both mutual understanding and reciprocal learning lead to sociocultural exchange and collaboration, implying that each party—the client and the nurse—is willing to communicate openly and contribute to resolving the problem. In this situation all participants are given the opportunity to express their ideas in an accepting environment. When dealing with a group or an organization, the culture of the organization, administrative relationships, organizational history, and politics all influence the communications. The consultant must acknowledge and

be aware of these factors to be effective in offering solutions to existing problems. Likewise, when working with an individual patient and family, the family's heritage, past health care practices, education, and economic levels must be clearly understood to establish an environment in which change can occur in that family (Rosenkoetter, 1997).

Consensual deliberation involves participants in a process where together the client and the consultant assess, plan, and implement decisions, using skills of listening, validating, and negotiating until a desirable outcome is reached. Progressive growth and development involve leaving the client with a strong sense of self-worth, an analysis of the problem that offers several alternatives to solving the problem, recommendations that can be achieved, and a vision for the future change (Rosenkoetter, 1997).

Certain principles are implied in all models, regardless of the model chosen in the consultative situation. The *process model* is considered to be the best approach because it involves the client in the problem solution. The capable consultant must possess the skills found in Box 24-4.

■ WHAT ARE THE ROLES OF THE CONSULTANT?

Nurse consultants can fill a variety of consulting roles, but each has as its goal to assist clients to empower themselves to make needed changes. Lippett and Lippett (1986) delineated a typology of eight consulting behaviors. Patterson et al. (1995) explained that the eight roles that consultants might adopt vary from highly directive to completely nondirective. Box 24-5 illustrates how the eight roles vary along this continuum.

Each of the roles described in Box 24-5 helps move the client to a new reality and therefore represents a tool for change. Bhola's (cf., 1994) theory of planned change is based on the assumption that people create their own reality (Tiffany & Lutjens, 1998). The consulting roles outlined above suggest the ways in which consultants work with clients to alter reality to achieve new goals. Schein's (1969) three models of consultation have implications for each of the consultant's roles.

BOX 2 4 - 4

Skills of Effective Consultants

Consultant Skills

- Good listening skills
- Fitting in with the mission and culture of the client
- Good teaching skills
- Ability to promote the client's independence
- Ability to provide good service
- Ability to respect confidences
- Ability to produce quality results
- Willingness to challenge the assumptions of the client about the problem
- Recognized expertise
- Objectivity
- Ability to deliver a product or report
- Ability to refrain from selling one's own ideas
- Ability to celebrate successes with clients

From Bader, G., & Stich, T. (1993). Using external consultants wisely. *Seminars for Nurse Managers, 1*(1), 22-25.

In the first of Schein's (1969) models, the consultant helps the client identify the problem and in this way serves more as an advisor. This is referred to as a *doctor-patient* or *medical model* because of the emphasis on problem diagnosis. The assumption is that the consultant is an expert who is better prepared than the client to diagnose the problem. The client is expected to accept the consultant's definition of the problem.

In the second model, the consultant functions as an advisor, either recommending solutions to a problem already identified by the organization or suggesting strategies for implementing a particular solution. The consultant prescribes recommended solutions or actions in this model. Schein (1969) called this the *purchase-of-expertise model.* It has also been referred to as an *engineering model* (Gibson, 1997).

Schein's (1969; 1989) *process model* emphasizes client empowerment through collaboration with the consultant. The consultant does not assume the responsibility for diagnosing and defining the problem but works with the client to jointly diagnose and define the issue. Neither does the consultant direct the client to a "best" solution but instead works with the client to identify a solution best suited to the norms and values of the client's organization. This model is thought to have the most lasting impact on or-

BOX 2 4 - 5

Continuum of Consultant Roles

Directive							**Nondirective**
Advocate	Information specialist	Trainer/ educator	Joint problem solver	Identifier of alternatives/ links to resources	Fact finder	Process counselor	Objective observer

From Patterson, J.E., Strumpf, N.E., & Evans, L.K. (1995). Nursing consultation to reduce restraints in a nursing home. *Clinical Nurse Specialist, 9*, 232; originally adapted from Lippitt, G.L., & Lippitt, R. (1986). *The consulting process in action* (2nd ed.). San Diego, Calif.: Pfeiffer.

ganizational effectiveness because the client develops new skills as a result of the consultation that can be used in other situations.

How Can Consultation Influence Change?

The theory of planned change articulated by Bennis, Benne, and Chin (1985) proposed that three basic approaches are available for managing change. The first of these is the *power-coercive approach,* in which managers or policy makers use their access to rewards and sanctions to insist on implementation of particular changes. *Empirical-rational strategies* for implementing change are those in which managers assume that by appealing to reason and presenting employees with logical information about the anticipated benefits of a change, that employees will willingly cooperate with the change. Gibson (1997) notes that managers with this belief are simply ignoring the realities of organizational life, in which individual and group norms and values, as well as organizational culture, play a critical role in determining employee responses to changes.

The third approach to managing change builds on an understanding of the importance of norms, values, and organizational culture. The *normative-reeducative strategy* for managing change emphasizes (1) identifying group norms that can either facilitate or hinder change pro-

cesses, and (2) developing educational strategies about the change that build on an understanding of the group's mores.

For example, if an organization is moving to a shared governance model but staff have long depended on management to develop schedules and policies, it would be useful to implement a series of workshops around the concept of self-governance and what that will mean to employees in terms of more responsibility for functions such as scheduling and recommending policies. It would be a mistake to begin with a series of classes on how to develop schedules or policies without moving through the feelings associated with taking on these responsibilities in the first place.

None of the consulting roles outlined by Lippitt and Lippitt are consistent with power-coercive approaches to managing change. However, each of the other roles is relatively more consistent with either the normative-reeducative approach or the empirical-rational approach to planned change. Patterson and her colleagues (1995) suggest that the choice of approaches depends in part on where the organization is in the change process and the organizational culture that exists. Box 24-6 lists the links between consulting roles and strategies for managing change.

An excellent example of an external consultant serving as a change agent is described by

---

B O X   2 4 - 6

Links Between Lippitt and Lippitt's Categorization of Consulting Roles and the Theory of Planned Change

Power-Coercive	Empirical-Rational	Normative-Reeducative
None	Fact finder	Objective observer
	Information specialist	Process counselor
	Identifier of alternatives/	Joint problem solver
	links to resources	Advocate
	Trainer/educator	

Patterson and her colleagues (1995). In this case, a clinical nurse specialist (CNS) worked with the administrators and staff of a nursing home to reduce restraint use among the residents. This work was part of a controlled clinical trial by Evans et al. (1992) that aimed to determine whether a formal educational program, education with consultation, or no intervention would be most effective in reducing restraint use among nursing home residents. This study followed implementation of the Nursing Home Reform Act (Omnibus Reconciliation Act, 1987), which stipulated that use of physical restraints be limited or eliminated.

The CNS spent 24 weeks working with administrators and staff on restraint reduction. The nursing home administrator identified the goal of reducing restraint use among the residents by 50%. The consultant's approach varied in how directive she was, based on the particular stage of the change process (Patterson, 1995). This is consistent with Schein's (1989) recommendation that consultants focus primarily on process consultation but also offer suggestions and advice at various points as requested by the client.

Restraint use was reduced during the intervention, although 6 months after the conclusion of the consultation, restraint use was increasing again at the nursing home. Patterson and her colleagues (1995) concluded that consultation was effective in initiating change but needed to be continued to maintain the change. They also speculated that a more directive approach to consultation was the most effective in a nursing home setting, since the staff were not familiar with the CNS role and did not have specialized education in gerontology. They observed that care routines were based primarily on habit as opposed to scientific evidence. Because of this, they reasoned that a more directive approach to consultation, emphasizing the roles of advocate, information specialist, and educator, would be the most effective. Thus many of the consul-

tant's interventions were consistent with the empirical-rational approach to planned change.

It may have been the case that these directive approaches were especially effective with initiating a change. However, less directive approaches to skill building and shared values around the importance of the change seem to be necessary for long-term change to be maintained. Stated in terms of Lewin's stages of change (1947a; 1947b), more directive approaches may be helpful in the "moving" stage and less directive approaches in the "refreezing" stage.

Another example of external consultation by advanced practice nurses is that provided by the Occupational Reproductive Health Nurse Consultant Practice within the Wisconsin Division of Health. Hewitt and Tellier (1996, p. 366) explain that "the consultant's primary responsibility is to provide advice and technical assistance to statewide agencies, organizations, industries, and individuals to promote the recognition and abatement of reproductive hazards in the workplace." This role includes many different types of clients, including organizations, professionals, and members of the public. The focus is on making changes in the workplace to promote a safe environment for individuals contemplating pregnancy.

Nurses who function in this capacity provide telephone and on-site workplace consultations, and specific recommendations for changes that both employers and employees should make to provide a healthy working environment and protect against exposure to teratogens or other reproductive health and safety hazards. An interesting feature of this model is the involvement that the nurse consultants seek from employees' health care providers. After obtaining the employee's consent, the nurse consultant makes recommendations for changes in the work situation directly to the employee's health care provider, who then contacts the employer requesting the changes. When employees decline to allow the nurse consultant to contact the employee's health care provider, the nurse consultant recommends to the employee that she contact her health care provider directly with the information.

■ HOW DOES THE PACE OF CHANGE INFLUENCE CONSULTATION?

The current health care environment is often described as "hyperturbulent" and "discontinuous." These terms suggest not only that is change occurring with increasing rapidity, but also that the changes themselves are profound and sometimes seem disjointed, contradictory, or both. This means that the stages of change do not last as long as they might have in years past and that there is little time for unfreezing (Lewin, 1947a; 1947b), getting rid of old ideas and behaviors, and refreezing (Lewin, 1947a; 1947b), or taking on new ideas and behaviors. However, it is important to note that unfreezing and refreezing are still important behavioral components of change. People need to become convinced of the need to change in a particular direction, and they need to have some sense of stability once a change has been introduced. Combined with a rapidly changing environment, these needs suggest that it is more important than ever for consultants to work with clients in identifying ways to maximize the unfreezing and refreezing stages.

These observations about hyperturbulence and discontinuity also indicate that sometimes people must work at maintaining old systems and initiating new systems at the same time. In fact, it is not unusual to be faced with working in ways that seem mutually contradictory. For example, in parts of the country in which managed care saturation is not very high, health care professionals and systems must simultaneously provide care for clients with fee-for-service and managed care third-party payment. Because the incentives are completely opposite in these two payment mechanisms, health professionals must constantly balance opposing systems. With a fee-for-service payment system, providers generate more revenues when more services are provided. In a managed care environment, more money is made (through savings, rather than revenue generation) when fewer costly services are provided. This means that in a market with less than about 30% managed care saturation, providers are constantly juggling two different sets of incentives while trying to provide the highest quality of care possible.

In the business world, people commonly think of changes in terms of product life cycle, or what happens as a new product is introduced to the market, gains increasing amounts of mar-

Key terms	
Term	**Definition**
Hyperturbulence	Increasingly rapid change
Discontinuous change	Disjointed or contradictory change
Product life cycle	Period of time during which a new product or service is developed, implemented, gains acceptance, enjoys popularity, and eventually declines
S curves	Sigmoid curves (Handy, 1994); pictorial representations of product life cycles

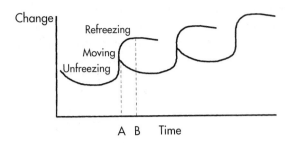

Figure 24-1 ▪ Life cycle of health care innovations. (Modified from Handy, C. [1994]. *The age of paradox.* Boston: Harvard Business School Press.)

ket share, and finally begins to lose market share as newer and more appealing products are introduced (Handy, 1994). We can think of change in health care in much the same way, depicting it with an S curve (Figure 24-1).

On the first curve in Figure 24-1, the downward slope of the S indicates that people are becoming dissatisfied with the status quo and are beginning to agree on the need for change. This corresponds with what Lewin refers to as unfreezing (1947a; 1947b). The upward slope of the curve represents the "moving" phase of the change process in which people are implementing the change and are developing strategies for making it work in the long run. The top of the curve indicates stability, or refreezing the new behavior (Lewin, 1947a; 1947b).

In a stable health care market, one change would follow another in a relatively orderly pattern, allowing people time to adjust to one way of working before learning another. Even in such a hypothetical environment, Handy (1994) points out that people must simultaneously do things in the old way while initiating a new behavior. Point *A* on the first curve occurs at the spot when some people are beginning to be dissatisfied with the current way of doing things and are beginning the unfreezing process. However, others are still adopting the current strategy, as indicated by the upward slope of the

curve between points *A* and *B*. Between *A* and *B* the organization is faced with maintaining a productive environment with people who are at radically different stages of the change process.

After point *B*, the slope of the curve begins to drop downward, suggesting that the initial behaviors are no longer effective. A new change process is well underway, as seen by the second curve. However, some participants are still content with the status quo represented by the first behavior. Handy (1994) argues that it is inevitable that individuals will be at different points in the process of change, and the challenge is to develop an environment in which all ideas and concerns are respected, while still making it possible to move ahead as necessary to meet new environmental demands.

For consultants, this suggests the importance of working with the client to determine how all parties feel about a change and identifying with the client ways to acknowledge concerns and fears when implementing a new way of functioning. It also suggests the importance of working with the client to accurately diagnose a need, and to determine where on the curve the organization or group is currently functioning. The client may be an individual, family, group, or organization.

In today's environment, hyperturbulence means that changes are occurring so rapidly that people do not have time to adjust to one way of doing things before they are faced with another. Figure 24-2 represents a hyperturbulent situation. The time period between points *A* and *B* is so short that many people are still learning one way of doing things while others became disillusioned with that approach some time earlier and still others are beginning to think that a third strategy may be desirable. This can lead to beliefs (fears) that the system is in chaos.

Figure 24-3 represents both hyperturbulence and discontinuity. In this situation, not only is change occurring rapidly, but the nature of the

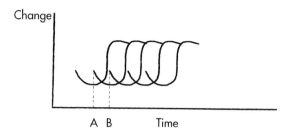

Figure 24-2 ■ Hyperturbulence. (Modified from Handy, C. [1994]. *The age of paradox.* Boston: Harvard Business School Press.)

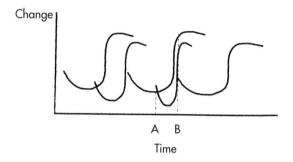

Figure 24-3 ■ Hyperturbulence and discontinuity. (Modified from Handy, C. [1994]. *The age of paradox.* Boston: Harvard Business School Press.)

changes is quite different. Some are radical departures from earlier ways of working, whereas others may require less time and psychic energy to adopt. The time period between points *A* and *B* on Figure 24-3 represents a particularly vulnerable period, because the organization or group has already been through multiple changes and three different changes are now occurring simultaneously.

An example of this type of situation is occurring in home health at this time. Home health services are still expanding as hospitals increasingly focus on shortening lengths of stay and discharging sicker patients. The Health Care Financing Administration (HCFA), however, has become concerned about fraud in home health

and is increasing regulatory oversight to prevent fraudulent use of tax dollars by home health agencies. Thus pressures are being brought to bear to provide care for sicker patients, while home health agencies are under pressure from other sources to carefully justify why care is needed by their patients. At the same time, increasing use of managed care is pushing more care into the home, but with an emphasis on health promotion and primary and secondary illness prevention rather than the tertiary prevention or rehabilitative focus for which home health has been reimbursed over the years. With these pressures in mind, home health agencies are developing new services, such as adult day care for frail elderly clients, to begin developing the capacity to meet the challenges of a new reimbursement environment. Nursing and therapy staff in these agencies must be skilled at managing these multiple and sometimes conflicting pressures.

This kind of situation may feel chaotic and result in lowered morale, distrust of consultants, and high turnover, thereby potentially reducing quality of care. McDaniel (1997) argues that chaos is inevitable and not necessarily a negative feature of the current environment. He suggests that the most important strategy is valuing the different perspectives that emerge in chaotic times because those perspectives can lead to novel interventions that might be more effective than earlier strategies and would not have otherwise been considered. The key is maintaining an environment of inclusiveness and openness, in which the emergence of ideas and concerns is nurtured and encouraged.

In a hyperturbulent environment in which change is discontinuous, consultants should understand that Schein's process and content models of consultation are not necessarily mutually exclusive (Rokwood, 1993) and that depending on the stage of the change process and the readiness of the clients, they should vary their strategies as necessary. So, for example, in a situation such as the one described by Patterson and her colleagues (1995) in the nursing home, the consultant gave direct recommendations at times when staff were unfamiliar with the principles of gerontologic nursing, and at other times, solicited input and worked together to develop strategies for reducing restraint use while acknowledging the legitimacy of staff concerns for client safety.

■ ETHICAL AND LEGAL ISSUES ASSOCIATED WITH CONSULTING

Key Ethical Issues

In addition to possessing characteristics and qualities previously described to be a successful consultant, one must operate from a set of clinical and consultative standards that includes ethical duties to clients served and principles that underlie one's practice as a consultant. Such principles will assist the nurse consultant in answering the following questions: Who is the client? What are the nurse consultant's responsibilities if the customer clearly favors advice that may be in conflict with the consultant's professional values, beliefs, or knowledge? How can conflict of interest be defined? What is the role of truth telling?

Of the three duties that apply to the nurse as consultant as outlined in the American Nurses Association *Code of Ethics* (1996, revised draft), accountability and confidentiality are not only ethical duties but legal requirements, whereas veracity is essential to the ongoing success of the nurse consultant (Box 24-7).

Accountability is defined in the ANA *Code for Nurses* (1996, revised draft) as "being answerable to someone for something someone has done." Accountability includes providing an explanation to self, the client, and the profession for what one has done as a nurse consultant. It is this duty that is the basis for developing a contractual agreement between the nurse and the client. Because of this contractual agreement the nurse consultant is answerable for performing the consultation according to the agreed terms, the time frame, use of resources, and performance standards. The nurse consultant is responsible for the delivery of competent, quality services and is accountable to self, client, and the profession for what has been done (Fry, 1996). When services are not provided as contracted, the profession and the client have legal recourse through the courts and state boards of nursing respectively.

In interactions with the client, all information is regarded as confidential. If the duty of *confidentiality* is not followed, the consulting client may not reveal information necessary to identify the "right problem," which then results

---

Key Terms

Term	Definition
Accountability	Ethical duty to provide an explanation for what one has done
Autonomy	Ethical principle that refers to individual freedom of action
Beneficence	Ethical principle that implies a duty to help others gain what is of benefit to them without obligation to risk self-welfare or interest in helping others
Confidentiality	Ethical duty to preserve the privacy of another's concerns, needs, and information
Justice	Ethical principle that holds that equals should be treated equally and those that are unequal should be treated differently
Veracity	Ethical duty to tell the truth and not lie or deceive others

in the consultant recommending inappropriate solutions (Fry, 1996). This then can lead to legal action by the client. The *Code for Nurses* (1996) indicates the nurse's duty to "safeguard the client's right to privacy by . . . protecting information of a confidential nature." This duty can be ignored only in situations where a client or organization is imposing a health risk to others, the community, or society. Such disclosures are usually dictated by law (e.g., a communicable disease outbreak or the violation of an OSHA standard by an agency).

The duty of *veracity* requires the nurse consultant to tell the truth. Such a duty implies that the nurse consultant respects the clients served and considers clients to be self-determining, autonomous persons. The nurse consultant must be truthful about the scope of the services he or she can offer and the limitations of the consultant's abilities. This duty implies the duty of keeping promises. It is implied in the client-consultant contract that the nurse consultant will communicate with the client and will be truthful about the problem, as well as in other interactions with the client. To be truthful will create an environment of trust and will establish positive relationships between client and consultant (Fry, 1996). A reputation for truthfulness will enhance the consultant's ability to be recognized as an expert and worthy consultant.

Schein's process consultative model (1969, 1989) supports the client's right to autonomy. The ethical principle of *autonomy* refers to client freedom of action and the belief in clients' capability to choose and act on plans they have selected. This principle is applied when the nurse consultant engages in the "consensus deliberation" described by Rosenkoetter (1997). Through facilitation and negotiation in the problem-solving process the nurse consultant shows respect for the clients served and gives the client the opportunity to influence the outcome of the problem-solving process. Contract negotiations establish the boundaries of

---

B O X   2 4 - 7

ANA Code for Nurses

1. The nurse provides services with respect for human dignity and the uniqueness of the client unrestricted by considerations of social or economic status, personal attributes, or the nature of health problems.
2. The nurse safeguards the client's right to privacy by judiciously protecting information of a confidential nature.
3. The nurse acts to safeguard the client and the public when health care and safety are affected by the incompetent, unethical, or illegal practice of any person.
4. The nurse assumes responsibility and accountability for individual nursing judgements and actions.
5. The nurse maintains competence in nursing.
6. The nurse exercises informed judgement and uses individual competence and qualifications as criteria in seeking consultation, accepting responsibilities, and delegating nursing activities to others.
7. The nurse participates in activities that contribute to the ongoing development of the profession's body of knowledge.
8. The nurse participates in the profession's efforts to implement and improve standards of nursing care.
9. The nurse participates in the profession's efforts to establish and maintain conditions of employment conducive to high quality nursing care.
10. The nurse participates in the profession's effort to protect the public from misinformation and misrepresentation and to maintain the integrity of nursing.
11. The nurse collaborates with members of the health professions and other citizens in promoting community and national efforts to meet the health needs of the public.

From American Nurses Association. (1985). *Code for nurses with interpretive statements.* Washington, D.C.: American Nurses Publishing, American Nurses Foundation/American Nurses Association.

the consultative relationship and provide for informed consent, a requirement of the principle of autonomy. Through the contract the client knows what to expect from the relationship. Applying the duty of confidentiality and protecting the privacy of the client also meets the requirement of the principle of autonomy (Fry, 1996; Swansburg, 1996).

The principle of *justice* indicates that the nurse consultant should give to the client what is owed, deserved, or legitimately claimed (Davis, 1982). If one has clearly delineated the terms of the relationship through the contract, fulfilling those terms is all that is required. In some instances clients may ask the consultant to go beyond the contractual agreement and to provide direct services or, for example, to extend the amount of time spent on solving the problem and planning strategies for implementation. That is not essential to applying the principle of justice. With new requests the consultant should take the opportunity to renegotiate the contract or remind the client of the terms of the contract and the time-limiting nature of the consulting relationship.

The principle of *beneficence* implies that the nurse ought to do good and prevent or avoid doing harm. It is the nurse consultant's responsibility through the contract to help the client solve the problem. If the consultant is unable to do so, it is best to avoid harm through recommending inappropriate solutions and to refer the client to another resource. It is the consultant's duty to benefit the client through appropriate nurse consultant interventions. In consultation one can apply the principle of beneficence by assisting the client in performing cost/benefit analysis of all possible alternatives that may be chosen to resolve the client's problem. This will offer the client the opportunity to weigh the benefits of certain alternatives while looking at the potential risks of choosing each alternative (Fry, 1996; Swansburg, 1996).

Legal Issues

Nurse consultants are accountable for adhering to certain standards of professional care in their practice as consultants. For example, the American Association of Legal Nurse Consultants (1995) published the *Scope and Standards of Legal Nurse Consulting Practice.* The *Standards of Practice* indicate the levels of professional service to which legal nurse consultants are held accountable.

Scott and Beare (1993, p. 332) note that

. . . in a malpractice case, the consultant who fails to meet the standard of care is liable in civil court for the tort of malpractice. To be liable for malpractice, four elements must be proved against the nurse: duty (nurse-client relationship), breach of duty, proximate cause, and damages. If any of these are not present, there cannot be a valid claim of malpractice.

A key strategy to guard against frivolous lawsuits is good communication and a good relationship with the client (Alvarez, 1993; Scott & Beare, 1993). A clearly written contract is the first step in establishing good communication between consultant and client, as well as the first step in establishing a trusting relationship. Consulting contracts should include the elements outlined in Box 24-8. A sample contract is included at the end of this chapter for review (Box 24-9).

Other aspects of the consulting relationship that should be developed to provide excellent service and minimize the likelihood of frivolous lawsuits include regular, open, and honest communication between the consultant and client. Alvarez (1993) notes that full and honest communication is a reciprocal process between consultant and client. The consultant cannot fully ensure that he or she will receive complete information from the client. The client may be embarrassed by organizational weaknesses or may choose to withhold critical information for political reasons. Alvarez cites the case of a nurse

B O X   2 4 - 8

Key Elements of a Consulting Contract

1. General statement of project goals
2. Consultant tasks and the types of consultant services
3. Client tasks and/or the supplies to be rendered
4. Special considerations
   a. Number of consultation sessions
   b. Time schedule for the project and final report
   c. Criteria for evaluation
   d. Frequency of communication between parties
   e. Audit of progress of work
   f. Conditions of termination
   g. Possible modification of contract
   h. Assurance of confidentiality
   i. Permission to use the client's name in advertising
   j. Description of the services to be subcontracted
   k. Limitation of consultant liability
   l. Description of process to resolve disagreements
5. Exact terms and conditions of payment of fees
6. Signatures of the contracting parties.

From Scott, L.D., & Beare, P.G. (1993). Nurse consultant and professional liability. *Clinical Nurse Specialist, 7,* 334.

consultant working with a small business that was expanding. The chief executive officer of the business resented certain state regulations and had chosen (1) to ignore them and (2) not to make that known to the nurse consultant. When state auditors determined that the business was not in compliance with the regulations, the nurse consultant was threatened with a lawsuit.

Alvarez (1993) also points out the liability implications of the fact that the nurse consul-

tant does not simply function to share expert knowledge. The ways in which that knowledge is shared, under what circumstances, and at which points in time all influence the effectiveness of the communication process. This relates to the model of consultation the nurse chooses to use. Nurse consultants who use more directive approaches or content models may anger clients and inadvertently create poor environments for communication. On the other hand, nurse consultants who use very nondirective approaches may similarly anger clients who want quick fixes, direct diagnoses, and recommendations for solutions. The communication context is important in maintaining an effective consulting relationship. The approach chosen will depend on several factors, including the people involved, the problem being addressed, and the history, culture, and communication patterns of the participants in the organization.

Another aspect of regular, open communication between consultant and client is that frequent communication will help both parties determine if the goals of the relationship are being met and, if not, allows for midcourse corrections if necessary. Scott and Beare (1993, p. 334) have observed that ". . . a satisfied client is less likely to seek legal action." Frequent progress reports help keep both the consultant and the client aware of the other's perceptions and needs (Bader & Stich, 1993).

In summary, consultation is about a helping relationship built on regular, trustworthy communication. The consultant possesses special expertise that the client believes will be helpful in solving a problem. Together, client and consultant develop a mutually satisfactory agreement about the terms of their relationship and collaborate on the execution of the plan. All professional and advanced practice nurses have opportunities to consult with others, whether as internal or external consultants. Sometimes

Sample Contract

O'Brien Consulting
and
HealthPointe Managed Care

This contract is for the purpose of engaging Charles O'Brien, RN, MSN of O'Brien Consulting as a consultant with HealthPointe Managed Care.

Goals:
1. Develop a Nursing Case Management Program for adults with cancer.
2. Assist HealthPointe Managed Care administrative staff with the adoption of a clinical information system to support the Nursing Case Management Program.
3. Work with the nursing staff at HealthPointe Managed Care to develop expertise in case management.

Consultant Tasks and Services:
Tasks:
• Assess the organization's readiness for a Nursing Case Management Program.
• Assess the need and potential demand in the community for a Nursing Case Management Program.
Services:
• Two inservice education programs for nursing staff on case management.
• Business Plan for a Nursing Case Management Program for adults with cancer.

Time Frame:
One inservice every three months; Business Plan for Nursing Case Management Program to be delivered at the end of six months.

Progress Reports:
To be delivered every three months.

Assurance of Confidentiality:
The consultant agrees that all information about HealthPointe Managed Care Company, its clients, staff, financial status, and strategic plans, is confidential and not to be shared with any outside party without the express written consent of HealthPointe Managed Care.

Conditions of Payment:
HealthPointe Managed Care agrees to pay Charles O'Brien in the amount of _____, payable on or before the first of every month during the term of the contract.

Signatures:

_____   _____
Charles O'Brien, RN, MSN   Barbara Redecker, MBA
O'Brien Consulting   Chief Executive Officer
                                         HealthPointe Managed Care

_____   _____
Date   Date

these roles are formal and involve exchange of payment for services rendered. Other times, consulting is less formal, occurring between colleagues engaged in problem solving. Regardless of the degree of formality involved, nurse consultants can make significant contributions to organizational change within the health care system and should exercise their responsibilities ethically and with an understanding of the legal issues involved.

■ KEY POINTS

- Consultation is a helping relationship based on special expertise and collaborative decision making. It is a powerful tool for planned change.
- Professional and advanced practice nurses have opportunities to consult with other health care professionals, consumers, and community agency representatives. Nurse scientists may consult with governmental agencies on policy issues.
- Consultation may be either internal to an organization or external, involving a consultant employed outside the target organization. A variety of considerations enter into the decision to contract with internal or external consultants.
- Schein's (1969) *process model* of consultation is most consistent with a collaborative and participatory approach to planned change that results in client empowerment.
- Nurse consultants need skills as effective listeners, teachers, and collaborators. Excellent skills in organizational assessment, understanding organizational culture, and project management are essential. Nurse consultants must be able to develop conclusions, write reports, and deliver agreed-on products.
- Consulting roles vary from highly directive to nondirective and include roles as advocate, information provider, teacher, collaborator,

identifier of resources, fact finder, counselor, and observer (Lippitt & Lippitt, 1986; Patterson et al., 1995).
- In times of hyperturbulent change, consultants work with clients to manage multiple, overlapping, and often contradictory changes.
- The consulting contract is the basis for informed consent by the client in the relationship. Ethical issues important in consulting include the principles of beneficence, nonmaleficence, and justice and the duty of veracity.
- Legal issues are related to truth telling and regular, open communication.

■ CRITICAL THINKING QUESTIONS

1. Pretend you were asked to consult with a group of clients to determine whether a health clinic should be developed in a high rise for the elderly or if the service should be contracted to an existing facility. Answer the following questions.
   A. What is needed?
   B. Why is it needed?
   C. What outcome is desired?
   D. What is the time frame?
   E. What are the obstacles to each approach?
   F. What resources are available?
   G. What type of change would be most comfortable? Why?
   H. Who is important to achieving the goal?
2. You are the internal consultant in the hospital, and you have been asked by staff to work with them on dealing with a difficult patient who is quite demanding.
   A. What are the pros and cons of using internal versus external consultants?
   B. What model would you use to deal with them and why?
   C. Develop a contract for its consultation.
   D. What are the anticipated outcomes of the consultation?

3. If you were an external consultant who was asked by the administration of an agency to determine why staff morale was low and you found out that the problem was the administrator, your client, how would you handle the situation? What ethical principles would you use? Why?

4. Review the sample contract on p. 604. To what extent does it include the essential elements of a consulting contract (see Box 24-8)? Explain any other items you think would be important to include and why. If you were Charles O'Brien, how would you begin working with HealthPointe Managed Care? Describe how you would organize your work and how you would engage the staff and administrators at the managed care company in the development of the new nursing case management program.

■ REFERENCES

Abrahm, L.L., Callahan, J., Rossetti, K., & Pierre, L. (1996). The impact of a hospital consultation team on the care of veterans with advanced cancer. *Journal of Pain and Symptom Management, 12*(1), 23-31.

Alvarez, C. (1993). Potential liability in good consultative practice. *Clinical Nurse Specialist, 7,* 330.

American Association of Legal Nurse Consultants. (1995). Scope and standards for legal nurse consulting practice. *Journal of Legal Nurse Consulting, 6*(4), 24-28.

American Nurses Association. (1986). *Clinical nurse specialists: Distribution and utilization.* Kansas City, Mo.: Author, Publication No. NP-69.

American Nurses Association. (1986 & 1996, revised). *Code for Nurses.* Washington, D.C.: Author.

Bader, G., & Stich, T. (1993). Using external consultants wisely. *Seminars for Nurse Managers, 1*(1), 22-25.

Bennis, W.G., Benne, K.D., & Chin, R. (1985). *The planning of change* (4th ed.). New York: Holt, Rinehart, & Winston.

Bhola, H.S. (1994). The CLER model: Thinking through change. *Nursing Management, 25*(5), 59-63.

Davis, A. (1982). Helping your staff address ethical dilemmas. *Journal of Nursing Administration, 12*(2):9-13.

Evans, L., Strumpf, N., Taylor, L, & Jacobsen, B. (1990-1992). Reducing restraints in nursing homes: A clinical trial. (Grant 1 RO1AGO8324). Bethesda, Md.: National Institute on Aging.

Fry, S. (1996). Ethics in community health nursing practice. In M. Stanhope & J. Lancaster (Eds.). *Community health nursing: Promoting health of aggregates, families, and individuals,* (4th ed.). St. Louis: Mosby, pp. 93-116.

Furlow, L. (1995). So what good are consultants anyway? *Journal of Nursing Administration, 25*(7/8), 13, 15.

Furlow, L., & Higman, D. (1995). Consultants: When to look for outside help. *Nursing Management, 26*(5), 49-51.

Gibson, J.L. (1997). *Managing organizational change and development.* Unpublished manuscript, Lexington, Ky.: University of Kentucky College of Business and Economics.

Handy, C. (1994). *The age of paradox.* Boston: Harvard Business School Press.

Hewitt, J.B., & Tellier, L. (1996). A description of an occupational reproductive health nurse consultant practice and women's occupational exposures during pregnancy. *Public Health Nursing, 13,* 365-373.

Ingersoll, G.L., & Jones, L.S. (1992). The art of the consultation note. *Clinical Nurse Specialist, 6,* 218-220.

Lewin, K. (1947a). Frontiers in group dynamics I. *Human Relations, 1,* 5-42.

Lewin, K. (1947b). Frontiers in group dynamics II. *Human Relations, 1,* 143-153.

Lippitt, G.L., & Lippitt, R. (1986). *The consulting process in action* (2nd ed.). San Diego, Calif.: Pfeiffer.

Marriner-Tomey, A. (1996). *A guide to nursing management* (5th ed). St. Louis: Mosby.

McDaniel, R.R. (1997). Strategic leadership: A view from quantum and chaos theories. *Health Care Management Review, 22*(1), 21-37.

Naylor, M.D., & Brooten, D. (1993). The roles and functions of clinical nurse specialists. *IMAGE: Journal of Nursing Scholarship, 25,* 73-78.

Patterson, J.E., Strumpf, N.E., & Evans, L.K. (1995). Nursing consultation to reduce restraints in a nursing home. *Clinical Nurse Specialist, 9,* 231-235.

Rokwood, G.F. (1993). Edgar Schein's process versus content consultation models. *Journal of Counseling and Development, 71,* 636-638.

Rosenkoetter, M. (1997). A framework for international health care consultations. *Nursing Outlook, 45*(4), 182-187.

Roy, D.L. (1997). Consulting in occupational health nursing. *American Association of Occupational Health Nursing Journal, 45*(1), 8-13.

Schein, E.H. (1969). *Process consultation: Its role in organizational development.* Reading, Mass.: Addison Wesley Longman.

Schein, E.H. (1989). Process consultation as a general model of helping. *Consulting Psychology Bulletin, 41,* 3-15.

Scholz, J. (1996). Nursing practice issues and answers. *Ohio Nurses Review, 71*(3), 16.

Scott, L.D., & Beare, P.G. (1993). Nurse consultant and professional liability. *Clinical Nurse Specialist, 7,* 331-334.

Sebastian, J.G., & Stanhope, M. (1996). Community health nurse manager and consultant. In M. Stanhope & J. Lancaster (Eds.). *Community health nursing: Promoting health of aggregates, families, and individuals* (4th ed.). St. Louis: Mosby, pp. 849-877.

Swansburg, R. (1996). *Management and leadership for nurse managers* (2nd. ed.). Sudbury, Mass.: Jones & Bartlett.

Tiffany, C.R., & Lutjens, L.R.J. (1998). *Planned change theories for nursing: Review, analysis, and implications.* Thousand Oaks, Calif.: Sage.

Energizing Yourself for Change

John G. Bruhn

INTRODUCTION

Leaders in nursing need to create new mind-sets for managing and leading change. Everyone knows that the future is basically unknowable, and herein lies the challenge; to plan ahead positively using the instability and uncertainty that change creates (Stacey 1992). It is important to relish the opportunities that change and uncertainty create, rather than try to restrain change and its effects and mold them into order and stability. The following poem emphasizes this point:

Enjoying Uncertainty
Not much is certain in this life.
No one knows whether they will see another
    sunrise or sunset.
No one knows whether or not they have just
    said their last goodbye.
There may not be another opportunity to
    forgive.
There may not be another chance to do a good
    deed, to say a kind word, to think a positive
    thought.
Maybe we need to learn to relish uncertainty.
                John G. Bruhn (1995)

This chapter outlines how nurses can become agents for change. A change agent is a leader with a vision. Change must be created and directed toward some purpose and goal. This requires knowledge about and careful selection of one or more appropriate strategies for positive change to occur. Several effective change strategies are presented and related to leadership, planning, and participation.

Change agents require several strong personal and professional abilities. Of special importance is how one becomes energized for change and becomes an inspiration for others to follow in bringing about desired change. A change agent, as a leader with vision, must be able to tap into the soul of the organization and its members to gain their collective acceptance of change.

Being an agent of change is not easy; satisfactions and achievements do not come quickly or easily. Therefore change agents must learn how to cultivate a strong support system and engage in revitalizing activities that prevent burnout and dropout. As professionals, nurses must be as skilled in surviving change as they are in creating and directing it.

609

After reading this chapter, you will be able to:

1. Describe the art and science of change leadership and what it means to be an agent of change
2. Discuss the tools of a change agent and how they are applied
3. Evaluate the relationship among leadership, vision, and change
4. Illustrate the use of spirit as a motivator for change
5. Develop a plan demonstrating how a nurse can be an active leader for positive change

■ THE ART AND SCIENCE OF CHANGE LEADERSHIP

Each person is a veteran in experiencing change. Some people cope with change better than others, but no one is an expert. This is because most change is unpredictable, complex, cumulative, and subtle. Therefore people often find themselves dealing with the effects of change rather than the origins of change. When change is dealt with effectively, it seems to be the result more of art than of science. Change is such a complex subject that there is no unitary science of change. There are, instead, theories and techniques learned from people's successes and failures that can be applied to coping with future change. This process is flawed because change never repeats itself in the same way. Indeed, change is tied closely to time. People change at the same time that they are attempting to understand and direct change.

Blue and Brooks (1997) discuss the interplay between changes in nursing practice, that is, new technology, organizational changes, and their impact on nursing education, and the impact of changes in nursing education on nursing practice. This symbiotic relationship makes it difficult to plan for and direct change in practice without also doing so in education. As nursing shifts from an acute care/cure focus to a disease prevention/health promotion model, nurses will become increasingly concerned with patient-nurse interaction in the process of changing behaviors of both patients and nurses (Blue & Brooks, 1997).

It is important that participants do not feel victimized by change and allow themselves to be defeated by it. Some people are fatalistic—so externally controlled that they believe themselves to be helpless in the hands of fate. However, people are less likely to become victims of change if they anticipate it, plan for it, direct it, and assume responsibility for the part of change that can be controlled. Being a change agent is a form of artistry; it requires seeing the whole picture and relationships among parts of the picture and being able to change those parts to shape a final outcome. When there is no artistry, change merely happens and the resulting picture may be a collage, not a design.

■ WHAT IT MEANS TO BE A CHANGE AGENT

Being a change agent is explicitly or implicitly a part of everyone's job description; how much people are involved in change and the scope of their responsibility for change is just a matter of degree. One thing is certain: no person's job is exactly the same day after day; people change their jobs and their jobs change them, even if they do not always recognize the subtleties of the changes.

Key terms	
Term	**Definition**
Change	Alteration of an existing field of forces
Change agent	Person who plans, introduces, and manages change in families, groups, organizations, or larger entities
Planned change	Change that is designed, directed, and targeted to have a desired effect
Intervention	Direct effort to change the current state of an organism, e.g., an intervention to stop or modify a behavior or life-style
Strategies for change	Using aspects of a culture to bring about constructive change
Placebo effect	Nonspecific psychologic or physiologic effect (positive, negative, or neutral) of a specific action such as treatment for a health condition

The focus here is on nurses whose major responsibility is to create and manage change. Agents of change can be creators of change; they are often called *visionaries,* trying to bring about positive change, or *traffic cops,* trying to moderate the effects of negative change. In reality, however, change agents cannot separate the aspects of change they want to deal with. The positive and negative aspects of change coexist, and visionaries and traffic cops are involved with both aspects of change.

A change agent is usually a strategist and a motivator of people. A change agent is often selected to bring about, or cause, one or more specific or targeted changes. All change involves motivating people to change as well as changing structures, procedures, or policies. A change agent usually develops a plan with ample input from those involved in the proposed change. The plan includes strategies, resources needed, timetables, expected outcomes, and responsibilities for carrying out specific aspects of the plan. A change agent can be a person, team, or group from inside or outside the organization or a mixture of insiders and outsiders. The larger and more complex the changes, the more agents of change need to be involved to ensure that the proposed changes are as uniform as possible. That means that as agents of change, nurses should be well qualified with respect to both personal and professional skills and should undergo a period of training regarding the proposed plan for change. This is an extremely important point, because it is often thought that anyone can create and monitor change—you just have "to do it." However, impulsive or ill-planned changes can be costly to organizations for years. It should also not be assumed that a job title automatically qualifies that person as an expert change agent.

Being a change agent involves a great deal of responsibility (Box 25-1). First, the would-be change agent needs to be willing to experience change. Second, it is impossible to create, monitor, and manage change alone—change management must be delegated. Third, change is not something that is created or mandated and then forgotten. The anticipated and unanticipated effects of change in an organization are forever a part of life for everyone in that organization. Fourth, being a change agent means assuming accountability. Not all change or its effects are good—mistakes are made, and unplanned events can alter changes planned or in process. Change agents must have broad shoulders and be willing to admit to, and learn from, mistakes.

Tips on Being an Effective Change Agent

1. You have to be willing to change.
2. Change management must be delegated.
3. The expected and unexpected effects of change are lasting.
4. Change agents must be accountable for what they do and do not do.
5. Change agents should involve others in their plan.
6. Change agents must be ethical and professional in their behavior.
7. Change agents should be full participants in the change process.

Fifth, some change agents are better at visioning, whereas others are better at managing; one's strengths and limitations should be recognized in building a plan. Change agents are not super people, and success or failure should not rest on the shoulders of a single person. This is not likely to happen if there is open involvement and acceptance by the majority of others who will be affected by the planned changes. Sixth, a change agent should always be ethical and professional. Change will always be resisted. It is sometimes easy to forget or ignore those people who are resisting change and instead cling to supporters. If this happens and dissidents do not have a voice, efforts can be sabotaged and the organization disrupted by a few. Finally, change agents should not be so naive as to assume that they alone are the sources for determining what changes are needed or how they should be managed. A change agent should be a full participant in change so as to experience, hear, and see the change process. As Warren Bennis (1993, p. 107) says, "The successful leader will not have the loudest voice, but the readiest ear. His or her real genius may well lie not in personal achievements, but in unleashing other people's talent."

■ **TOOLS OF A CHANGE AGENT**
The Self as a Tool

The most powerful tool in creating change is one's self—an individual's personality, beliefs, values, and priorities and how these are reflected in daily behavior. Others cannot be asked to do what the change agent is not willing to do. Knaus (1994) says that the path of change should begin with oneself and be a journey of self-discovery. Insights about creating and managing changes in others will be gained first by understanding one's own perspective of change. An understanding of what people value most and least and how receptive they are to changing their values and priorities is the first step in becoming an effective agent of change.

What people are willing or not willing to change is deeply rooted in their personal value systems. If people believe that what happens to them is essentially beyond their control and determined by fate (externally controlled), they will be less likely to be convinced, for example, that not smoking cigarettes or that wearing a seat belt in a car will help to extend their lives. Indeed, health educators have shown that the more externally controlled (as opposed to internally controlled) individuals are, the less likely they are to engage in preventive health behaviors. Anthony Robbins (1991, p. 114) says, "We have to believe, *I can* change it."

Hartmann (1991) conceived that willingness to change is related to the boundaries people create in their minds, which become part of their personalities. He sees boundaries as a way people organize their lives. Thus individuals who develop "thick" boundaries are more territorial and perhaps more inflexible than people with "thin" boundaries. Boundaries influence opinions and judgments as well as decision making and actions. As such, boundaries are closely aligned with values and self-concepts (Bruhn et al., 1993).

The ability to modify or change one's own behavior is connected with patterns of thinking and feeling about oneself. People with an optimistic perspective, a strong sense of coherence, a spirit of engagement in life, confidence in their own abilities to make changes, and a basic trust in other people, tend to be healthier and, one might conjecture, more receptive to change (Kabat-Zinn, 1990). People who have insight into health-promoting and change-receptive behaviors in themselves will be able to understand sources of strength and resistance in others and will be able to use themselves more effectively as tools for change.

A Realistic Plan

Too often leaders of change have a plan but do not share it and encourage input from others; or the plan is short-term and therefore short-sighted; or the plan is someone else's idea and the leader does not feel ownership for it; or the plan is static and not periodically revisited and revised. *The point is that change happens and most of us end up managing and directing the effects of change that often have been created by the lack of planning.* Planning is often thought of as a waste of time because the plan is not used or followed after a substantial investment of time. When people do plan, they tend to plan in 5-year blocks, almost as if they can stop at 5-year intervals to generate the next plan. In addition, planning is often based on the philosophy of the current leadership in an organization. As leaders change, their enthusiasm for planning and directing change varies.

All change cannot be contained, directed, and managed. Unplanned change will continue to happen inside and outside of the unit of concern. What is key in planned change is to target certain changes and their impact to create a desired effect (Figure 25-1). The more complex

(too many changes at once) and less specific (too broad) the change, the more difficult it is to create successful change effects (Bruhn, 1988a).

Targeted change is purposeful. Change is an intervention (Bruhn, 1991). The most common type of intervention is usually directed toward individuals or families. Examples of interventions are those focused on weight control, a healthy diet, smoking cessation, stress control, abstinence from drugs and alcohol, and unprotected sex. These all involve changing harmful behaviors that are embedded in people's lifestyles and values. Health behaviors, good and bad, are all interrelated (Langlie, 1977).

Langlie, in her examination more than 20 years ago of 11 preventive health behaviors, found that behaviors fell into two sets: indirect preventive health behaviors, such as seat belt use, nutrition habits, medical check-ups, and immunizations; and direct preventive health behaviors, such as driving behavior, personal hygiene, and nonsmoking. She reported that people who engage in one set of preventive health behaviors are not necessarily likely to engage in the other. Furthermore, there are somewhat different predictors for each type of behavior. A strong sense of control over one's health status, perceptions that preventive actions are worthwhile, and membership in a higher socioeconomic group tend to predict indirect preventive health behavior. Conversely, women and older people are likely to exhibit direct preventive health behavior. Similarly, Harris and Guten (1979) found that an average respondent in their study practiced between 5 and 19 specific behaviors aimed at health promotion. They identified five types of health-promoting activities: health practices, safety practices, preventive health care, environmental hazard avoidance, and substance avoidance. These authors, like Langlie, found that health protective behavior is not unidimensional. People who sought preventive examina-

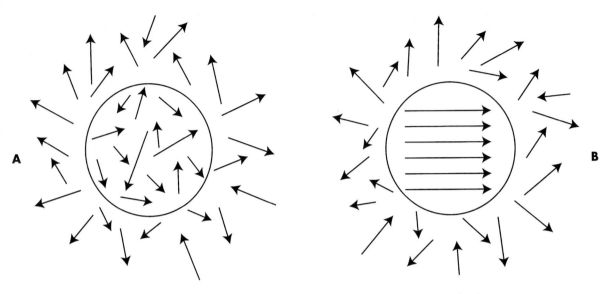

Figure 25-1 ■ A, Unplanned change. B, A single planned (targeted) change.

tions or who practiced certain nutritional habits were generally not much more likely to engage in other preventive practices than were individuals who did not have preventive examinations or practice good nutrition.

The complexity and interrelatedness of health behavior illustrates the need for a plan for change. A plan should have several common steps regardless of whether the change is targeted for an individual or an organization (Box 25-2). The six stages outlined to guide the planning of an intervention are not discrete stages, nor do they necessarily follow sequentially. Several stages may overlap, and depending on the target for change, several stages may precede the order suggested in Box 25-2. The important point is that there should be some degree of order to planned change and accountability on the part of all parties involved in the change.

Principles and Strategies

Bennis et al. (1985) suggest that self-knowledge and skill and capacity in establishing, maintaining, and terminating mutually helpful relationships with clients are the only instrumentation a change agent needs. Another way of looking at change strategies is to view the process of creating change as similar to that of problem solving. Creating change requires the ability to identify forces or variables surrounding a problem and to develop a strategy for manipulating these variables. Bennis and his colleagues (1985) state that three principles should guide the selection of a strategy for change:

1. Change must ultimately affect the culture of the person or unit. That means that change agents must consider the value system and social structure of those who will be involved in the change.

C A S E   S T U D Y

"Too Much All at Once"

Harry had a mild heart attack at age 52. He had been about 100 lbs. overweight, smoked cigarettes, did not exercise, worked at a stressful job, and was facing a merger at work when the attack occurred. He was told by his physician that he would have to make substantial changes in his lifestyle. Sent home for 6 weeks, he was given the following instructions: "Follow a low-fat diet, start walking daily, start a smoking cessation program, start a stress control program, and develop a hobby to divert some of your work fixation." Who was Harry's change agent? Such a segmented, uncoordinated plan of rehabilitation, which gave full responsibility to a depressed patient concerned about possible death and the young family he would leave behind, was doomed to fail. It did. Harry was overwhelmed. He became even more depressed and frustrated. He was unclear about which behavior change was most important and did not have time to engage in them all with equal vigor, so he tried to do them all as time permitted.

Although this case may represent an extreme one, "one that wouldn't happen in my hospital or clinic," it did happen. It points out the complexity and interrelatedness of behavior change in one person. There is usually a standard prescription for behavior change in cardiac patients, but unless the regimen involves the patient's family and "fits" with the family and patient's values and beliefs, it is likely to be yet another source of frustration and stress. Who is the change agent when rehabilitation involves a team? Who determines what is a success, and what kind or level of behavior change can be considered successful in Harry's case?

A nurse can make a difference in this case by applying the methods and principles of health behavior research and change theory as well as the interaction model of patient health behavior. Of particular importance is the nurse's perspective that considers the importance of engaging the patient and the family and that also includes an appreciation for the totality of the patient in the rehabilitation process.

2. Change agents must be prepared to work with the healthy part of a system, recognize forces of resistance, and attempt to include them in the change. The change agent cannot be obsessed with "getting everyone on board."

3. Any change program involves a set of core values that are reflected in the change strategies. An essential value is reciprocity, based on the acknowledgment that change is a two-way process.

These three principles are integrated into a flow diagram illustrating the process for creating change (Figure 25-2). The change agent is the central focus of the process. The change agent must integrate the external and internal forces favorable to the change, thus building a support system for change while selecting strategies for unlearning old behaviors and learning new behaviors that are appropriate for the culture or setting of the targeted change. This entire process must be reciprocal, or two-way, between the change agent and the target of change, enabling the strategies for change to be modified as necessary while the change is in process. This represents a huge juggling act for the change agent. Continual antipathy exists between forces favoring and opposing change in any setting. Working with the positive forces does not ensure success for the planned change.

O'Toole (1996) advocates a values-based approach to leading change. He suggests that creating change using dictatorial, manipulative, or paternalistic methods is outmoded. O'Toole

Stages in Planned Intervention to Create Change

Stage 1   **Assessment**
Who is the target of change? What is the degree of receptiveness of the target to change? What specifically is to be changed? What is the social and cultural support for current behavior? What are the obstacles to change?

Stage 2   **Target behaviors and timetable**
Which and how many behaviors are to be changed? Over what time frame? What will be called a successful outcome? Does the target of change understand his or her responsibility and accountability?

Stage 3   **Support system and obstacles**
Who, and to what degree, supports the planned change? Who opposes it and why? Is the support system strong enough to support change? How can the obstacles be turned into support?

Stage 4   **Techniques for change**
What methods or techniques will be used to create change? Why were the particular methods chosen? What are the alternative plans should these techniques fail?

Stage 5   **Outcome and follow-up**
The intervention should be assessed periodically, and the change effort should be followed over time. Who is responsible for follow-up?

Stage 6   **Closing the loop**
Use follow-up and the assessment of the effectiveness of change to create new changes.

proposes that a leader who has the welfare of followers at heart will get the best results. Such a leader creates an organization that encourages change and self-reevaluation and fosters an atmosphere of open-mindedness and new thinking in which assumptions can be challenged and goals reassessed.

There are many effective strategies for change, and most are used in combination with one or more others (Box 25-3). Researchers in behavioral medicine who are attempting to modify behaviors such as obesity, smoking, and alcohol and drug abuse or treat complex conditions such as asthma, hypertension, and stress have, in general, found that multicomponent programs work better than those that focus on changing single factors. The results of using multicomponent programs are not uniformly

positive. Many researchers have used a "throw in everything but the kitchen sink" approach. This is tempting when researchers and change agents are under pressure to bring about a positive outcome. Indeed, change agents need to be aware that their presence and involvement may be a factor (and may be more important than the carefully selected strategies) in creating change. This so-called *placebo effect* is difficult to plan for but demonstrates how carefully change agents and their behavior may be observed and may be a possible factor in the outcome of planned change.

Professionalism and Ethics

One of the essential tools of a change agent is professionalism. Creating change and providing a direction for it is a serious responsibility be-

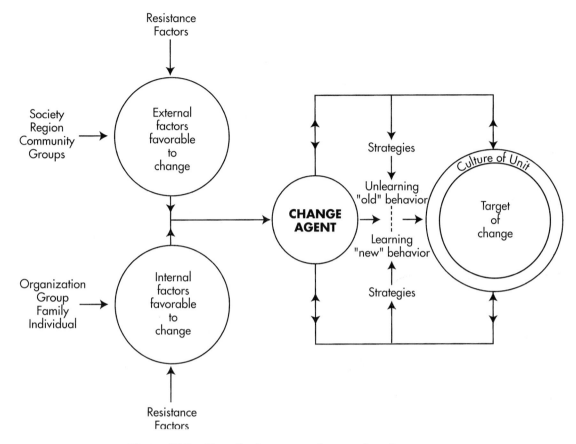

Figure 25-2 ■ Hypothetic process for creating change.

cause it involves changing beliefs and values. People do not give up or trade their beliefs or values easily. A change agent causes people to question their beliefs and values and consider alternatives. It is important, therefore, that change agents do not deprecate the beliefs and values of others or assume that these can easily be given up. It is important that change agents do not give the impression that they believe their beliefs and values are superior to those targeted for change. It is important that change agents be visible and identifiable so that change does not become something created and directed by unknown forces. Change agents need

to be accountable for the negative as well as the positive effects of change. That is why it is important for change agents to view change and its process as a partnership in which all parties share responsibility for the outcome. Change agents need to abide by a code of ethics. No tricks will lead to successful change. Strategies of change should be based on the ethics of informed consent. People need to know what to expect. Change involves control; often those who are not in control feel powerless and victimized. Their fears are heightened when the familiar changes and what will replace it is uncertain. Change agents should not work

BOX 25-3

Some Strategies for Change

- Knowledge/information
  (on why change is needed and how it might happen)
- Group pressure
  (support from others for change)
- Role modeling
  (other persons or groups who benefitted by change)
- Self-help and support groups
  (change is easier when others also share its difficulties)
- Rewards and incentives
  (to help motivate people to act)
- Participation and involvement
  (to make those affected by change help to shape it)
- Alliances, partnerships, coalitions
  (to broaden the base of change)
- Redefining boundaries
  (to restructure roles and responsibilities as a result of change)
- Redistributing power and status
  (how people relate to each other needs reexamination as goals and tasks change)
- Using espoused values
  (to build change around cherished values)
- Building individual or group pride and identity
  (people can feel good about change when it has obvious benefits)
- Selling a new vision by examining basic values
  (when people strongly agree on certain values, they are usually receptive to finding ways to further strengthen these values)

to control or suppress anxiety during the change process. Those involved in change need an outlet for their fears and feelings. Change agents should also be bound by an ethic of minimizing surprise. Although positive outcomes usually are expected, not all of the side effects of change can be forecast. Risks associated with change should not be kept secret. Finally, change agents should do what they said they would do. Often, the desire to see change happen is so strong that not all aspects of the change, or the expected end result, are fully communicated to those who are being changed. It is critical that the change agent be open and honest about the rationale and expectations of the change.

There are three kinds of change: (1) closed; (2) contained; and (3) open-ended (Stacy, 1992). The principal features of closed change are the clearly understandable and predictable consequences of events. In contained change, it is possible to predict only what probably will happen. Open-ended change involves the greatest risk and uncertainty and is the most difficult for change agents to direct. Often it is impossible to state what caused a particular result or what all of its consequences will be. Change agents should not let the flexibility and uncertainty of open change create a laissez-faire attitude about their ethical responsibilities. The more open and broad-based the planned change, the greater the agents' need to adhere to a strict code of ethics.

■ LEADERSHIP, VISION, AND CHANGE
Creating Change

Change agents are leaders. Whether they are carrying out their own vision or the vision of another, change agents must have the big picture of where a unit is going. Nanus (1992) points out that vision is the key to leadership. Vision is a realistic, credible, attractive future for your organization (Nanus, 1992). However small or large a change in an organization, it ultimately affects the vision and direction of the organization. All change creates conflict and is disruptive to an organization. This is why it is important for organizational leaders and change agents to gain acceptance from the majority of organizational members. Everyone involved must go through change and live with the results. Nanus (1992, p. 9) says

> Sooner or later, the time will come when an organization needs redirection or perhaps a complete transformation, and then the first step should always be a new vision, a wake-up call to everyone involved with the organization that fundamental change is needed and is on the way.

The role of the change agent is to tie change to the organizational mission and vision. Planned change is thereby limited to a purpose and not indiscriminate.

Sometimes there is little time for change. Some organizations, like individuals, are not proactive and hence are faced with change only when their backs are to the wall. This is not the best situation in which to plan change. When change is precipitated by a crisis and the process is accelerated because of a time shortage, the acceptance process often is aborted and employees feel that change is being imposed on them without their participation and input. Change and survival, however, are often limited.

Managing Change

Managing change requires skills different from those needed for creating change. Often, change agents create change and leave its management to others. However, the management of change is the key to its success. The greatest vision and leadership for new ideas are only as good as the people who implement them and see them in operation. Bennis (1993) discusses several ways to avoid disaster during periods of change. A key factor in the success of change is "knowing the territory." Too often, change agents operate from a vision or a paper plan; if they do not know the organization, significant problems can arise in the implementation of the plan. The management of change needs to be delegated. If responsibility and accountability

are shared, the likelihood is greater that any change will be successful. If the management of change is not decentralized, the likelihood is greater that those who resist the changes will find ways of sabotaging them. Without a commitment from the supporters of the change, there will be little support to sustain changes that are denigrated by the resisters.

There must, however, be a type of ombudsperson who oversees the management of change—to keep it going. Because employees come and go in any organization, the need to train new employees as well as to integrate them in the changing culture is continual. "Old" employees will do their own orientation of new employees. It is important to the organization not to permit the growth of two distinct cultures—those who oppose change and those who welcome it. Change agents can help prevent this by providing continual opportunities for dialogue and input among all employees and organizational leaders.

■ SPIRIT, HOPE, AND CHANGE
Using Spirit and Hope as Motivators for Change

Bolman and Deal (1995; 1997) note that each organization needs to evolve for itself a sense of its ethical and spiritual core. The core beliefs and values of an individual or organization will determine how change is viewed and embraced. The spirit or soul of an organization is what gives it a purpose, a reason for existing. This is unique to every organization, just as it is for individuals. All organizations have a spirit, but it is more apparent in some than in others. Bolman and Deal (1997) describe spirited organizations as those that emphasize quality, excellence, creativity, and service. These organizations are always changing something to enhance their competitiveness. Change is an accepted ethic. On the other hand, organizations may have spirit, but it is embedded in tradition—in a pride of being the same. As a result, such organizations find themselves the target of mergers, takeovers, or declining business. Having spirit means caring about the future and attempting to be a step ahead of it.

Spirit, if it is the core of an organization, pervades all aspects of the organization. Employees are ready for change and relish it. Change agents should not only be spirited themselves but be able to tap into organizational spirit to help use it as a basis for change. Change creates conflict, and spirit can be a great antidote for conflict. The change agent, however, cannot be expected to *give* spirit to others; the change agent can only capture it when it exists and make it work for positive change (Bolman & Deal, 1995).

Just as spirit is important for organizational change, hope is an important motivator for individual change. Hope appears to foster health (Ornstein & Sobel, 1987). There is a fair amount of research, both animal and human, on the phenomenon of learned helplessness. Schmale and Iker (1971) studied whether patients' attitudes of hopefulness or hopelessness could predict cervical cancer. The researchers were able to correctly predict 68% of the cancer patients based on their hopeless attitudes. Beliefs and expectations are powerful. If persons perceive that they have the ability to control or change their symptoms (i.e., have self-efficacy), they are more likely to improve. The best predictor, for example, in managing arthritis symptoms was how likely persons thought they would be to improve. Arthritis self-management classes were organized to maximize patients' sense of self-efficacy. Patients were encouraged to set their own goals and to break them down into achievable steps to ensure success.

Hope, a belief in oneself, and a willingness to change are important correlates of good health and well-being, as well as longevity and recovery from illness (Ornstein & Sobel, 1987). Beliefs,

feelings, and expectations have been referred to as the "pharmacy within." The nurse can be a key person in helping patients to mobilize their own self-healing capabilities through social support and a connected patient-nurse relationship.

Preparing Oneself for Change

Knaus (1994) discusses several personal "blockers" to change. These include complaining, complacency, avoiding conflict, learned helplessness, distrust, and fear. One of the key underlying reasons people resist change is a fear that they might lose their job or that their job might be reengineered so that they will no longer be qualified for it. The author is reminded of the dean of a school at a large university who had a computer on his desk. He never used it, stating that he had only a few more years until retirement. The computer on his desk was a symbol of change that he recognized as the future, but he feared that if he turned it on, it would reveal incompetencies that he would have to deal with. To avoid coping with technology, he became an advocate of the need for original sources of data (books) in the library.

An administrator once said that 20% of his employees talk about change and do something about it, 60% talk about change and point out its value while others carry it out, and the remaining 20% fear change and avoid and resist it, hoping to remain anonymous in the sea of change that surrounds them. The biggest challenge to a change agent is the middle group, those who think change is great for the other person. There is a "level of readiness" for change that needs to be determined, tapped into, and developed. Often this requires individual attention. For example, persons who would not take a class on how to operate a computer might respond positively when offered individual lessons in contrast to a group setting where their limited knowledge would be known to everyone.

It is said to be easier to introduce technologic change that requires minimal reengineering or learning new skills as compared with change that requires the development of new personal habits and necessitates major personal retooling. Whatever the scope of change, it takes energy, both psychic and physical. It is not uncommon to hear "I'm too old to learn that" or "What's wrong with the way I am doing it now?" as reasons not to expend the necessary energy to change. Usually, strong incentives or rewards are needed to entice people to change, retire early, or seek other career options. One of the challenges confronting a change agent is "preparing" a client for change.

The change agent's own spirit and the spirit of the organization for which he or she works are key motivators for change. Change agents not only must be energetic, positive, and creative, but they must be sensitive to the sources of resistance in their workplace. Change need not be an ordeal. Everyone is a survivor of change. Change can be made to work for us if we become more active in shaping it.

■ SURVIVING THE JOB OF CHANGE AGENT
Knowing Oneself

Change is stressful and unsettling even if it is not unique to an individual and does not involve him or her personally. Everyone is surrounded by change every moment of every day—usually change that they were not consulted about and over which they have no control, for example, the repair of potholes and detours, changes in the hours of a favorite food store, power outages, or the sudden illness of a family member. People know how to adapt to changes they have experienced before. The closer a change comes to affecting or challenging people's life-style, beliefs, or values, the more disturbed they become. Changes in health or workplace are particularly stressful, since these are direct threats to a person's livelihood. Change is so much a part of our culture that we relish opportunities "to get off the treadmill," to avoid creating more change when there is so much of it going on. Not all change is good, and if people do not attempt to direct it, they will remain complaining receptacles of it. Many things that people do they do not do well. Hence, the question "Can't we do this a little better?" This is the underlying premise of continuous quality improvement.

Whether they recognize it or not, all people are change agents. Each one causes change at some level to happen every day. People become aware of their role as change agents when they participate in something "big," such as a wedding or graduation. Emotion is involved in such changes, and these changes precipitate additional changes. It is important to learn more about how people adapt to change—how they are affected by change of various types and magnitudes. The more insightful people become about how they cope with change, the better appreciation they will have of how change affects others. When people are put in a position of creating changes that will affect others, it is hoped that they will not forget their own experiences with change.

Not everyone should deliberately assume the role of change agent. Before an individual assumes responsibilities for change beyond his or her own life, that individual should do a careful self-assessment. The following questions are helpful in developing self-knowledge and making appropriate decisions about assuming larger roles with respect to change:

- What are my strengths? What do I do best?
- What level of responsibility do I feel most comfortable in assuming?
- How do I handle change in my own life?
- How do I handle crises, my own and others'?
- How well do I work in situations of ambiguity and uncertainty?
- How effective am I in handling many issues and problems simultaneously?

- How well do I handle failure?
- Do I perform best when handling details, or when I am visioning, planning, and implementing?
- Am I a person with energy, enthusiasm, and a positive attitude?

The answers to these questions can help in making the decision as to whether to become or continue to be a change agent. Oliver Wendell Holmes (1906, p. 88) said:

> I find the great thing in this world is not so much where we stand, as in what direction we are moving: to reach the port of heaven, we must sail sometimes with the wind, and sometimes against it—but we must sail, and not drift, not lie at anchor.

Change agents are never at anchor.

Renewal and Revitalization

Being a change agent is like working in a critical care or coronary care unit: it is taxing in body, mind, and spirit. It is not uncommon for agents of change to become frustrated, angry, or depressed or to feel hopeless, drained, and burned out. Pritchett and Pound (1995) offer several practical ways to handle the stress of change (Box 25-4). They note that there are three key "drivers of change"—people, technology, and information. All three of these "drivers" are outside the control of change agents, but they do have control of how they react to these sources of stress. Change agents must assume responsibility for monitoring their own need for renewal and revitalization (Malone, 1997; Canavan, 1997). As Lyth (1991) points out, institutions have an extraordinary capacity to sustain their most important characteristics over time, even when significant change has occurred. Therefore it is less likely for an individual to change an institution than to fit into it. This points out the limitations of change agents in bringing about major, permanent changes in in-

---

B O X   2 5 - 4

How Much Stress Do You Create for Yourself?

Three major sources of stress are changes in our environment, conflictual relationships, and internally created emotional pressures and conflicts.

Most often, the greatest source of stress is the pressure and anxiety that we create with our own thoughts and feelings. We do this in various ways:

- **Worrying** about situations we can't control
- **Being perfectionists**—expecting too much of ourselves or others
- **Being self-critical**—focusing on our faults, not strengths
- **Expecting others**, not ourselves, to provide our emotional security
- **Making assumptions** that we know how others feel and what they want from us, instead of asking them
- **Feeling powerless**—failing to see available choices
- **Hurrying**—expecting ourselves to perform better and faster
- **Comparing** our achievements, or lack of them, with those of others
- **Being pessimistic**—expecting the worst from life
- **Expecting problem-free** living

Prescription

Stress can be an opportunity, depending on how we perceive it and the options we choose. There is no stress-free life, so we need to create opportunities, not obstacles, in our lives.

---

stitutions with long histories and strong traditions. Therefore change agents should not take their jobs too seriously.

There are only three universal bits of advice to assist change agents in their renewal and revitalization. The first is "Know your limitations." Everything is not within your control; therefore be concerned about those things you can control. Second, a sense of humor is essential. A sense of humor helps to keep difficulties and failures in perspective. Change will happen no matter what—it is best to achieve a balance between the two. Third, change agents and health professionals constantly give of themselves to others and often do poorly themselves those things they advise others to do. Remember that change will prevail far beyond the life of any one person. There are no Nobel prizes for change agents. Therefore, while creating and managing change, change agents must create and manage meaningful, satisfying lives for themselves.

Becoming Risk-Sensitive

Morgan (1997) notes that for successful double-loop learning to occur, organizations and individuals must support change and risk-taking. They have to embrace the idea that in rapidly changing circumstances with high degrees of uncertainty, problems and errors are inevitable. They have to promote an openness that encourages dialogue and the expression of conflicting points of view. All of this raises levels of anxiety, yet individuals and organizations have to be willing to find new ways of coping with the anxiety of change for new action to emerge. "To stay alive and lively, we need a steady diet of risk" (Keyes, 1985).

Most risks are chosen rather than imposed. In making choices about whether to take a risk, people are supposed to go through a rational process of assessing the costs and benefits of the risk and weighing its alternatives. Most risk assessment, however, is based on incomplete information and estimates (Bruhn, 1988b). Change agents should be risk-sensitive persons if they are going to create and direct change that has risks associated with it. Not all risks involve negative consequences. Indeed, stress provides an opportunity for professional growth (Bruhn, 1989). Individuals perceive stress differently.

One person's stress might be another person's stimulus (see Box 25-4). Nevertheless, stress does motivate people to take some action. Health professionals create stress by the way they choose to perceive it and the options they choose to take to resolve it. Personal and professional growth are impossible unless options are perceived and considered. Change must be seen as an opportunity rather than as an obstacle, and the capacity must be developed to pull back and correct a course of action rather than see it through to the end. Too often, change agents are their own worst enemies—that is, they see accomplishment as a fixed state (and, it is hoped, a positive one).

Carl Rogers said that the good life is a process, not a state of being (Rogers, 1961, p. 27). It is a direction, not a destination. This should be the personal and professional ethic for change agents.

■ KEY POINTS

- Change agents need to become energized for change to become an inspiration for others in bringing about desired change.
- Nurses need to be as skilled in surviving change as they are in creating and directing it.
- We are changing at the same time we are attempting to understand and direct change.
- Being a change agent is artistry; it requires seeing the whole picture and relationships among parts of the picture.
- A change agent can be a person, team, or group from inside or outside an organization, or a mixture of insiders and outsiders.
- A change agent should be a full participant in change so as to experience, hear, and see the change process.
- The most powerful tool in creating change is oneself.
- There are many effective strategies for change, and most are used in combination with each other.

- Change agents need to abide by a code of ethics.
- Managing change requires skills different from those for creating change.
- Not everyone should assume the role of change agent. Careful self-assessment is needed.
- Change agents should be risk-sensitive persons.
- Creating change is a serious responsibility because it causes people to question their beliefs and values.

■ CRITICAL THINKING QUESTIONS

1. Discuss why there is no science of change.
2. Differentiate approaches a nurse might take in creating change in an individual patient versus in an organization.
3. What are some possible reasons a patient might not make an expected change?
4. What does it mean to create successful change? Describe an example of successful change.
5. How do the strategies of change relate to nursing principles and practice?
6. What is meant by a values-approach to change?
7. Discuss the differences in skills needed to create change and manage change.
8. How can nurses use spirit and hope to create change?

■ REFERENCES

Bennis, W. *An invented life.* (1993). Reading, Mass: Addison-Wesley.

Bennis, W.G., Benne, K.D., & Chin, R. (Eds.). (1985). *The planning of change* (4th ed.). New York: Holt, Rinehart, & Winston.

Blue, C.L., & Brooks, J.A. (1997). Relevance of health behavior research for nursing. In D.S. Gochman (Ed.). *Handbook of health behavior research IV* (pp. 75-102). New York: Plenum.

Bolman, L.G., & Deal, T.E. (1995). *Leading with soul.* San Francisco: Jossey-Bass.

Bolman, L.G., & Deal, T.E. (1997). *Reframing organizations* (2nd ed.). San Francisco: Jossey-Bass.

Bruhn, J.G. (1988a). Lifestyle and health behavior. In D.S. Gochman (Ed.). *Health behavior: Emerging research perspectives* (pp. 71-86). New York: Plenum.

Bruhn, J.G. (1988b). Creating risk-sensitive persons: The roles of choice and chance in staying healthy. *Southern Medical Journal, 81*(5), 624-629.

Bruhn, J.G. (1989). Job stress: An opportunity for professional growth. *The Career Development Quarterly, 37,* 306-315.

Bruhn, J.G. (1991). Health promotion and clinical sociology. In H.M. Rebach & J.G. Bruhn (Eds.). *Handbook of clinical sociology* (pp. 197-216). New York: Plenum.

Bruhn, J.G. (1995). *Life is an inside job.* Privately printed.

Bruhn, J.G., Levine, H.G., & Levine, P.L. (1993). *Managing boundaries in the health professions.* Springfield, Ill.: Charles C. Thomas.

Canavan, K. (1997). Nurses strive to balance changes in health care with stresses of home life. *The American Nurse, 29*(1), 14.

Harris, D.M., & Guten, S. (1979). Health protective behavior: An explanatory study. *Journal of Health and Social Behavior, 20,* 17-29.

Hartman, E. (1991). *Boundaries in the mind.* New York: Basic Books.

Holmes, O.W. (1906). *The autocrat of the breakfast table.* London: J.M. Dent & Sons.

Kabat-Zinn, J. (1990). *Full catastrophe living.* New York: Delta.

Keyes, R. (1985). *Chancing it: Why we take risks.* Boston: Little, Brown.

Knaus, W.J. (1994). *Change your life now: Powerful techniques for positive change.* New York: John Wiley.

Langlie, J.K. (1977). Social networks, health beliefs, and preventive health behavior. *Journal of Health and Social Behavior, 18,* 244-260.

Lyth, I.M. (1991). Changing organizations and individuals: Psychoanalytic insights for improving organizational health. In M.F.R. Kets de Vries and Associates (Eds.). *Organizations on the couch: Clinical perspectives on organizational behavior and change* (pp. 361-378). San Francisco: Jossey-Bass.

Malone, B. (1997). Managing stress is the art of balance. *The American Nurse, 29*(1), 4.

Morgan, G. (1997). *Images of organization* (2nd ed.). Thousand Oaks, Calif.: Sage.

Nanus, B. (1992). *Visionary leadership.* San Francisco: Jossey-Bass.

Ornstein, R., & Sobel, D. (1987). *The healing brain.* New York: Simon & Schuster.

O'Toole, J. (1996). *Leading change.* New York: Ballantine Books.

Pritchett, P., & Pound, R. (1995). *A survival guide to the stress of organizational change.* Dallas: Pritchett & Associates.

Robbins, A. (1991). *Awaken the giant within.* New York: Simon & Schuster.

Rogers, C.R. (1961). *On becoming a person.* Boston: Houghton Mifflin.

Schmale, A., & Iker, H. (1971). Hopelessness as a predictor of cervical cancer. *Social Science and Medicine, 5,* 95-100.

Stacey, R.O. (1992). *Managing the unknowable: Strategic boundaries between order and chaos in organizations.* San Francisco: Jossey-Bass.

Index